Essentials of Pharmacology f
Pain Medicine, and Critical C

Alan David Kaye • Adam M. Kaye
Richard D. Urman

Editors

Essentials of Pharmacology for Anesthesia, Pain Medicine, and Critical Care

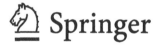 Springer

Editors
Alan David Kaye, MD, PhD
Departments of Anesthesiology
and Pharmacology
LSU Health Sciences Center
New Orleans, LA
USA

LSU Interim Hospital
and Ochsner Kenner Hospital
New Orleans, LA
USA

Adam M. Kaye, PharmD
Department of Pharmacy Practice
Thomas J. Long School of Pharmacy
and Health Sciences
University of the Pacific
Stockton, CA
USA

Richard D. Urman, MD, MBA
Department of Anesthesiology
Perioperative and Pain Medicine
Brigham and Women's Hospital
Harvard Medical School
Boston, MA
USA

Ambulatory Care Center
Brigham and Women's Hospital
Chestnut Hill, MA
USA

Center for Perioperative Management
and Medical Informatics
Department of Anesthesiology
Perioperative and Pain Medicine
Brigham and Women's Hospital
Boston, MA
USA

ISBN 978-1-4614-8947-4   ISBN 978-1-4614-8948-1   (eBook)
DOI 10.1007/978-1-4614-8948-1
Springer New York Heidelberg Dordrecht London

Library of Congress Control Number: 2014948072

Printed on acid-free paper

Springer is part of Springer Science+Business Media (www.springer.com)

Adam and I wish to thank our parents, Florence Feldman and Joel Kaye, for their love and support. We also want to thank our stepparents, Andrea Kaye and the late Gideon Feldman, along with the Gittelman family for always helping and treating us with love and kindness over our lifetime. All three of us wish to thank Dr. Jonathan Jahr and Dr. Karina Gritsenko, MD, for their extra help in the preparation of this book. This book has been the largest project I have undertaken in many decades. I wish to dedicate this book to everyone interested to learn about anesthesia and pharmacology. I also wish to dedicate this book to my family: my wife Dr. Kim Kaye, my son Aaron, and my daughter Rachel. I also wish to thank my pharmacology and anesthesia mentors, Dr. Alan W. Grogono, MD; Dr. Philip J. Kadowitz, PhD; and Dr. Bobby D. Nossaman, MD, for allowing me to complete my PhD in pharmacology while serving my full-time duties at Tulane Medical Center many years ago.

Alan D. Kaye, MD, PhD

I would like to dedicate this book to my wife Beth Kaye and daughter Jessica Kaye and thank them from the bottom of my heart for their patience and love. I would like to thank James W. Blankenship, PhD, Emeritus Professor, Department of Physiology and Pharmacology, for stimulating my interest while a student at the Thomas J. Long School of Pharmacy and Health Sciences, University of the Pacific. Most importantly, I would like to thank my older and wiser brother Alan Kaye for being my first teacher and best friend.

Adam M. Kaye, PharmD

This book covers extensive amount of material highly relevant to the practice of anesthesiology, pain, and critical care medicine. I would like to thank my colleagues, students, and mentors for encouraging me to undertake this massive project. I hope that current and future generations of practitioners and trainees will benefit from my efforts. I would like to thank my wife Zina Matlyuk, MD, for her editorial assistance and advice. I wish to dedicate this book to Zina, my daughters Abigail and Isabelle, and my parents Dennis and Tanya Urman.

Richard D. Urman, MD, MBA

Foreword

The word *pharmacology* is derived from the Greek φάρμακον, *pharmakon*, and -λογία, *-logia*, "study of." Strangely φάρμακον meant "poison" in classic Greek but came to mean "drug" in the modern language. But what is a drug? It can be described as anything manufactured, natural, or endogenous that exerts some physiological cellular. Pharmacology is the study of the interactions between a living organism and substances that have an impact on normal or abnormal function.

The division between food and herbs is somewhat blurred as the latter preparations are not governed by the Food and Drug Administration but rather held to the standards of the food industry where trials of effectiveness and universal testing of safety are not required. However, the word "drug" is believed to originate from an old French word "drogue" and later from the Dutch "droge-vate," which referred to the drying or preserving barrels used to store plants for medicinal use (in other words, drugs and herbs are the same thing). Indeed, today about 30 % of our medicines derive directly from herbs, the only difference being that drugs have specified amounts of active ingredients and herbs are not regulated as to content.

Some of our earliest medical texts have centered on medicinal therapies. The *Yellow Emperor's Classic of Internal Medicine*, collected around 2600 BC, describes plants and foods that are applicable to the maintenance of health and the treatment of specifically diseased organs. Writing in the first century AD, Pedanius Dioscorides (circa 40–90 AD), a Greek physician, pharmacologist, and botanist, authored a 5-volume encyclopedia about some 600 herbal medicines that was the standard reference for 1,500 years. During the Renaissance the book was read in Latin, Greek, and Arabic. Before that, in the seventh century AD, Paulus Aeginata, also Greek, in a monumental act of plagiarism (although he does give some acknowledgements), collected all the works of Hippocrates, Galen, Dioscorides, and Aretaeus, among others, and produced seven books, the last of which is over 600 pages long and is devoted entirely to herbal remedies. In all of these works, many of the drugs we use today such as opium, aspirin, cannabis, castor oil, mandragora (atropine, scopolamine), cocaine, physostigmine, and digitalis among many others are listed. It is to the efforts of William Withering to understand the effects of this last herb, digitalis, from the purple foxglove, that we see the foundations of pharmacology. In his text,

An Account of the Foxglove, Withering relates how he achieved the potion from an old lady in Shropshire and sent samples to his colleagues to gauge under which circumstances the extract would relieve lower extremity edema and other signs of heart failure.

One of the frightening experiences the new resident in anesthesia has is encountering the sometimes bewildering array of medications that can take patients to the door of death and then (hopefully) bring them back. With an aging population come more comorbidities and the risk of drug interactions increases. Ever-increasing complexity of machines, requirements for monitoring, and mandated data collection all add to the stress of the perioperative period. The ability to turn to a concise yet easy to read comprehensive text on the drugs we use daily is something to be treasured and an immense help for the practitioner. In this, the latest of a long line of pharmaceutical texts, Drs. Kaye and Urman are to be congratulated on gathering together such a wide range of authors from many different venues and perspectives. The coverage of topics within *Essentials of Pharmacology* is indeed encyclopedic. It is my hope that this book will allow practitioners of anesthesia to embrace the topic of pharmacology and thus gain confidence in the knowledge that their patients will be cared for appropriately and safely.

New York, NY, USA   Elizabeth A.M. Frost, MD

Preface

In many academic papers that we have read and written over the years, drugs are described in abstract and theoretical ways. These drugs might possess novel mechanisms or improved duration of activity. These agents might be less toxic or possess reduced side effects. Clearly, drugs dramatically affect our life spans, including our quality of life. As the years have gone by, we have a much greater appreciation for their wonders.

It was not long ago that our life spans were much shorter. Tens of thousands of people died due to plague, an organism easily treated with sulfonamides. It is an astonishing fact that dysentery was the single greatest cause of death of Confederate and Union soldiers during our epic Civil War. Some of our greatest figures in history had shortened lives related to what we would now consider very treatable states. George Washington probably died of acute bacterial epiglottis. The poet Lord Byron died prematurely from an epileptic seizure. Harry Houdini probably died from acute appendicitis. Arthur Ashe died, in part, from transmission of the human immune deficiency virus. Thousands of people die each year from NSAID-mediated silent gastrointestinal bleeding.

Principally during the last 50 years, we have dramatically increased our understanding of disease states, and the technology to detect these states has also grown significantly. Drug development has resulted in an increasing longevity, reduced pain, and enhanced quality of life. On a daily basis in every community, an anesthesiologist is called to a code with a patient appearing lifeless and without hope and delivers atropine, epinephrine, sodium bicarbonate, and calcium, and the patient is ultimately rescued and stabilized. These drug-mediated miracles are commonplace and routine in our practices.

In the last decade, we have seen complete cataloging of the entire human genome and an increase in drug targets from five hundred to well over one thousand. No longer is it a guaranteed death sentence to have human immune deficiency virus, many types of cancers, or sepsis. There is now new hope in drug targeting for vascular atherosclerosis, diabetes mellitus, cardiomyopathy, many cancers, and even Alzheimer's disease. We find ourselves constantly at a new beginning with drugs, including in our fields of anesthesia and pain medicine. Structural activity relationships and complex three-dimensional analyses of therapeutic targets have produced further advances. Freudenberg received a patent for a cyclodextrin structure in 1953; while, in 2014, we appreciate the role of a cyclodextrin-structured agent, sugammadex, in neuromuscular drug reversal. Forty years ago, we first identified an opiate receptor. In recent years, we have made substantial increases in understanding of endogenous opiates and subgroup opioid receptors throughout the body. With these understandings, our future will ultimately see better targeting agents for acute and chronic pain states. It is an exciting time filled with hope in modern medicine and in our field. Anesthesia has never been safer, thanks, in part, to drug development.

In this book, we have attempted to cover all pharmacological considerations in the field of anesthesiology in a slightly different way. The first section of the book covers basic drugs, including an introduction, mechanisms, drug class, structure, drug interactions, side effects, black box warnings, and clinical pearls. The second section looks at pharmacological considerations in each anesthesia-related subspecialty. The third section is timely and describes interesting and provocative current topics that directly influence how we practice anesthesiology. The final section is devoted to new vistas in many aspects of both anesthesiology and pain management.

History affords us lessons and clues to be better prepared for our present and futures. We must remain critical about expectations regarding quality and standardization of our drugs in order to maintain appropriate bioavailability and therapeutic outcomes. An appreciation of current black box warnings in the United States is given a special focus in this book. We must be leaders as many people within our hospitals suddenly are finding it their business to influence our practices and decision making. It is a golden age for drugs, and we should continue to improve the quality of life on this planet. Let us all be up to the challenge one patient at a time.

New Orleans, LA, USA   Alan David Kaye, MD, PhD, DABA, DABPM, DABIPP
Stockton, CA, USA   Adam M. Kaye, PharmD, FASCP, FCPhA
Boston, MA, USA   Richard D. Urman, MD, MBA, CPE

Contents

Contributors

Jacqueline Volpi Abadie, MD Department of Anesthesiology, Alton Ochsner Clinic, New Orleans, LA, USA

Andrew Abe, PharmD Drug Information Center, University of Kansas, Lawrence, KS, USA

Alexis Appelstein, DO Department of Anesthesiology, Montefiore Medical Center, Albert Einstein College of Medicine, Bronx, NY, USA

Melinda Aquino, MD Department of Anesthesiology, Montefiore Medical Center, Albert Einstein College of Medicine – Yeshiva University, Bronx, NY, USA

Tod Aust, MD Department of Anesthesiology, David Geffen School of Medicine at UCLA, Los Angeles, CA, USA

Amir Baluch, MD Metropolitan Anesthesia Consultants, Dallas, TX, USA

Ratan K. Banik, MD, PhD Department of Anesthesiology, Montefiore Medical Center, Albert Einstein College of Medicine, Bronx, NY, USA

Mary Bekhit, MD Department of Anesthesiology, Ronald Reagan UCLA Medical Center, Los Angeles, CA, USA

Honorio T. Benzon, MD Department of Anesthesiology, Northwestern University Feinberg School of Medicine, Chicago, IL, USA

Jay S. Berger, MD, PhD Department of Anesthesiology, Montefiore Medical Center, Albert Einstein College of Medicine, Bronx, NY, USA

Jeff Bernstein Department of Anesthesiology, Montefiore Medical Center, Albert Einstein College of Medicine, Bronx, NY, USA

Subarna Biswas, MD Department of Surgery, UCLA Medical Center,
Los Angeles, CA, USA

M. Dustin Boone, MD Department of Anesthesia, Harvard Medical School,
Boston, MA, USA

Department of Anesthesia, Critical Care and Pain Medicine,
Beth Israel Deaconess Medical Center, Boston, MA, USA

Mark V. Boswell, MD, PhD, MBA Department of Anesthesiology
and Perioperative Medicine, University of Louisville School of Medicine,
Louisville, KY, USA

Michelle Braunfeld UCLA Department of Anesthesiology,
David Geffen School of Medicine at UCLA, Los Angeles, CA, USA

Ethan O. Bryson, MD Departments of Anesthesiology and Psychiatry,
The Mount Sinai School of Medicine, New York, NY, USA

Maria Bustillo, MD Department of Anesthesiology, Montefiore Medical Center,
Albert Einstein College of Medicine, Bronx, NY, USA

Patrick Chan, PharmD, PhD Department of Pharmacy Practice and
Administration, Western University of Health Sciences, Pomona, CA, USA

Ming Chen, MD Department of Anesthesiology, Hubei Women and Children's
Hospital, Wuhan, China

Mingbing Chen, MD Department of Anesthesiology, Tulane University Medical
Center, New Orleans, LA, USA

Mabel Chung, MD Department of Anesthesiology, Montefiore Medical Center,
Albert Einstein College of Medicine, Bronx, NY, USA

Molly Chung, MD Department of Anesthesiology, David Geffen School
of Medicine at UCLA, Ronald Reagan UCLA Medical Center,
Los Angeles, CA, USA

Roy Esaki, MD, MS Department of Anesthesiology, Perioperative
and Pain Medicine, Stanford University School of Medicine, Stanford,
CA, USA

Ryan Field, MD Department of Anesthesiology and Perioperative Care,
School of Medicine, University of California–Irvine, Irvine, CA, USA

Aaron M. Fields, MD Department of Anesthesiology, Tripler Army Medical
Center, Honolulu, HI, USA

Charles Fox, MD Department of Anesthesiology, LSU Health Science
Center Shreveport, Shreveport, LA, USA

Scott D. Friedman, MD Department of Anesthesiology, Tulane University
School of Medicine, New Orleans, LA, USA

Elizabeth A.M. Frost, MD Department of Anesthesiology,
Icahn School of Medicine at Mount Sinai, New York, NY, USA

Julie A. Gayle, MD Department of Anesthesiology, Louisiana State University
Health Sciences Center, New Orleans, LA, USA

Andrew Ghobrial, MD Department of Anesthesiology, David Geffen School
of Medicine at UCLA, Los Angeles, CA, USA

Rudolph R. Gonzales Jr., RN, MSN, CNOR, CRCST, CHL Sterile Processing
Services, North Texas Veterans Administration Health Care System,
Dallas, TX, USA

Justo Gonzalez, MD Department of Anesthesiology, Montefiore Medical Center,
Albert Einstein College of Medicine, Bronx, NY, USA

Gabriel Goodwin Department of Anesthesiology, Montefiore Medical Center,
Albert Einstein College of Medicine, Bronx, NY, USA

Basavana Gouda Goudra, MD, FRCA, FCARCSI Department of Clinical
Anesthesiology and Critical Care, Perelman School of Medicine, Philadelphia,
PA, USA

Department of Anesthesiology and Critical Care Medicine,
Hospital of the University of Pennsylvania, Philadelphia, PA, USA

Philip Gregory, PharmD Center for Drug Information
and Evidence-Based Practice, Creighton University, Omaha, NE, USA

Karina Gritsenko, MD Department of Anesthesiology,
Montefiore Medical Center, Albert Einstein College of Medicine,
Yeshiva University, Bronx, NY, USA

Department of Family and Social Medicine, Montefiore Medical Center,
Albert Einstein College of Medicine, Yeshiva University, Bronx, NY, USA

Darren Hein, PharmD Center for Drug Information and Evidence-Based
Practice, Creighton University, Omaha, NE, USA

David Hirsch, MD Department of Anesthesiology, Tulane Medical Center,
New Orleans, LA, USA

Joe C. Hong, MD UCLA Department of Anesthesiology,
Ronald Reagan UCLA Medical Center, Los Angeles, CA, USA

Richard Hong Department of Anesthesiology,
Ronald Reagan UCLA Medical Center, Los Angeles, CA, USA

Eric Hsu, MD Anesthesiology Pain Medicine Center,
UCLA–School of Medicine, University of California, Los Angeles, USA

Jonathan S. Jahr, MD Department of Anesthesiology,
David Geffen School of Medicine at UCLA, Ronald Reagan UCLA Medical Center,
Los Angeles, CA, USA

Judy Johnson, MD Department of Anesthesiology, Louisiana State University, New Orleans, LA, USA

Rebecca Johnson, MD Department of Anesthesiology, Tulane Medical Center, New Orleans, LA, USA

Vilma Joseph Department of Anesthesiology, Montefiore Medical Center, Albert Einstein College of Medicine, Bronx, NY, USA

Sunitha Kanchi Kandadai, MD Department of Anesthesiology and Perioperative Medicine, University of Louisville School of Medicine, Louisville, KY, USA

Heesung Kang, MD Department of Anesthesiology, Montefiore Medical Center, Albert Einstein College of Medicine of Yeshiva University, Bronx, NY, USA

Jeffrey A. Katz, MD Department of Anesthesiology, Northwestern University Feinberg School of Medicine, Chicago, IL, USA

Adam M. Kaye, PharmD Thomas J. Long School of Pharmacy and Health Sciences, University of the Pacific, Stockton, CA, USA

Alan David Kaye, MD, PhD Department of Anesthesiology, Tulane Medical Center, New Orleans, LA, USA

Department of Anesthesiology, Louisiana State University Health Sciences Center, New Orleans, LA, USA

Hanjo Ko, MD Department of Anesthesiology and Perioperative Medicine, Brigham and Women's Hospital, Boston, MA, USA

Boleslav Kosharskyy, MD Department of Anesthesiology, Albert Einstein School of Medicine – Yeshiva University, Montefiore Medical Center, Bronx, NY, USA

Angelika Kosse, MD Department of Anesthesiology, Montefiore Medical Center, Albert Einstein College of Medicine of Yeshiva University, Bronx, NY, USA

Valeriy Kozmenko, MD Department of Anesthesiology, Louisiana State University Health Sciences Center, New Orleans, LA, USA

Timothy Ku, MD Department of Anesthesiology, Tulane Medical Center, New Orleans, LA, USA

Richard Lancaster, MD Department of Anesthesiology, Tulane Medical Center, New Orleans, LA, USA

Robyn Landy, MD Department of Anesthesiology, Montefiore Medical Center, Albert Einstein College of Medicine, Bronx, NY, USA

Meghan Brooks Lane-Fall, MD, MSHP Department of Anesthesiology and Critical Care, University of Pennsylvania, Philadelphia, PA, USA

Rebecca Lintner, MD Department of Anesthesiology,
Montefiore Medical Center, Albert Einstein College of Medicine,
Bronx, NY, USA

Henry Liu, MD Department of Anesthesiology, Tulane Medical Center,
New Orleans, LA, USA

Joyce C. Lo, MD Department of Anesthesiology, Pain, and Perioperative Care,
Stanford University School of Medicine, Palo Alto, CA, USA

Alex Macario, MD, MBA Department of Anesthesiology, Perioperative and Pain
Medicine, Stanford University School of Medicine, Stanford, CA, USA

Laura Mayer, MD Department of Anesthesiology,
David Geffen School of Medicine at UCLA, Ronald Reagan UCLA Medical Center,
Los Angeles, CA, USA

Brian McClure Department of Anesthesiology,
Tulane University School of Medicine, New Orleans, LA, USA

John S. McNeil, MD Department of Anesthesia, Harvard Medical School,
Boston, MA, USA

Department of Anesthesia, Critical Care and Pain Medicine,
Beth Israel Deaconess Medical Center, Boston, MA, USA

Christopher K. Merritt, MD Department of Anesthesiology, Louisiana State
University, New Orleans, LA, USA

Matthew T. Murrell, MD, PhD Department of Anesthesiology,
Weill Cornell Medical College, New York, NY, USA

Kaveh Navab, MD Department of Anesthesiology,
David Geffen School of Medicine at UCLA, Los Angeles, CA, USA

Gundappa Neelakanta, MD Department of Anesthesiology,
Ronald Reagan UCLA Medical Center, David Geffen School of Medicine at UCLA,
Los Angeles, CA, USA

Vanessa Ng, MD Department of Anesthesiology, Montefiore Medical Center,
Albert Einstein College of Medicine, Bronx, NY, USA

Hamid Nourmand, MD Department of Anesthesiology,
David Geffen School of Medicine at UCLA, Ronald Reagan UCLA Medical Center,
Los Angeles, CA, USA

Brian O'Gara, MD Department of Anesthesia, Harvard Medical School,
Boston, MA, USA

Department of Anesthesia, Critical Care and Pain Medicine,
Beth Israel Deaconess Medical Center, Boston, MA, USA

Beverley A. Orser Department of Physiology, University of Toronto, Toronto, ON, Canada

Department of Anesthesia, Sunnybrook Health Sciences Centre, Toronto, ON, Canada

Department of Anesthesia, University of Toronto, Toronto, ON, Canada

Pamela P. Palmer, MD, PhD AcelRx Pharmaceuticals, Inc., Redwood City, CA, USA

Neesa Patel, MD Department of Anesthesiology, UCLA - Santa Monica Medical Center and Orthopedic Hospital, Santa Monica, CA, USA

Department of Anesthesiology, Ronald Reagan UCLA Medical Center, Los Angeles, CA, USA

Department of Anesthesiology, David Geffen School of Medicine, University of California, Los Angeles, CA, USA

John Pawlowski Division of Thoracic Anesthesia, Beth Israel Deaconess Medical Center, Boston, MA, USA

Amit Prabhakar, MD, MS Department of Anesthesiology, Louisiana State University Health Sciences Center, New Orleans, LA, USA

Shamantha Reddy, MD Department of Anesthesiology, Montefiore Medical Center, Albert Einstein College of Medicine, Bronx, NY, USA

Jillian Redgate, RD, CNSC Nutrition and Food Services, VA Greater Los Angeles Healthcare System, Los Angeles, CA, USA

James Riopelle, MD Department of Anesthesiology, Louisiana State University Health Sciences Center, New Orleans, LA, USA

Mike A. Royal, MD, MBA, JD AcelRx Pharmaceuticals, Inc., Redwood City, CA, USA

Alireza Sadoughi, MD Department of Anesthesiology, UCLA - Santa Monica Medical Center and Orthopedic Hospital, Santa Monica, CA, USA

Department of Anesthesiology, David Geffen School of Medicine, University of California, Los Angeles, CA, USA

Tarang Safi, MD Department of Anesthesiology, Montefiore Medical Center, Albert Einstein College of Medicine, Yeshiva University, Bronx, NY, USA

Orlando J. Salinas, MD Department of Anesthesiology, Louisiana State University, New Orleans, LA, USA

Jun Sasaki, MD UCLA Department of Anesthesiology, David Geffen School of Medicine at UCLA, Los Angeles, CA, USA

John J. Savarese, MD Department of Anesthesiology, Weill Cornell Medical College, New York, NY, USA

Michelle Schlunt, MD Department of Anesthesiology, Loma Linda University, Loma Linda, CA, USA

Shahzad Shaefi, MD Department of Anesthesia, Harvard Medical School, Boston, MA, USA

Department of Anesthesia, Critical Care and Pain Medicine, Beth Israel Deaconess Medical Center, Boston, MA, USA

Naum Shaparin, MD Department of Anesthesiology, Albert Einstein School of Medicine – Yeshiva University, Montefiore Medical Center, Bronx, NY, USA

Department of Family and Social Medicine, Albert Einstein School of Medicine – Yeshiva University, Montefiore Medical Center, Bronx, NY, USA

Andrew Sim, MD Department of Anesthesiology, Montefiore Medical Center, Albert Einstein College of Medicine, Bronx, NY, USA

Preet Mohinder Singh, MD, DNB Department of Anesthesia, All India Institute of Medical Sciences, New Delhi, India

Sumit Singh, MD, UCLA Department of Anesthesiology, David Geffen School of Medicine at UCLA, Los Angeles, CA, USA

Nutrition and Food Services, VA Greater Los Angeles Healthcare System, Los Angeles, CA, USA

Allison Spinelli, MD Department of Anesthesiology, Montefiore Medical Center, Albert Einstein College of Medicine, Bronx, NY, USA

My Tu, MD Department of Anesthesiology, Albert Einstein School of Medicine – Yeshiva University, Montefiore Medical Center, Bronx, NY, USA

James A. Uchizono, PharmD, Phd Department of Pharmaceutics and Medicinal Chemistry, University of the Pacific, Stockton, CA, USA

Richard D. Urman, MD, MBA Department of Anesthesiology, Perioperative and Pain Medicine, Brigham and Women's Hospital, Harvard Medical School, Boston, MA, USA

Center for Perioperative Management and Medical Informatics, Brigham and Women's Hospital, Boston, MA, USA

Elizabeth Valentine, MD Department of Anesthesiology and Critical Care, Perelman School of Medicine at the University of Pennsylvania, Philadelphia, PA, USA

Tricia Vecchione, MD Department of Anesthesiology, Montefiore Medical Center, Albert Einstein College of Medicine, Bronx, NY, USA

Angela Vick, MD Department of Anesthesiology, Montefiore Medical Center, Albert Einstein College of Medicine, Yeshiva University, Bronx, NY, USA

Kumar Vivek, MD Department of Anesthesiology, Montefiore Medical Center, Albert Einstein College of Medicine, Bronx, NY, USA

Jackie V. Abadie, MD Department of Anesthesiology, Alton Ochsner Clinic, New Orleans, LA, USA

Amaresh Vydyanathan, MD, MS Department of Anesthesiology, Montefiore Medical Center, Albert Einstein College of Medicine, Yeshiva University, Bronx, NY, USA

Adrienne B. Warrick, MD Department of Anesthesiology, Montefiore Medical Center, Albert Einstein College of Medicine – Yeshiva University, Bronx, NY, USA

Victor Xia, MD Department of Anesthesiology, Ronald Reagan UCLA Medical Center, David Geffen School of Medicine at UCLA, Los Angeles, CA, USA

Hong Yan Department of Anesthesiology, Wuhan Central Hospital, Wuhan, China

Michael Yarborough, MD Department of Anesthesiology, Tulane Medical Center, New Orleans, LA, USA

Michelle You Department of Anesthesiology, David Geffen School of Medicine at UCLA, Ronald Reagan UCLA Medical Center, Los Angeles, CA, USA

Agnieszka A. Zurek Department of Physiology, University of Toronto, Toronto, ON, Canada

Part I
Basic Pharmacologic Principles

Chapter 1
Pharmacokinetics and Pharmacodynamics of Anesthetics

Patrick Chan and James A. Uchizono

Contents

Introduction

Our understanding of the numerous barriers and cascades that govern drug kinetic and dynamic behavior of clinical response(s) continues to grow in complexity as the inextricable link between pharmacokinetics (PK) and pharmacodynamics (PD) becomes increasingly apparent. Colloquially, PK is described as "what the body

P. Chan, PharmD, PhD (✉)
Department of Pharmacy Practice and Administration,
Western University of Health Sciences, Pomona, CA, USA
e-mail: chanp@westernu.edu

J.A. Uchizono, PharmD, PhD
Department of Pharmaceutics and Medicinal Chemistry,
University of the Pacific, Stockton, CA, USA
e-mail: juchizono@pacific.edu

A.D. Kaye et al. (eds.), *Essentials of Pharmacology for Anesthesia,*
Pain Medicine, and Critical Care, DOI 10.1007/978-1-4614-8948-1_1,
© Springer Science+Business Media New York 2015

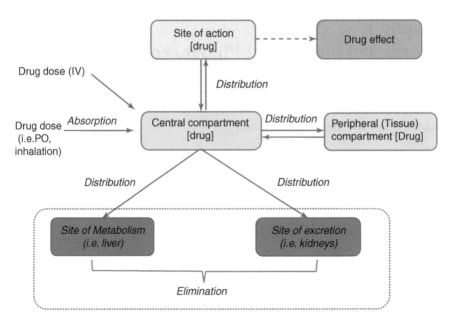

Fig. 1.1 The relationship among the pharmacokinetic processes of absorption, distribution, metabolism, and excretion with the central, peripheral, and site of action compartments

does to the drug" and PD is described as "what the drug does to the body." The key element to those phrases is "what is changing?": In PK, it is the drug concentration; in PD, it is the "body" or the physiological and pharmacological systems and cascades that convert drug concentrations into responses. More precisely, PK encompasses all of the kinetic processes from the drug released from its dosage form (e.g., i.v., p.o., i.m., extended release) to the delivery of the drug to its site or tissue responsible for initiating the translation of drug concentration/exposure into a response (shown as the solid arrows in Fig. 1.1). And where PK ends, PD begins by explaining the time-course translation/transduction of drug concentration into a "biological signal" or "messenger" (e.g., intracellular Ca^{2+} concentration) that ultimately leads to the end desired response or effect (e.g., increased pain relief) (shown as the broken line arrow in Fig. 1.1).

Upon closer examination, PK includes even the kinetics of drug released from the dosage form prior to absorption—such as drug being transferred from syringe to systemic circulation (i.e., i.v. bolus) or the complex disintegration, solvation, and dissolution of drug released by an advanced drug delivery system (ADDS) into the gastrointestinal (GI) tract milieu for permeation (passive diffusion and active or facilitated transport) across the GI endothelial barrier to the systemic circulation. Additional terms associated with the PK of a drug include absorption, distribution, excretion, and metabolism (see Fig. 1.1). A general term describing the sum of drug excretion and metabolism is elimination. An even more general PK term, disposition, describes the kinetic time course of drug distribution, excretion, and metabolism. The input function of drug (e.g., i.v. bolus, p.o.) combined with the disposition is the drug PK. *Most importantly, clinicians can generally only control the input function of drugs, while the "body" or physiology controls the disposition.*

An essential hypothesis of PK is that there is a quantitative relationship between drug concentration and pharmacological effect [1]. Clinical PK incorporates the fundamentals of PK to dose calculations, infusion rates, predictions of drug concentrations, dosing intervals, and time to eliminate the drug from the body. The primary objective of clinical PK is to maximize efficacy while minimizing toxicities, through a process called therapeutic drug monitoring (TDM). A complete TDM protocol entails monitoring-defined therapeutic endpoints (which include plasma drug concentration if appropriate) and adverse reactions. Adjustments of doses can be guided by TDM to provide individualized regimens. Clinical PK can be affected by numerous covariates, such as age, genetics, gender, race, comorbid disease states, and concomitant medications, resulting in drug interactions. These factors should be considered into the dosing regimen for each patient.

Absorption

The absorption of a drug is largely dependent on the route of delivery. Drugs can be administered by depot type of routes: oral, inhaled, subcutaneous, intramuscular, sublingual, rectal, intraocular, intranasal, vaginal, and transdermal. Although intravenous and intra-arterial technically do have an aspect of absorption (i.e., release of drug from a syringe or i.v./i.a. bag), these routes deliver drug directly into the systemic circulation and are a special subset of PK input (i.e., instantaneous absorption processes having a bioavailability of 1.0). The physicochemical properties (i.e., solubility, pKa, ionization, polarity, molecular weight, partition coefficient) play a critical role in the absorption of drugs. The route of delivery impacts the rate of absorption as well as the extent of absorption. Bioavailability is defined as the rate and extent of drug absorption or the percentage or fraction of the parent compound that reaches systemic (plasma) circulation. The bioavailability of the same drug in the same patient may be different depending on the route of administration. Drug references frequently provide the bioavailabilities of drugs and are typically denoted as F. The extent of absorption, but not the rate, can be described by the parameter area under the curve (AUC). In an acute setting, the rate of absorption, generally k_a, tends to be more important, whereas the extent of absorption tends to be more important in chronic use medications. The salt factor (S) is the fraction of a dose that is the active base form of the drug and pragmatically can be viewed as an attenuation of F (e.g., "effective dose" = F*S*dose). Probably, the most frequently used routes of administration of drugs in anesthesiology are oral, intravenous/intra-arterial, inhaled, and local (epidural, interscalene, etc.).

The absolute bioavailability, F, is determined by comparing the availability for any given extravascular (e.v.) route of administration measured against an i.v. point of reference of availability of the drug administered intravenously (Eq. 1.1):

Table 1.1 Partition coefficients of commonly used inhaled anesthetics

	Isoflurane	Sevoflurane	Desflurane	Nitrous oxide
Blood/gas partition coefficient	1.46	0.69	0.42	0.47
Brain/blood partition coefficient	1.6	1.70	1.29	1.1
Muscle/blood partition coefficient	2.9	3.13	2.02	1.2
Fat/blood partition coefficient	45	47.5	27.2	2.3

$$F = \frac{\text{AUC}_{e.v.} / \text{Dose}_{e.v.}}{\text{AUC}_{i.v} / \text{Dose}_{i.v.}} \tag{1.1}$$

Since anesthetics and pain management medications can be delivered via numerous routes of administration, the value of F is important in determining the "effective dose" for these e.v. drugs. The physicochemical properties, previously mentioned, of the drug affect the drug's ability to partition from lipid to aqueous phases, and therefore, F. Food, drug interactions, and gastrointestinal (GI) motility can all affect drug solubility and absorption. First-pass metabolism, which is pre-systemic metabolism of the drug, can occur in the GI tract and the liver prior to reaching systemic circulation. All of these factors can affect F and the route will sometimes dictate the countersalt needed, thus affecting S, as well.

For inhaled anesthetics, three major factors influencing absorption are solubility in the blood, alveolar blood flow, and the partial pressure gradient between alveolar gas and venous blood. The solubility of inhaled anesthetics in blood is described by blood/gas partition coefficients (Table 1.1). The inhaled anesthetics are absorbed almost completely and rapidly through the lungs. A lower blood/gas partition coefficient indicates a more rapid onset and dissipation of anesthetic action.

Volume of Distribution

The volume of distribution V_d is a PK parameter characterizing the extent of drug distribution into the tissue from the blood. The physicochemical properties of a drug, plasma protein binding, and tissue binding influence V_d. It has also been termed *apparent* volume of distribution because it does not correlate with an actual physiological volume compartment in the human body, but rather, it is the inferred volume in which the drug appears to be dissolved. It is inferred because as Eq. 1.2 shows, the clinician knows the dose given and Cp (drug plasma concentration) is measured; the V_d is inferred or calculated from the two values of dose and Cp. The lower limit for nearly all drugs is 3 L or the actual average volume of human plasma. As the apparent or inferred volume of distribution increases in size, the interpretation begins to focus on the distribution of drug into extravascular tissues. The apparent or inferred V_d can be calculated using Eq. 1.2:

$$V_d = \frac{\text{Dose}_{\text{i.v.}}}{\text{Cp}} \tag{1.2}$$

If the plasma concentration Cp of a drug is small immediately following a single-bolus dose, this generally indicates substantial drug permeation into the tissue(s), and the resultant V_d is >40–80 L, indicating extensive distribution into the tissue. In contrast, if V_d is small (close to 3 L), a large fraction of the drug is assumed to reside in the blood plasma, thus suggesting a little amount of drug has permeated into the extravascular tissue(s). While V_d provides insight as to whether the drug is residing in the blood or tissue, its value does not determine which specific tissue compartment the drug permeates into.

V_d is useful in determining the loading dose necessary to achieve a targeted Cp. The usual loading dose equation is Loading Dose = $V_d \times \text{Cp}_{\text{target}}$. For drugs that have a large V_d, a greater loading dose is necessary to achieve the targeted Cp. Drugs with a small V_d require a reduced loading dose to obtain the targeted Cp.

As shown in Table 1.1, the inhaled anesthetics have high brain/blood, muscle/blood, and fat/blood partition coefficients. In particular, most inhaled anesthetics distribute extensively into the fat tissues.

Clearance

Clearance is an independent PK parameter quantifying the rate the body is able to eliminate a drug. More specifically, clearance is the volume of blood that is completely cleared of the drug per unit time. The units are in volume/time, usually liters per hour (L/h) or milliliters per minute (mL/min). While the liver is primarily responsible for drug metabolism and the kidneys are primarily responsible for parent drug and metabolite excretion (filtration and secretion), other routes of elimination include the chemical decomposition, feces, skin, and lungs. Hepatic metabolism and elimination are components of drug clearance. Total clearance is characterized by Eq. 1.3:

$$\text{Cl}_{\text{Total}} = \text{Cl}_{\text{Hepatic}} + \text{Cl}_{\text{Renal}} + \text{Cl}_{\text{Other}} \tag{1.3}$$

Total clearance Cl_{Total} is used in most dose calculations without taking into account the specific route of elimination. Clearance is an important parameter because it controls the steady-state concentration Cp_{ss} as shown in Eq. 1.4:

$$\text{Cp}_{\text{ss}} = \frac{(S)(F)(\text{Dose}/\tau)}{\text{Cl}} \tag{1.4}$$

S is the salt factor, F is the bioavailability, and tau (τ) is the dosing interval.

Metabolism

Drug metabolism occurs primarily in the liver, though metabolism can also occur at other sites such as the gastrointestinal wall, kidneys, and blood-brain barrier. Metabolism can be characterized as phase I or phase II reactions. Phase I reactions include oxidation, epoxidation, dealkylation, and hydroxylation reactions catalyzed by the cytochrome P450 enzyme system. A majority of the cytochrome P450 enzymes reside in the microsomes of hepatocytes where it metabolizes the highest number of substrates (chemical, drugs, and pollutants) in the body. Phase II reactions are glucuronidation and sulfation processes.

Many drug interactions involve the cytochrome P450 enzyme system. Certain drugs, termed inducers, may increase the activity of specific cytochrome P450 isozymes, leading to increased metabolism of drugs which are substrates of that particular isozyme. The reduction in plasma concentration of the drug substrates may lead to decreased therapeutic effects. Other drugs are inhibitors of cytochrome P450 enzymes, decreasing the metabolism of drugs that are substrates. The increase in substrate plasma concentration may result in not only enhanced pharmacological effects but also enhanced toxicological effects. Clinicians are encouraged to consider dosing adjustments based on known drug interactions to achieve therapeutic effects while minimizing adverse reactions.

Excretion

Excretion frequently refers to the irreversible clearance of a drug typically through the kidneys. The three major physiological processes occurring in the kidneys governing renal excretion are glomerular filtration, active secretion, and reabsorption. The glomerular filtration of an adult patient may be estimated by the Cockcroft-Gault equation [3] (Eq. 1.5):

$$Cl_{Cr}\left(mL\,/\,min\right)=\frac{\left(140-age\right)\times IBW}{72\times SCr}\left(Multiplied\,by\,0.85\,if\,female\right) \quad (1.5)$$

Cl_{Cr} is the creatinine clearance in mL/min, the age of the patient is in years, SCr is the serum creatinine, and IBW is the ideal body weight of the patient in kilograms (kg). For female patients, the resultant Cl_{Cr} is multiplied by 85 % to account for lower muscle mass typically exhibited by females. The Cockcroft-Gault equation utilizes serum creatinine, which is a by-product of muscle metabolism and is freely filtered by the glomerulus. Creatinine is not actively secreted nor is it reabsorbed. For drugs that are primarily eliminated via the renal route, dose adjustments may be made on the basis of creatinine clearance (Cl_{Cr}) and are provided by drug package inserts or drug information references.

Elimination Rate Constant and Half-Life

The dependent parameter K is a first-order rate constant. It is a function of V_d and Cl. K can be described as the percentage or fraction of the amount of drug that is cleared from the body per unit time. The units are typically expressed as 1/h (hr^{-1}) or 1/min (min^{-1}). As shown in Eq. 1.6, K can be viewed as a proportionality constant between V_d and Cl:

$$K = \frac{Cl}{V_d} \qquad (1.6)$$

A large K value indicates rapid elimination of the drug. If two drug concentrations are drawn within the same dosing interval, K can be determined using Eq. 1.7 [4]:

$$K = \frac{Ln\left(Cp_1 / Cp_2\right)}{\Delta t} \qquad (1.7)$$

Ln is natural log and Δt is the time elapsed between Cp_1 and Cp_2. The determination of K is integral to calculating half-life, $t_{1/2}$, as shown in Eq. 1.8:

$$t_{1/2} = \frac{Ln(2)}{K} = \frac{(V_d) * Ln(2)}{Cl} \qquad (1.8)$$

Equation 1.8 also shows the relationship among $t_{1/2}$ and V_d and Cl. The $t_{1/2}$ is the amount of time it takes for the drug currently in the body to reduce by 50 %. The $t_{1/2}$ can also predict the amount of time it takes for a patient to achieve steady-state drug concentrations (assuming no loading dose and the same dose was administered at the same interval). For example, after one $t_{1/2}$, Cp is 50 % of the final steady-state Cp_{ss}. Under these conditions, a patient is considered to be clinically at steady state if the drug concentration is >90 % of the true steady-state level. As shown in Table 1.2, it would take approximately 3.3 half-lives for a patient to achieve 90 % of

Table 1.2 The number of half-lives and the expected percent of true steady-state concentration Cp_{ss} or percent of drug eliminated

Number of $t_{1/2}$	Percent of Cp_{ss} or percent eliminated
1	50
2	75
3	87.5
4	93.8
5	96.9
6	98.5
7	99.2

the true steady state. Conversely, it would take 3.3 half-lives for a patient to eliminate 90 % of the drug once the administration of the drug has ceased. To note, $t_{1/2}$ determines the dosing interval, but V_d and Cl determine the size of the dose.

Pharmacodynamics

The time-course conversion of drug concentration (Ce) into a pharmacological effect (response) is pharmacodynamics. The *biosensor process* is the detection of the drug's presence, Ce. Frequently, the *biosensor process* is the receptor system on the cell's surface. The white and black *biosensor process* rectangles indicate that the drug (Ce) either stimulates (white) or inhibits (black) the zero-order and first-order constants k_{in} or k_{out}, respectively. The *biosignal* is similar to the second messenger, in that it directs the end response. While the pathway in between the *biosignal* and the *response* can contain nonlinear and time-varying processes (circadian, drug-induced—such as drug tolerance), it still is the *biosignal* that is responsible for the end response. Alterations of k_{in} or k_{out} are frequently the sites for the nonlinearities or time-varying processes. This model is known as an "indirect" model and is relatively general; the most important aspect of this model is that a change in Cp is not instantaneously realized as a change in response (Fig. 1.2). Somewhere along the pathway of D, drug, diffusing out of Cp in to Ce or in the translation of D binding

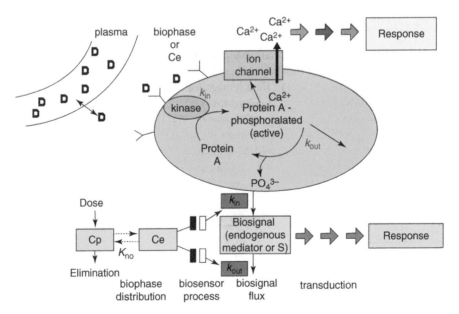

Fig. 1.2 The indirect model (*bottom*) is laid over a generic diagram of how cells (*top*) generally convert drug (*D*) into a pharmacological or physiological response (*response*). In this example, phosphorylated protein A acts as the biosignal responsible for the end response

Fig. 1.3 Comparison of three different values of γ for the same E_{max} model with baseline. E_0, E_{max}, and EC_{50} are kept constant for all three plots to show the behavior of γ

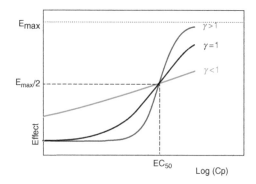

to the receptors to produce the response, there is a rate-limiting step that causes the response to lag behind changes in Cp.

A subset model of the indirect model is the direct model. In the direct model, the pharmacodynamic system very rapidly converts the Ce concentration of drug to response relative to the rate at which the Ce or Cp steady state is achieved. Or in other words, there is no time lag, as in the indirect model, between changes in Cp or Ce and response. Typical direct models have the form of $E = E_0 \pm \dfrac{E_{max}Cp^{\gamma}}{EC_{50}^{\gamma} + Cp^{\gamma}}$, where E_0 is the endogenous baseline (i.e., value of E in the absence of drug), E_{max} is the maximal effect achievable, EC_{50} is the concentration of drug that produces ½ of the E_{max} response, and γ is the Hill coefficient. When $\gamma > 1$, the PD is said to have positive cooperativity; when $\gamma < 1$, the PD has negative cooperativity; and when $\gamma = 1$, the PD has no cooperativity (see Fig. 1.3 for a comparison of γ).

In the more commonly used model, notice that as "dose" or the x-axis changes, the effect or response instantaneously changes. Another way to view this relationship between "dose" and "response" is to assume that the "dose" or "log (Cp)" has reached steady state or equilibrium before the effect has been measured. The direct model can still be used to simulate drug tolerance by either attenuating E_{max} or increasing EC_{50} as a function of Cp or Ce. The utility of this model cannot be overstated as it has provided many researchers and clinicians with useful pharmacodynamic insights.

Therapeutic Range and Therapeutic Monitoring

Most drugs have established therapeutic ranges. Therapeutic ranges are typically expressed as a range of drug plasma concentrations that achieve an optimal effect while minimizing adverse reactions. However, drugs that require constant monitoring of drug concentrations are ones that have narrow therapeutic ranges, a low threshold for serious adverse reactions, or must reach a minimum plasma concentration to achieve an effect.

Table 1.3 Minimal alveolar concentration of commonly used inhaled anesthetics

	Isoflurane	Sevoflurane	Desflurane	Nitrous oxide
MAC in O_2 in adults	1.15	1.71	6.0	104

In anesthesiology, the minimum alveolar concentration (MAC; Table 1.3) of inhaled anesthetics is used as the target to achieve the necessary therapeutic effect. MAC is the amount of inhaled anesthetic required to inhibit physical movement in response to a noxious stimuli in 50 % of patients [5]. MAC values can also be used to compare the relative potencies between two inhaled anesthetic agents.

The continuous monitoring of plasma concentrations of intravenous anesthetics is not performed due to practicality. The half-lives and durations of action of most intravenous anesthetics are relatively short. It may take several hours for the laboratory to determine anesthetic concentrations. Therefore, anesthetic concentrations do not provide rapid feedback for clinicians to make necessary adjustments to doses during the course of surgery or medical intervention. Thus, monitoring of intravenous anesthetics is reliant on the signs and symptoms of anesthesia for the attainment of therapeutic efficacy and respiratory depression and blood pressure for toxicology.

Table 1.4 summarizes the pharmacokinetic (distribution, metabolism, and renal excretion) and pharmacodynamic properties (onset of action and duration of action) of various anesthetic agents.

Drug Tables (Tables 1.5 and 1.6)

The mechanism of action, indications, contraindications, cautions, pregnancy category, clinical pearls, dosing options, drug interactions, and side effects of commonly-used anesthetic agents are presented in Table 1.5 Lidocaine, with its numerous routes of delivery and dosing options, are presented in Table 1.6.

Table 1.4 Pharmacokinetic and pharmacodynamic properties of anesthetic agents

	Distribution	Metabolism	Renal excretion	Onset of action	Duration of action
Isoflurane	Distributes quickly and extensively to the brain, heart, liver, kidneys, and lungs [6] Does not distribute well into adipose tissue	0.17 % of isoflurane is metabolized by the liver	Rapidly eliminated by lungs	7–10 min [7]	
Sevoflurane	Distributes well to the brain [8] Does not distribute well into adipose tissue	3–5 % hepatic via CYP2E1	Rapidly eliminated by lungs Exhaled gases, up to 3.5 %, excreted renally as inorganic fluoride	1.2 min [9]	4–14 min
Desflurane	Not available	0.02 % [10]	Rapidly eliminated by lungs <0.02 % as metabolite through urine	Single agent, 5–16 min [11] With oxygen, 2–3 min [11] With NO$_2$, 1.5–2 min [11]	
Nitrous oxide	0.5 blood/gas partition coefficient [12]	<0.004 %	Rapidly eliminated by lungs	2–5 min	
Xenon		Minimum [115]			
Thiopental	Distributes well into adipose tissue; 6–12 times blood	Primarily to inactive metabolites, but pentobarbital (active) is also formed		30–60 s	10–30 min [65]

(continued)

Table 1.4 (continued)

	Distribution	Metabolism	Renal excretion	Onset of action	Duration of action
Methohexital	Distributes quickly into brain, within 30 s; redistribution occurs within 30 min into less vascular areas	Extensive [13]	Less than 1 % excreted unchanged in urine	2–45 s [14]	4–8 min after doses of 45–125 mg [15]
	Does not distribute well into adipose tissue				15–30 min after higher doses of 240–310 mg [15]
Propofol	Rapid distribution: 1–8 min [16]	Rapid and extensive by cytochrome P4502B6 [17]	<0.3 % excreted unchanged; 88 % excreted as metabolite	30 s (10–50 s); onset is infusion rate related [18]	3–10 min
Etomidate	Rapid distribution [116]	Extensive by cytochrome P450	2 % excreted unchanged in urine	30–60 s	3–5 min
Ketamine	Rapid distribution into highly perfused tissues [19]	Extensive by cytochrome P450	4 % excreted unchanged in urine	IV: 30 s IM: 3–4 min	IV: 5–10 min IM: 12–25 min
Chloroprocaine	Rapid distribution into highly perfused tissues	Plasma cholinesterases	Undergoes renal excretion	6–12 min	1 h
Procaine	Not available	Rapid by cholinesterase	2 % excreted unchanged in urine		1 h

Drug	Volume of distribution	Metabolism	Excretion	Onset	Duration
Lidocaine	1.5 L/kg	90 % by cytochrome P450 1A2 [20]; two active metabolites: monoethylglycinexylidide (MEGX) and glycinexylidide (GX)	10 % excreted unchanged in urine	Dental: <2 min / Local: 2–4 min	2 h
Prilocaine	0.7–4.4 L/kg	Undergoes hepatic metabolism [21]	Undergoes renal excretion [21]	2–3 min	1 h
Bupivacaine	2.5 L/kg	Extensive hepatic metabolism	6 % excreted unchanged in urine [22]	5–10 min [23]	1.5–8 h
Ropivacaine	36–60 L	Extensive hepatic metabolism by cytochrome P450 1A2	1 % excreted unchanged in urine	Brachial: 15–30 min / Cesarean: 2.5–25 min / Epidural: 6–8 min [24]	1.5–8 h
Mepivacaine	Extensively distributes into liver, lung, heart, and brain	Extensive hepatic metabolism by hydroxylation and N-demethylation	5–10 % excreted unchanged in urine	Epidural: 5–15 min / Nerve block: 10–20 min	2 h
Articaine	1–2 L/kg	Primarily hepatic by carboxylesterase	2–5 % excreted unchanged in urine [25]	1–6 min	1 h
Tetracaine	Not available	Extensive by plasma esterases		Topical: 30 s / Topical, liposomal: 30 min / Spinal: 3–5 min / Epidural: 8–20 min	Topical: 2.5 h / Topical, liposomal: 2.5 h / Spinal: 2–3 h / Epidural: 7.5–10.5 h
Levobupivacaine	54–66.9 L [26]	Extensive by hepatic metabolism	Undetectable unchanged drug in urine		
Etidocaine	134 L [27]	Extensive by hepatic metabolism	<10 % excreted unchanged in urine	Infiltration, nerve block, retrobulbar: 2–5 min [28] / Epidural: 15–30 min [29]	Infiltration, nerve block: 4–10 h / Epidural: 6–10 h

Table 1.5 Drug information of anesthetic agents

Drug name, mechanism of action, indication	Contraindication, caution, pregnancy category, breast feeding	Clinical pearls	Dosing options	Drug interactions and side effects
Isoflurane (Florane™, Terrell™) [7, 30]	*Contraindications*: (1) known sensitivity to isoflurane, (2) patients at risk for malignant hyperthermia	Low blood/gas partition coefficient, producing rapid induction and recovery from anesthesia	Induction: 1.5–3 % with O_2 or O_2/nitrous oxide mix; anesthesia obtained within 7–10 min	*Drug interactions* [31]:
MOA: modulation of $GABA_A$ receptors, potentiating inhibitory synaptic transmission [32]	*Caution*: (1) hyperkalemia, (2) malignant hyperthermia	Pungent odor may limit rate of induction	Maintenance: 1–2.5 % with NO; additional 0.5–1 % with O_2 only	clarithromycin, class I and III antiarrhythmics, dolasetron, droperidol, fluconazole, fluoxetine, haloperidol, hydromorphone, ondansetron, oxycodone, quetiapine, risperidone, St. John's wort, telithromycin, tricyclic antidepressants, ziprasidone

| Indications: induction and maintenance of anesthesia | Pregnancy category: C

Breast feeding: infant risk has not been ruled out | Good cardiovascular stability; not proarrhythmic

Lower incidence of hepatotoxicity [34] | MAC [7, 33]: | Concurrent use with neuromuscular-blocking agents (atracurium, cisatracurium, pancuronium) may result in prolongation of neuromuscular-blocking effects

Side effects:
Common: nausea, vomiting, hypotension, cough, excessive salivation, headache
Serious: bradycardia, cardiac arrest, myocardial infarction, hyperkalemia, malignant hyperthermia, decreased liver function, hepatic necrosis, liver failure, seizure, myoglobinuria, renal failure, respiratory depression [7] |

MAC [7, 33]:

Age	100% O_2	70% NO_2
26±4	1.28	0.56
44±7	1.15	0.50
64±5	1.05	0.37

(continued)

Table 1.5 (continued)

Drug name, mechanism of action, indication	Contraindication, caution, pregnancy category, breast feeding	Clinical pearls	Dosing options	Drug interactions and side effects
Sevoflurane (Ultane™, Sojourn™) [35, 36] MOA: modulation of GABA_A receptors, potentiating inhibitory synaptic transmission [39] Indication: general anesthesia	*Contraindication*: patients at risk for malignant hyperthermia *Caution*: (1) hyperkalemia, (2) malignant hyperthermia *Pregnancy category: B* *Breast feeding*: infant risk has not been ruled out	Low blood/gas partition coefficient, producing rapid induction and recovery from anesthesia FDA limits its use to 2 MAC hours (1 MAC for 2 h or 2 MACs for 1 h) due to its by-product, compound A, that has caused renal injury in rat models [40] Not as pungent as isoflurane or desflurane Good cardiovascular stability	0.5–3 % concentration with or without concomitant use of nitrous oxide [37] <table><tr><td>Age (yrs)</td><td>With O₂</td><td>With 65% NO₂/3 5% O₂</td></tr><tr><td>0-1mo</td><td>3.3%</td><td>–</td></tr><tr><td>1-6mos</td><td>3.0%</td><td>–</td></tr><tr><td>6mos-3yrs</td><td>2.8%</td><td>2.0%*</td></tr><tr><td>3-12</td><td>2.5%</td><td>–</td></tr><tr><td>25</td><td>2.6%</td><td>1.4%</td></tr><tr><td>40</td><td>2.1%</td><td>1.1%</td></tr><tr><td>60</td><td>1.7%</td><td>0.9%</td></tr><tr><td>80</td><td>1.4%</td><td>0.7%</td></tr></table>*60/40% used	*Drug interactions* [38]: hydromorphone, oxycodone, St. John's wort *Side effects*: *Common*: bradycardia, hypotension, nausea, vomiting, somnolence, agitation, cough, interrupted breathing, shivering *Serious*: AV block, hemorrhage, QT prolongation, torsades de pointes, hyperkalemia, malignant hyperthermia, hepatic necrosis, liver failure, hypersensitivity, seizure, laryngeal spasm, respiratory depression

Age (yrs)	With O_2	With 65% NO_2/3 5% O_2
0-1mo	3.3%	–
1-6mos	3.0%	–
6mos-3yrs	2.8%	2.0%*
3-12	2.5%	–
25	2.6%	1.4%
40	2.1%	1.1%
60	1.7%	0.9%
80	1.4%	0.7%

*60/40% used

Desflurane (Suprane™) [41, 42]	Contraindication: patients at risk for malignant hyperthermia	Induction: initiate with 3 % in O_2 or nitrous oxide/O_2 and increase by 0.5–1 % every 2–3 breaths or as tolerated (up to 11 %) until loss of consciousness [41]	Drug interactions [45]: cisatracurium, hydromorphone, oxycodone, St. John's wort
MOA: modulation of GABA$_A$ receptors, potentiating inhibitory synaptic transmission [43]	Pregnancy category: B	Concentrations exceeding 12 % have been reported to be safe [44]	Side effects:
Indication: general anesthesia	Breast feeding: infant risk has not been ruled out	Maintenance: 2.5–8.5 % with or without concomitant NO_2	Common: hypotension, salivation, nausea, vomiting, cough [48]
			Serious: bradycardia, cardiac arrest, heart failure, hypertension, malignant hypertension, shock, sinus arrhythmia, torsades de pointes, hyperkalemia, pancreatitis, hepatic necrosis, liver failure, rhabdomyolysis, nephrotoxicity, interrupted breath, laryngeal spasm

MAC [46, 47]

Age	With O_2	With 60% NO_2
18-30	7.25%	4%
31-65	6%	2.8%

(continued)

Table 1.5 (continued)

Drug name, mechanism of action, indication	Contraindication, caution, pregnancy category, breast feeding	Clinical pearls	Dosing options	Drug interactions and side effects
Nitrous oxide [49, 50]	*Contraindication*: patients receiving nitrous oxide for longer than 24 h	Used primarily in combination with other anesthetics to reduce their dose and therefore side effects; 70 % NO_2 reduces MAC of other anesthetics by 60 % (GG)	Induction: NO_2 with at least 25–30 % O_2; premedicate with narcotic analgesics or barbiturates	
MOA: noncompetitive antagonist activity at the NMDA receptor, potentiating inhibitory synaptic transmission (double-check if it is inhibitory) [51, 52]	*Caution*: patients at risk for gas embolism, pneumothorax, or ileus	Must be administered with at least 25–30 % O_2	Maintenance: 30–70 % NO_2 with O_2	*Drug interactions*: no known significant drug interactions
In addition to anesthesia, also has analgesia and anxiolytic properties	*Pregnancy category*: not established	Less effective in areas of high altitude		*Side effects: frequency not defined* [53]: arrhythmias, hypotension, pulmonary hypertension, hypothermia, malignant hyperthermia, abdominal distension, nausea, vomiting, anemia, vitamin B_{12} deficiency, megaloblastic erythropoiesis, methemoglobinemia, myelosuppression, pancytopenia, increased liver enzymes, jaundice, neuropathy, increased intracranial pressure, seizure, spastic paraparesis, spinal cord disease, abnormal vision, psychotic disorder, increased sputum production
Indications: (1) general anesthesia (2) relief of severe pain	*Breast feeding*: infant risk has not been ruled out	Analgesia is produced at concentrations as low as 20 % (GG)		

Xenon			
MOA: noncompetitive antagonist activity at the NMDA/glutamate receptor, potentiating inhibitory synaptic transmission [51]	Contraindication: hypersensitivity to xenon	Does not potentiate duration of neuromuscular-blocking agents [54]	Drug interactions [55]: no known drug interactions
Indication: general anesthesia	Caution: patients at risk for gas embolism, pneumothorax, or ileus [56]	Production costs are high [57]	Side effects:
	Pregnancy category: not teratogenic	Not detrimental to environment [58]	Common: nausea and vomiting (substantial)
	Breast feeding: infant risk has not been ruled out	Does not affect renal, hepatic, coagulation, platelet, or immune system function [58, 59]	Serious: increased pulmonary resistance [60, 61]
		Does not induce malignant hyperthermia [62]	
		Contains analgesic properties [63]	
		More effective than nitrous oxide on cardiovascular function [64]	

(continued)

Table 1.5 (continued)

Drug name, mechanism of action, indication	Contraindication, caution, pregnancy category, breast feeding	Clinical pearls	Dosing options	Drug interactions and side effects
Intravenous anesthetics				
Thiopental (Pentothal™) [65, 66]	*Contraindications:* acute intermittent porphyria and variegate porphyria	Duration is very short, therefore not recommended in surgical procedures lasting longer than 15 min	Slow induction: 50–75 mg slow IV, single dose at 20–40 s intervals [65]	*Drug interactions* [67]: benzodiazepines, carisoprodol, metaxalone, methocarbamol, opioid analgesics, quetiapine
MOA: GABA$_A$ receptor agonist, opening Cl channels and causing depolarization, resulting in increased inhibitory synaptic transmission [68]	*Caution:* (1) severe cardiovascular shock, (2) hypotension or shock, (3) conditions in which hypnotic effect may be prolonged or potentiated, (4) status asthmaticus, (5) endocrine insufficiency, (6) increased intracranial pressure, (7) ophthalmoplegia, (8) respiratory impairment or obstruction		Rapid induction: 210–280 mg (3–4 mg/kg) IV divided in 2–4 doses	*Side effects:*
Indications: (1) general anesthesia, (2) regional anesthesia; adjunct	Pregnancy category: C		Maintenance: 25–50 mg IV repeat PRN or continuous IV of 0.2 % or 0.4 % solution	*Common:* injection site reaction
	Breast feeding: compatible with breast feeding		Dosing in obese (BMI ≥30) (40) Loading TBW / Maintenance IBW	*Serious:* myocardial infarction, hemolytic anemia, anaphylaxis, radial neuropathy, apnea, laryngeal spasm, respiratory depression
			Renal failure (GFR <10 mL/ min): 75 % of usual dose Hepatic insufficiency: no dosing adjustment needed [70]	

Methohexital (Brevital™) [71, 72]	Contraindication: latent porphyria	Induction: 50–120 mg (or 1–1.5 mg/kg) in 1 % solution administered at a rate of 1 mL over 5 s [73]	Drug interactions [74]: benzodiazepines, carisoprodol, metaxalone, methocarbamol, opioid analgesics, quetiapine
MOA: GABA$_A$ receptor agonist, opening Cl channels and causing depolarization, resulting in increased inhibitory synaptic transmission	Caution: (1) anemia, (2) cardiovascular disease, (3) hepatic impairment, (4) obesity, (5) pulmonary disease, (6) renal impairment, (7) seizure disorder	Maintenance: (1) 20–40 mg in 1 % solution administered every 4–7 min, PRN, or (2) 3 mL continuous drip of 0.2 % solution/min (1 drop/s); for longer surgical procedures, gradually reduce rate of administration	Side effects:
Indications: (1) general anesthesia prior to other anesthetic agents; (2) adjunct to inhaled anesthetic agents; (3) adjunct with other parenteral agents, typically narcotic analgesics, to supplement less potent inhaled anesthetics; (4) for short procedures and inducing hypnotic state	Pregnancy category: C	Procedural sedation (unlabeled dose): I.V.: 0.75–1 mg/kg; can redose 0.5 mg/kg every 2–5 min as needed [75]	Common: hypotension, injection site pain, spasmodic movement, cough, hiccoughs, laryngeal spasm
	Breast feeding: compatible with breast feeding		Serious: cardiac arrest, shock, thrombophlebitis, anaphylaxis, seizure, cardiorespiratory arrest, respiratory depression
	BBW: should only be administered in hospitals or ambulatory care settings with continuous monitoring of respiratory function; resuscitative drugs, age- and size-appropriate intubation equipment, and trained personnel experienced in handling their use should be readily available		

(continued)

Table 1.5 (continued)

Drug name, mechanism of action, indication	Contraindication, caution, pregnancy category, breast feeding	Clinical pearls	Dosing options	Drug interactions and side effects
Propofol (Diprivan™) [76, 77]	*Contraindications:* (1) allergies to eggs, egg products, soybeans, or soy products (Abraxis brand), (2) allergies to soy or peanut (Fresenius Propoven)	Propofol should be administered within 4 h of its removal from sterile packaging due to risk of bacterial growth	*Healthy adults <55 years* [76] Induction: 50 mg IV every 10 s until onset (2–2.5 mg/kg); dose adjust according to age and surgery type	*Drug interactions* [78]: bupivacaine, hydromorphone, lidocaine, meclizine, oxycodone, St. John's wort, zolpidem
MOA: $GABA_A$ receptor agonist, opening Cl channels and causing depolarization, resulting in increased inhibitory synaptic transmission [79]	*Caution:* (1) elderly, debilitated, or ASA III/IV patients, (2) seizure history	Patients may still recover rapidly after long duration of use	Maintenance: 100–200 mcg/kg/min IV (6–12 mg/kg/h); dose adjust according to age and surgery type; may administer 20–50 mg IV PRN	*Side effects:*

| Indications: (1) general anesthesia, (2) monitored anesthesia care sedation, (3) sedation for mechanically ventilated patient in ICU | *Pregnancy category*: B

Breast feeding: infant risk has not been ruled out | Less nausea and vomiting than other anesthetic agents (Micromedex)

Short half-life allows for flexibility in controlling sedation depth | *Pediatric*
Induction (3–16 years): 2.5–3.5 mg/kg IV over 20–30 s
Maintenance (2 months–16 years): 125–300 mcg/kg/min IV (7.5–18 mg/kg/h)
Geriatric
Induction: 20 mg IV every 10 s (1–1.5 mg/kg)
Maintenance: 50–100 mcg/kg/min (3–6 mg/kg/h)
Debiliated, ASA-PS III–IV patients
Induction: 20 mg IV every 10 s until onset (1–1.5 mg/kg)
Maintenance: 50–100 mcg/kg/min (3–6 mg/kg/h)
Cardiac patients
Induction: 20 mg IV every 10 s until onset (0.5–1.5 mg/kg)
Maintenance: (1) if propofol is the primary agent, 100–150 mcg/kg/min IV with opioid as adjuvant, or (2) if opioid is the primary agent, propofol 50–100 mcg/kg/min
Neurosurgical patients
Induction: 20 mg IV every 10 s (1–2 mg/kg)
Maintenance: 100–200 mcg/kg/min (6–12 mc/kg/h) IV | *Common*: injection site pain, nausea, vomiting, involuntary movement

Serious: bradycardia, heart failure, hypertension, pancreatitis, anaphylaxis, seizure, acute renal failure, priapism, apnea, respiratory acidosis |

(continued)

Table 1.5 (continued)

Drug name, mechanism of action, indication	Contraindication, caution, pregnancy category, breast feeding	Clinical pearls	Dosing options	Drug interactions and side effects
Etomidate (Amidate™) [58, 80, 81] MOA: modulation of $GABA_A$ receptors, potentiating inhibitory synaptic transmission (6281035) Indications: (1) general anesthesia, (2) adjunct to subpotent anesthetic agents during maintenance of anesthesia of short procedures	Contraindication: hypersensitivity to etomidate Caution: (1) elderly, especially with hypertension, (2) renal impairment Pregnancy category: C Breast feeding: infant risk has not been ruled out	Rapid recovery with wide therapeutic window Minimal effects on cardiovascular and respiratory function [83] Does not cause histamine release [84]	Induction (>10 years): 0.3 mg/kg (0.2–0.6 mg/kg) injected over 30–60 s [52] Maintenance, adjunct: 0.01–0.02 mg/kg/min IV; dosage must be individualized Smaller increments may be administered as adjunct to subpotent anesthetic agents such as nitrous oxide for short procedures	Drug interactions [82]: St. John's wort Common: injection site pain, nausea, vomiting Serious: hypotension, myoclonus
Ketamine (Ketalar™) [85, 86] MOA: noncompetitive NMDA receptor antagonist, blocking glutamate binding [87]	Contraindication: in patients in whom a significant elevation of blood pressure would constitute a serious hazard Caution: (1) alcohol intoxication or history of alcohol abuse	Useful in pediatric and uncontrollable patients Has anesthetic, analgesic, and sedative properties	Induction: (1) 1–4.5 mg/kg infused over 60 s, (2) 1–2 mg/kg/IV infused at 0.5 mg/kg/min, (3) 6.5–13 mg/kg IM Additionally, diazepam 2–5 mg administered in separate syringe over 60 s can be used (<15 mg total) [88]	Drug interactions [86]: hydromorphone, oxycodone, St. John's wort, tramadol Side effects:

Indications: (1) general anesthesia, (2) adjunct to subpotent anesthetic agents during maintenance of anesthesia of short procedures	Pregnancy category: A	Diazepam frequently administered as adjunct to prevent psychological manifestations (dreamlike observations, emergence delirium)	Maintenance: increments of 50–100 % of induction dose may be repeated PRN	Common: hypertension, tachycardia, psychiatric sign or symptom upon emergence from anesthesia
	Breast feeding: compatible with breast feeding by WHO; infant risk has not been ruled out by Micromedex	Larger doses will require longer recovery times		Serious: bradycardia, arrhythmias, hypotension, anaphylaxis, apnea, laryngeal spasm, pulmonary edema, respiratory depression
Local anesthetics				
Chloroprocaine (Nesacaine™) [89, 90]	Contraindication: hypersensitivity to chloroprocaine	Effective in labor and delivery due to rapid onset of action and low systemic toxicity	Procedure [89] Mandibular: 2–3 mL of 2 % solution (40–60 mg total)	Drug interactions [90]: St. John's wort

(continued)

Table 1.5 (continued)

Drug name, mechanism of action, indication	Contraindication, caution, pregnancy category, breast feeding	Clinical pearls	Dosing options	Drug interactions and side effects
MOA: blocks sodium channels on nerve membranes, decreasing rate of nerve conduction related to pain transmission	*Caution*: neurological disease, spinal deformities, septicemia, severe hypertension	Not recommended for spinal administration	Infraorbital: 0.5–1 mL of 2 % solution (10–20 mg total)	*Side effects*:
Indication: local anesthesia	*Pregnancy category*: C		Brachial plexus: 30–40 mL of 2 % solution (600–800 mg total)	*Common*: dizziness
	Breast feeding: infant risk has not been ruled out		Digital, without epinephrine: 3–4 mL of 1 % solution (30–40 mg total)	*Serious*: cardiac arrest, negative cardiac inotropic effect, ventricular arrhythmia, anaphylaxis, immune hypersensitivity reaction, chondrolysis of articular cartilage, arachnoiditis, CNS depression, CNS stimulation, loss of consciousness, seizure, hypoventilation, respiratory arrest
			Pudendal: 10 mL each side of 2 % solution (400 mg total)	
			Paracervical 3 per each of 4 sites of 1 % solution (up to 120 mg total)	
			Pediatric (>3 years)	
			Infiltration: 0.5–1 % solution; max 11 mg/kg	
			Nerve block: 1–1.5 % solution; max 11 mg/kg	
			Max dose without epinephrine: 11 mg/kg not to exceed 800 mg total	
			Max dose with epinephrine (1:200,000): 15 mg/kg not to exceed 1,000 mg total	

			Drug interactions [92]: St. John's wort
Procaine (Novocain™) [91, 92]		Local infiltration: 350–600 mg, administered as diluted solution (140–240 mL of a 0.25 % solution or 70–120 mL of a 0.5 % solution)	Side effects:
Contraindication: hypersensitivity to procaine, drugs of a similar chemical structure, or para-aminobenzoic acid (PABA) or its derivatives	Slow onset		
MOA: blocks sodium channels on nerve membranes, decreasing rate of nerve conduction related to pain transmission	Addition of epinephrine as adjunct may be warranted for vasoconstrictive effect	Peripheral nerve block: 0.5 % (up to 200 mL), 1 % (up to 100 mL), or 2 % (up to 50 mL)	Common: nausea, vomiting, nervousness, dizziness, blurred vision
Caution: (1) severe disturbances of cardiac rhythm, shock, heart block, or hypotension, (2) hepatic disease		Epinephrine: 0.5–1 mL of epinephrine 1:1,000 per 100 mL may be added for (1:200,000–1:100,000) during local infiltration and peripheral nerve block	
Indication: production of local or regional analgesia and anesthesia and peripheral nerve block			Serious: negative cardiac inotropic effect, hypotension, hypertension, bradycardia, ventricular arrhythmias, cardiac arrest, urticaria, edema, tremors, seizures, respiratory arrest
Pregnancy category: C		Max dose: 1,000 mg/treatment	
Breast feeding: infant risk has not been ruled out			

(continued)

Table 1.5 (continued)

Drug name, mechanism of action, indication	Contraindication, caution, pregnancy category, breast feeding	Clinical pearls	Dosing options	Drug interactions and side effects
Lidocaine (Xylocaine™) [93–96]	*Contraindications*: (1) hypersensitivity to local amide anesthetic, (2) myasthenia gravis, (3) shock, (4) cardiac conduction disease, (5) severe liver disease, (6) severe kidney disease, (7) concurrent systemic use of dronedarone, saquinavir, or dihydroergotamine		See Table 1.6.	*Drug interactions*: amiodarone, amprenavir, arbutamine, atazanavir, class I antiarrhythmics, class III antiarrhythmics, cobicistat, darunavir, delavirdine, dihydroergotamine, dronedarone, etravirine, fosamprenavir, fosphenytoin, lopinavir, metoprolol, nadolol, phenytoin, propofol, propranolol, saquinavir, succinylcholine, St. John's wort
MOA: blocks sodium channels on nerve membranes, decreasing rate of nerve conduction related to pain transmission [97]	*Caution*: (1) acutely ill and debilitated patients			*Side effects*:
Indication: local anesthesia	*Pregnancy category*: B *Breast feeding*: infant risk is minimal			*Common*: hypotension, nausea *Serious*: cardiac arrest, cardiac arrhythmias, methemoglobinemia, anaphylaxis

Drug / MOA / Indications	Contraindications / Caution	Description	Dosing	Side effects / Drug interactions
Prilocaine (Citanest™) [21, 98] MOA: blocks sodium channels on nerve membranes, decreasing rate of nerve conduction related to pain transmission Indications: (1) local anesthetic nerve block, (2) local anesthetic dental infiltration	Contraindications: (1) hypersensitivity to prilocaine or local amide anesthetic, (2) congenital or idiopathic methemoglobinemia Caution: (1) hepatic disease, (2) impaired cardiovascular function Pregnancy category: B	No cross-sensitivity in patients allergic to procaine, tetracaine, or benzocaine	Adults local anesthetic dental infiltration/local anesthetic nerve block: 1–2 mL (40–80 mg) 4 % solution with or without epinephrine Max dose calculated based on weight (8 mg/kg) up to 15 mL (600 mg) within a 2-h period	Drug interactions [21]: class I antiarrhythmics, class III antiarrhythmics, propranolol, St. John's wort Side effects:
Bupivacaine (Marcaine HCL™, Marcaine Spinal™, Sensorcaine™, Sensorcaine-MPF™) [99, 100]	Breast feeding: infant risk has not been ruled out Black box warning: 0.75 % solution not recommended for obstetrical anesthesia	Long-acting useful in local or regional anesthesia for surgical, dental, diagnostic, and obstetrical procedures	Pediatrics local anesthetic dental infiltration/local anesthetic nerve block (age up to 10 years): 1 mL (40 mg) of 4 % solution Max dose calculated based on weight (6.6–8.8 mg/kg) Local: 10–30 mL intrapleural bolus of 0.25 %, 0.375 %, or 0.5 % every 4–8 h	Common: bradycardia, hypotension, muscle twitch, tremor, confusion, dizziness, lightheadedness, somnolence, blurred vision, diplopia, tinnitus, apprehension, euphoria, feeling nervous, abnormal sensation Serious: cardiac arrest, vomiting, methemoglobinemia, anaphylaxis, loss of consciousness, seizure, respiratory arrest Drug interactions [100]: propofol, propranolol, St. John's wort, verapamil

(continued)

Table 1.5 (continued)

Drug name, mechanism of action, indication	Contraindication, caution, pregnancy category, breast feeding	Clinical pearls	Dosing options	Drug interactions and side effects
MOA: blocks sodium channels on nerve membranes, decreasing rate of nerve conduction related to pain transmission	*Contraindications:* (1) hypersensitivity to bupivacaine or local amide anesthetic; (2) severe hemorrhage, hypotension, shock, or arrhythmias; (3) local infection at site of proposed lumbar puncture	Analgesic properties of bupivacaine may reduce postoperative analgesic requirements [101]	Local: 0.375 % bupivacaine with epinephrine at 6 mL/h after 20 mL loading dose intrapleural	*Side effects:*
Indications: (1) local anesthesia, (2) regional anesthesia, (3) dental procedure anesthesia, (4) eye procedure anesthesia	*Caution:* (1) history of chondrolysis, (2) concurrent use of monoamine oxidase inhibitors (MAOI) or antidepressants (triptyline or imipramine types), (3) less than 18 years, (4) hepatic disease, (5) impaired cardiovascular function		Regional: 6.25–18.75 mg/h epidural continuous infusion, as a 0.0625–0.125 % solution	*Common:* hypotension

Pregnancy category: C	Dental procedure: 1.8–3.6 mL of 0.5 % solution (9–18 mg) with epinephrine; a second dose (9 mg) may be administered; max 90 mg total	*Serious*: bradycardia, heart block, ventricular arrhythmias, bacterial meningitis, immune hypersensitivity reaction, chondrolysis of articular cartilage, CNS stimulation, CNS depression, cranial nerve disorder paraplegia, seizure, respiratory arrest
Breast feeding: infant risk is minimal	Procedures on eye: complete motor blockade, 2–4 mL (15–30 mg) of 0.75 % solution	
	Local infiltration: 0.25 % solution up to max doses (max 225 mg with epinephrine or 175 mg without epinephrine)	
	Local sacral epidural: moderate to complete blockade, 15–30 mL of 0.5 % solution (75–150 mg) or 0.25 % solution (37.5–75 mg), repeated once every 3 h PRN	
	Regional epidural: partial to moderate motor blockade, 10–20 mL (25–50 mg) of a 0.25 % solution; moderate to complete motor blockade, 10–20 mL (50–100 mg) as a 0.5 % solution; complete motor blockade, 10–20 mL (75–150 mg) as a 0.75 % solution; repeat once every 3 h PRN	

(continued)

Table 1.5 (continued)

Drug name, mechanism of action, indication	Contraindication, caution, pregnancy category, breast feeding	Clinical pearls	Dosing options	Drug interactions and side effects
			Regional (obstetrical) hyperbaric spinal, bupivacaine in dextrose formulation only; normal vaginal delivery, 0.8 mL (6 mg) bupivacaine in dextrose as 0.75 % solution; Cesarean section, 1–1.4 mL (7.5–10.5 mg) bupivacaine in dextrose as 0.75 % solution	
			Regional hyperbaric spinal, bupivacaine in dextrose formulation only; lower extremity and perineal procedures, 1 mL (7.5 mg) bupivacaine in dextrose as 0.75 % solution; lower abdominal procedures, 1.6 mL (12 mg) bupivacaine in dextrose as 0.75 % solution; upper abdominal surgery, 2 mL (15 mg) bupivacaine in dextrose, in horizontal position	
			Regional peripheral nerve block: moderate to complete motor blockade, 5–37.5 mL (25–175 mg) of 0.5 % solution or 5–70 mL (12.5–175 mg) of 0.25 % solution, repeat every 3 h PRN	

Ropivacaine (Naropin™) [102, 103]	Less cardiotoxic than bupivacaine [104]	Regional sympathetic nerve block: 20–50 mL (50–125 mg) of 0.25 % solution, repeat once every 3 h PRN	*Drug interactions* [103]: bupivacaine, St. John's wort
MOA: blocks sodium channels on nerve membranes, decreasing rate of nerve conduction related to pain transmission	*Contraindication:* (1) hypersensitivity to ropivacaine or local amide anesthetic	Local anesthetic lumbar epidural block for Cesarean section: 20–30 mL of 0.5 % solution (100–150 mg) or 15–20 mL of 0.75 % solution (113–150 mg)	*Side effects:*
	Caution: (1) elderly patients with heart disease, (2) cardiovascular impairment, (3) concurrent use of class I or III antiarrhythmics, (4) hepatic disease, (5) hypotension, hypovolemia, or heart block	Epidural anesthesia for surgical procedure: 15–30 mL (75–150 mg) of 0.5 % solution	
Indications: (1) local anesthetic lumbar epidural block for Cesarean section, (2) epidural anesthesia for surgical procedure, (3) local anesthetic nerve block for surgical procedure, (4) postoperative pain	*Pregnancy category:* B	Local anesthetic field block for surgical procedure: 1–40 mL of 0.5 % solution (5–200 mg)	*Common:* bradycardia, hypotension, pruritus, nausea, vomiting, backache, headache, paresthesia, fever
	Breast feeding: infant risk has not been ruled out	Local anesthetic nerve block for surgical procedure: 35–50 mL of 0.5 % solution (175–250 mg), 10–40 mL of 0.75 % solution (75–300 mg)	*Serious:* cardiac arrest, chondrolysis of articular cartilage, Horner's syndrome

(continued)

Table 1.5 (continued)

Drug name, mechanism of action, indication	Contraindication, caution, pregnancy category, breast feeding	Clinical pearls	Dosing options	Drug interactions and side effects
Mepivacaine (Carbocaine™, Polocaine™, Polocaine-MPF™, Polocaine Dental™) [105, 106] MOA: blocks sodium channels on nerve membranes, decreasing rate of nerve conduction related to pain transmission	*Contraindication*: (1) hypersensitivity to mepivacaine or local amide anesthetic *Caution*: (1) hepatic impairment; (2) renal impairment; (3) cardiovascular impairment; (4) debilitated, elderly, or acutely ill; (5) inflammation or sepsis at site of injection	NOT for use in spinal anesthesia	Cervical, brachial, intercostal, and pudendal nerve block: 5–40 mL (50–400 mg) of 1 % solution or 5–20 mL (100–400 mg) of 2 % solution [105] Transvaginal block (paracervical plus pudendal): up to 30 mL both sides (up to 300 mg both sides) of 1 % solution [105]	*Drug interactions* [106]: propranolol, St. John's wort, verapamil *Side effects*:

Indications: (1) local anesthesia; (2) epidural block; (3) anesthetic injection into brachial plexus; (4) anesthetic injection into pudendal nerve; (5) local anesthesia, intercostal nerve block; (6) local anesthesia, cervical region nerve block; (7) paracervical block; (8) regional anesthesia; (9) pain management	*Pregnancy category*: C *Breast feeding*: infant risk has not been ruled out	Paracervical block: up to 20 mg both sides (up to 200 mg both sides) of 1 % solution [105] Caudal and epidural block: 15–30 mL (150–300 mg) of 1 % solution or 10–25 mL (150–375 mL) of 1.5 % solution or 10–20 mL (200–400 mg) of 2 % solution [105] Infiltration: up to 40 mg (up to 400 mL) of 1 % solution [105] Therapeutic block (pain management): 1–5 mL (10–50 mg) of 1 % solution or 1–5 mL (20–100 mg) of 2 % solution [105]	*Common*: anxiety, chills, dizziness, excitation, restlessness, tremors, incontinence, tinnitus, sneezing *Serious*: cardiac arrest, bradycardia, heart block, hypotension, ventricular arrhythmia, bacterial meningitis, immune hypersensitivity reaction, chondrolysis of articular cartilage, cranial nerve disorder, seizure, respiratory arrest

(continued)

Table 1.5 (continued)

Drug name, mechanism of action, indication	Contraindication, caution, pregnancy category, breast feeding	Clinical pearls	Dosing options	Drug interactions and side effects
Articaine and epinephrine (Articadent™, Orabloc™, Septocaine™, with epinephrine) [107, 108]	*Contraindication:* (1) hypersensitivity to articaine or local amide anesthetic	First FDA approval in 30 years of a new local dental anesthetic providing complete pulpal anesthesia for approximately 1 h	Infiltration: 0.5–2.5 mL (20–100 mg) of 4 % solution	*Drug interactions* [108]: bucindolol, carteolol, carvedilol, digoxin, dihydroergotamine, entacapone, halothane, isocarboxazid, labetalol, levobunolol, linezolid, metipranolol, nadolol, penbutolol, phenelzine, pindolol, propranolol, rasagiline, sotalol, tertatolol, timolol, tranylcypromine, tricyclic antidepressants
MOA: blocks sodium channels on nerve membranes, decreasing rate of nerve conduction related to pain transmission	*Caution:* (1) hepatic impairment; (2) renal impairment; (3) cardiovascular impairment; (4) debilitated, elderly, or acutely ill; (5) concomitant use of MAO inhibitors, tricyclic antidepressants, nonselective beta-blockers, phenothiazines, or butyrophenones		Nerve block: 0.5–3.4 mL (20–136 mg) of 4 % solution	*Note:* all drug interactions due to epinephrine in formulation
Indication: (1) local, infiltrative, or conductive anesthesia in both simple and complex dental procedures	*Pregnancy category:* C		Oral surgery: 1–5.1 mL (40–204 mg) of 4 % solution	*Side effects:*
	Breast feeding: infant risk has not been ruled out		Max dosage adults and pediatrics: 7 mg/kg (0.175 mL/kg) or 3.2 mg/lb body weight	*Common:* hypotension, pain *Serious:* cardiac arrest, negative inotrope, syncope, ventricular arrhythmia, injection site necrosis, immune hypersensitivity reaction

Tetracaine (Pontocaine™, [109, 110]) Blocks sodium channels on nerve membranes, decreasing rate of nerve conduction related to pain transmission Indications: (1) for rapid- and short-acting ophthalmic anesthesia, (2) spinal anesthesia	Contraindication: (1) hypersensitivity to tetracaine hydrochloride, ester-type local anesthetics, or para-aminobenzoic acid (PABA) or its derivatives Caution: (1) acutely ill, elderly ill, or debilitated patients, (2) cardiac disease, (3) concomitant use of sulfonamides, (4) shock, (5) cardiovascular disease, (6) hyperthyroidism (Lexicomp) Pregnancy category: C Breast feeding: infant risk has not been ruled out	Ophthalmic procedures: 1 drop into the eyes PRN Perineal: 5 mg Perineal and lower extremities: 10 mg Costal margin: 15 mg; doses up to 20 mg may be given, but are reserved for exceptional cases Low spinal (saddle block): 2–5 mg	Drug interactions [110]: no known significant drug interactions Side effects: Common: stinging, burning, and conjunctival redness, hypotension, nausea, vomiting Serious: allergic corneal reaction, apnea

(continued)

Table 1.5 (continued)

Drug name, mechanism of action, indication	Contraindication, caution, pregnancy category, breast feeding	Clinical pearls	Dosing options	Drug interactions and side effects
Levobupivacaine (Chirocaine™) [111]	*Contraindication:* (1) hypersensitivity to levobupivacaine or local amide anesthetic	Slow onset of action	Local: 60 mL (150 mg) of 0.25 % solution	*Drug interactions* [112]: St. John's wort
MOA: blocks sodium channels on nerve membranes, decreasing rate of nerve conduction related to pain transmission	*Caution:* (1) hepatic impairment		Local, retrobulbar: 5 mL of 0.5 % solution	*Side effects:*
Indications: (1) local anesthesia, (2) regional anesthesia, (3) obstetrical pain, (4) postoperative pain	*Pregnancy category:* C		Regional, peribulbar infiltration: 5–15 mL (37.5–112.5 mg) of 0.75 solution	*Common:* pruritis, nausea, vomiting, dizziness, fever
	Breast feeding: infant risk has not been ruled out		Regional, peripheral block: 30 mL or 0.4 mL/kg of 0.25–0.5 % solution	*Serious:* cardiac arrest, arrhythmias, hypotension, apnea
			Regional, epidural (surgical): 10–20 mL (50–150 mg) of 0.05–0.75 % solution	
			Regional, epidural (Cesarean section): 10–20 mL of 0.5 % solution (100–150 mg)—avoid using 0.75 % solution	

Etidocaine (Duranest) [113]	Indication: (1) local, infiltrative, or conductive anesthesia in both simple and complex dental procedures	Contraindication: (1) hypersensitivity to articaine or local amide anesthetic	First FDA approval in 30 years of a new local dental anesthetic providing complete pulpal anesthesia for approximately 1 h	Infiltration: 0.5–2.5 mL (20–100 mg) of 4 % solution	Drug interactions [114]: bucindolol, carteolol, carvedilol, digoxin, dihydroergotamine, entacapone, halothane, isocarboxazid, labetalol, levobunolol, linezolid, metipranolol, nadolol, penbutolol, phenelzine, pindolol, propranolol, rasagiline, sotalol, tertatolol, timolol, tranylcypromine, tricyclic antidepressants
	MOA: blocks sodium channels on nerve membranes, decreasing rate of nerve conduction related to pain transmission	Caution: (1) hepatic impairment; (2) renal impairment; (3) cardiovascular impairment; (4) debilitated, elderly, or acutely ill; (5) concomitant use of MAO inhibitors, tricyclic antidepressants, nonselective beta-blockers, phenothiazines, or butyrophenones	Contains epinephrine	Nerve block: 0.5–3.4 mL (20–136 mg) of 4 % solution	Note: all drug interactions due to epinephrine in formulation
		Pregnancy category: C		Oral surgery: 1–5.1 mL (40–204 mg) of 4 % solution	Side effects:
		Breast feeding: infant risk has not been ruled out		Max dosage: adults and pediatrics, 7 mg/kg (0.175 mL/kg) or 3.2 mg/lb body weight	Common: hypotension, pain
					Serious: cardiac arrest, negative inotrope, syncope, ventricular arrhythmia, injection site necrosis, immune hypersensitivity reaction

Table 1.6 Dosing options of lidocaine

Adults (>16 years)	Dose
Abdominal	1.5–2 mL (75–100 mg) of 5 % solution with glucose 7.5 %
Brachial block	15–20 mL (225–300 mg) of 1.5 % solution
Cataract surgery	2 % gel applied topically 3–5 times 15–20 min prior to surgery
	2 drops of 4 % solution instilled into both eyes 6 times (i.e., 60, 50, 40, 30, 20, 10 min) prior to surgery
Cervical block	5 mL (50 mg) of 1 % solution
Dental block	1–5 mL of 2 % solution with epinephrine 1:50,000 or 1:100,000 using smallest effective volume; max dose with epinephrine is 7 mg/kg; max dose without epinephrine is 4.5 mg/kg
Eye procedure	2 drops of 3.5 % ophthalmic gel to the eye; reapply as necessary
Intercostal block	3–5 mL (30–50 mg) of 1 % solution
Lumbar epidural block	25–30 mL (250–300 mg) of 1 % solution; test dose of 2–3 mL of 1.5 % solution should be given at least 5 min prior to administering total volume; do not repeat max dose for at least 90 min for continuous epidural
Obstetrical low spinal block	1 mL (50 mg) for normal vaginal delivery of 5 % solution; 1.5 mL (75 mg) for Cesarean section of 5 % solution
Paravertebral block	3–5 mL (30–50 mg) of 1 % solution
Pudendal block	10 mL (100 mg) of 1 % solution; do not repeat for 90 min
Regional block	10–60 mL (50–300 mg) intravenous regional infiltration of 5 % solution; max dose is 4 mg/kg
Percutaneous infiltration	1–60 mL (5–300 mg) of 0.5 or 1 % solution
Retrobulbar infiltration	3–5 mL (120–200 mg) of 4 % solution
Surgical block	1.5–2.0 mL (75–100 mg) of 5 % solution
Topical	Single application not to exceed 5 g of 5 % ointment (250 mg of lidocaine); approximately 6 in. length of ointment from tube; max dose is 17–20 g of ointment (850–1,000 mg of lidocaine) per day
Hepatic impairment	Doses and infusion rates should be reduced

References

1. Buxton ILO, Benet LZ. Chapter 2. Pharmacokinetics: the dynamics of drug absorption, distribution, metabolism, and elimination. In: Brunton LL, Chabner BA, BC K, editors. Goodman & Gilman's the pharmacological basis of therapeutics. New York: McGraw-Hill; 2011.
2. Wagner JG, Northam JI. Estimation of volume of distribution and half-life of a compound after rapid intravenous injection. J Pharm Sci. 1967;56(4):529–31. Epub 1967/04/01.
3. Cockcroft DW, Gault MH. Prediction of creatinine clearance from serum creatinine. Nephron. 1976;16(1):31–41. Epub 1976/01/01.
4. Gibaldi M, Perrier D. Pharmacokinetics, vol. 8. 2nd ed. New York: M. Dekker; 1982. p. 494.
5. Eger 2nd EI, Saidman LJ, Brandstater B. Minimum alveolar anesthetic concentration: a standard of anesthetic potency. Anesthesiology. 1965;26(6):756–63. Epub 1965/11/01.
6. Eger 2nd EI. The pharmacology of isoflurane. Br J Anaesth. 1984;56 Suppl 1:71S–99. Epub 1984/01/01.
7. Product information: FORANE(R) inhalation liquid, isoflurane inhalation liquid. Deerfield: Baxter Healthcare Corporation; 2010.
8. Strum DP, Eger 2nd EI. Partition coefficients for sevoflurane in human blood, saline, and olive oil. Anesth Analg. 1987;66(7):654–6. Epub 1987/07/01.
9. Saito S, Goto F, Kadoi Y, Takahashi T, Fujita T, Mogi K. Comparative clinical study of induction and emergence time in sevoflurane and enflurane anaesthesia. Acta Anaesthesiol Scand. 1989;33(5):389–90. Epub 1989/07/01.
10. Sutton TS, Koblin DD, Gruenke LD, Weiskopf RB, Rampil IJ, Waskell L, et al. Fluoride metabolites after prolonged exposure of volunteers and patients to desflurane. Anesth Analg. 1991;73(2):180–5. Epub 1991/08/01.
11. Wrigley SR, Fairfield JE, Jones RM, Black AE. Induction and recovery characteristics of desflurane in day case patients: a comparison with propofol. Anaesthesia. 1991;46(8):615–22. Epub 1991/08/01.
12. Stenqvist O. Nitrous oxide kinetics. Acta Anaesthesiol Scand. 1994;38(8):757–60. Epub 1994/11/01.
13. Hudson RJ, Stanski DR, Burch PG. Pharmacokinetics of methohexital and thiopental in surgical patients. Anesthesiology. 1983;59(3):215–9. Epub 1983/09/01.
14. O'Leary J. A clinical investigation of methohexital sodium. Med J Aust. 1962;49(1):594–5. Epub 1962/04/21.
15. Dhuner KG, Peterhoff V. Clinical trials with methohexital. A new ultra-short-acting barbiturate for intravenous anesthesia. Acta Chir Scand. 1962;123:339–42. Epub 1962/05/01.
16. Schuttler J, Stoeckel H, Schwilden H. Pharmacokinetic and pharmacodynamic modelling of propofol ('Diprivan') in volunteers and surgical patients. Postgrad Med J. 1985;61 Suppl 3:53–4. Epub 1985/01/01.
17. Oda Y, Hamaoka N, Hiroi T, Imaoka S, Hase I, Tanaka K, et al. Involvement of human liver cytochrome P4502B6 in the metabolism of propofol. Br J Clin Pharmacol. 2001;51(3):281–5. Epub 2001/04/12.
18. McCollum JS, Dundee JW, Halliday NJ, Clarke RS. Dose response studies with propofol ('Diprivan') in unpremedicated patients. Postgrad Med J. 1985;61 Suppl 3:85–7. Epub 1985/01/01.
19. White PF, Way WL, Trevor AJ. Ketamine–its pharmacology and therapeutic uses. Anesthesiology. 1982;56(2):119–36. Epub 1982/02/01.
20. Orlando R, Piccoli P, De Martin S, Padrini R, Floreani M, Palatini P. Cytochrome P450 1A2 is a major determinant of lidocaine metabolism in vivo: effects of liver function. Clin Pharmacol Ther. 2004;75(1):80–8. Epub 2004/01/30.
21. Prilocaine. In: DRUGDEX system [internet database]. Greenwood Village: Thomson Reuters (Healthcare) Inc. Updated periodically.
22. Reynolds F. Metabolism and excretion of bupivacaine in man: a comparison with mepivacaine. Br J Anaesth. 1971;43(1):33–7. Epub 1971/01/01.

23. Moore DC, Bridenbaugh LD, Bridenbaugh PO, Tucker GT. Bupivacaine. A review of 2,077 cases. JAMA J Am Med Assoc. 1970;214(4):713–8.
24. Brockway MS, Bannister J, McClure JH, McKeown D, Wildsmith JA. Comparison of extradural ropivacaine and bupivacaine. Br J Anaesth. 1991;66(1):31–7. Epub 1991/01/01.
25. van Oss GE, Vree TB, Baars AM, Termond EF, Booij LH. Pharmacokinetics, metabolism, and renal excretion of articaine and its metabolite articainic acid in patients after epidural administration. Eur J Anaesthesiol. 1989;6(1):49–56. Epub 1989/01/01.
26. Thomas JM, Schug SA. Recent advances in the pharmacokinetics of local anaesthetics. Long-acting amide enantiomers and continuous infusions. Clin Pharmacokinet. 1999;36(1):67–83. Epub 1999/02/16.
27. Burm AG. Clinical pharmacokinetics of epidural and spinal anaesthesia. Clin Pharmacokinet. 1989;16(5):283–311. Epub 1989/05/01.
28. Jensen OT, Upton LG, Hayward JR, Sweet RB. Advantages of long-acting local anesthesia using etidocaine hydrochloride. J Oral Surg. 1981;39(5):350–3. Epub 1981/05/01.
29. Axelsson K, Nydahl PA, Philipson L, Larsson P. Motor and sensory blockade after epidural injection of mepivacaine, bupivacaine, and etidocaine–a double-blind study. Anesth Analg. 1989;69(6):739–47. Epub 1989/12/01.
30. Isoflurane. In: DRUGDEX System [Internet database]. Greenwood Village: Thomson Reuters (Healthcare) Inc. Updated periodically.
31. Isoflurane. In: DRUG-REAX® system [internet database]. Greenwood Village: Thomson Healthcare. Updated periodically.
32. Grasshoff C, Antkowiak B. Effects of isoflurane and enflurane on GABAA and glycine receptors contribute equally to depressant actions on spinal ventral horn neurones in rats. Br J Anaesth. 2006;97(5):687–94. Epub 2006/09/16.
33. Eger 2nd EI, Stevens WC, Cromwell TH. The electroencephalogram in man anesthetized with forane. Anesthesiology. 1971;35(5):504–8. Epub 1971/11/01.
34. Wade JG, Stevens WC. Isoflurane: an anesthetic for the eighties? Anesth Analg. 1981;60(9):666–82. Epub 1981/09/01.
35. Product information: ULTANE(R) inhalation liquid, sevoflurane inhalation liquid. North Chicago: Abbott Laboratories (per FDA); 2012.
36. Sevoflurane. In: DRUGDEX system [internet database]. Greenwood Village: Thomson Reuters (Healthcare) Inc. Updated periodically.
37. Product information: sevoflurane, USP – volatile liquid for inhalation. Deerfield: Baxter Healthcare Corporation; 2008.
38. Sevoflurane. In: DRUG-REAX® system [internet database]. Greenwood Village: Thomson Healthcare. Updated periodically.
39. Wu J, Harata N, Akaike N. Potentiation by sevoflurane of the gamma-aminobutyric acid-induced chloride current in acutely dissociated CA1 pyramidal neurones from rat hippocampus. Br J Pharmacol. 1996;119(5):1013–21. Epub 1996/11/01.
40. Stabernack CR, Eger 2nd EI, Warnken UH, Forster H, Hanks DK, Ferrell LD. Sevoflurane degradation by carbon dioxide absorbents may produce more than one nephrotoxic compound in rats. Canadian journal of anaesthesia. J Can Anesth. 2003;50(3):249–52.
41. Product information: SUPRANE(R) liquid for inhalation, desflurane liquid for inhalation. Deerfield: Baxter Healthcare Corporation; 2005
42. Desflurane. In: DRUGDEX system [internet database]. Greenwood Village: Thomson Reuters (Healthcare) Inc. Updated periodically.
43. Nishikawa K, Harrison NL. The actions of sevoflurane and desflurane on the gamma-aminobutyric acid receptor type A: effects of TM2 mutations in the alpha and beta subunits. Anesthesiology. 2003;99(3):678–84. Epub 2003/09/10.
44. Fletcher JE, Sebel PS, Murphy MR, Smith CA, Mick SA, Flister MP. Psychomotor performance after desflurane anesthesia: a comparison with isoflurane. Anesth Analg. 1991;73(3):260–5. Epub 1991/09/01.
45. Desflurane. In: DRUG-REAX® system [internet database]. Greenwood Village: Thomson Healthcare. Updated periodically.

46. Rampil IJ, Lockhart SH, Zwass MS, Peterson N, Yasuda N, Eger 2nd EI, et al. Clinical characteristics of desflurane in surgical patients: minimum alveolar concentration. Anesthesiology. 1991;74(3):429–33. Epub 1991/03/01.
47. Caldwell JE. Desflurane clinical pharmacokinetics and pharmacodynamics. Clin Pharmacokinet. 1994;27(1):6–18. Epub 1994/07/01.
48. Sakai EM, Connolly LA, Klauck JA. Inhalation anesthesiology and volatile liquid anesthetics: focus on isoflurane, desflurane, and sevoflurane. Pharmacotherapy. 2005;25(12):1773–88. Epub 2005/11/25.
49. Sweetman SC, editor. Martindale: the complete drug reference. [online] London: Pharmaceutical Press. http://www.medicinescomplete.com. Accessed 30 Mar 2013.
50. Nitrous oxide. In: DRUGDEX system [internet database]. Greenwood Village: Thomson Reuters (Healthcare) Inc. Updated periodically.
51. Yamakura T, Harris RA. Effects of gaseous anesthetics nitrous oxide and xenon on ligand-gated ion channels. Comparison with isoflurane and ethanol. Anesthesiology. 2000;93(4):1095–101. Epub 2000/10/06.
52. Mennerick S, Jevtovic-Todorovic V, Todorovic SM, Shen W, Olney JW, Zorumski CF. Effect of nitrous oxide on excitatory and inhibitory synaptic transmission in hippocampal cultures. J Neurosci. 1998;18(23):9716–26. Epub 1998/11/21.
53. Micromedex healthcare series: nitrous oxide. Greenwood Village: Thomson Reuters (Healthcare) Inc. Updated periodically.
54. Kunitz O, Baumert JH, Hecker K, Beeker T, Coburn M, Zuhlsdorff A, et al. Xenon does not prolong neuromuscular block of rocuronium. Anesth Analg. 2004;99(5):1398–401; table of contents. Epub 2004/10/27.
55. Derwall M, Coburn M, Rex S, Hein M, Rossaint R, Fries M. Xenon: recent developments and future perspectives. Minerva Anestesiol. 2009;75(1–2):37–45. Epub 2008/05/14.
56. Senno A, Schweitzer P, Merrill C, Clauss R. Arteriovenous fistulas of the internal mammary artery. Rev Lit J Cardiovasc Surg. 1975;16(3):296–301. Epub 1975/05/01.
57. Hanne P, Marx T, Musati S, Santo M, Suwa K, Morita S. Xenon: uptake and costs. Int Anesthesiol Clin. 2001;39(2):43–61. Epub 2001/08/17.
58. Sanders RD, Ma D, Maze M. Xenon: elemental anaesthesia in clinical practice. Br Med Bull. 2004;71:115–35. Epub 2005/02/25.
59. Reinelt H, Marx T, Kotzerke J, Topalidis P, Luederwald S, Armbruster S, et al. Hepatic function during xenon anesthesia in pigs. Acta Anaesthesiol Scand. 2002;46(6):713–6. Epub 2002/06/13.
60. Zhang P, Ohara A, Mashimo T, Imanaka H, Uchiyama A, Yoshiya I. Pulmonary resistance in dogs: a comparison of xenon with nitrous oxide. Can J Anaesth. 1995;42(6):547–53.
61. Prielipp RC. An anesthesiologist's perspective on inhaled anesthesia decision-making. Am J Health Syst Pharm. 2010;67(8 Suppl 4):S13–20. Epub 2010/04/14.
62. Baur CP, Klingler W, Jurkat-Rott K, Froeba G, Schoch E, Marx T, et al. Xenon does not induce contracture in human malignant hyperthermia muscle. Br J Anaesth. 2000;85(5):712–6. Epub 2000/11/30.
63. Petersen-Felix S, Luginbuhl M, Schnider TW, Curatolo M, Arendt-Nielsen L, Zbinden AM. Comparison of the analgesic potency of xenon and nitrous oxide in humans evaluated by experimental pain. Br J Anaesth. 1998;81(5):742–7. Epub 1999/04/08.
64. Lachmann B, Armbruster S, Schairer W, Landstra M, Trouwborst A, Van Daal GJ, et al. Safety and efficacy of xenon in routine use as an inhalational anaesthetic. Lancet. 1990;335(8703):1413–5. Epub 1990/06/16.
65. Product information: PENTOTHAL(R) IV injection, thiopental sodium IV injection. Lake Forest: Hospira, Inc; 2004.
66. Thiopental. In: DRUGDEX system [internet database]. Greenwood Village: Thomson Reuters (Healthcare) Inc. Updated periodically.
67. Thiopental. In: DRUG-REAX® system [internet database]. Greenwood Village: Thomson Healthcare. Updated periodically.
68. Higashi H, Nishi S. Effect of barbiturates on the GABA receptor of cat primary afferent neurones. J Physiol. 1982;332:299–314. Epub 1982/11/01.

69. Wada DR, Bjorkman S, Ebling WF, Harashima H, Harapat SR, Stanski DR. Computer simulation of the effects of alterations in blood flows and body composition on thiopental pharmacokinetics in humans. Anesthesiology. 1997;87(4):884–99. Epub 1997/11/14.

70. Pandele G, Chaux F, Salvadori C, Farinotti M, Duvaldestin P. Thiopental pharmacokinetics in patients with cirrhosis. Anesthesiology. 1983;59(2):123–6. Epub 1983/08/01.

71. Product information: BREVITAL(R) SODIUM intravenous injection, rectal injection, intramuscular injection, methohexital sodium intravenous injection, rectal injection, intramuscular injection. Rochester: JHP Pharmaceuticals; 2009.

72. Methohexital. In: DRUGDEX system [internet database]. Greenwood Village: Thomson Reuters (Healthcare) Inc. Updated periodically.

73. Product information: Brevital(R), methohexital. Indianapolis: Eli Lilly and Company; 2001.

74. Methohexital. In: DRUG-REAX® system [internet database]. Greenwood Village: Thomson Healthcare. Updated periodically.

75. Bahn EL, Holt KR. Procedural sedation and analgesia: a review and new concepts. Emerg Med Clin North Am. 2005;23(2):503–17. Epub 2005/04/15.

76. Product information: DIPRIVAN(R) IV injectable emulsion, propofol IV injectable emulsion. Schaumburg: APP Pharmaceuticals LLC; 2008.

77. Propofol. In: DRUGDEX system [internet database]. Greenwood Village: Thomson Reuters (Healthcare) Inc. Updated periodically.

78. Propofol. In: DRUG-REAX® system [internet database]. Greenwood Village: Thomson Healthcare. Updated periodically.

79. Hara M, Kai Y, Ikemoto Y. Propofol activates GABAA receptor-chloride ionophore complex in dissociated hippocampal pyramidal neurons of the rat. Anesthesiology. 1993;79(4):781–8. Epub 1993/10/01.

80. Product information: AMIDATE (etomidate) injection, solution. Lake Forest: Hospira, Inc; 2011.

81. Etomidate. In: DRUGDEX System [Internet database]. Greenwood Village, Colo: Thomson Reuters (Healthcare) Inc. Updated periodically.

82. Etomidate. In: DRUG-REAX® system [internet database]. Greenwood Village: Thomson Healthcare. Updated periodically.

83. Morgan M, Lumley J, Whitwam JG. Etomidate, a new water-soluble non-barbiturate intravenous induction agent. Lancet. 1975;1(7913):955–6. Epub 1975/04/26.

84. Doenicke A, Lorenz W, Beigl R, Bezecny H, Uhlig G, Kalmar L, et al. Histamine release after intravenous application of short-acting hypnotics. A comparison of etomidate, Althesin (CT1341) and propanidid. Br J Anaesth. 1973;45(11):1097–104.

85. Product information: KETAMINE HYDROCHLORIDE injection, solution. Rockford: Mylan Institutional, LLC; 2012.

86. Ketamine. In: DRUGDEX system [internet database]. Greenwood Village: Thomson Reuters (Healthcare) Inc. Updated periodically.

87. Anis NA, Berry SC, Burton NR, Lodge D. The dissociative anaesthetics, ketamine and phencyclidine, selectively reduce excitation of central mammalian neurones by N-methyl-aspartate. Br J Pharmacol. 1983;79(2):565–75. Epub 1983/06/01.

88. Product information: KETAMINE HYDROCHLORIDE injection. Bedford: Bedford Laboratories; 2012.

89. Product information: NESACAINE – chloroprocaine hydrochloride injection. Wilmington: AstraZeneca; 2004.

90. Chloroprocaine. In: DRUGDEX system [internet database]. Greenwood Village: Thomson Reuters (Healthcare) Inc. Updated periodically.

91. Product information: novocaine (procaine hydrochloride) injection, solution. Lake Forest: Hospira, Inc.; 2004.

92. Procaine. In: DRUGDEX system [internet database]. Greenwood Village: Thomson Reuters (Healthcare) Inc. Updated periodically.

93. Lidocaine. In: Lexi-comp online. Hudson: Lexi-Comp, Inc.

94. Product information: XYLOCAINE (lidocaine hydrochloride) injection, solution. Schaumburg: APP Pharmaceuticals, LLC; 2011.
95. Lidocaine. In: DRUGDEX System [Internet database]. Greenwood Village, Colo: Thomson Reuters (Healthcare) Inc. Updated periodically.
96. Product information: lidocaine hydrochloride and dextrose – lidocaine hydrochloride anhydrous and dextrose monohydrate injection, solution. Lake Forest: Hospira, Inc.; 2010.
97. Strichartz GR. The inhibition of sodium currents in myelinated nerve by quaternary derivatives of lidocaine. J Gen Physiol. 1973;62(1):37–57. Epub 1973/07/01.
98. Product information: prilocaine hydrochloride – prilocaine hydrochloride injection, solution. Louisville: Novocol Pharmaceutical of Canada, Inc.; 2010.
99. Product information: marcaine spinal – bupivacaine hydrochloride injection, solution. Lake Forest: Hospira, Inc.; 2011.
100. Bupivacaine. In: DRUGDEX system [internet database]. Greenwood Village: Thomson Reuters (Healthcare) Inc. Updated periodically.
101. Moore PA. Bupivacaine: a long-lasting local anesthetic for dentistry. Oral Surg Oral Med Oral Pathol. 1984;58(4):369–74. Epub 1984/10/01.
102. Product information: NAROPIN (ropivacaine hydrochloride monohydrate) injection, solution. East Schaumburg: APP Pharmaceuticals; 2009.
103. Ropivacaine. In: DRUGDEX system [internet database]. Greenwood Village: Thomson Reuters (Healthcare) Inc. Updated periodically.
104. Raeder JC, Drosdahl S, Klaastad O, Kvalsvik O, Isaksen B, Stromskag KE, et al. Axillary brachial plexus block with ropivacaine 7.5 mg/ml. A comparative study with bupivacaine 5 mg/ml. Acta Anaesthesiol Scand. 1999;43(8):794–8.
105. Product information: carbocaine (mepivacaine hydrochloride) injection, solution. Lake Forest: Hospira, Inc.; 2010.
106. Mepivacaine. In: DRUGDEX system [internet database]. Greenwood Village: Thomson Reuters (Healthcare) Inc. Updated periodically.
107. Product information: articadent – articaine hydrochloride and epinephrine bitartrate injection, solution. Cambridge: Novocol Pharmaceutical of Canada, Inc.; 2009.
108. Articaine. In: DRUGDEX system [internet database]. Greenwood Village: Thomson Reuters (Healthcare) Inc. Updated periodically.
109. Product information: tetracaine hydrochloride – tetracaine hydrochloride solution. Fort Worth: Alcon Laboratories, Inc.; 2010.
110. Tetracaine. In: DRUGDEX system [internet database]. Greenwood Village: Thomson Reuters (Healthcare) Inc. Updated periodically.
111. Levobupivacaine. In: DRUGDEX system [internet database]. Greenwood Village: Thomson Reuters (Healthcare) Inc. Updated periodically.
112. Levobupivacaine. In: DRUG-REAX® system [internet database]. Greenwood Village: Thomson Healthcare. Updated periodically.
113. Etidocaine. In: DRUGDEX system [internet database]. Greenwood Village: Thomson Reuters (Healthcare) Inc. Updated periodically.
114. Etodicaine. In: DRUG-REAX® system [internet database]. Greenwood Village: Thomson Healthcare. Updated periodically.
115. Aziz TS. Xenon in anesthesia. Int Anesthesiol Clin. 2001;39(2):1–14. Epub 2001/08/17.
116. Van Hamme MJ, Ghoneim MM, Ambre JJ. Pharmacokinetics of etomidate, a new intravenous anesthetic. Anesthesiology. 1978;49(4):274–7. Epub 1978/10/01.

Chapter 2
A Review of Mechanisms of Inhalational Anesthetic Agents

Elizabeth A.M. Frost

Contents

Introduction

Long before the discovery of intravenous techniques, man has inhaled vapors to mitigate pain. Smoking cannabis and opium to achieve both pleasurable sensations and decreased consciousness has been described for over 3,000 years. Theodoric, a thirteenth-century monk and surgeon, devised a balanced anesthetic of opium, mulberry, hyoscyamine, hemlock, mandragora, woody ivy, dock, and water hemlock. These ingredients were to be boiled on a sponge, with or without the addition of alcohol, until dried out. The sponge could be rehydrated and inhaled until the

E.A.M. Frost, MD
Department of Anesthesiology, Icahn School of Medicine at Mount Sinai,
New York, NY, USA
e-mail: elzfrost@aol.com, elizabeth.frost@mountsinai.org

A.D. Kaye et al. (eds.), *Essentials of Pharmacology for Anesthesia,*
Pain Medicine, and Critical Care, DOI 10.1007/978-1-4614-8948-1_2,
© Springer Science+Business Media New York 2015

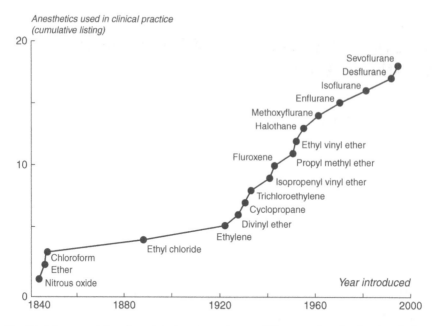

Anesthetics used in clinical practice (cumulative listing)

Fig. 2.1 Many agents have been introduced over the past 170 years only to be abandoned after a few years

patient became unconscious and surgery could commence. Reversal from the hypnotic state was by inhalation from a sponge soaked in vinegar [1]. And while use of the *spongia somnifera* was largely abandoned by the end of the Middle Ages, ether and chloroform were to become the children of alcohol. Paracelsus discovered the hypnotic effect of ether around 1540, and the first surgical use was credited to Crawford Long in 1842 [2]. The first public demonstration of ether was on October 16, 1846, in Boston in what is now known as the "Ether Dome" [3]. As cautery became integral to surgical technique during the twentieth century, anesthetic agents that did not explode had to be found. The halogenated anesthetics were born. Nitrous oxide, a weak agent, was discovered by Joseph Priestly in 1772 [4]. It was widely used as a recreational drug for over 40 years but later found places both in dentistry and as an analgesic or anesthetic-sparing component of balanced techniques.

Drug Class

Inhaled anesthetics that have been used in clinical practice and the time of their introduction are shown in Fig. 2.1. Many of these agents have fallen by the wayside because of toxicity or flammability. Those that remain may be classified as:

Potent Agents
Halothane, enflurane, isoflurane, sevoflurane, and desflurane

Others
Nitrous oxide and xenon

An inhalational anesthetic is a chemical compound possessing general anesthetic properties that can be delivered via inhalation. Agents of significant contemporary clinical interest include volatile anesthetic agents such as isoflurane, sevoflurane, and desflurane as well as certain anesthetic gases such as nitrous oxide and xenon. These agents are liquid at room temperature but evaporate easily for administration by inhalation through vaporizers. They are all hydrophobic, dissolving better in oil than in water.

Other gases that produce general anesthesia by inhalation include nitrous oxide and xenon (cyclopropane is no longer used). They are stored in gas cylinders and administered using flow meters. Xenon is odorless with a rapid onset. It is expensive and requires special equipment to administer and monitor. At 80 % concentration it has anesthetic capabilities. Nitrous oxide, even at 80 % concentration, does not produce a surgical depth of anesthesia at standard atmospheric pressure and is thus used in combinations with other agents.

At hyperbaric pressures, gases such as nitrogen and inert gases like argon and krypton have some anesthetic effect. When inhaled at high partial pressures (>4 bar, at depths below about 30 m in scuba diving), nitrogen can cause nitrogen narcosis [5, 6]. However, the minimum alveolar concentration (MAC) for nitrogen requires pressures of about 20–30 atm (bar). Argon has about twice the anesthetic potency of nitrogen per unit of partial pressure.

Mechanism of Action

The mechanism of action of volatile anesthetic agents is unknown and has been debated for years. While intravenous agents appear to act on a single molecular target, inhaled drugs seem to act at multiple sites. There are thus many theories surrounding the site(s) of action of inhaled anesthetics.

As early as 1847 Ernst von Bibra and Emil Harless suggested that ether acts by dissolving and removing the fatty fraction of brain cells [7]. This hypothesis governed the thinking of the mechanism of action for over 100 years. Meyer proposed that anesthetic potency is related to lipid solubility in 1899. By comparing the potency (defined as the reciprocal of the molar concentration required to induce anesthesia in tadpoles, with the olive oil/water partition coefficient), Meyer proposed a relationship between lipid solubility and effectiveness [8]. Two years later Overton presented a similar theory [8, 9]. The Meyer-Overton theory, as it became known, correlated lipid solubility of inhaled agents and suggested that it is the

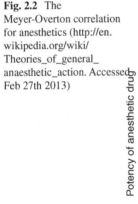

Fig. 2.2 The Meyer-Overton correlation for anesthetics (http://en.wikipedia.org/wiki/Theories_of_general_anaesthetic_action. Accessed Feb 27th 2013)

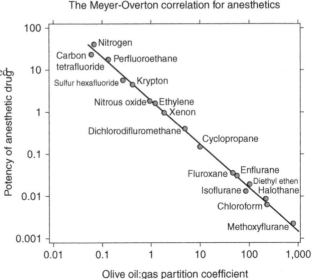

Fig. 2.3 Anesthetic agents with larger molecules cause greater expansion and disruption of the lipid bilayer and thus should be more potent

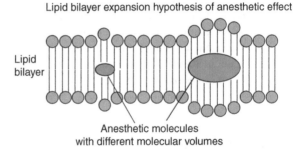

number of dissolved molecules rather than the specific agent that causes anesthesia (Fig. 2.2). The correlation does hold true for a wide range of inhaled agents with lipid solubilities ranging over four to five orders of magnitude if olive oil is used as the oil phase and can be correlated even more closely if octanol [10] or a fully hydrated fluid lipid bilayer is used as the "oil" phase [11]. These conclusions offer a single mechanism in that as anesthetic agents are dissolved in the lipid bilayers, neurons malfunction at some critical level. Adding to this theory, Mullins felt that molecular volumes should also be added to the equation: the greater the volume, the more potent [12]. By 1973, Miller et al. suggested a critical volume or lipid bilayer expansion hypothesis, supposing that hydrophobic anesthetic molecules gather in neuronal lipid membranes causing distortion and expansion [13]. Membrane thickening could reversibly alter function of ion channels, neuronal density, and fluidity, resulting in anesthesia (Fig. 2.3).

For almost 100 years, the Meyer-Overton hypothesis was taught and accepted with few additions such as including changes in lateral phase separations, bilayer thickness, curvature, and several other parameters [14, 15]. But as more agents were synthesized, it became apparent that there were at least four weaknesses in the single-mechanism theory [16]:

1. Stereoisomers may have the same or similar oil/gas partition coefficients but differ greatly in anesthetic potency. While these enantiomers have identical physicochemical effects in the lipid bilayer, in vivo anesthetic action may be far from similar. Although there is identical partition in the lipid layer, there are differential effects on ion channels and synaptic transmission [17]. Thus the primary target for anesthetic agents may not be the achiral (a molecule that is superimposable on its mirror image) lipid bilayer itself but rather stereoselective binding sites on membrane proteins that provide a chiral environment for specific anesthetic-protein docking interactions [17].
2. General anesthetics stop movement in response to noxious stimulation by depression of spinal cord function and amnesia through higher cerebral depression. Many drugs have high lipid solubility but only exert one function of anesthesia, i.e., they allow amnesia but maintain movement. These nonimmobilizers appear to affect different molecular targets rather than simply the bilipid layer [18].
3. The Meyer-Overton theory notes that increasing the chain length increases lipid solubility and hence anesthetic potency. However, at a certain chain length, varying between about 13 for the n-alcohols and between 6 and 10 for the n-alkanes, anesthetic potency disappears [19, 20].
4. Changes in membrane density and fluidity caused by anesthetics are very small, and even increases in temperature of 1 °C can have the same effect without loss of consciousness.

Despite these apparent flaws, the correlation of lipid solubility and anesthetic action remains compelling, and a more recent lipid hypothesis has been offered [21]. Mohr et al. suggest that anesthetic effect is caused by solubilization in the bilayer resulting in a redistribution of membrane lateral pressure. Each bilayer membrane has a distinct profile of distribution of lateral pressures, which are large and vary with depth. Membrane proteins, especially ion channels, are sensitive to changes in this lateral pressure distribution profile, which shifts the conformational equilibrium of certain membrane proteins such as ligand-gated ion channels. This mechanism also appears to be nonspecific because potency is determined not by chemical structure but by position and orientation distribution within the bilayer. However, the exact molecular mechanism remains unclear. A lattice statistical thermodynamic model suggests that incorporation of amphiphilic and other active solutes like general anesthetics into the bilayer increases lateral pressure selectively near the aqueous interfaces, compensated by a decrease in lateral pressure toward the center of the bilayer [22]. As a channel tries to open in response to a nerve impulse, the cross-sectional area of the protein closer to the aqueous interface increases. Any increase in lateral pressure shifts the protein conformational equilibrium back to the closed state. Opening of the ion channel in a postsynaptic ligand-gated membrane protein may then be inhibited [22].

It is thus clear that not simply lipids but also the lipid/protein interface is critical to anesthetic action. Franks and Lieb showed a correlation between anesthetic action and soluble proteins. Luciferases and cytochrome P450 can be inactivated by inhaled anesthetics [23]. Thus, these drugs may interact with hydrophobic protein sites as well as membrane proteins through nonspecific interactions, using the lipid bilayer as a mediator. Indeed, anesthetics may alter the function of many cytoplasm signaling proteins including protein kinase C as well as the ion channels. But anesthetics appear to bind more selectively to proteins, involving relatively few, mainly neurotransmitter-gated ion channels. Also the Cys-loop receptors are targets and include inhibitory receptors (GABA A, GABA C, glycine) and excitatory receptors (acetylcholine and 5-HT3 serotonin receptors) [24].

Thus while an understanding of the mechanism of action of inhalation anesthetics is still not understood, it is clearly not a single, unified effect but one that involves both lipids and proteins and especially inhibition of ion channels. Although argon is an inert gas, it, too, can have anesthetic properties suggesting that the mechanism of action of volatile anesthetics may in part be physical, causing swelling of nerve cell membranes from gas solution in the lipid bilayer. However, other theories suggest that inhaled anesthetic agents disrupt synaptic transmission by interference with the release of neurotransmitters from presynaptic nerve terminals, either enhancing or depressing transmission. Or the reuptake of neurotransmitters may be altered by a change in the binding to the postsynaptic receptor sites. Or the ionic conductance change that follows activation of the postsynaptic receptor by neurotransmitters may be affected. Both pre- and postsynaptic effects have been described. Direct interaction with the neuronal plasma membrane is very likely, and indirect action via production of a second messenger also remains possible.

Indications

Inhalational anesthesia remains the most commonly employed means to surgical analgesia today.

Enflurane, halothane, isoflurane, desflurane, and nitrous oxide are indicated for the induction and maintenance of general anesthesia. Methoxyflurane is no longer used because of nephrotoxicity. Cyclopropane and ether have been abandoned due to explosion risk. Enflurane is less used because of the advent of the more agreeable agents such as sevoflurane (less pungent) and desflurane (shorter acting). Halothane has also been replaced in large measure by sevoflurane in developed countries; it is still used in many areas for financial reasons. Inhalation anesthetic agents are rarely used alone and other drugs such as opiates, muscle relaxants, and benzodiazepines among others are frequently administered to induce or supplement anesthesia. Because of its weak anesthetic potency and poor muscle relaxant properties, nitrous oxide must be supplemented with another anesthetic or adjunct (such as a barbiturate, benzodiazepine, opioid analgesic, or another inhalation anesthetic) and/or a neuromuscular blocking agent. It is often administered together with another inhalation anesthetic to decrease the requirement for the more potent anesthetic. It may also be used in low dose for procedures not requiring loss of consciousness.

The main indications for the use of inhalation agents are outlined in Table 2.1.

Table 2.1 Some of the situations where conditions might dictate use of specific inhalation agents

Indications	Reason	Preferred agent
Children	IV access traumatic	Sevoflurane
Cardiothoracic cases	Chest open/controlled ventilation	Sevoflurane/isoflurane
Neurosurgical procedures	Control of intracranial dynamics	Isoflurane/desflurane/sevoflurane
Drug addict	Limited IV access	Isoflurane/desflurane/sevoflurane
Short, painful procedures	Quick onset/offset	Desflurane
Patient insistence/refusal of regional techniques	Preference	Isoflurane/sevoflurane/desflurane
Emergency situations	Need for rapid anesthesia	Desflurane/sevoflurane

Several studies have shown that desflurane does not adversely impact intracranial dynamics in patients with space-occupying lesions and allows faster awakening for neurologic assessment [25]. As such, desflurane is an acceptable agent for neurosurgery. However, as many of these procedures tend to be extremely long, expense must be considered along with the substitution of isoflurane with desflurane toward the end of the case.

Clinical Pearls

Desflurane has the lowest blood and fat and lean tissue solubilities of all potent inhaled anesthetic agents. It enters and leaves the blood and tissues more rapidly and is indicated in outpatient settings after an intravenous induction where rapid emergence is desirable. Its higher price limits its use in many countries. Sevoflurane is also expensive but less pungent and is better tolerated when an intravenous induction may not be possible. Isoflurane is cheaper and preferable for long cases or when rapid emergence and extubation are not expected. It and halothane, which is also less irritating to the airway, are widely used worldwide where cost is a major factor.

A study of seven healthy volunteers showed that the inhalation of 1.5MAC desflurane after thiopental 5 mg/kg resulted in transient sympathetic hyperactivity [26]. The up to 2.5-fold changes to blood pressure, heart rate, and sympathetic nerve activity were not seen with isoflurane. The authors advised caution in administering higher doses of desflurane to patients with cardiac compromise.

Dosing Options

Isoflurane and sevoflurane boil near 50 °C and have a vapor pressure near 200 mmHg. In contrast, desflurane boils near room temperature and has a higher vapor pressure (close to 1 atm). These properties necessitate that desflurane be packaged in sealed

Table 2.2 The relation of MAC-awake and MAC-BAR for commonly used inhalation agents is shown along with the effects of the addition of nitrous oxide

MAC, MAC-awake, and MAC-BAR				
MAC in subjects ages 30–55				
	In O_2 (%)	In 60–70 % N_2O (%)	MAC-awake (%)	MAC-BAR
Desflurane	6.00	2.83	2.42	1.45 MAC
Sevoflurane	1.71	0.66	0.61	2.24 MAC
Halothane	0.77	0.29	0.41	1.3 MAC
Isoflurane	1.15	0.50	0.39	1.3 MAC
Nitrous oxide	104	–	67	
Methoxyflurane	0.16	0.07		

Adapted from Barash et al. *Clin Anesth.* (1992), Daniel et al. *Anesthesiology.* (1998), Jones et al. *Anesth Analg.* (1990), Katoh et al. *Anesthesiology.* (1999), Katoh et al. *Br J Anaesth.* (1992), Roizen et al. *Anesthesiology.* (1981), Stoelting et al. *Anesthesiology.* (1970)

Table 2.3 Some of the conditions that affect dosing requirements for inhalation agents

Increased dosing requirements	Decreased dosing requirements
Chronic alcohol abuse	Acute alcohol abuse
Infant (highest at 6 months)	Geriatric patient
Red hair	Anemia (Hb < 5 g)
Hypernatremia	Hyponatremia
Febrile condition	Hypercarbia
Hypermetabolic states	Hypoxia
No adjuvant agents	Pregnancy

bottles that can withstand a high pressure of 80 lb psi and also require new vaporizer technology to administer appropriate anesthetic capability.

Dosing depends on several factors including MAC-awake and MAC-BAR. MAC-awake, initially determined in dogs in which the tails were clamped, is the alveolar concentration at which 50 % of subjects respond appropriately to command. MAC-BAR is the concentration of an inhaled anesthetic that blocks the sympathetic response (increased blood pressure and/or heart rate) in 50 % of patients to a noxious stimulus, such as a skin incision. The ratio of MAC-awake to MAC-BAR is between 0.3 and 0.5 for potent inhalation agents. Thus, MAC must be exceeded by a factor of 1.3 in order to assure sufficient surgical anesthesia for most patients. At 1.3 times MAC, movement is prevented in about 95 % of patients. The importance of the ratio of MAC-awake to MAC lies in the relation of MAC-awake and amnesia. The addiction of nitrous oxide reduces the values for MAC-awake and MAC-BAR. The concept of MAC is that equilibration of the alveolar concentration of the gas equals the blood concentration and thereafter represents the partial pressure of the anesthetic in the central nervous system (CNS) and is therefore a useful index of anesthetic potency (Table 2.2).

Other factors that alter the dosing requirements of inhalation anesthetics are shown in Table 2.3

Drug Interactions

Given that the average patient receives five to ten drugs during anesthesia, it is remarkable that there are not many drug interactions attributed to inhalation agents. Perhaps the most relevant is the rapid rise in alveolar uptake when nitrous oxide is added to a potent gas. When a constant concentration of a potent anesthetic is inspired, the increase in alveolar concentration is accelerated by concomitant administration of nitrous oxide, because alveolar uptake of the latter creates a potential subatmospheric intrapulmonary pressure that leads to increased tracheal inflow (the second gas effect) [27]. As noted above, the common practice of developing a balanced anesthetic technique with the addition of opioids, benzodiazepines, and barbiturates to inhalation agents results in a decreased requirement for the latter. The precise mechanism whereby this effect is realized is unclear but may be related to a decrease in postsynaptic transmission by the intravenous drugs. A synergistic effect is also seen with the neuromuscular blocking agents and the potent inhalants, necessitating a lower dose of pancuronium, vecuronium, and atracurium.

Potent inhaled anesthetics all cause hypotension in a dose-dependent manner. Antihypertensive drugs act in different ways: some deplete catecholamine stores such as beta blockers which increases the degree of hypotension. Thiazides cause hypokalemia and hypovolemia increasing the risk of dysrhythmias and hypotension. Calcium channel blockers inhibit cardiac conduction and may induce cardiac arrest in conjunction with inhaled anesthetics. Angiotensin-converting enzyme (ACE) inhibitors inhibit the enzyme that cleaves angiotensin I to form angiotensin II. Not only does vasodilation occur, concentrations of angiotensin II and noradrenalin decrease and levels of bradykinin and nitric oxide increase. Aldosterone and antidiuretic hormone secretion are reduced, thus reducing salt and water reabsorption by the kidney. All these actions can result in severe hypotension (vasoplegic syndrome) during anesthesia with inhaled agents [28]. Treatment is with vasopressin and the nitric oxide blocker and guanylate cyclase inhibitor, methylene blue [29].

Black Box Warnings

At present, given the inhalation agents that are in general use, there are few if any black box warnings. However, based on very rare occurrences, mainly under experimental conditions, the following warnings have been issued:

1. An exothermic reaction occurs when sevoflurane is exposed to CO_2 absorbents. This reaction is increased when the CO_2 absorbent becomes desiccated, such as after an extended period of dry gas flow through the CO_2 absorbent canisters. Rare cases of extreme heat, smoke, and/or spontaneous fire in the anesthesia breathing circuit have been reported during sevoflurane use in conjunction with the use of desiccated CO_2 absorbent, specifically those containing potassium hydroxide (e.g. Baralyme). KOH containing CO_2 absorbents are not recommended for use with sevoflurane. An unusually delayed rise or unexpected

decline of inspired sevoflurane concentration compared to the vaporizer setting may be associated with excessive heating of the CO_2 absorbent and chemical breakdown of sevoflurane.

As with other inhalational anesthetics, degradation and production of degradation products can occur when sevoflurane is exposed to desiccated absorbents. When a clinician suspects that the CO_2 absorbent may be desiccated, it should be replaced. The color indicator of most CO_2 absorbents may not change upon desiccation. Therefore, the lack of significant color change should not be taken as an assurance of adequate hydration. CO_2 absorbents should be replaced routinely regardless of the state of the color indicator. (http://www.rxlist.com/ultane-drug/side-effects-interactions.htm accessed Feb 27th 2013)

2. Malignant hyperthermia (MH), a disease inherited through autosomal dominance, is a potentially fatal complication of general anesthesia triggered by volatile anesthetics. MH may also occur with several other muscle disease such as multiminicore myopathies and central core disease. Although sevoflurane was initially considered to be a weak trigger, a recent study found no evidence to support the postulate [30]. Thus use of all potent inhalation anesthetics is contraindicated in patients with a history of MH. Inheritance of the defect should be excluded for all patients with a family history of MH. Restriction of inhaled anesthetic use does not appear to extend to the many mitochondrial diseases.

Clinical Pearl

Recovery from Inhalational Anesthetics

Desflurane will always give the quickest recovery owing to its lowest solubility and most minimal metabolism. Studies have shown a 50 % quicker recovery versus isoflurane. Desflurane is modestly quicker versus sevoflurane for cases of short duration and, again, has shown 50 % quicker recovery in cases greater than 3 h.

Chemical Structures

**Chemical Structure
2.1** Sevoflurane

**Chemical Structure
2.2** Isoflurane

References

1. Raper HR. Man against pain. New York: Prentice-Hall; 1945. p. 7–18.
2. Long CW. An account of the first use of sulphuric ether by inhalation as an anaesthetic in surgical operations. South Med Surg J. 1849;5:705–13.
3. Warren JC. The influence of anaesthesia on the surgery of the nineteenth century, being the address of the president before the American Surgical Association1847; 18–20. Boston, Privately Printed 1906.
4. Keys TE. The history of surgical anesthesia. Huntington: Krieger Pub Co; 1978. p. 14.
5. Fowler B, Ackles KN, Porlier G. Effects of inert gas narcosis on behavior—a critical review. Undersea Biomed Res. 1985;12(4):369–402.
6. Rogers WH, Moeller G. Effect of brief, repeated hyperbaric exposures on susceptibility to nitrogen narcosis. Undersea Biomed Res. 1989;16(3):227–32.
7. Harless E, von Bibra E. Die Ergebnisse der Versuche über die Wirkung des Schwefeläthers. Erlangen. 1847.
8. Meyer HH. Zur Theorie der Alkoholnarkose Arch. Exp Pathol Pharmacol. 1899;42:2–4.
9. Overton CE. Studien über die Narkose zugleich ein Beitrag zur allgemeinen Pharmakologie. Jena: Gustav Fischer; 1901.
10. Franks NP, Lieb WR. Where do general anaesthetics act? Nature. 1978;274(5669):339–42.
11. Taheri S, Halsey MJ, Liu J, Eger EI, Koblin DD, Laster MJ. What solvent best represents the site of action of inhaled anesthetics in humans, rats, and dogs? Anesth Analg. 1991;72(5):627–34.
12. Mullins LI. Some physical mechanisms in narcosis. Chem Rev. 1954;54(2):289–323.
13. Miller KW, Paton WD, Smith RA, Smith EB. The pressure reversal of general anesthesia and the critical volume hypothesis. Mol Pharmacol. 1973;9(2):131–43. PMID 4711696.
14. Janoff AS, Miller KW. A critical assessment of the lipid theories of general anaesthetic action. Biol Membr. 1982;4(1):417–76.
15. Trudell JR. A unitary theory of anesthesia based on lateral phase separations in nerve membranes. Anesthesiology. 1977;46(1):5–10. PMID 12686.
16. Cameron JW. The molecular mechanisms of general anaesthesia: dissecting the GABAA receptor. Contin Educ Anaesth Crit Care Pain. 2006;6(2):49–53.
17. Franks NP, Lieb WR. Stereospecific effects of inhalational general anesthetic optical isomers on nerve ion channels. Science. 1991;254(5030):427–30. PMID 1925602.
18. Eger 2nd EI, Koblin DD, Harris RA, Kendig JJ, Pohorille A, Halsey MJ, Trudell JR. Hypothesis: inhaled anesthetics produce immobility and amnesia by different mechanisms at different sites. Anesth Analg. 1997;84(4):915–8. PMID 9085981.
19. Pringle MJ, Brown KB, Miller KW. Can the lipid theories of anesthesia account for the cut off in anesthetic potency in homologous series of alcohols? Mol Pharmacol. 1981;19(1):49–55.
20. Liu J, Laster MJ, Taheri S, Eger EI, Koblin DD, Halsey MJ. Is there a cutoff in anesthetic potency for the normal alkanes? Anesth Analg. 1993;77(1):12–8. PMID 8317717.
21. Mohr JT, Gribble GW, Lin SS, Eckenhoff RG, Cantor RS. Anesthetic potency of two novel synthetic polyhydric alkanols longer than the n-alkanol cutoff: evidence for a bilayer-mediated mechanism of anesthesia? J Med Chem. 2005;48(12):4172–6. PMID 15943489.
22. Lerner RA. A hypothesis about the endogenous analogue of general anesthesia. Proc Natl Acad Sci U S A. 1997;94(25):13375–7. PMID 9391028.
23. Franks NP, Lieb WR. Do general anaesthetics act by competitive binding to specific receptors? Nature. 1984;310(16):599–601. PMID 6462249.
24. Eckenhoff RG, Johansson JS. Molecular interactions between inhaled anesthetics and proteins. Pharmacol Rev. 1997;49(4):343–67.
25. Kaye A, Kucera IJ, Heavner J, Gelb A, et al. the comparative effects of desflurane and isoflurane on lumbar cerebrospinal fluid pressure in patients undergoing craniotomy for supratentorial tumors. Anesth Analg. 2004;98(4):1127–32.
26. Eberrt TJ, Muzi M. Sympathetic hyperactivity during desflurane anesthesia in healthy volunteers. A comparison with isoflurane. Anesthesiology. 1993;79(3):444–53.

27. Korman B, Mapleson WW. Concentration and second-gas effects in the water analogue. B J A. 1998;81:837–43.
28. Croft R, Cook G, Washington S. Angiotensin-converting enzyme inhibitors in the perioperative period. Br J Hosp Med (Lond). 2012;73(2):118.
29. Lavigne D. Vasopressin and methylene blue: alternate therapies in vasodilatory shock. Semin Cardiothorac Vasc Anesth. 2010;14(3):186–9.
30. Migita T, Mukaida K, Kobayashi M, Hamada H, Kawamoto M. The severity of sevoflurane-induced hyperthermia. Acta Anaesthesiol Scand. 2012;56(3):351–6.

Chapter 3
Pharmacokinetics, Pharmacodynamics, and Physical Properties of Inhalational Agents

Hanjo Ko, Alan David Kaye, and Richard D. Urman

Contents

H. Ko, MD (✉)
Department of Anesthesiology and Perioperative Medicine,
Brigham and Women's Hospital, Boston, MA, USA
e-mail: hko3@partners.org

A.D. Kaye, MD, PhD
Department of Anesthesiology, Tulane Medical Center, New Orleans, LA, USA

Department of Anesthesiology, Louisiana State University
Health Sciences Center, New Orleans, LA 70112, USA
e-mail: alankaye44@hotmail.com

R.D. Urman, MD, MBA
Department of Anesthesiology, Perioperative and Pain Medicine, Brigham and Women's
Hospital, Harvard Medical School, Boston, MA, USA

Center for Perioperative Management and Medical Informatics,
Brigham and Women's Hospital, Boston, MA, USA
e-mail: urmanr@gmail.com

A.D. Kaye et al. (eds.), *Essentials of Pharmacology for Anesthesia,*
Pain Medicine, and Critical Care, DOI 10.1007/978-1-4614-8948-1_3,
© Springer Science+Business Media New York 2015

While there are multiple inhalational agents discovered over the past few decades, only three remain particularly relevant today in the United States. This chapter will review major properties of sevoflurane, desflurane, isoflurane, nitrous oxide, and halothane in clinical practice as well as the basic pharmacodynamics and pharmacokinetics of inhalational agents.

Pharmacodynamics Properties of Inhalational Agents

Despite multiple attempts of identifying the physiological site of actions of inhalational agents in the past, which have centered around $GABA_A$ receptor modulation, the exact mechanism remains to be a mystery (see Chap. 2 for further details). Clinically, the pharmacodynamics properties of inhalational agents focus on the concept of minimum alveolar concentration (MAC). MAC is defined as the alveolar concentration that prevents movement in 50 % of patients in response to surgical stimuli. Another way to think of MAC is the equivalent of a median effective dose, i.e., ED_{50}. ED_{95} is roughly 1.3 MAC of any inhalational agents, while 0.3–0.4 MAC is often defined as MAC_{awake}, which represents the return of response to verbal command during emergence. $MAC_{intubation}$ is roughly 2.0 MAC which designates the concentration at which no movement or cough occurs during endotracheal intubation. MAC_{BAR} is about 1.6–1.7 MAC and represents inhibition of autonomic response to surgical incision.

MACs of various inhalational agents are additive, while other physiological effects (such as the effect of myocardial depression) are not. For example, the amount of myocardial depression is greater with 1 MAC of sevoflurane than the combination of 0.5 MAC of nitrous oxide and 0.5 MAC of sevoflurane.

There are several factors that modify the MAC requirement in each individual, such as age and the presence of alcohol (Table 3.1). During clinical practice, one must take these factors into consideration so that the depth of anesthesia can be titrated appropriately to minimize hemodynamic disturbance.

Table 3.1 Factors that affect MAC

Factors that affect MAC		Factors that do not affect MAC
Increased MAC	Decreased MAC	Gender
Red hair	Elderly patients	Duration of anesthesia
Hyperthermia	Hypothermia	Thyroid function
Hyponatremia	Hypernatremia	Hypokalemia/hyperkalemia
Chronic alcohol abuse	Acute alcohol intoxication	Hypertension/hypotension unless
Cyclosporine	Opioids	MAP<40 mmHg
	Lidocaine	
	Benzodiazepines	
	Ketamine	
	PaO_2 <38 mmHg	

Pharmacokinetics of Inhalational Agents

The delivery of inhalational agents to its target site of action (i.e., brain) can be divided into three major components: F_i (inspired gas concentration), F_A (alveolar gas concentration), and F_a (arterial gas concentration). The elimination of inhalational agents depends mainly on exhalation (and as a result, factors contributing to exhalation).

Delivery of Inhalational Agents

F_i (Inspired Gas Concentration)

For inspired gas concentration, it is determined by rate of fresh gas flow, the amount of breathing circuit volume, and any absorption from the circuit. The higher the fresh gas flow, the smaller the breathing circuit volume, and the lesser the absorption from the circuit, the closer the inspired gas concentration is to the set fresh gas concentration.

F_A (Alveolar Gas Concentration)

For alveolar gas concentration, it is influenced by (1) uptake, (2) ventilation, and (3) the concentration effect. The relationship of F_i and F_A can be illustrated by the alveolar tension curve.

Uptake

The inhalational agent is first taken up by the pulmonary circulation. The greater the uptake from the pulmonary circulation, the lesser the inhalational agent is able to reach to alveoli, which leads to slower rate of the rise of the alveolar concentration ($F_A/F_i < 1.0$). Since the alveolar partial pressure is proportional to alveolar gas concentration, the slower the rise of alveolar concentration, the longer it takes for the alveolar partial pressure to reach to clinical effect. As a result, the greater the uptake of the inhalational agent, the slower the rate of induction.

There are four factors that determine the amount of update: (1) blood/gas solubility, (2) alveolar blood flow, (3) the difference in partial pressure between alveolar gas and venous blood, and (4) the barometric pressure (see Eq. 3.1) where λ represents blood/gas solubility, Q represents cardiac output which is then related to alveolar blood flow, and ($P_a - P_v$) represents the difference in partial pressure between alveolar gas and venous blood:

$$Uptake = \frac{\lambda \times Q \times (P_a - P_v)}{Barometric\ pressure}. \tag{3.1}$$

The less soluble the inhalation agent is (such as nitrous oxide), the faster the rise of alveolar concentration, which leads to faster induction. The higher the alveolar blood flow is (such as in patients of higher cardiac output), the greater the uptake of the inhalational agent, which leads to slower induction. The greater the difference in the partial pressure between alveolar gas and venous blood is, the greater the uptake, which leads to slower induction. Finally, barometric pressure also plays a role in the amount of uptake, and uptake is greater in San Diego than in Denver, for example.

In terms of the amount of uptake by the tissue, it depends highly on the type of tissues and the temporal relationship is best illustrated by the alveolar tension curve. One can categorize tissues into vessel-rich, muscle, fat, and vessel-poor groups. The vessel-rich group (such as the brain, heart, liver, kidneys, and endocrine organs) is the first to reach equilibrium between arterial and tissue partial pressures, while the fat group takes days to reach equilibrium. The tail portion of the alveolar tension curve demonstrates such effect as the rate of rise slows as the muscle/fat group slowly reaches equilibrium. The alveolar tension curve also demonstrates the effect of blood/gas solubility on the rate of rise of F_A/F_i since desflurane (an agent of low blood/gas solubility) rises much quicker than halothane (an agent which is highly soluble).

Ventilation

One can speed up the onset of inhalational agent by increasing the minute ventilation as one constantly replaces anesthetic agent taken up by the pulmonary circulation with higher inspired gas concentration. Such effect is more pronounced with soluble agents such as isoflurane since its speed of onset is influenced by the uptake the most.

Concentration Effect

As one increases the concentration of inspired gas, one not only increases the alveolar concentration but also increases the rate of F_A/F_i rise (see Fig. 3.1). Such effect is termed concentration effect, which is in reality a combination of two contributing factors: (1) concentrating effect and (2) augmented inflow effect. The concentrating effect states that a higher inspired concentration results in a disproportionately higher alveolar concentration. The augmented inflow effect shows that the higher the inspired concentration, the higher the amount of inhalational agent will replace the equal volume of uptake from pulmonary circulation to avoid alveolar collapse.

Finally, the second gas effect is the concentration effect of one gas upon another. The combination of nitrous oxide and another inhalational agent is a typical example of second gas effect although this is insignificant in clinical practice.

Fig. 3.1 Alveolar tension curves of several anesthetics (*Graphs* are redrawn from the data of Yasuda et al. [16])

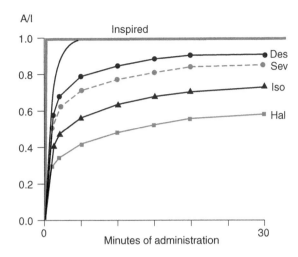

F_a (Arterial Gas Concentration)

For arterial gas concentration, it is determined by ventilation/perfusion mismatch. Mismatch acts as a restriction to arterial and/or alveolar flow and therefore will slow the induction.

Elimination of Inhalational Agents

Several factors affect the elimination of inhalational agents. For example, for agents that undergo extensive metabolism (such as halothane), they tend to have a faster elimination. While the exact molecular pathway has not been identified with certainty, it appears that cytochrome P-450 (especially CYP 2E1 subgroup) plays a major rule in the metabolism of certain inhalational agents. However, the most important element of elimination is via the respiratory system. The same factors that speed up induction are the same factors that fasten elimination such as elimination of rebreathing, high fresh gas flow, low anesthetic-circuit volume, low blood/gas solubility, high cerebral blood flow, and high minute ventilation. Nevertheless, one should keep in mind that emergence from anesthesia is a more complicated topic than elimination of inhalational agents itself and that it also depends on other factors such as the duration of anesthetics. For instance, emergence is faster after short anesthetics than after long anesthetics. In addition, in patients with significant amount of fat or muscle group, these compartments serve as a reservoir of inhalational agents during emergence.

Diffusion hypoxia is a specific phenomenon for nitrous oxide. The elimination of nitrous oxide is extremely rapid, which leads to lower concentration of alveolar oxygenation and carbon dioxide. The lower oxygenation itself leads to hypoxia, while the lower carbon dioxide in the alveoli decreases respiratory drive and hinders ventilation. As a result, after discontinuing nitrous oxide, it is recommended to provide supplemental oxygen to avoid diffusion hypoxia. Clinically, one does not often observe diffusion hypoxia since it is a common practice to provide supplemental oxygen after discontinuation of anesthetics.

Properties of Modern Inhalational Agents

Sevoflurane

The sweet smell as well as its least pungent odor makes sevoflurane (2,2,2-trifluoro-1-[trifluoromethyl]ethyl fluoromethyl ether) an ideal agent for inhalation induction. This is particular true in the pediatric population where mask induction is often required. Furthermore, sevoflurane itself can produce adequate muscle relaxation for intubation following inhalation induction.

Similar to other inhalational agents, sevoflurane depresses myocardial contractility, depresses respiration, reverses bronchospasm, and causes slight increases in cerebral blood flow and intracranial pressure [1–3].

However, there are specific properties related to sevoflurane. For example, the liver microsomal enzyme p-450 (especially the 2E1 isoform) metabolizes sevoflurane 10–25 times the rate that of isoflurane or desflurane, which leads to an increase in inorganic fluoride (F^-). Inorganic fluoride has the potential to cause nephrotoxicity, but no clinically significant renal dysfunction has been associated with sevoflurane thus far. Another factor in sevoflurane metabolism is the production of compound A (fluoromethyl-2,2-difluoro-1-[trifluoromethyl]vinyl-ether) via the degradation of sevoflurane through alkali such as barium hydroxide lime or soda lime, which is another proven (at least in rats) nephrotoxin. Risks of accumulation of compound A include high respiratory gas temperature, low-flow anesthesia, dry barium hydroxide absorbent (Baralyme), high sevoflurane concentration, and long anesthetic duration. Even though most studies have not demonstrated any clinical significant association between postoperative renal dysfunction and sevoflurane usage, some clinicians advocate the fresh gas flow to be at least 2 L/min for anesthetics lasting more than a few hours and that sevoflurane should not be used in patients with preexisting renal impairment.

Desflurane

Desflurane (1,2,2,2-tetrafluoroethyl difluoromethyl ether) requires a special vaporizer given that its vapor pressure at 20 °C reaches 681 mmHg, which boils at room temperature at high altitudes. Desflurane possesses the lowest blood/gas coefficient of all modern inhalational agents, has minimal metabolism, and allows for wake-up times of approximately 50 % less than those compared to isoflurane and 50 % quicker wake-up time when compared to sevoflurane in cases greater than 3 hours. However, switching from isoflurane to desflurane toward the end of anesthesia does not significantly fasten recovery or discharge [4, 5]. Compared with sevoflurane, desflurane is associated with similar incidence of emergence delirium in the pediatric population [6, 7].

While the cardiovascular properties of desflurane are similar to other inhalational agents, including dose-dependent decreases in systemic vascular resistance and cardiac output, a rapid increase in desflurane concentration can lead to transient elevation in heart rate, blood pressure, and catecholamine levels, known as transient sympathetic hyperactivity [8–10]. Even though desflurane is a bronchodilator, the pungency, increase in secretion production, and potential for airway irritation all can lead to laryngospasm, breath-holding, coughing, and sequelae related to increased salivation. It should be noted that in clinical trials, there was no significant increase in airway events when compared with sevoflurane [11].

Desflurane degradation can lead to potentially clinically significant carbon monoxide poisoning, which can be detected by arterial blood gas or lower than expected pulse oximetry reading. Timely exchange of dried-out absorbent or use of calcium hydroxide can help minimize this rare side effect.

Isoflurane

Isoflurane maintains cardiac output by an increase in heart rate due to partially preserved baroreflexes and transient increased level of plasma norepinephrine similar to desflurane. It also dilates coronary arteries, which could potentially lead to coronary steal syndrome. The theory is that the dilation of normal coronary arteries can divert blood away from fixed stenotic lesions, which can then cause regional myocardial ischemia. Such phenomenon, however, has not been proven consistent in several outcome studies and remains one of the theoretical concerns.

In contrast to other inhalational agents, isoflurane was the agent of choice during neurosurgical procedures until three studies were performed at the Mayo Clinic, Cleveland Clinic, and Tulane Medical Center which demonstrated that desflurane provided no significant changes in cerebrospinal fluid pressures while affording quicker recovery postoperatively [12, 13]. Isoflurane, as with all inhalation agents, causes dose-dependent reduction in cerebral metabolic oxygen requirements and can produce burst suppression, which provides a certain degree of neuroprotection during cerebral ischemia [14]. Nevertheless, it is true that isoflurane, similar to other inhalational agents, increases cerebral blood flow and intracranial pressure when administered at concentration greater than 1 MAC. This affects can be attenuated, in part, with hypocarbia [15].

Isoflurane is metabolized to trifluoroacetic acid, but no evidence of renal dysfunction has been observed even during prolonged sedation.

Nitrous Oxide

Nitrous oxide has been one of the oldest inhalational agents that are still widely used today. It is colorless, odorless, nonexplosive, and nonflammable (although it is capable of supporting combustion).

The characteristics of nitrous oxide are quite different from other inhalational agents. For example, nitrous oxide stimulates the sympathetic nervous system. An increase in arterial blood pressure, cardiac output, and heart rate can be observed in the clinical setting due to higher level of endogenous catecholamine levels. It also constricts the pulmonary vascular smooth muscle, which leads to higher pulmonary vascular resistance and, therefore, should be avoided in patients with pulmonary hypertension. In addition, nitrous oxide does not provide any muscle relaxation. In fact, it can lead to skeletal muscle rigidity although it is safe to use nitrous oxide in patients with malignant hyperthermia.

The use of nitrous oxide has also been associated with increased incidence of postoperative nausea and vomiting; however, this has remained controversial since other studies have failed to demonstrate such association in pediatric population where nitrous oxide is frequently employed during inhalation induction.

The pharmacokinetics of nitrous oxide deserves special attention since it irreversibly oxidizes the cobalt atom in vitamin B_{12}. This leads to inhibition of enzymes that are vitamin B_{12} dependent such as methionine synthetase, which is necessary for myelin formation, and thymidylate synthetase, which is necessary for DNA synthesis. There have been reports of bone marrow depression including megaloblastic anemia and neurological deficits including peripheral neuropathy and pernicious anemia, following prolonged exposure of nitrous oxide. In addition, there is an association between nitrous oxide and teratogenicity, and nitrous oxide is often avoided in pregnant patients.

The low solubility of nitrous oxide makes it a good candidate for faster recovery. However, it is still more soluble than nitrogen, and its physical properties can lead to expansion of air-containing cavities. This can be detrimental in a number of patients, including those who have air embolism, pneumothorax, acute intestinal obstruction, tension pneumocephalus following dural closure or pneumoencephalography, pulmonary air cysts, intraocular air bubbles, and tympanic membrane grafting.

The high MAC of nitrous oxide makes it impossible to be the sole inhalational agent to achieve surgical anesthesia, and its use is often combined with other more potent inhalational agents. The addition of 65 % nitrous oxide can often decrease the MAC of the volatile anesthetic gas by approximately 50 %. However, given the need of high concentration, it is not ideal for patients who require high inspired oxygen concentration to avoid hypoxemia.

Halothane

Halothane is the least expensive inhalational agent with reasonable safety profile and hence is still used worldwide. It is rarely utilized in the United States at present as most facilities retired the drug when sevoflurane came to market in the late 1990s.

It is metabolized to a much greater degree than the newer inhalation agents, resulting in delayed emergence and metabolic products that can result in morbidity and in mortality.

One of the most notable disadvantages of halothane is the existence of halothane hepatitis, which leads to elevated liver function test, jaundice, encephalopathy, and fulminant liver failure. Risk factors include patients who are exposed to multiple anesthetics using halothane, middle-aged obese women, and patients with familial predisposition or with personal history. Multiple mechanisms of halothane hepatitis have been proposed. For example, the hepatic damage observed in halothane hepatitis can be replicated in animal models under hypoxic condition. In the absence of oxygen, halothane undergoes reductive metabolism, which may produce hepatotoxic end products, especially when animals are pretreated with cytochrome p-450 inducers such as phenobarbital. Another possible mechanism involves an immune-mediated response since certain signs of halothane hepatitis do not appear until days later such as eosinophilia, rash, and fever. It is therefore theorized that certain liver microsomal proteins are modified by the metabolite of halothane, trifluoroacetic acid, and later become triggering antigens. Given the severity of halothane hepatitis, it is advised not to use halothane in patients who have evidence of hepatic dysfunction following previous exposure.

Halothane causes direct myocardial depression by (1) interfering with sodium-calcium exchange and intracellular calcium utilization, which leads to higher right atrial pressure, (2) inhibition of baroreflex which would have otherwise increased heart rate in response to hypotension, and (3) slowing of sinoatrial node conduction, which may lead to junctional rhythm. Halothane also sensitizes the myocardium to catecholamines, which can lead to significant arrhythmias. For example, the combination of halothane and aminophylline has lead to significant ventricular arrhythmias.

Similar to other inhalational agents, halothane causes bronchodilation and is the most potent bronchodilator of all the inhalational agents. It also increases apneic threshold, increases intracranial pressure, decreases renal blood flow, and decreases hepatic blood flow.

	Sevoflurane	Desflurane	Isoflurane	Nitrous oxide	Halothane
MAC	2.05	6.0	1.15	104	0.75
Vapor pressure	160	664	240	39,000	244
Blood/gas coefficient	0.65	0.45	1.4	0.47	2.5
Brain/blood coefficient	1.7	1.3	1.6	1.1	1.9
Fat/blood coefficient	47	27	45	2.3	51
Cardiac output	↓	No change or ↓	No change	No change	↓
Cerebral metabolic rate	↓↓	↓↓	↓↓	↑	↓
Cerebral blood flow	↑	↑	↑	↑	↑↑↑

(continued)

	Sevoflurane	Desflurane	Isoflurane	Nitrous oxide	Halothane
Direct cerebral vasodilation	Yes	Yes	Yes	Yes	Yes
Renal blood flow	↓	↓	↓↓	↓↓	↓↓
Hepatic blood flow	↓	↓	↓	↓	↓↓
Metabolism (%)	5	<0.1	0.2	0.004	15–20
CO_2 absorbent stability	Compound A formation; heat production	CO formation when dry	CO formation when dry	Yes	CO formation when dry
Pungency	No	Yes	Yes	No	No
Neuromuscular nondepolarizing blockade	↑↑	↑↑↑	↑↑↑	↑	↑↑

Chemical Structures

3.1 Sevoflurane

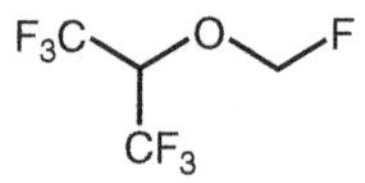

3.2 Desflurane

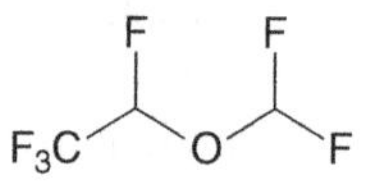

3.3 Isoflurane

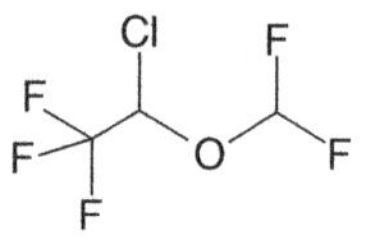

3.4 Nitrous oxide

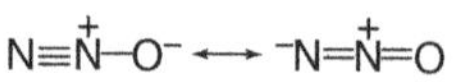

3.5 Halothane

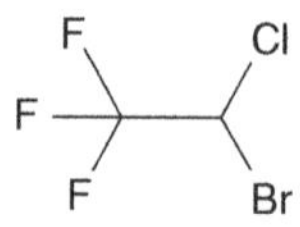

References

1. Newbreg LA, Milide JH, Michenfelder JD. The cerebral metabolic effects of isoflurane at and above concentrations that suppress cortical electrical activity. Anesthesiology. 1983;59:23–8.
2. Scheller MS, Tateishi A, Drummond JC, Zornow MH. The effects of sevoflurane on cerebral blood flow, cerebral metabolic rate for oxygen, intracranial pressure, and the electroencephalogram are similar to those of isoflurane in the rabbit. Anesthesiology. 1998;68:548–51.
3. Lutz LJ, Milde JH, Milde LN. The cerebral functional, metabolic, and hemodynamic effects of desflurane in dogs. Anesthesiology. 1990;73:125–31.
4. Wilhelm W, Kuster M, Larsen B, Larsen R. Desflurane and isoflurane. A comparison of recovery and circulatory parameters in surgical interventions. Anaesthesist. 1996;45:37–46.
5. Morgan GE, Mikhail MS, Murray MJ. Clinical anesthesiology, 4th ed. Lange Medical Books. 2005; p. 173.
6. Mayer J, Boldt J, Rohm KD, Scheuemann K, Suttner SW. Desflurane anesthesia after sevoflurane inhaled induction reduces severity of emergence agitation in children undergoing minor ear-nose-throat surgery compared with sevoflurane induction and maintenance. Anesth Analg. 2006;102:400–4.
7. Locatelli BG, Ingelmo PM, Emre S, Meroni V, Minardi C, Frawley G, Benigni A, Di Marco S, Spotti A, Busi I, Sonzogni V. Emergence delirium in children: a comparison of sevoflurane and desflurane anesthesia using the paediatric anesthesia emergence delirium scale. Paediatr Anaesth. 2013;23:301–8.
8. Weiskopf RB, Eger EI, Noorani M, Daniel M. Repetitive rapid increases in desflurane concentration blunt transient cardiovascular stimulation in humans. Anesthesiology. 1994;81:843–9.
9. Weiskopf RB, Eger EI, Daniel M, Noorani M. Cardiovascular stimulation induced by rapid increases in desflurane concentration in humans results from activation of tracheopulmonary and systemic receptors. Anesthesiology. 1995;83:1173–8.
10. Ebert TJ, Muzi M. Sympathetic hyperactivity during desflurane anesthesia in healthy volunteers. A comparison with isoflurane. Anesthesiology. 1993;79:444–53.
11. Eshima RW, Maurer A, King T, Lin BK, Heavner JE, Bogetz MS, Kaye AD. A comparison of airway responses during desflurane and sevoflurane administration via a laryngeal mask airway for maintenance of anesthesia. Anesth Analg. 2003;96:701–5.
12. Kaye A, Jucera IJ, Heavner J, Gelb A, Anwar M, Duban M, Arif AS, Craen R, Chang CT, Trillo R, Hoffman M. The comparative effects of desflurane and isoflurane on lumbar cerebrospinal fluid pressure in patients undergoing craniotomy fur supratentorial tumors. Anesth Analg. 2004;98:1127–32.
13. Ornstein E, Young WL, Fleischer LH, Ostapkovich N. Desflurane and isoflurane have similar effects on cerebral blood flow in patients with intracranial mass lesions. Anesthesiology. 1993;79:498–502.
14. Miura Y, Grocolt HP, Bart RD, Pearistein RD, Dexter F, Warner DS. Differential effects of anesthetic agents on outcome from near-complete but not incomplete global ischemia in the rat. Anesthesiology. 1998;89:391–400.
15. Adams RW, Cuchiara RF, Gronert GA, Messick JM, Michenfelder JD. Isoflurane and cerebrospinal fluid pressure in neurosurgical patients. Anesthesiology. 1981;54:97–9.
16. Yasuda N, Lockhart SH, Eger 2nd EI, et al. Comparison of kinetics of sevoflurane and isoflurane in humans. Anesth Analg. 1991;72:316–24.

Chapter 4
Principles of Total Intravenous Anesthesia

Basavana Gouda Goudra and Preet Mohinder Singh

Contents

B.G. Goudra, MD, FRCA, FCARCSI (✉)
Department of Anesthesiology and Critical Care Medicine,
Hospital of the University of Pennsylvania, 3400 Spruce Street,
680 Dulles, Philadelphia, PA, USA

Department of Clinical Anesthesiology and Critical Care,
Perelman School of Medicine, Philadelphia, PA, USA
e-mail: goudrab@uphs.upenn.edu

P.M. Singh, MD, DNB
Department of Anesthesia, All India Institute of Medical Sciences,
New Delhi 110029, India

A.D. Kaye et al. (eds.), *Essentials of Pharmacology for Anesthesia,*
Pain Medicine, and Critical Care, DOI 10.1007/978-1-4614-8948-1_4,
© Springer Science+Business Media New York 2015

Anesthesiology, like any other specialty in medicine, is continuously evolving. Perhaps the most important changes are driven by applications of physics leading to improved monitoring, as well as by advances in pharmacology (e.g., improved understanding of drug targets). TIVA (total intravenous anesthesia) is an extension of the concept of balanced anesthesia using real-time pharmacokinetic modeling, delivering all anesthetic drugs via intravenous route targeted to achieve optimal operating conditions with maximal patient comfort and safety. However, there is a natural reluctance among physicians, in general, and anesthesiologists, in particular, to change their practice unless the advantages are striking or the established techniques are proven unsafe. This is probably the main reason why intravenous anesthesia is not being embraced as fondly as one might have expected. Coupled with this, the issues related to modalities of administration are not yet perfected and the pharmacological principles on which they are based are constantly evolving. The aim of the chapter is to explore briefly the intricacies of intravenous anesthesia, examine the potential advantages, briefly review the disadvantages, and wrap up with the areas where it is inevitable and areas where it is immensely useful.

Basics of Total Intravenous Anesthesia (TIVA)

The idea of injecting drugs to produce sleep is older than inhalational anesthesia. Opium is known to have been injected intravenously in 1665 by Elscholtz [1]. However, total intravenous anesthesia where an anesthesiologist does not administer any inhalational anesthetic to induce or maintain anesthesia and relies entirely on intravenous anesthetic agents to achieve the twin objectives – hypnosis and analgesia – is relatively new. The phenomenal increase in this new way of maintaining anesthesia (intravenous induction has been the standard since the discovery of barbiturates in the 1930s) is largely because of the availability of propofol and remifentanil. We are also seeing resurgence in the use of ketamine as an analgesic and co-anesthetic with propofol [2]. Better understanding of pharmacokinetics and the availability of "smart" intravenous anesthesia infusion systems incorporating pharmacokinetic model(s) are other reasons for this increase. One of the reasons why TIVA is still not as popular in the USA as in Europe is nonavailability of these "smart" pumps.

An understanding of the pharmacokinetic/pharmacodynamic modeling of intravenous anesthetics and opiates is essential for safe practice of TIVA. The various models extrapolate drug concentrations in distinct population subgroups eliminating extreme dose response variations for intravenous drug-based infusions. Technology is available to adapt this knowledge into clinical practice with the availability of specialized infusion devices (pumps) that incorporate these models. These pumps aim to improve predictability and eliminate interindividual variability. However, it has to be borne in mind that, with inhalational anesthesia, the end-tidal gas concentrations are *measured* and this is in turn used to guide anesthesia depth, although relationship between end-tidal gas concentrations and brain concentrations is never investigated [3]. With TIVA, the plasma (or effect site) concentrations are *estimated*. Total intravenous anesthesia aims to achieve and maintain therapeutic plasma or "effect site" concentration of an intravenous anesthetic with an appropriate analgesic (administered as a continuous infusion or bolus and infusion with or without supplemental regional blockade). Among the available intravenous drugs, propofol is widely tested and accepted – both pharmacokinetically and pharmacodynamically. With TIVA, the aim is to replace the inhalational agents (nitrous oxide and halogenated vapors) with intravenous agents to achieve hypnosis and analgesia. Although intubation can be performed in the majority of the cases without skeletal muscle relaxants, use of relaxants may be guided by the anesthetic (e.g., rapid sequence) or the surgical requirements. This chapter discusses the various aspects of total intravenous anesthesia in general and target-controlled infusion in particular. For the ease of understanding, target-controlled infusion systems are discussed first.

Target-Controlled Infusion Technique

In a target-controlled infusion-based system, the anesthesia practitioner aims to administer a bolus (loading dose) followed by an infusion (variable) of an anesthetic in order to achieve and maintain a predetermined plasma (or effect site) concentration. Just as one uses a vaporizer to achieve and hold on to a required end-tidal concentration of an inhalational anesthetic, in intravenous anesthesia the practitioner uses a manual- or computer-based infusion device to achieve and maintain an appropriate drug concentration. However, we can measure and display the inhalational anesthetic concentration and such a luxury is not available with intravenous anesthesia delivery systems. As a result the practitioner has to rely on the knowledge of pharmacokinetics from previous studies and the ability of the pumps to do calculations using the inbuilt pharmacokinetic models to accurately predict and maintain a user-selected concentration. The concentration could be of the plasma or effect site (brain/target effect organ) [4]. The absence of a method to measure the plasma concentration in real time is a factor that can discourage anesthesiologists who would like to start practicing intravenous anesthesia. The very fact that there are multiple models which can predict these concentrations indicates the imprecision of the excising systems. There can be two different dosing regimens (infusing different amount of drug) for the same target plasma concentration or same amount of drug administered and yet different models predicting different concentrations. To compound this is the issue of pharmacodynamic variability that can be as much as threefold. However, these concerns should be offset by the fact that data for propofol-based dosing is acquired from huge sample sizes and the likelihood of predicted concentrations being significantly different than measured concentrations is small. On similar grounds, measured end-tidal concentration of inhalation anesthetic does not necessarily tell us anything about brain concentration and importantly; the pharmacodynamic variability still remains unaddressed. Thus, in contrast to popular thinking, both gas anesthesia and TIVA suffer similar limitations of dose response variability [5].

All target-controlled infusion (TCI) systems assume that the body handles the drugs administered in a particular and predictable way and exploit this behavior to

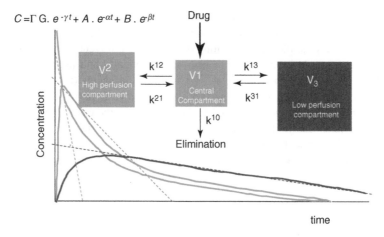

$$C = \Gamma\ G.\ e^{-\gamma t} + A . e^{-\alpha t} + B . e^{\beta t}$$

Fig. 4.1 Three-compartment open model

design the delivery. TCI systems are available for propofol, remifentanil, alfentanil, and sufentanil. An "open" system is one that allows the user to use more than one model for a given drug and also more than one drug in the same pump. These pumps also allow the user to choose between many commercially available syringes of different sizes and many identify the syringe. This is in contrast to the "closed" TCI system (Diprifusor, AstraZeneca, London, UK) that only allows the Marsh pharmacokinetic model to chose and a prefilled syringe to administer propofol [6].

Most of the pharmacokinetic models that explain the behavior of commonly used intravenous anesthetics and opiates are based on either two or three compartments (Fig. 4.1). It is important to bear in mind that the existence of these compartments is entirely theoretical. All drugs are injected into a central compartment (blood/tissue, where the mixing is assumed to happen instantly), from which they diffuse into either one (e.g., ketamine, dexmedetomidine) [7, 8] or two (e.g., propofol, remifentanil, sufentanil, and alfentanil) peripheral compartments, which gives us the two or three compartmental models [9]. The assumption is based on the rate of decay of concentration of these drugs (measured plasma concentration) after a single bolus administration. The elimination could happen in an organ-independent process that occurs in all compartments (e.g., remifentanil) or depend on a specific organ(s). The fall in the plasma concentration is dictated both by redistribution and elimination. Both these processes start immediately after drug administration. The correct depiction of the number of pharmacokinetic compartments adds additional safety margin of accurately predicting possible drug effect site concentrations even with variations in hemodynamic and body compositions seen in practical settings [10]. If the various compartmental volumes and inter-compartmental distribution rate constants and elimination are known, it is possible to predict the plasma concentration at any given time. Conversely it is possible to design a system that can infuse the drug to

Table 4.1 Anesthetic drugs and pharmacokinetic models

Drug	Model
Propofol	Modified Marsh and Schneider
Remifentanil	Minto
Sufentanil	Gepts
Alfentanil	Maitre
Ketamine	Domino

attain and maintain a user-desired plasma concentration (or effect site concentration) with the knowledge of these volumes and constants [11].

Developments are being made to deploy mathematical models for predicting pharmacodynamic effects of anesthetic drugs to counter interindividual variability. Using hypothetical "bio-phase compartment model" estimates of drug administration and onset of clinical effects is already under clinical investigation and is likely to improve predictability of dosage requirement for TCI [11]. Using effect site concentration-based TCI rather than plasma concentration can eliminate hysteresis (delay between peak concentration and peak clinical effect) and predict clinical onset times better.

The pharmacokinetic models that have been widely studied and adapted by TCI pump manufacturers are shown in Table 4.1.

Most of the understanding of TCI comes from the commonly used models of Marsh or Schneider for propofol and of Minto for remifentanil.

There are few drawbacks with these commercially available TCI pumps, mainly due to the shortcomings of the currently available pharmacokinetic models.

1. All these models are derived from the blood concentrations of drugs measured in population samples. As a result, the predictions are only estimates. We are all aware of the fact that drug behavior can be influenced by age, weight, gender, enzyme state, and comorbidity. The pharmacokinetics can also change during the course of administration depending on the blood loss and the type and volume of fluid administered.
2. Even if the model predicts the drug concentration accurately, there is the problem of pharmacodynamic variability that needs to be addressed. Pharmacodynamic variability could be more important than the pharmacokinetic variability and could be as much as threefold [12].

It is also important to bear in mind that the Pk/Pd (pharmacokinetic and pharmacodynamic) models that are used in these pumps are from the data of healthy volunteers for single drug infusion alone. None of them are based on combined remifentanil-propofol anesthesia, which is the most popular TCI-based total intravenous anesthesia technique. As a result the drug interaction between these two is not taken into account in any of these models [13]. These drugs when combined not only can alter pharmacokinetics but also distort individual pharmacodynamics, thus altering predictability of TCIs [3]. It is impossible to design a model that takes into account every conceivable factor influencing pharmacokinetics. It is not dissimilar to the MAC (minimum alveolar concentration) values of inhalational agents that were worked on a single inhalational anesthetic agent and not with opioids or other co-anesthetics.

Manual Infusion Technique

The aim of manual infusion techniques is same as that of target controlled. We aim at a plasma therapeutic concentration, assisted by mental mathematics to decide the initial bolus and the subsequent infusion rates for a desired target concentration (and clinical effect). Analogous to inhalational anesthesia, it requires experience to choose the appropriate loading doses and infusion rates for different patients and surgical procedures. Addition of any drugs (some of them are a necessity, e.g., opioid either remifentanil or alfentanil) adds another layer of complexity. The drug infusion rates and the need for any additional boluses is usually guided by the intensity of surgical stimulation and accompanying hemodynamic response.

Irrespective of the infusion technique chosen, it is important to bear in mind that technical problems like unnoticed IV (intravenous) line disconnection or accidental infiltration into interstitial or subcutaneous space can lead to awareness. In the commonest propofol-remifentanil-based TIVA, tachycardia and hypertension (or even movement in a non-paralyzed patient) due to loss of remifentanil effect might be seen first. This is due to the shorter and predictable context-sensitive halftime of remifentanil. Depending on the duration of infusion, it can take 10–20 min for the effects of propofol to wear off [14]. A gas can be introduced if a disconnection or infiltration is noticed, while efforts are being made to secure another intravenous access.

Practical Conduct of Intravenous Anesthesia

At the outset, any contraindications to TIVA must be ruled out. Allergy to propofol or any of the components will obviate its use. A strong opioid like remifentanil, sufentanil, or alfentanil is almost mandatory especially if muscle relaxants are to be avoided. An IV cannula is essential to initiate and maintain TIVA. As a result children and adults who need inhalational agents to insert IV are not candidates for TIVA although, following inhalation induction, one can switch over to intravenous agents (after securing IV access). Excessive preoperative anxiety warrants need of a sedative anxiolytic (e.g., midazolam), although this may prolong wake-up times after termination of the infusions. The bolus dose is dictated by the lean body mass, age, sex, and comorbidity. With 1.5–2 µg/kg of remifentanil over 2 min, one normally would require 2–2.5 mg/kg (bolus over 2 min) of propofol. With this dose, intubation can be achieved without relaxants or placement of a LMA can be done in 1–2 min after end of bolus dose. If TCI system is being used, target an initial propofol concentration of 5–6 µg/ml and remifentanil of 4–5 ng/ml [15]. Time to peak effect of propofol is around 2 min. It is important to bear in mind that there could be substantial bradycardia and hypotension at induction. Frequently preempting this with a small dose of pressor (like ephedrine) may be required [16]. It is especially advised in the young/healthy/ASA I who have predilection to bradycardia (due to heightened vagal tone) and very elderly who often show hypotension. The latter is because of heightened pharmacodynamic response to both propofol and remifentanil with insufficient sympathetic compensation [17].

To compensate for the rapid fall in the plasma propofol concentration after initial bolus (mainly due to redistribution), higher infusion rates are required in the first 10–15 min of anesthesia. However, due consideration should be given to prolonged periods of absent stimulation depending on the surgeon, surgery, and the country practices. In USA typically these times are 10–15 min. One would be tempted to cut the infusion rates during this period; however, it is important to supplement bolus 1–2 min before incision to bring up the plasma concentrations. Otherwise, there could be patient movement that would be perceived as awareness by the surgeons and nurses. However, the incidence of awareness is rare with intravenous anesthesia, barring technical issues or equipment malfunction [18]. After the initial surgical stimulation, depending on the surgical procedure and the hemodynamic responses, infusion rates (or target concentrations) can be titrated accordingly.

Context-Sensitive Halftimes

Context-sensitive halftime is defined as the time required for drug plasma concentration to decrease by 50 % after cessation of the drug infusion. The context here is the duration for which the drug infusion is run. The timing of the cessation of infusion (at the end of surgery) should be guided by the context-sensitive halftime of the drug in question. As remifentanil washout is context insensitive, due to rapid metabolism, minimal redistribution, and inactive metabolites, its plasma half-life is typically 2–3 min irrespective of the duration of infusion. However, with propofol, there is prolongation of the 50 % plasma decrement times after prolonged infusions, and this has to be taken into consideration while reducing and stopping its infusion. It is also known that elimination half-life of a drug often fails to predict the context-sensitive halftime as factors other than elimination half-life (redistribution, active metabolites, etc.) also play a significant role in the fall of drug concentration post infusion. For example, the context-sensitive halftime for propofol is significantly shorter than midazolam, despite the fact that it has much longer elimination half-life (around 400 min versus 170 min for midazolam) [19]. Clinical utility of this translates into the fact that concerns of delayed respiratory depression using intravenous opioids must not be guided by longer half-lives rather by context-sensitive halftime. Clinical results prove that despite much longer half-life of sufentanil when compared to alfentanil, the context-sensitive halftime of sufentanil is much shorter and thus alfentanil is more liable to cause delayed respiratory depression despite shorter elimination half-life [20]. If significant postoperative pain is expected, it is important to address this either with nerve block or alternate analgesic before turning off remifentanil infusion because of shorter context-sensitive halftime.

Although halftimes predict time for drop in the plasma concentrations by half, they do not necessarily reflect "wake-up" times. Most patients respond to verbal commands even at concentrations close to half of the plasma anesthetic concentrations. However, some patients may wake up at concentrations more than 50 % of anesthetic concentrations, and others may not wake up at concentrations even significantly below 50 %. Coadministration of any benzodiazepines and opioids with longer context-sensitive halftime is another factor affecting wake-up times. Although it is more practical to administer opioids with shorter context-sensitive halftimes (like remifentanil) especially for long cases, opioids with long context-sensitive halftimes (sufentanil, alfentanil) can be administered intelligently to achieve shorter recovery times especially in surgeries with long skin closure times. A good knowledge of pharmacokinetics is essential. Empirically the infusion rate for short periods after initial bolus is approximately the product of elimination clearance and target plasma concentration [19].

Advantages of TCI over Manual Infusion Schemes for TIVA

Enormous variability in the pharmacokinetics and pharmacodynamics among intravenous anesthetic agents would mean that no model can accurately predict the plasma concentrations. Even if there is a way of accurately estimating or measuring the plasma levels, the variable response needs to be addressed. Pharmacodynamic variability can be anticipated and allowance made in some situations like elderly or existing narcotic use (or abuse). But there are many situations like changing surgical stimulation that cannot be always anticipated or quantified accurately. Anesthesia providers try to match the depth of anesthesia with the intensity of surgical stimulation. Sometimes it is impossible to find any factors to explain very high propofol/remifentanil concentrations required to maintain acceptable hemodynamic parameters or depth of anesthesia as measured by EEG (electroencephalography)-based monitoring. Apparent lighter levels as evidenced by patient movement may punctuate a perfectly smooth conduct of anesthesia. This could be annoying and alarming to the surgeon and may even disrupt the surgical procedure. BIS (bispectral index) may be capable of reflecting this; however, unfortunately only after the event has occurred. Fortunately these events are almost never reported as awareness in the absence of technical administration problems. These problems cannot be adequately addressed by a model of any complexity or microprocessor of any speed.

Advantages of using TCI pumps for the administration of TIVA are

1. These pumps make the whole process of setting up and conduct of intravenous anesthesia easy and convenient by taking away the need for doing calculations. Considering that one of the objections to the practice of TIVA is complicated and time consuming setting up, these pumps certainly address this issue. They might also eliminate the possibility of erroneous drug dose infusion due to the possibility of miscalculations.
2. TCI pumps come with many added safety features that are not available in ordinary continuous infusion systems, like indication of line occlusion or disconnection (sudden fall in the resistance to infusion).
3. They aid learning and teaching. TCI practice helps anesthesia practitioners to understand relation between plasma (or effect site) concentrations and clinical effect. They help us to understand compartment pharmacology better. It allows

one to work with numbers akin to end-tidal gas concentrations, although these are not measured, but calculated.

4. These pumps reduce the number of changes the user has to make to the rates of infusion. This can make them user-friendly and increase safety by eliminating requirement of constant manual readjustments, leading to possibility of an error. The anesthesiologist can concentrate on other aspects of patient care rather than being constantly preoccupied with the device.

Choice of Opioid

A question frequently asked is "Can TIVA be practiced safely without the use of remifentanil as an analgesic?" The answer is a qualified yes. Avoiding remifentanil increases use of muscle relaxant and drugs for controlling hemodynamic responses. Remifentanil in the clinical doses is an excellent agent to produce controlled hypotension. Any analgesic other than remifentanil requires the use of additional muscle relaxants to avoid patient movement and facilitate intubation. For example, although, remifentanil is almost equipotent to fentanyl, the infusion rates required similar for clinical effect for fentanyl are four to five times ("cardiac" anesthetic doses) higher [21]. These higher doses, if run for longer durations, result in drug accumulation, thus leading to residual or prolonged effects. Moreover, fentanyl is context sensitive unlike remifentanil, with significant halftime prolongation at the cessation of intermediate to long periods of infusion. Fentanyl might be an acceptable choice for short procedures [22]. However, if large component of analgesia is provided using neuroaxial blockade or plexus/peripheral nerve blockade, then one can safely perform TIVA with smaller infusion doses of remifentanil or fentanyl. None of the available opioids allow rapid titration like remifentanil which makes it the drug of choice for procedures like awake fiberoptic intubation (with or without propofol) and many endoscopy procedures [23]. The reader is referred to [24] for an excellent review on remifentanil.

Cost of TCI-Based Anesthesia

Presumed increased cost of anesthetic agents has been a common factor among many anesthesiologists for their reluctance to change practice. Many do not see the benefits significant enough to merit a change in their time-tested methods of anesthesia practice. The often quoted "it is how you do and not what you do that matters" concept may not be all that true in this case as the benefits of TIVA are far too obvious to ignore and cannot be simulated with gases.

Suttner et al. evaluated the direct cost of 60 patients undergoing elective laparoscopic cholecystectomy [25]. They compared the cost of three techniques – propofol administered with TCI device and remifentanil; manual infusion of propofol, N_2O, and remifentanil; and propofol-fentanyl induction with isoflurane, N_2O, and fentanyl maintenance. They concluded that the propofol-remifentanil technique, although was associated with the highest intraoperative costs, had the fewest postoperative side effects. The postoperative benefits were significantly shorter period of time spent in PACU (postanesthesia care unit) and lesser incidence of postoperative nausea and vomiting both in the PACU and surgical wards. However, both Suttner and others [26] have found a roughly fourfold increase in the direct costs of total intravenous anesthesia.

Most of these studies on cost issues were done with diprivan than generic propofol. Many benefits of TIVA can have significant indirect cost savings if implemented appropriately. For example, a streamlined discharge system from day surgery as soon as the patients meet the criteria for discharge can free up the space to improve through-put. The surgical centers can be closed at scheduled times if the patients can be dis-charged as scheduled. If these benefits lead to increases in surgical volume and reduced overtime payment to staff, then the cost savings are significant. Analysis including functional recovery, additional nursing costs and costs related to PONV (postoperative nausea vomiting), when evaluated in totality favors TIVA practice [27, 28]. However, without a coordinated approach these hidden financial benefits cannot be realized [28].

Drawbacks of Inhalational Anesthesia

It is needless to say that if the FDA existed prior to 1930, or the rules and safety concerns were as stringent, then many of the inhalational agents and nitrous oxide would not have been introduced. Many of the toxic effects of inhalational agents are still being uncovered [7–16]. Recent evidence suggests increased neuronal apopto-sis associated with sevoflurane exposure and thus may affect long-term intellect of neonates being exposed to general anesthesia using sevoflurane [29]. Dr Wei and Dr Eckenhoff, at the Hospital of the University of Pennsylvania [30], have been look-ing at the neurotoxic effects of inhalational anesthetics for many years. Isoflurane is known to induce neurodegeneration mediated via inositol 1,4,5-triphosphate recep-tors in a rat model. Repeated exposure to isoflurane can herald early onset alzheim-er's disease in genetically predisposed individuals [31].

Exposure to even trace concentration of inhalational agents can cause genetic damage [32]. It is speculated that there is increased incidence of spontaneous abor-tions in women exposed to trace gas concentrations [33]. Halothane-induced hepa-titis and triggering of malignant hyperthermia by inhalational agents are well known. However, there is as yet no case for discontinuation of inhalational agents on the basis of existing evidence. If in the future TIVA becomes standard of care, it will be for a multitude of factors rather than any single factor.

Advantages of TIVA

A summary of the possible advantages of TIVA can be found in Table 4.2, among them the important ones are fewer admissions, significantly fewer side effects at 24 h follow-up, earlier discharge, better patient satisfaction, faster recovery, less

Table 4.2 TIVA clinical perspective

Advantages	Disadvantages
Smooth induction and maintenance	Needs special equipment (programmed infusion pumps)
Smooth patient emergence	No real-time concentrations measured – only estimates
Significantly reduced postoperative nausea vomiting	Context-sensitive halftime vary with the duration of infusion – thus predictability of offset varies
No exposure of vapors to anesthesiologist	Higher incidence of apnea if surgery planned under spontaneous ventilation
Environment friendly	Propofol infusion syndrome (prolonged infusions)
Special role in lowering intracranial pressure (ICP) – propofol decreases ICP, lowers brain metabolic rate	Higher direct cost vs. inhalational anesthesia
Only valid anesthesia technique in malignant hyperthermia and myopathies	Lack of familiarity compared to conventional inhalation techniques
Preferred method in surgeries requiring SSEP, MEP (minimal suppression unlike inhalation technique)	
Convenient method in airway surgeries	
Studies document higher patient satisfaction scores	

nausea and vomiting, no pollution, less emergence airway problems, reduced muscle relaxant requirements, usefulness in malignant arrhythmia, and reduced intraocular pressure.

Future of TIVA

Some of the advantages of TIVA are real and some are perceived. For example, reduction in PONV even in high-risk surgeries like middle ear operation is well known. Many ENT surgeons request for TIVA as it is known to reduce intraoperative blood loss. Neurosurgical procedures benefit from TIVA due to better hemodynamic stability, lesser postoperative coughing, and ability to assess neurological status rapidly. Certain procedures like bronchoscopy and gastrointestinal endoscopy are frequently done under TIVA. Due to increasing number and complexity (ERCP, removal of polyps, endoscopic ultrasound, endoscopic mucosal resection) of these outpatient procedures and requirement of rapid turnover, most of these procedures are being done under TIVA. A review of target-controlled infusion and patient-controlled sedation in GI endoscopy can be found at [34]. Many bronchoscopic procedures due to shared airway can be done only under TIVA. Even procedures like fiberoptic intubations especially taking long times are better done under TIVA. Due to intermittent ventilation with gases and longer desaturation times (due to 100 % oxygen), there is increased risk awareness especially in paralyzed patients. With TIVA there is one less thing to worry about due to continuous delivery of anesthetic agents. Concerns are being raised about environmental safety of inhalational agents due to their ozone depletion and greenhouse gas effect. TIVA is not only anesthesia provider friendly (no self-inhalation) but also environment friendly [35].

Rapid wake-up times and early discharge are debatable. Comparable wake-up times can be achieved with sevoflurane/desflurane and remifentanil. Early discharge is only financially relevant if it leads to increases in case turnover and reduction of staffing. This can only be achieved with a coordinated effort and better administration than any single anesthesia technique.

Chemical Structures

**Chemical Structure
4.1** Propofol

**Chemical Structure
4.2** Remifentanil

**Chemical Structure
4.3** Desflurane

**Chemical Structure
4.4** Fentanyl

References

1. Nagelhout JJ, Plaus K. Nurse anesthesia. Philadelphia: Elsevier Health Sciences; 2009.
2. Guit JB, Koning HM, Coster ML, Niemeijer RP, Mackie DP. Ketamine as analgesic for total intravenous anaesthesia with propofol. Anaesthesia. 1991;46(1):24–7.
3. Minto CF, Schnider TW. Contributions of PK/PD modeling to intravenous anesthesia. Clin Pharmacol Ther. 2008;84(1):27–38.
4. Shafer SL, Stanski DR. Defining depth of anesthesia. Handb Exp Pharmacol. 2008;182: 409–23.
5. Absalom AR, Mani V, De Smet T, Struys MMRF. Pharmacokinetic models for propofol–defining and illuminating the devil in the detail. Br J Anaesth. 2009;103(1):26–37.
6. Bressan N, Moreira AP, Amorim P, Nunes CS. Target controlled infusion algorithms for anesthesia: theory vs practical implementation. Conf Proc IEEE Eng Med Biol Soc. 2009;2009: 6234–7.
7. Hijazi Y, Bodonian C, Bolon M, Salord F, Boulieu R. Pharmacokinetics and haemodynamics of ketamine in intensive care patients with brain or spinal cord injury. Br J Anaesth. 2003; 90(2):155–60.
8. Iirola T, Ihmsen H, Laitio R, Kentala E, Aantaa R, Kurvinen J-P, et al. Population pharmacokinetics of dexmedetomidine during long-term sedation in intensive care patients. Br J Anaesth. 2012;108(3):460–8.
9. Levitt DG, Schnider TW. Human physiologically based pharmacokinetic model for propofol. BMC Anesthesiol. 2005;5(1):4.
10. Masui K, Upton RN, Doufas AG, Coetzee JF, Kazama T, Mortier EP, et al. The performance of compartmental and physiologically based recirculatory pharmacokinetic models for propofol: a comparison using bolus, continuous, and target-controlled infusion data. Anesth Analg. 2010;111(2):368–79.
11. Bienert A, Wiczling P, Grześkowiak E, Cywiński JBJ, Kusza K. Potential pitfalls of propofol target controlled infusion delivery related to its pharmacokinetics and pharmacodynamics. Pharmacol Rep. 2012;64(4):782–95.
12. Sear JW, Glen JB. Propofol administered by a manual infusion regimen. Br J Anaesth. 1995;74(4):362–7.
13. Kim HS, Park HJ, Kim CS, Lee JR. Combination of propofol and remifentanil target-controlled infusion for laryngeal mask airway insertion in children. Minerva Anestesiol. 2011;77(7): 687–92.
14. Russell D, Wilkes MP, Hunter SC, Glen JB, Hutton P, Kenny GN. Manual compared with target-controlled infusion of propofol. Br J Anaesth. 1995;75(5):562–6.
15. Ithnin F, Lim Y, Shah M, Shen L, Sia ATH. Tracheal intubating conditions using propofol and remifentanil target-controlled infusion: a comparison of remifentanil EC50 for Glidescope and Macintosh. Eur J Anaesthesiol. 2009;26(3):223–8.
16. Maruyama K, Nishikawa Y, Nakagawa H, Ariyama J, Kitamura A, Hayashida M. Can intravenous atropine prevent bradycardia and hypotension during induction of total intravenous anesthesia with propofol and remifentanil? J Anesth. 2010;24(2):293–6.
17. Ouattara A, Boccara G, Lemaire S, Köckler U, Landi M, Vaissier E, et al. Target-controlled infusion of propofol and remifentanil in cardiac anaesthesia: influence of age on predicted effect-site concentrations. Br J Anaesth. 2003;90(5):617–22.
18. Nordström O, Engström AM, Persson S, Sandin R. Incidence of awareness in total i.v. anaesthesia based on propofol, alfentanil and neuromuscular blockade. Acta Anaesthesiol Scand. 1997;41(8):978–84.
19. Bailey JM. Context-sensitive half-times: what are they and how valuable are they in anaesthesiology? Clin Pharmacokinet. 2002;41(11):793–9.
20. Hughes MA, Glass PS, Jacobs JR. Context-sensitive half-time in multicompartment pharmacokinetic models for intravenous anesthetic drugs. Anesthesiology. 1992;76(3): 334–41.

21. Bürkle H, Dunbar S, Van Aken H. Remifentanil: a novel, short-acting, mu-opioid. Anesth Analg. 1996;83(3):646–51.
22. Coskun D, Celebi H, Karaca G, Karabiyik L. Remifentanil versus fentanyl compared in a target-controlled infusion of propofol anesthesia: quality of anesthesia and recovery profile. J Anesth. 2010;24(3):373–9.
23. Mingo OH, Ashpole KJ, Irving CJ, Rucklidge MWM. Remifentanil sedation for awake fibre-optic intubation with limited application of local anaesthetic in patients for elective head and neck surgery. Anaesthesia. 2008;63(10):1065–9.
24. Komatsu R, Turan AM, Orhan-Sungur M, McGuire J, Radke OC, Apfel CC. Remifentanil for general anaesthesia: a systematic review. Anaesthesia. 2007;62(12):1266–80.
25. Suttner S, Boldt J, Schmidt C, Piper S, Kumle B. Cost analysis of target-controlled infusion-based anesthesia compared with standard anesthesia regimens. Anesth Analg. 1999;88(1): 77–82.
26. Alhashemi JA, Miller DR, O'Brien HV, Hull KA. Cost-effectiveness of inhalational, balanced and total intravenous anaesthesia for ambulatory knee surgery. Can J Anaesth. 1997;44(2): 118–25.
27. Sung YF, Reiss N, Tillette T. The differential cost of anesthesia and recovery with propofol-nitrous oxide anesthesia versus thiopental sodium-isoflurane-nitrous oxide anesthesia. J Clin Anesth. 1991;3(5):391–4.
28. Sneyd JR, Holmes KA. Inhalational or total intravenous anaesthesia: is total intravenous anaesthesia useful and are there economic benefits? Curr Opin Anaesthesiol. 2011;24(2): 182–7.
29. Dong Y, Zhang G, Zhang B, Moir RD, Xia W, Marcantonio ER, et al. The common inhalational anesthetic sevoflurane induces apoptosis and increases beta-amyloid protein levels. Arch Neurol. 2009;66(5):620–31.
30. Tang J, Eckenhoff MF, Eckenhoff RG. Anesthesia and the old brain. Anesth Analg. 2010;110(2):421–6.
31. Wei H, Liang G, Yang H, Wang Q, Hawkins B, Madesh M, et al. The common inhalational anesthetic isoflurane induces apoptosis via activation of inositol 1,4,5-trisphosphate receptors. Anesthesiology. 2008;108(2):251–60.
32. Wrońska-Nofer T, Palus J, Krajewski W, Jajte J, Kucharska M, Stetkiewicz J, et al. DNA damage induced by nitrous oxide: study in medical personnel of operating rooms. Mutat Res. 2009;666(1–2):39–43.
33. Boivin JF. Risk of spontaneous abortion in women occupationally exposed to anaesthetic gases: a meta-analysis. Occup Environ Med. 1997;54(8):541–8.
34. Goudra BG, Mandel JE. Target-controlled infusions/patient-controlled sedation. Tech Gastrointest Endosc. 2009;11(4):181–7.
35. Sulbaek Andersen MP, Nielsen OJ, Wallington TJ, Karpichev B, Sander SP. Medical intelligence article: assessing the impact on global climate from general anesthetic gases. Anesth Analg. 2012;114(5):1081–5.

Chapter 5
Perioperative Considerations in Pharmacology

Angela Vick, Amaresh Vydyanathan, Tarang Safi, and Karina Gritsenko

Contents

A. Vick, MD (✉) • A. Vydyanathan, MD, MS • T. Safi, MD
Department of Anesthesiology, Montefiore Medical Center,
Albert Einstein College of Medicine, Yeshiva University, Bronx, NY, USA
e-mail: avick@montefiore.org; avydyana@montefiore.org; tasafi@montefiore.org

K. Gritsenko, MD
Department of Anesthesiology, Montefiore Medical Center,
Albert Einstein College of Medicine, Yeshiva University, Bronx, NY, USA

Department of Family and Social Medicine, Montefiore Medical Center,
Albert Einstein College of Medicine, Yeshiva University, Bronx, NY, USA
e-mail: karinagritsenko@googlemail.com

A.D. Kaye et al. (eds.), *Essentials of Pharmacology for Anesthesia,*
Pain Medicine, and Critical Care, DOI 10.1007/978-1-4614-8948-1_5,
© Springer Science+Business Media New York 2015

Introduction

Although anesthesiologists are adept at caring for the perioperative patient and the many physiologic aberrations resulting from surgery and anesthesia, management of perioperative pharmacology presents its own diverse set of challenges. Pharmacologic considerations for the perioperative period include the impact of (1) variable responses based on the patient's genotype and/or phenotype, (2) preexisting diseases and drug therapies, (3) interactions with herbal supplementation, and (4) the physiologic changes associated with anesthesia. Many surgical patients are on chronic medications for comorbidities unrelated to the diagnosis that brought them to the OR. Anesthesiologists must be aware of both the effects of withdrawing chronic medications and the potential for interactions between "home" medications and the many drugs administered during the perioperative period. In addition to pharmacologic interactions, patient-specific factors like weight and genetic makeup will also impact the anesthetic plan. This chapter will discuss these factors, as well as anesthetic implications of commonly used medications, including herbal supplements. The side effects of nicotine and other aspects of cigarette smoking will also be discussed due to its prevalence and important anesthetic implications. Finally, the impact of anesthesia and surgery on human physiology and subsequent effects on drug metabolism will be reviewed.

Patient-Specific Factors

Weight

The alteration in pulmonary mechanics secondary to obesity requires modification in anesthetic management during the perioperative period. The obese patient's decreased pulmonary reserve (generally a restrictive pattern of lung disease) and propensity to desaturate quickly due to low functional residual capacity [1] and potentially challenging airway [2] make the administration of medications causing respiratory depression, such as opioids, a reason for concern. The risks increase postoperatively when other anesthetic agents remain in the patients system and lead to synergistic respiratory depression. Obstructive sleep apnea, commonly associated with obesity, further increases this risk [2]. Evidence-based recommendations are scarce, but experts agree that a multimodal pharmacologic approach for analgesia which includes NSAIDs and regional techniques should be utilized for the obese patient in order to decrease the opioid requirement. In addition to modifications in technique, these patients require careful perioperative monitoring, and the use of sedation scores and continuous pulse oximetry should be considered [3].

Another perioperative implication to consider in obese patients is the determination of the body weight calculation that should be used for various anesthetic agents. Experimental studies have used a variety of calculations to assess body weight and pharmacokinetics, and these have included total body weight (TBW), lean body weight (LBW), and ideal body weight (IBW) [4]. LBW values for a given obese

Table 5.1 Body weight to be used for corresponding medications

Drug	Weight used for dosing
Propofol	
Induction	IBW
Maintenance	TBW
Fentanyl	TBW
Sufentanil	TBW
Remifentanil	IBW
Alfentanil	IBW
Morphine	IBW
Midazolam	TBW
Rocuronium	IBW
Vecuronium	IBW
Succinylcholine	TBW

IBW ideal body weight, *TBW* total body weight

individual are greater than those in IBW nomograms. The calculation of LBW requires an estimate of the fractional fat mass (FM_{frac}) and is then as follows: TBW – (FM_{frac} × weight). Obesity affects drug distribution and elimination, particularly for lipid-soluble drugs. Commonly used anesthetic agents are briefly discussed and summarized in Table 5.1: *Inhaled anesthetics*: Modern volatile agents have low lipid solubility and are thus only minimally affected by obesity. *IV anesthetics*: Induction doses of propofol should utilize ideal body weight, and although highly lipid soluble, it does not accumulate in morbidly obese patients; thus, actual or total body weight can be used for infusions [5, 6]. Fentanyl, sufentanil, and midazolam doses are calculated using lean body weight, while ideal body weight is used for the administration of remifentanil, morphine, and alfentanil. *Neuromuscular relaxants* (*NMRs*): The depolarizing agent succinylcholine is dosed based on total body weight, while the steroid-based nondepolarizers, rocuronium and vecuronium, utilize ideal body weight [7]. The NMRs atracurium and cisatracurium, benzylisoquinoline class, are associated with prolonged duration of action if dosed on body weight [8, 9].

Genetic, Phenotypic, and Cultural Differences

Numerous genetic polymorphisms lead to individual patient variations in enzyme activity. These variations alter responses to anesthetics and adjuncts used perioperatively. A common polymorphism is the genetic mutation leading to a dysfunctional form of the enzyme pseudocholinesterase which is responsible for the metabolism of succinylcholine [10]. Often found incidentally in the operating room, a single dose of succinylcholine may result in prolonged decreased muscle strength [10]. If suspected, then the patient should be tested with findings reported to future anesthesia providers. Another genetically mediated complication associated with succinylcholine is malignant hyperthermia (MH) [11]. Once identified, prompt treatment with dantrolene and the avoidance of further exposure to "triggers" (volatile anesthetics and succinylcholine) can be lifesaving [11]. Additional perioperative drugs are subject to genomic polymorphisms which may alter their efficacy and safety. One example is codeine whose action is primarily dependent on the metabolism to its active metabolite, morphine. CYP2D6, the cytochrome P450 enzyme responsible for the conversion of codeine to morphine, is associated with genetic polymorphisms that range from "poor metabolizers" who get little analgesic effect to "ultrarapid metabolizers" who are at risk for opioid toxicity. Unfortunately, there is no reliable phenotype that identifies to which group a patient belongs, so judicious use is recommended especially in those naïve to the drug [12].

Ethnic and physical phenotypic characteristics have been associated with changes in anesthesia requirements perioperatively. One phenotype shown to change anesthetic requirement perioperatively is red hair. These patients have a higher than expected minimum alveolar concentration (MAC) [13]. Other differences among patients may be cultural rather than genetic. Lower negative behavioral changes (including anxiety, apathy, and eating disturbances) are reported by Spanish-speaking Hispanics when compared to English-speaking whites [14]. These findings are important for the anesthesia provider to consider as suboptimal treatment may take place if these subtle characteristics are ignored [14].

Cardiovascular Medications

Hypertension is one of the most common diseases in the United States [15], and antihypertensive therapy is often prescribed. The anesthetic implications of this group of medications are numerous and mainly positive. This is appreciated when one examines the mortality reduction seen in high-risk patients who maintain beta-blocker and/or alpha-2 agonist therapy into the perioperative period [16, 17]. Alpha-2 agonists also have analgesic, sedative, and anti-shivering properties, which lower anesthetic requirements [18]. However, signs of hypovolemia and/or anemia may be masked by the drugs blunting of the normal compensatory sympathetic discharge mechanism. As a result, the anesthesia provider may fail to recognize intravascular volume depletion [19]. Investigation into the length of administration, compliance, and the timing of the patient's last dose is an important part of the pre-assessment. A patient may become tachycardic or severely hypertensive if either beta-blockers or alpha-2 agonists are abruptly discontinued. This rebound effect must be considered by the anesthesia provider in the differential for tachycardia or hypertension in the perioperative period [20].

Other antihypertensive medications commonly used include the angiotensin receptor blockers (ARB), angiotensin-converting enzyme (ACE) inhibitors, and diuretics. These drugs deplete intravascular volume which may increase hypotensive episodes shortly after the induction of general anesthesia – necessitating the need for more vigorous fluid resuscitation intraoperatively [21]. Furthermore, some diuretics (i.e., thiazides and loop diuretics) can cause hypokalemia leading to hyperpolarization of the neuromuscular membrane and, thus, potentiating the effects of non-depolarizing neuromuscular blockers [22]. The effects of these medications should be considered in the anesthetic plan.

Pulmonary Meds

Asthma affects millions in the United States [23]. Inhaled bronchodilators, including beta-2 agonists and anticholinergics, are often prescribed for the asthmatic. Side effects include tachycardia, but the benefits far outweigh the risks. First, both inhaled beta-2 agonists and anticholinergics have been shown to decrease perioperative pulmonary complications and should be continued into the perioperative period [24]. Second, the duration of treatment and frequency of use of these medications may indicate disease severity allowing for adjustments to the anesthetic plan.

Corticosteroids (both oral and inhaled) are prescribed for asthma and chronic obstructive pulmonary disease (COPD). Like bronchodilators, patients should continue their inhaled corticosteroids perioperatively to reduce pulmonary complications [25]. Maintenance of steroid therapy also reduces the incidence of acute adrenal insufficiency due to suppression of the hypothalamic-pituitary-adrenal (HPA) axis from chronic steroid use [26, 27]. A commonly used intravenous anesthetic agent, etomidate, can cause adrenal suppression and is best avoided with long-standing corticosteroid therapy [28]. Because of its cardiovascular stability, its use may be unavoidable, and patients should be monitored for signs of adrenal insufficiency and receive additional steroids [29]. "Stress dosing" of asthmatic patients taking oral steroids (the intravenous administration of the normal daily requirement, approximately 150 mg of hydrocortisone in divided doses) is controversial and depends upon many factors including therapy duration, route of administration, and dose of corticosteroid as well as degree of surgical stress expected [30, 31]. An additional stress dose of corticosteroids should be provided to patients who are on replacement therapy for primary adrenal insufficiency. Patients without primary adrenal insufficiency who have taken a therapeutic dose of steroids on the day of surgery may be observed and given additional corticosteroid as necessary [32]. Supplemental perioperative steroids are not indicated for patients on inhaled corticosteroids.

Estrogen-Containing Medications

Surgery is a known risk factor for thromboembolic events [33]. The anesthetic implications of estrogen-containing medications include their propensity to further increase this risk [34]. Estrogen is commonly found in oral contraceptive pills (OCPs) and hormone replacement therapy (HRT). Selective estrogen receptor modulators (SERMs) act at the estrogen receptor and carry the same risk as the former two classes of estrogen-containing drugs. Patients undergoing procedures associated with a high risk for thromboembolic events may benefit from discontinuing estrogen-containing medications preoperatively – at least 6 weeks prior to surgery [35]. However, this may be difficult for patients on OCPs without other means of birth control and for those on SERMs for treatment of breast cancer. A discussion with the surgeon regarding the risks and benefits of discontinuing these medications preoperatively may be warranted.

Antiplatelets

Many patients with peripheral arterial disease (PAD) are prescribed antiplatelet medications. These agents decrease thromboembolic events, particularly in patients undergoing coronary artery bypass and surgery for PAD [36]. The two commonly used classes of antiplatelet medications are cyclooxygenase inhibitors (i.e., aspirin) and P2Y12 inhibitors (i.e., clopidogrel). If a patient is taking aspirin, the risks and benefits of continuing aspirin perioperatively should be weighed. The risk is increased bleeding intraoperatively, while the benefit is a reduced risk of thromboembolism. Unless a bleeding complication would yield catastrophic results as with surgeries involving the posterior chamber of the eye, middle ear, and intracranial and intramedullary spine, patients who are at a moderate risk for cardiovascular thrombotic events in the perioperative period should continue taking aspirin [37]. Neuraxial blocks are not contraindicated in patients on aspirin [38]. If aspirin must be discontinued, it should be done 7 days prior to surgery to ensure its effects have receded.

P2Y12 receptor blockers such as clopidogrel and ticlopidine are commonly used in patients with coronary stents. After stent placement, dual antiplatelet therapy is required for a minimum duration during which time discontinuation of the medications can increase risk of stent thrombosis [37]. Elective surgery should be delayed as stent thrombosis is a catastrophic complication [37]. When the risk of hemorrhage outweighs the benefits of P2Y12 blocker therapy and the surgical procedure is urgent or emergent, P2Y12 receptor blockers should be stopped briefly and resumed shortly thereafter [39]. Ideally, in order to fully regain platelet function, clopidogrel should be stopped for at least 7 days and ticlopidine stopped for at least 14 days prior to surgery [40]. These patients may benefit from multidisciplinary management involving the anesthesia providers and the patients' cardiologist and surgeon. Neuraxial blocks are contraindicated in patients taking P2Y12 receptor antagonists due to the high risk for developing epidural hematomas and can only be safely used if the drug is stopped for a sufficient time for platelet function to be regained [41].

Psychotropic Medications

Antidepressants

Antidepressant medications are a commonly used class of medications and carry significant anesthetic implications. Most common and severe are the interactions seen with the use of vasopressors. The main classes of antidepressants in common use are tricyclic antidepressants (TCAs), serotonin reuptake inhibitors (SSRIs), and monoamine oxidase (MAO) inhibitors. TCAs work by inhibiting norepinephrine and serotonin uptake at the synaptic cleft. Intuitively, concomitant perioperative use of sympathomimetic drugs could lead to an exaggerated sympathetic response [42]. Therefore, the use of direct and indirect sympathomimetic drugs should be carefully titrated and monitored. Furthermore, anesthetic agents that can augment sympathetic activity (e.g., ketamine, pancuronium) should be used with caution. MAO inhibitors prevent the enzyme monoamine oxidase from metabolizing catecholamines. Secondarily, administration of indirect sympathomimetics to patients taking this class of antidepressants can lead to a massive and life-threatening catecholamine surge [43]. In addition, MAO inhibitors administered with meperidine increases the risk of serotonin syndrome, presenting as agitation, headaches, fever, seizures, and possibly coma and death. Further, abrupt cessation of TCAs can cause withdrawal symptoms, while cessation of either MAO inhibitors or TCAs can precipitate acute depressive episodes. Serotonin reuptake inhibitors (SSRIs) inhibit serotonin reuptake at synaptic clefts. SSRIs have anesthetic implications by way of their antiplatelet actions causing potential for increased blood loss intraoperatively. Conversely, the antiplatelet activity carries potential protective effects in patients with ischemic heart disease [44].

Mood Stabilizers and Antipsychotics

These classes of medications are seen in patients with severe psychiatric illnesses. The major mood-stabilizing medication with significant anesthetic implications is lithium which is the treatment of choice for bipolar disorder. Complications of lithium therapy include nephrogenic diabetes insipidus and hypothyroidism [45, 46]. Investigation for these conditions should be considered preoperatively as both of these complications have major perioperative implications. Furthermore, lithium potentiates the effect of non-depolarizing neuromuscular junction blockers, and their use should be carefully titrated in these patients [47]. Conversely, valproic acid (sometimes used as second line treatment for bipolar disorder) antagonizes non-depolarizing muscle relaxants necessitating increased dosing [48].

Many antipsychotic medications work by inhibiting dopaminergic transmission in the brain [49]. Both first- and second-generation antipsychotics are associated with an increased risk of sudden death when taken in the perioperative period [50]. This may be secondary to the increased risk of arrhythmias associated with the QT prolongation seen with the use of these medications – especially when used in conjunction with volatile anesthetics and some antibiotics such as quinolones and erythromycin [51, 52]. Despite these concerns, cessation of antipsychotics preoperatively may not be a feasible option in some as acute withdrawal from antipsychotics can precipitate psychoses or the neuroleptic malignant syndrome [53]. This provides a challenge for the anesthesia provider, and thus consultation with a psychiatrist is recommended preoperatively.

Table 5.2 Herbal medication or remedy and its potential effects and implication on the anesthetic plan

Herbal remedy	Associated effect and anesthesia implication
Ephedra	Increase in risk for myocardial infarction and stroke – should be stopped at least 24 h preop. It should be considered a less pure and natural ephedrine
Garlic	Increases bleeding risk – should be stopped at least 7 days preop
Ginkgo	Increases bleeding risk – should be stopped at least 36 h preop
Ginseng	Can precipitate hypoglycemia, increase bleeding risk – should be stopped at least 7 days preop
Kava	Has sedative effects and can decrease mood with association of depression. Coadministration with sedatives such as benzodiazepines and barbiturates can enhance sedation. Dozens of reported cases of kava-mediated liver injury, including fatal hepatotoxicity
St. John's wort	19 million prescriptions a year in the United States and in Europe. Can lower effect of several drugs by induction of cytochrome p450 enzymes – should be discontinued at least 5 days preop. Theoretical concern of interaction with meperidine and serotonin syndrome
Valerian	Has sedative effects. Associated with withdrawal symptoms. Taper weeks preop
Echinacea	Associated with allergic reaction and immune stimulation

Opioids

Patients who chronically take opioids will develop tolerance to their analgesic effects. These patients will thus require higher doses of analgesics in the perioperative period [54]. Preoperatively, these patients are advised to maintain opioid use to optimize perioperative care and avoid withdrawal symptoms [55]. The use of adjuvant analgesic therapy as well as regional techniques may be invaluable in the perioperative care of these patients. Obtaining a preoperative pain management consult to guide perioperative pain regimen may help improve postoperative patient recovery and satisfaction. Tolerance to some opioid effects is not observed (e.g., miosis, constipation). Therefore, using pupil size in an anesthetized patient to determine the degree of narcosis is still plausible in these patients [56].

Herbal Medications

Herbal medications are becoming an increasingly important part of medical care of patients. Common herbal remedies include ephedra, garlic, ginkgo, ginseng, kava, St. John's wort, valerian, and echinacea. All these herbal medications have associated side effects that impact the perioperative care of patients. Table 5.2 enumerates the side effects and anesthetic concerns with commonly encountered herbal medications. Of note, there are no reported benefits to the use of herbal medications in the perioperative period. In fact, there are reports of increased morbidity, and it is generally recommended to stop the use of herbal medications 2–3 weeks prior to elective surgery given that the half-life of these agents in any single preparation is typically unknown [57].

Smoking

Smoking remains very prevalent despite exposure-associated deleterious effects affecting multiple organ systems [58]. There are numerous anesthetic implications to consider in patients reporting a history of cigarette smoking. The nicotine contained in cigarettes can cause an increase in sympathetic tone, leading to an elevated blood pressure, heart rate, and myocardial oxygen requirement and increase in peripheral vascular resistance [59]. In addition to the effects of nicotine, cigarettes also contain carbon monoxide, which causes a leftward shift in the oxygen hemoglobin curve, increases propensity for cardiac arrhythmias, and decreases intracellular oxygen content. There is also an associated increased risk of arterial thrombosis [59, 60]. Given the half-life of carboxyhemoglobin on room air, cessation of smoking should be at least 12 h prior to anesthesia induction. However, as the increased mucus production, ciliary inactivation, and increased bronchial/laryngeal hyperactivity recover only 4–6 weeks after smoking cessation, full benefits including a decrease in incidence of pulmonary complications are seen only when cessation of smoking occurs at least 8 weeks prior to surgery [61]. Other effects of smoking on the patients receiving anesthesia include a decrease in pain tolerance, decreased incidence of postoperative nausea and vomiting (PONV), and increased incidence of infections secondary to impaired immunity [62].

Regional or MAC anesthesia is preferred if appropriate as it may reduce the incidence of postoperative pulmonary complications. The anesthesia provider must be aware of the increased airway reactivity in these patients that may necessitate avoidance of irritant inhalational agents like desflurane and consideration of extubation in a deeper plane if patients exhibit extreme bronchial reactivity [63]. Postoperative pulmonary function should be optimized with deep breathing exercises [64].

Perioperative Physiology and Its Pharmacologic Impact

Alterations in thermoregulation, intravascular fluid volume, and plasma protein concentrations as a result of anesthetic management impact drug metabolism. The vasodilatory effects of volatile anesthetics and regional anesthetics as well as the sympatholytic effects of potent opioids such as fentanyl act to decrease thermoregulation. Opioids also directly inhibit the hypothalamic thermogenic process, an effect which is exploited in the postoperative period to prevent patient discomfort secondary to shivering. With the loss of thermoregulation, core temperature may fall by several degrees in a cold operating room. The resultant hypothermia leads to decreased drug metabolism and, subsequently, to increased drug concentration and effect. For example, plasma concentrations of propofol are increased by 30 % in patients who are 3 °C hypothermic [65]. Hypothermia also decreases volatile anesthetic requirements or MAC (minimal alveolar concentration) and prolongs the effects of neuromuscular relaxants. Likewise, effects on cardiac output secondary to volatile anesthetics and intravascular fluid shifts impact the pharmacokinetics of distribution and elimination. Plasma protein, electrolyte, and drug concentrations may be affected by inadequate or excessive intravenous fluid administration. Additionally, the choice of fluid used may change the patient's acid-base physiology resulting in changes in drug ionization or ion trapping as with the hyperchloremic metabolic acidosis associated with the administration of large volumes of 0.9 % sodium chloride solution or normal saline for resuscitation. Perioperative physiologic alterations create a dynamic milieu and an obligation for the anesthesia provider to fully integrate his or her knowledge of pharmacologic principles into the anesthetic plan for the management of the surgical patient.

Conclusion

The perioperative plan including the choice of anesthetic care is determined in consideration of patient safety and satisfaction. A thorough understanding of patient-related factors as well as knowledge of their medication regimen is essential in this regard. We discussed the commonly used medications taken by patients as well as some intrinsic patient-specific factors and its associated anesthetic implications. In addition, collaborative efforts with the patient's primary care physician/specialists may be necessary to optimize their perioperative care.

Chemical Structures

Chemical Structure
5.1 Propofol

Chemical Structure
5.2 Rocuronium bromide

References

1. Pelosi P. Perioperative management of obese patients. Best Pract Res Clin Anesthesiol. 2010; 24(2):211.
2. El-Orbany M, Woehick HJ. Difficult mask ventilation. Anesth Analg. 2009;109(6):1870–80.
3. Schug SA. Postoperative pain management of the obese patient. Best Pract Res Clin Anesthesiol. 2011;25(1):73–81.
4. Green B, Duffull SB. What is the best size descriptor to use for pharmacokinetic studies in the obese? Br J Clin Pharmacol. 2004;58(2):119–33.
5. Servin F, Farinotti R, Haberer JP, Desmonts JM. Propofol infusion for maintenance of anesthesia in morbidly obese patients receiving nitrous oxide. A clinical and pharmacokinetic study. Anesthesiology. 1993;78:657–65.
6. Ingrande J, Brodsky JB, Lemmens HJ. Lean body weight scalar for the anesthetic induction dose of propofol in morbidly obese subjects. Anesth Analg. 2011;113(1):57–62.
7. Baerdemaeker L. Pharmacokinetics in obese patients. Contin Educ Anesth Crit Care Pain. 2004;4:152–5.
8. Leykin Y, Pellis T, Lucca M, Lomangino G, Marzano B, Gullo A. The effects of cisatracurium on morbidly obese women. Anesth Analg. 2004;99:1090.
9. Kirkegaard-Nielsen H, Helbo-Hansen HS, Lindholm P, Severinsen IK, Pedersen HS. Anthropometric variables as predictors for duration of action of atracurium-induced neuromuscular block. Anesth Analg. 1996;83:1076–80.
10. Hodgkin WE, Giblett ER. Complete pseudocholinesterase deficiency: genetic and immunologic characterization. J Clin Investig. 1965;44(3):486–93.
11. Dong-Chan K. Malignant hyperthermia. Kor J Anesthesiol. 2012;63(5):391–401.
12. Crews KR, et al. Clinical Pharmacogenetics Implementation Consortium (CPIC) guidelines for codeine therapy in the context of *Cytochrome P450 2D6 (CYP2D6)* genotype. Clin Pharmacol Ther. 2012;91(2):321–6.
13. Liem EB, Lin CM, Suleman MUI, Doufas AG, Gregg RG, Veauthier JM, et al. Anesthetic requirement is increased in redheads. Anesthesiology. 2004;01:279–83.
14. Fortier MA, Tan ET, Mayes LC, Wahi A, Rosenbaum A, Strom S, Santistevan R, Kain ZN. Ethnicity and parental report of postoperative behavioral changes in children. Paediatr Anaesth. 2012;23:422–8.
15. Yoon SS, Ostchega Y, Louis T. Recent trends in the prevalence of high blood pressure and its treatment and control, 1999–2008. NCHS data brief, no 48. Hyattsville, MD: National Center for Health stats 2010.
16. Lindenauer PK, Pekow P, Wang K, Mamidi DK, Gutierrez B, et al. Perioperative beta-blocker therapy and mortality after major noncardiac surgery. N Engl J Med. 2005;28;353(4): 349–61.
17. Wijeysundera DN, Naik JS, Beattie WS. Alpha-2 adrenergic agonists to prevent perioperative cardiovascular complications: a metaanalysis. Am J Med. 2003;114:742–52.
18. Hayashi Y, Maze M. Alpha 2 adrenoceptor agonists and anaesthesia. Br J Anaesth. 1993;71(8):108–18.
19. Neideen T, Lam M, Brasel KJ. Preinjury beta blockers are associated with increased mortality in geriatric trauma patients. J Trauma. 2008;65:1016–20.
20. Metz S, Klein C, Morton N. Rebound hypertension after discontinuation of transdermal clonidine therapy. Am J Med. 1987;82:17.
21. Kataja JHK, Kaukinen S, Viinamaki OVK, et al. Hemodynamic and hormonal changes in patients pretreated with captopril for surgery of the abdominal aorta. J Cardiothorac Vasc Anesth. 1989;3:425–32.
22. Miller RD, Roderick LL. Diuretic-induced hypokalaemia, pancuronium neuromuscular blockade and its antagonism by neostigmine. Br J Anaesth. 1978;50:541–4.
23. Centers for Disease Control and Prevention. Vital signs. 2011. www.cdc.gov/vitalsigns/asthma/index.html

24. Warner DO, Warner MA, Barnes RD, et al. Perioperative respiratory complications in patients with asthma. Anesthesiology. 1996;85:460–7.
25. Kabalin CS, Yarnold PR, Grammer LC. Low complication rate of corticosteroid-treated asthmatics undergoing surgical procedures. Arch Intern Med. 1995;155:1379.
26. Todd GR, Acerini CL, Ross-Russell R, et al. Survey of adrenal crisis associated with inhaled corticosteroids in the United Kingdom. Arch Dis Child. 2002;87:457.
27. Lipworth BJ. Systemic adverse effects of inhaled corticosteroid therapy: a systematic review and meta-analysis. Arch Intern Med. 1999;159:941.
28. Wagner RL, White PF, Kan PB, et al. Inhibition of adrenal steroidogenesis by the anesthetic etomidate. N Engl J Med. 1984;310:1415.
29. Murray H, Marik PE. Etomidate for endotracheal intubation in sepsis: acknowledging the good while accepting the bad. Chest. 2005;127:707.
30. Livanou T, Ferriman D, James VH. Recovery of hypothalamo-pituitary-adrenal function after corticosteroid therapy. Lancet. 1967;2:856.
31. Westerhof L, Van Ditmars MJ, Der Kinderen PJ, et al. Recovery of adrenocortical function during long-term treatment with corticosteroids. Br Med J. 1972;2:195.
32. Marik PE, Varon J. Requirement of perioperative stress doses of corticosteroids: a systematic review of the literature. Arch Surg. 2008;143(12):1222–6.
33. Kakkar AK, Cohen AT, Tapson VF, ENDORSE Investigators, et al. Venous thromboembolism risk and prophylaxis in the acute care hospital setting (ENDORSE survey): findings in surgical patients. Ann Surg. 2010;251:330–8.
34. Cushman M, Kuller LH, Prentice R, et al. Estrogen plus progestin and risk of venous thrombosis. JAMA. 2004;292:1573–80.
35. Zambouri A. Preoperative evaluation and preparation for anesthesia and surgery. Hippokratia. 2007;11(1):13–21.
36. Prevention of pulmonary embolism and deep vein thrombosis with low dose aspirin: Pulmonary Embolism Prevention (PEP) trial. Lancet 2000;355:1295.
37. Douketis JD, Spyropoulos AC, Spencer FA, et al. Perioperative management of antithrombotic therapy: antithrombotic therapy and prevention of thrombosis, 9th ed: American College of Chest Physicians Evidence-Based Clinical Practice Guidelines. Chest. 2012;141:e326S.
38. Horlocker TT, Wedel DJ, Schroeder DR, Rose SH, Elliott BA, McGregor DG, Wong GY. Preoperative antiplatelet therapy does not increase the risk of spinal hematoma associated with regional anesthesia. Anesth Analg. 1995;80(2):303–9.
39. Llau JV, Lopez-Forte C, Sapena L, Ferrandis R. Perioperative management of antiplatelet agents in noncardiac surgery. Eur J Anaesthesiol. 2009;26:181–7.
40. Smart S, Aragola S, et al. Antiplatelet agents and anesthesia. Contin Educ Anaesth Crit Care Pain. 2007;7(5):157–61.
41. Horlocker T, Wedel D. Regional anesthesia in the anticoagulated patient: defining the risks (The second ASRA Consensus Conference on Neuraxial Anesthesia and Anticoagulation). Reg Anesth Pain Med. 2003;28(3):172–97.
42. Barar FS, Boakes AJ, Benedikter LB, Laurence DR, Prichard BN, Teoh PC. Interactions between catecholamines and tricyclic and monoamine oxidase inhibitor antidepressive agents in man. Br J Pharmacol. 1971;43(2):472P–3.
43. Stack CG, Rodgers P, Linter SP. Monoamine oxidase inhibitors and anesthesia. Br J Anaesth. 1988;60(2):222–7.
44. Andrade C, Sandarsh S, Chethan KB, Nagesh KS. Serotonin reuptake inhibitor antidepressants and abnormal bleeding: a review for clinicians and reconsideration of mechanisms. J Clin Psychiatry. 2010;71:1565–75.
45. Kurt AS. Lithium-induced nephrogenic diabetes insipidus. J Am Board Fam Pract. 1999;12:43–7.
46. Henry C. Lithium side-effects and predictors of hypothyroidism in patients with bipolar disorder: sex differences. J Psychiatry Neurosci. 2002;27(2):104–7.
47. Hill GE, Wong KC, Hodges MR. Lithium carbonate and neuromuscular blocking agents. Anesthesiology. 1977;46(2):122–6.

48. Kim, et al. Effects of valproic acid and magnesium sulphate on rocuronium requirement in patients undergoing craniotomy for cerebrovascular surgery. Br J Anesth. 2012;109:407–12.
49. Miller R. Mechanisms of action of antipsychotic drugs of different classes, refractoriness to therapeutic effects of classical neuroleptics, and individual variation in sensitivity to their actions: Part I. Curr Neuropharmacol. 2009;7(4):302–14.
50. Ray WA, Chung CP, Murray KT, et al. Atypical antipsychotic drugs and the risk of sudden cardiac death. N Engl J Med. 2009;360:225.
51. Glassman AH, Bigger Jr JT. Antipsychotic drugs: prolonged QTc interval, torsade de pointes, and sudden death. Am J Psychiatry. 2001;158(11):1774–82.
52. Viskin S, Justo D, Halkin A, Zeltser D. Long QT syndrome caused by noncardiac drugs. Prog Cardiovasc Dis. 2003;45(5):415–27.
53. Amore M, Zazzeri N. Neuroleptic malignant syndrome after neuroleptic discontinuation. Prog Neuropsychopharmacol Biol Psychiatry. 1995;19:1323–34.
54. Rozen D, DeGaetano NP. Perioperative management of opioid-tolerant chronic pain patients. J Opioid Manag. 2006;2:353–63.
55. Lewis N, Williams J. Acute pain management in patients receiving opioids for chronic and cancer pain. Contin Educ Anesth, Crit Care Pain. 2005;5:127–9.
56. Collett B-J. Opioid tolerance: the clinical perspective. Br J Anaesth. 1998;81:58–68.
57. Kaye AD, Clarke R, Sabar R, Kaye AM. Herbal medications survey. J Clin Anesth. 2000;12:468–71.
58. Trichopolos D, Kalandidi A, Sparros L, Macmahon B. Lung cancer and passive smoking. Int J Cancer. 1981;27:1–4.
59. Katz LN. Cigarette smoking and cardiovascular diseases: report by the American Heart Association. Circulation 1960;22:160–6.
60. Hung J, Lam J, Lacoste L, Letchacovski G. Cigarette smoking acutely increases platelet thrombus formation in patients with coronary artery disease taking aspirin. Circulation. 1995;92:2432–6.
61. Vassallo R, Ryu JH. Tobacco smoke-related diffuse lung diseases. Semin Respir Crit Care Med. 2008;29(6):643–50.
62. Whalen F, Sprung J, Burkle CM, Schroeder DR, Warner DO. Recent smoking behavior and postoperative nausea and vomiting. Anesth Analg. 2006;103(1):70–5.
63. Rodrigo C. The effects of cigarette smoking on anesthesia. Anesth Prog. 2000;47(4):143–50.
64. Westerdahl E, Lindmark B, Eriksson T, Friberg O, Hedenstierna G, Tenling A. Deep-breathing exercises reduce atelectasis and improve pulmonary function after coronary artery bypass surgery. Chest J. 2005;128(5):3482–8.
65. Leslie K, Sessler DI, Bjorksten AR, Moayeri A. Mild hypothermia alters propofol pharmacokinetics and increases the duration of action of atracurium. Anesth Analg. 1995;80:1007–14.

Part II
Drug Classes

Chapter 6
Anesthetic Induction Agents

David Hirsch, Charles Fox, and Alan David Kaye

Contents

Introduction

Induction agents have a variety of roles in the practice of anesthesiology. Most commonly, they are used to promote induction of general anesthesia or to provide sedation in the intensive care setting or for monitored anesthesia care. In recent years, propofol, etomidate, and ketamine have evolved as the principal induction agent in clinical practice [1–3].

D. Hirsch, MD (✉)
Department of Anesthesiology, Tulane Medical Center, New Orleans, LA, USA
e-mail: dhirsch2@tulane.edu

C. Fox, MD
Department of Anesthesiology, LSU Health Science Center Shreveport, Shreveport, LA, USA
e-mail: cfox1@lsuhsc.edu

A.D. Kaye, MD, PhD
Department of Anesthesiology, Tulane Medical Center, New Orleans, LA, USA

Department of Anesthesiology, Louisiana State University Health Sciences Center,
New Orleans, LA 70112, USA
e-mail: alankaye44@hotmail.com

A.D. Kaye et al. (eds.), *Essentials of Pharmacology for Anesthesia,*
Pain Medicine, and Critical Care, DOI 10.1007/978-1-4614-8948-1_6,
© Springer Science+Business Media New York 2015

Nonbarbiturate Induction Agents

Propofol

Propofol is one of the most commonly used agents for the induction of anesthesia. It is a substituted isopropylphenol (2,6-diisopropyl-phenol) that is chemically distinct from other intravenous induction agents [5].

Drug Class and Mechanism of Action

Propofol's suggested mechanism of action is through an interaction with gamma-aminobutyric acid type A ($GABA_A$), which is the principal inhibitory neurotransmitter in the CNS [1]. When the GABA receptor is activated, transmembrane chloride conduction is potentiated, which hyperpolarizes the postsynaptic cell membrane and causes functional inhibition of the neuron. Propofol's interaction with the GABA complex theoretically decreases the rate of dissociation of GABA from its receptor, which increases the conduction of the chloride channel causing hyperpolarization of the cell membrane [5, 6].

Indications

Propofol provides quick onset and offset making it the drug of choice for complete and rapid emergence. Propofol may also be used as a continuous infusion in the settings of procedural deep sedation or intraoperative monitored anesthesia care and/or instances where total IV anesthetic is required or for sedation purposes in the intensive care unit (ICU). Propofol has strong antiemetic properties, which make it very useful in both the inpatient and outpatient setting. Propofol decreases CBF, $CMRO_2$, and ICP. At a similar dosage rate, Propofol has amnestic properties similar to midazolam [1].

Dosing Options

Induction
The induction dose for adults is 1–2.5 mg/kg IV which gives a blood level of 3–8 µg/ml. Induction typically occurs around 30 s with a duration of 3–5 min. This level should produce unconsciousness depending on age and associated medications. Increased age, premedication (usually with benzodiazepines or opioids), and reduced cardiovascular reserve all decrease dosing needs. Children require a larger induction dose, usually around 2.5–3.5 mg/kg IV. Emergence typically occurs with a plasma concentration of 1–1.5 µg/ml [1].

Intravenous Sedation
Propofol's short context sensitive half-life, combined with its short distribution half-life, makes it a very useful drug for IV sedation. Typically, the conscious sedation dose is 25–100 µg/kg/min and is easily titratable [17]. Propofol is also commonly used as a sedative during mechanical ventilation in the ICU setting. This provides control of stress responses and is beneficial due to its amnestic as well as anticonvulsant properties.

Drug Interactions

Potentiates CNS depressants.

Ethanol and Sodium Oxybate
Contraindicated secondary to risk of respiratory and central nervous system depression and psychomotor impairment: additive effects

Succinylcholine
May potentiate risk of severe bradycardia: mechanism unknown [1, 4]

Side Effects

> **Black Box Warnings**
> Notne

- Most common: pain on injection (can be reduced with an opioid or coadministration with lidocaine
- Allergic reactions/anaphylactic reactions
- Propofol infusion syndrome: associated with long-term use of propofol, >4 mg/kg for more than 24 h, causing metabolic acidosis as well as possible cardiac failure, rhabdomyolysis, and renal failure. Treatment is supportive as well as discontinuation of propofol infusion.
- Bradycardia/asystole
- Profound hypotension
- Thrombosis
- Hyperlipidemia
- Seizures
- Bacterial growth [3].

Fospropofol

Water-soluble prodrug of propofol is established to improve the side effect profile of propofol. These water-soluble derivatives aim to decrease bacterial growth, hyperlipidemia, as well as pain on injection. Fospropofol has a similar profile to propofol; however, induction and awakening times are both elongated as it must be converted to the active form of propofol first. Fospropofol is currently only approved for monitored anesthetic care [7, 9].

Etomidate

Etomidate is a rapid-acting IV induction agent that is most useful for its cardiovascular stability. It has anesthetic as well as amnestic properties; however, unlike other induction agents, it produces no analgesic effects [12].

Drug Class and Mechanism of Action

Etomidate is a carboxylated imidazole derivative with two isomers. However, the preparation used for IV induction contains only the D-isomer, as this is the only one that is pharmacologically active [3]. The imidazole containing nucleus of etomidate makes it lipid soluble at a physiologic pH but water-soluble at an acidic pH. It is chemically different than other induction agents but is thought to act in a manner similar to propofol and benzodiazepines by producing CNS depression. Like propofol, it enhances the inhibitory effects of the $GABA_A$ receptor [1].

Indications

The most common indication for etomidate is for rapid IV induction in patients with impaired cardiac function or reserve, especially poor contractility [16]. It is very useful for rapid sequence intubation as it has a similar onset to propofol or the now discontinued thiopental. The advantage of this agent is that there is preservation of all of cardiovascular parameters within 10 % of baseline. Arterial blood pressures decreases are absent or minimal and are usually due to small decreases in systemic vascular resistance [14]. Etomidate very rarely decreases either heart rate or cardiac output [13, 15]. This also makes it useful for intubation in patients with a cardiac history or hemodynamic status that is unknown. Myoclonic movements during induction with etomidate are common and are theoretically caused by simultaneous excitatory and inhibitory actions on the corticothalamic fibers. Concurrent opioid administration can exacerbate the myoclonus activity; however; neuromuscular blockers administration can conceal this phenomenon. Etomidate is also a potent cerebral vasoconstrictor causing decreased ICP as well as CBF, yet it has not been shown to have neuroprotective qualities [17].

Dosing Options

The current suggested induction dose for etomidate is 0.3 mg/kg IV with a range of 0.2–0.6 mg/kg IV [1]. Unconsciousness usually occurs around 30 s with a duration of 3–5 min. Awakening, like induction, is very rapid and residual respiratory depression is uncommon. Postoperative nausea and vomiting are both slightly elevated compared to propofol. While theoretically etomidate would be ideal for long-term IV sedation, it is rarely used due to a dose-dependent adrenocortical suppression. Etomidate is also cautioned in patients with sepsis or hemorrhage due to suppression of the "stress" response [10]. For pediatric patients, the same dose (0.3 mg/kg IV) is indicated in children greater than 10 years old. For pediatric patients, less than 2 years old, etomidate is not currently recommended. Currently, research has shown that this dosage is likely safe in all pediatric patients greater than 2 years old for rapid sequence intubation when hemodynamic stability is paramount [8].

Drug Interactions

Potentiates CNS depressants.
    Use with hypertensive agents may cause exaggerated hypotension.

Side Effects

- *Adrenocortical suppression*: inhibits the conversion of cholesterol to cortisol by inhibiting 11 beta-hydroxylase. Inhibition lasts 4–8 h after an induction dose of etomidate [10, 11].
- *Pain on injection.*
- *Myoclonic movements.*
- *Nausea.*
- *Dysrhythmias* [17].

Ketamine

Ketamine is unique as an IV induction agent in that it produces a dissociative anesthesia as well as possesses strong analgesic properties. This dissociative anesthesia causes a characteristic cataleptic state where the patient's eyes remain open with a slow nystagmic gaze. The patient is typically noncommunicative with varying purposeful skeletal movements as well as hypertonia [1].

Drug Class and Mechanism of Action

Ketamine is a highly lipid soluble and partially water-soluble phencyclidine derivative [21]. Ketamine possesses two stereoisomers, the positive S causing more intense analgesia, though only the racemic mixture is available in the USA. Ketamine functions by interacting with N-methyl-D-aspartate (NMDA) receptors, opioid receptors, monoaminergic receptors, muscarinic receptors, and voltage-sensitive calcium channels [18]. While this causes ketamine's mechanism of action to be very complex, its most potent actions occur through the excitatory NMDA channel. Ketamine acts as a noncompetitive antagonist of the NMDA calcium receptor. It also interacts with the phencyclidine-binding receptor site leading to increased inhibition of the NMDA receptor [19]. This inhibitory action also produces analgesia by disrupting pain transmission in the spinal cord through the NMDA receptors in the dorsal horn [1]. In the peripheral system, ketamine seemingly has an antagonistic effect at the muscarinic receptors causing anticholinergic symptoms such as emergence delirium, bronchodilation, and sympathomimetic response [20].

Dosing Options

Induction with ketamine is produced by doses of 1–2 mg/kg IV or 4–6 mg/kg IM [2]. Unlike both propofol and etomidate, ketamine does not cause pain at the ejection site. Induction time is usually 45–60 s with IV administration and 2–4 min after IM administration. It is recommended to hold paralytic until induction is noted. Induction dose tends to last 5–15 min however; return to full mental capacity can require another hour. Emergence is further delayed with repeated dosing or continued infusion. Ketamine associated amnesia tends to last around 60–90 min with retrograde amnesia unlikely. Ketamine is useful for its relatively rapid IM induction properties with children or noncompliant patients. Unlike other induction agents, ketamine is also useful in hypovolemic patients for its cardiac-stimulating properties. However, if catecholamine stores are depleted, ketamine can cause myocardial depression. For anesthesia maintenance, the recommended dose is 0.1–0.5 mg/kg IV or 0.5–4.5 mg/kg as needed [21]. For IM maintenance, dosing is 3.25–13 mg/kg IM as needed. It is recommended to administer adjuvant benzodiazepine as well as an antisialogogue when using ketamine to pretreat reemergence phenomenon and increased salivation, respectively. Ketamine is typically given at 0.2–0.8 mg/kg IV in small boluses when additional analgesia is needed. This is especially helpful during use of regional anesthesia when additional pain control is needed. Ketamine is commonly used during cesarean section for this reason; as it does not produce any associated depression of the newborn. During general anesthesia, a continuous infusion (3–5 ug/kg/min) can help provide sufficient analgesia as well [1].

Drug Interactions

- *CNS depressants* may cause additive effects.
- *Monoamine oxidase inhibitor*: additive effects secondary to increased levels of catecholamine, theoretically SSRI and TCA, have a similar interaction [20].

Side Effects/Black Box Warnings

Black Box Warnings (www.fda.gov)
- There is a 12 % incidence of emergence phenomenon.
- Patients can appear confused or excited with or without vivid imagery, hallucinations, or delirium which can last up to 24 h postoperatively.
- These effects are decreased with diazepam coadministration and doses should be reduced with elderly (>65 years old) or pediatric (<15 years old) patients [18].
- It is recommended to use small doses of short-acting barbiturates in cases where severe emergence phenomenon is exhibited in patients.

- Avoid in schizophrenia or other hallucination-associated disease states as risk of psychosis is also increased.
- *Hypertension/tachycardia*: contraindicated in hypertensive crisis, acute myocardial infarction, aortic dissection, or recent use of methamphetamine.
- *Hypersalivation*: pretreatment with antisialogogue is useful.
- *Increased ICP/intraocular pressure*: contraindicated in glaucoma or acute global injury.
- *Cognitive impairments*: chronic use.
- *Nausea/vomiting.*
- *Tonic/clonic movements* [17].

Summary

After nearly 60 years of barbiturates primarily providing induction of general anesthesia, propofol with the advantage of quicker recovery has become the most popular iv induction agent worldwide. Etomidate, providing cardiovascular stability, is an attractive agent for any patient with limited cardiac reserve. Ketamine, owing to its high lipid solubility, can be delivered intramuscularly for the population of patients that will not allow for iv placement or a mask induction.

Chemical Structures

Chemical Structure
6.1 Propofol

Chemical Structure
6.2 Ketamine

Chemical Structure
6.3 Etomidate

References

1. Stoelting RK, Miller RD. Basics of anesthesia. 5th ed. Philadelphia: Churchill Livingstone, Elsevier; 2007.
2. Calvey TN, Williams NE. Principles and practice of pharmacology for anaesthetists. Oxford: Blackwell Science; 1997.
3. Cass TN, Cass L. Pharmacology for anaesthetists. Edinburgh: Churchill Livingstone; 1994.
4. Tramèr MR, Moore RA, McQuay HJ. Propofol and bradycardia: causation, frequency and severity. Br J Anaesth. 1997;78(6):642–51.
5. Trapani G, Altomare C, Liso G, Sanna E, Biggio G. Propofol in anesthesia. Mechanism of action, structure-activity relationships, and drug delivery. Curr Med Chem. 2000;7(2):249–71.
6. Trapani G, Latrofa A, Franco M, Altomare C, Sanna E, Usala M, Biggio G, Liso G. Propofol analogues. Synthesis, relationships between structure and affinity at GABA$_A$ receptor in rat brain, and differential electrophysiological profile at recombinant human GABAA receptors. J Med Chem. 1998;41(11):1846–54.
7. Garnock-Jones KP, Scott LJ. Fospropofol. Drugs. 2010;70(4):469–77.
8. Zuckerbraun NS, Pitetti RD, Herr SM, et al. Use of etomidate as an induction agent for rapid sequence intubation in a pediatric emergency department. Acad Emerg Med. 2006;13(6):602–9.
9. Fechner J, Ihmsen H, Hatterschild D, Jeleazcov C, Schiessl C, Vornov JJ, et al. Comparative pharmacokinetics and pharmacodynamics of the new propofol prodrug GPI 15715 and propofol emulsion. Anesthesiology. 2004;101(3):626–39.
10. Cuthbertson BH, Sprung CL, Annane D, Chevret S, Garfield M, Goodman S, Laterre PF, Vincent JL, et al. The effects of etomidate on adrenal responsiveness and mortality in patients with septic shock. Intensive Care Med. 2009;35(1):1868–76.
11. Hildreth AN, Mejia VA, Maxwell RA, Smith PW, Dart BW, Barker DE. Adrenal suppression following a single dose of etomidate for rapid sequence induction: a prospective randomized study. J Trauma. 2008;65(3):573–9.
12. Morgan M, Lumley J, Whitwam JG. Etomidate, a new water-soluble non-barbiturate intravenous induction agent. Lancet. 1975;321:955–6.
13. Latson TW, McCarroll SM, Mirhej MA, Hyndman VA, Whitten CW, Lipton JM. Effects of three anesthetic induction techniques on heart rate variability. J Clin Anesth. 1992;4:265–76.

14. du Cailar J, Bessou D, Griffe O, Kienlen J. Hemodynamic effects of etomidate. Ann Anesthesiol Fr. 1976;17:1223–7.
15. Ebert TJ, Muzi M, Berens R, Goff D, Kampine JP. Sympathetic responses to induction of anesthesia in humans with propofol or etomidate. Anesthesiology. 1992;76:725–33.
16. Bovill JG. Intravenous anesthesia for the patient with left ventricular dysfunction. Semin Cardiothorac Vasc Anesth. 2006;10:43–8.
17. Peck TE, Hill SA, Williams M. Pharmacology for anaesthesia and intensive care. 3rd ed. Cambridge: Cambridge University Press; 2008. p. 111.
18. Bergman SA. Ketamine: review of its pharmacology and its use in pediatric anesthesia. Anesth Prog. 1999;46(1):10–20.
19. Hirota K, Lambert D. Ketamine: its mechanism(s) of action and unusual clinical uses. Br J Anaesth. 1996;77(4):441–4.
20. Reich D, Sivay G. Ketamine: an update on the first twenty-five years of clinical experience. Can J Anesth. 1989;36:2.
21. Clements JA, Nimmo WS, Grant IS. Bioavailability, pharmacokinetics and analgesic activity of ketamine in humans. J Pharm Sci. 1982;71(5):539–42.

Chapter 7
Analgesics: Opiate Agonists, Mixed Agonists/ Antagonists, and Antagonists for Acute Pain Management

Orlando J. Salinas and Christopher K. Merritt

Contents

O.J. Salinas, MD (✉) • C.K. Merritt, MD
Department of Anesthesiology, Louisiana State University, New Orleans, LA, USA
e-mail: osalin@lsuhsc.edu; christopherkmerritt@yahoo.com

A.D. Kaye et al. (eds.), *Essentials of Pharmacology for Anesthesia,*
Pain Medicine, and Critical Care, DOI 10.1007/978-1-4614-8948-1_7,
© Springer Science+Business Media New York 2015

Introduction

Opioid analgesics represent one of the mainstays in management of acute pain. They are employed in the treatment of moderate to severe pain commonly as part of a multimodal therapy approach. In selecting opioids pharmacokinetics plays an important role since most opioids can be best described as pharmacodynamic equals with respect to their efficacy at receptors and propensity to produce ventilatory depression [1].

Opiate Agonists

Drug Class and Mechanism of Action

Opioid analgesics consist of four classes of drugs that include phenanthrenes, phenylpiperidines, benzomorphans, and phenylheptamines [2]. Hydromorphone, codeine, oxymorphone, oxycodone, and hydrocodone all belong to the phenanthrene class of drugs and are considered "semisynthetic" (derived from modification of the morphine molecule) opioids. Morphine is a naturally occurring (not semisynthetic or synthetic) compound derived from the opium poppy. While codeine exists naturally in the poppy, its concentrations are so low that commercially codeine is synthesized from the morphine. The majority of clinically relevant opioids act primarily on mu receptors and are referred to as mu agonists [2]. Morphine is the prototypical phenanthrene mu agonist against which all others are compared to. Fentanyl is related structurally to meperidine, the first synthetic opioid. Fentanyl and its congeners sufentanil, alfentanil, and remifentanil all belong to the phenylpiperidine class. Fentanyl is derived from meperidine, and sufentanil, alfentanil, and remifentanil are derived from rather complex manipulation of fentanyl's structure. Fentanyl and its congeners are often referred to as "synthetic opioids." The modulation of nociceptive (painful) stimuli within the CNS is thought to occur between the afferent (ascending) pathways (spinothalamic tract) and the efferent (descending) pathways (reticulospinal tract) that are considered inhibitory or "modulating" [3]. The opioid analgesics bind to opioid receptors located within the brain, spinal cord, peripheral nerves, and gastrointestinal tract [4]. These receptors include mu, kappa, and delta among others. Receptor subtypes (mu1, mu2, etc.) appear in the literature but conflicting data about their existence persists because it is unclear if these subtypes are coded for by specific genes or if they are a result of posttranslational protein modification [5]. Opioid receptors are G protein-coupled receptors. Their activation by endogenous peptides (endorphins, enkephalins, and dynorphins) or analgesic opioids activates transmembrane G proteins resulting in a cascade of events that ultimately decreases neuronal excitability and hyperpolarizes the neuron with the net effect being primarily inhibitory [6]. The release of excitatory neurotransmitters such as substance P is consequently decreased [7]. Opioid metabolism can produce active metabolites as in the case of morphine and meperidine (described below). Most opioids are metabolized in the liver by either phase 1 (modification) metabolism or phase 2 (conjugation) metabolism or both. In phase 1 metabolism cytochrome P450 (CYP) performs hydrolysis or oxidative modifications of the opioid molecule. In phase 2 metabolism an opioid molecule is conjugated (joined) with a hydrophilic substance (glucuronic acid) and eventually eliminated from the body primarily by the kidney [8].

Indications/Clinical Pearls

Opioids can be given by a wide variety of routes. These include oral, intranasal, transbuccal (sublingual), transdermal, and rectal routes of administration. More common methods of opioid administration for acute pain, especially in the perioperative setting, have been intramuscular, intravenous, and neuraxial (intrathecal and epidural). These methods offer rapid onset and better titratability [9]. Emerging technologies for sublingual (sufentanil) and transdermal (fentanyl) administration appear promising. Opioid agonist analgesics are indicated in the treatment of mild, moderate, or severe acute pain. Mild acute pain can be treated with oral opioids such as hydrocodone, oxymorphone, and oxycodone [10–12]. These drugs are frequently given after moderate to severe pain symptoms have subsided and discharge from the recovery room or facility is anticipated. They are often combined with an NSAID such as aspirin or acetaminophen and their dosing is usually limited by the nonopioid content. Oral opioids are subject to extensive first-pass effect in the liver and are not a first-line choice for moderate to severe acute pain because their bioavailability is low [13]. Intramuscular injections (morphine, hydromorphone) have been a popular route of administering opioid analgesics. Serum concentrations of opioids may vary greatly with this modality as uptake is erratic and dependent on perfusion of the site [13]. Despite these drawbacks, intramuscular injections of opioids can be considered in select situations (lack of IV access). Intravenous opioids (morphine, hydromorphone, fentanyl) are commonly used perioperatively and in intensive care units to treat moderate to severe acute pain. The sedation associated with morphine typically precedes its analgesic effect. This is an important clinical consideration to avoid "stacking" doses which may result in oversedation and respiratory depression. Morphine is conjugated (metabolized) in the liver with glucuronic acid into morphine-3-glucuronide (M3G) and morphine-6-glucuronide (M6G) prior to renal excretion. M6G is a potent mu receptor agonist, whereas M3G is pharmacologically inactive. The accumulation of M6G may produce respiratory embarrassment in patients with renal disease. Hydromorphone is a logical choice for renal patients because its metabolism does not produce (M6G). Hydromorphone metabolism generates an active metabolite (hydomorphone-3-glucuronide) that may exhibit excitatory properties [14]. Patient-controlled analgesia (PCA) allows patient titration of the opioid against their own pain requirements and eliminates the drawbacks associated with PRN dosing such as staff availability and subjective staff interpretations of patient's pain. PCA requires patient cooperation and thus appropriate selection of candidates for PCA therapy is indicated. Patient acceptance of PCA has been high, and studies demonstrate less total drug consumption with improved postoperative respiratory function when compared to patients receiving conventional as needed or scheduled dosing by trained staff [15, 16]. Continuous ("basal rate") PCA infusions have been shown to produce a higher incidence of respiratory depression particularly in opioid-naïve patients, and their use in this group is not recommended [14]. Morphine, hydromorphone, fentanyl, and sufentanil are all common choices for intravenous PCA. Fentanyl and sufentanil have no active metabolites and have been used with success in patients receiving intravenous PCA. Sufentanil provides better analgesia with less respiratory depression than fentanyl when used for intravenous PCA [14]. Intrathecal and epidural opioids provide excellent analgesia and rapid onset. Morphine, fentanyl, and sufentanil are commonly used for this purpose. Morphine's lack of lipid solubility provides extended analgesia for 12–24 h. This property makes one-time dosing or repeat dosing through an epidural catheter with morphine convenient. Fentanyl and sufentanil provide analgesia for about 2 h when administered neuraxial. They are commonly given together with a local anesthetic (ropivacaine, lidocaine) to speed onset of spinal analgesia. Their short duration of effect compared with morphine limits their usefulness as primary modalities for postoperative analgesia when administered as a single-shot injection; however, epidural PCA with either sufentanil or fentanyl via an epidural catheter has been used with success in patients requiring postoperative analgesia.

Dosing Options

Intramuscular

Morphine 10–15 mg, onset of action in 15–30 min and a peak analgesic effect in 30–90 min, repeat every 2–3 h prn. *Hydromorphone* 1–4 mg, onset of action about 20–30 min, repeat every 2–3 h prn.

Intravenous

Morphine 2.5–15 mg, onset of action 15 min, repeat every 3–4 h prn. *Hydromorphone* 0.2–1.0 mg, onset of action 15 min, repeat every 2–3 h prn. *Fentanyl* 20–50 mcg, onset of action 5–10 min, repeat every 1–1.5 h prn.

PCA

Morphine 0.5–2.5 mg bolus, 6–10 min lockout interval, 1–2 mg/h continuous infusion. *Hydromorphone* 0.05–0.25 mg bolus, 10–20 min lockout interval, 0.2–0.4 mg/h continuous infusion. *Fentanyl* 20–50 mcg bolus, 5–10 min lockout interval, 10–100 mcg/h continuous infusion. *Sufentanil* 2–5 mcg bolus, 4–10 min lockout interval, 2–8 mcg/h continuous infusion.

Drug Interactions

All sedatives potentiate the effects of the mu agonists when administered concomitantly. Drugs that induce liver enzymes (cytochrome P450) (rifampin, carbamazepine, and phenytoin) or inhibit macrolide antibiotics (e.g., erythromycin), azole antifungal agents (e.g., ketoconazole), and protease inhibitors (e.g., ritonavir) may require increasing or decreasing the dose of opioid, respectively. Meperidine is absolutely contraindicated for use with monoamine oxidase inhibitors.

Side Effects/Black Box Warnings

Opioid agonists all demonstrate dose-dependent respiratory depression. Morphine can produce delayed depression of ventilation when administered as a neuraxial analgesic. This effect may occur 6–12 h after epidural dosing reflecting the cephalad spread of morphine within the subarachnoid space. Opioid-induced bradycardia, vasodilation, and hypotension occur secondary to stimulation of the vagal nucleus and are most commonly observed with fentanyl and its congeners [17]. Muscle rigidity ("chest-wall rigidity") is more common after the administration of fentanyl and its congeners. Ventilation with a bag and mask may be impossible. These effects can be reversed with muscle relaxants or by administering an opioid antagonist such as naloxone. Opioids cause nausea/vomiting by stimulating the chemoreceptor trigger zone in the area postrema of the fourth ventricle in the brain. Opioid-induced nausea and vomiting may also be exacerbated by stimulation of the vestibular apparatus, contributing to the higher incidence of vomiting observed in ambulatory patients [18]. Histamine release is seen with morphine after rapid bolus administration but not with fentanyl or sufentanil [19]. Opioids can cause decreased peristalsis, constipation, and biliary colic (sphincter muscle spasm). Other side effects include pruritus, miosis (Edinger-Westphal nucleus stimulation), and urinary retention. Pruritus is the most common side effect of neuraxial analgesia. Normeperidine is a metabolite of meperidine with a long half-life that can accumulate with repeated doses. Toxicity from normeperidine can manifest as restlessness, tremors, myoclonus, seizures, and delirium. Meperidine has also caused fatal reactions in patients taking monoamine oxidase (MAO) inhibitors. The American Pain Society does not recommend using meperidine to treat acute pain [14]. It is, however, still used for acute pain management despite national recommendations against its continued use [20]. All opioids cross the placenta, and fetal respiratory depression is not uncommon.

Opioid Agonists/Antagonists

Drugs in this category include butorphanol, buprenorphine, nalbuphine, and pentazocine. They produce potent analgesia and sedation, but without the euphoria (buprenorphine is an exception described below) associated with pure mu agonists like morphine. Patients taking these drugs do not exhibit difficulty concentrating ("mental cloudiness") as seen with morphine. In fact they may appear sedated but are capable of having a lucid conversation when prompted to do so. With the exception of buprenorphine, these drugs can conveniently be considered "kappa agonists" [21].

Drug Class and Mechanism of Action

Butorphanol, buprenorphine, and nalbuphine are members of the phenanthrene class of opioids. Pentazocine is alone among opioids in the benzomorphan class of drugs. All these drugs exhibit agonist and antagonist effects at opioid receptors. They bind mu receptors but are much less efficacious ("weak agonists") than the pure mu agonists (morphine). When bound to mu receptors, they can displace pure mu agonists and precipitate withdrawal symptoms in opioid-dependent patients. Additionally, they can induce a sense of dysphoria in patients because they are agonists at kappa receptors (buprenorphine is an exception) which limit their abuse potential as compared with the pure agonist opioids. Buprenorphine binds to mu receptors with very high affinity and less efficacy (compared to morphine) and is slow to dissociate from the receptor [2]. Its high affinity and slow dissociation properties have important clinical considerations described below. It is antagonistic at kappa receptors [2, 21]. Buprenorphine is unique in the agonist/antagonist group because it induces morphine-like euphoria ("mood elevation") in patients receiving this drug. This mood elevation effect is a result of its greater efficacy at mu receptors as compared to the other agonists/antagonists.

Indications/Clinical Pearls

The agonist/antagonist opioids are indicated for the treatment of moderate to severe pain. They are usually given by intramuscular or intravenous routes and exhibit a "ceiling effect" which manifests as a lack of pharmacologic response from repeated dosing beyond a certain point. Traditionally their perceived benefit was the lower likelihood of respiratory depression, but some studies have demonstrated dose-dependent respiratory depression similar to morphine until the "ceiling effect" is reached [21]. In any event, even enormous doses of these drugs rarely produce apnea in normal patients [21]. Butorphanol has been traditionally used in obstetrics due to its perceived benefit of less respiratory depression. Pentazocine has a higher incidence of dysphoria as compared with the other receptor agonists/antagonists and is generally not as well tolerated by patients. Pentazocine can also increase heart rate and circulating levels of catecholamines which is not seen with butorphanol, nalbuphine, or buprenorphine [21]. Buprenorphine has the highest abuse potential within this group due to its morphine-like properties. Small doses of naloxone may be added to preparations of this drug to decrease the likelihood of abuse.

Dosing Options

Intramuscular

Butorphanol 1–4 mg every 3–4 h prn. *Buprenorphine* 0.3–0.6 mg every 6 h prn. *Nalbuphine* 10 mg every 3–6 h prn.

Intravenous

Butorphanol 0.5–2 mg every 3–4 h prn. *Buprenorphine* 0.3 mg repeat every 6 h prn. *Nalbuphine* 10 mg every 3–6 h prn.

Side Effects/Black Box Warnings

Drug interactions are the same as for mu agonists. Large doses of naloxone may not completely reverse buprenorphine-induced respiratory depression in susceptible patients, and thus there exists no reliable method of reversing the hypoventilation observed during buprenorphine overdose [2, 21]. The agonists/antagonists in general produce symptoms similar to the pure agonists (respiratory depression, pruritus, urinary retention), but these symptoms tend to be less severe in nature, hence the appeal of these drugs. All of these drugs may precipitate opioid withdrawal when given to opioid-dependent patients and should be used with caution in this group.

Opioid Antagonists

Naloxone, naltrexone, and nalbuphine are pure mu receptor antagonists with no agonist activity.

Drug Class and Mechanism of Action

Naloxone is derived from modification to the phenanthrene oxymorphone. Nalmefene and naltrexone are structurally similar to naloxone. They have a high affinity for opioid receptors (mu, kappa, delta) resulting in the displacement of opioid agonists from their binding sites.

Indications/Clinical Pearls

These drugs are used primarily to reverse the side effects of the mu agonists. They can also reverse effects of the kappa agonists (butorphanol, nalbuphine) reflecting their antagonism at that receptor site. Naloxone is commonly used to treat respiratory depression associated with opioid agonists. It can be given intravenous, intramuscular, or subcutaneous, but intravenous provides the most rapid onset of action. Its short duration of action (30–45 min) can result in the return of respiratory depression. This can be avoided by repeat boluses or a continuous infusion. Nalmefene has the primary advantage of a longer duration of action compared to naloxone. Nalmefene has an elimination half-time of about 10 h in contrast to one hour for naloxone. These drugs need to be titrated when attempting to counter the respiratory depression caused by opioid analgesics.

Dosing Options

The usual dose for opioid-induced respiratory depression is a 1–4 mcg/kg bolus intravenously. Alternatively an infusion of 3–5 mcg/kg/h may be considered.

Side Effects/Black Box Warnings

The side effects of opioid antagonists resemble sympathetic stimulation. Careful titration of antagonists will reduce these side effects. Rapid bolusing of large doses may produce tachycardia, hypertension, pulmonary edema, and cardiac dysrhythmias. Fatal outcomes have been reported.

Summary

Opioid agents continue to be major drugs utilized in acute pain management after surgical procedures. An appreciation for the different pharmacology of these drugs and an appreciation for the development of newer delivery systems into the future will ultimately reduce potential risks and aid in the overall management of patients postoperatively.

Chemical Structures

7.1 Morphine

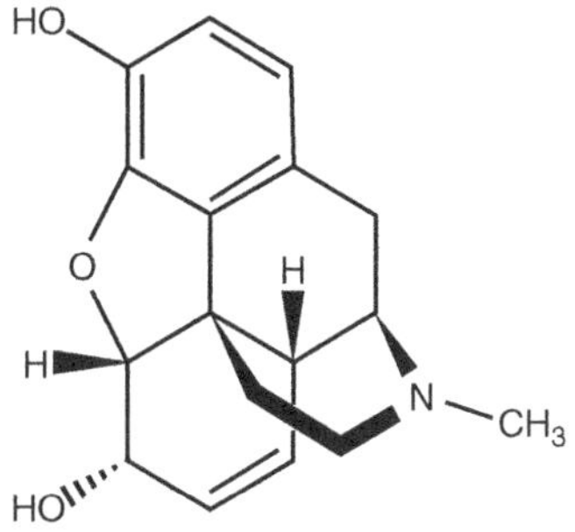

7.2 Hydromorphone

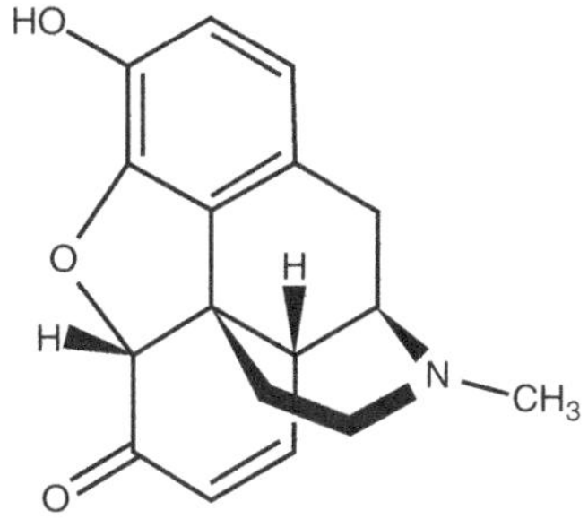

7.3 Fentanyl

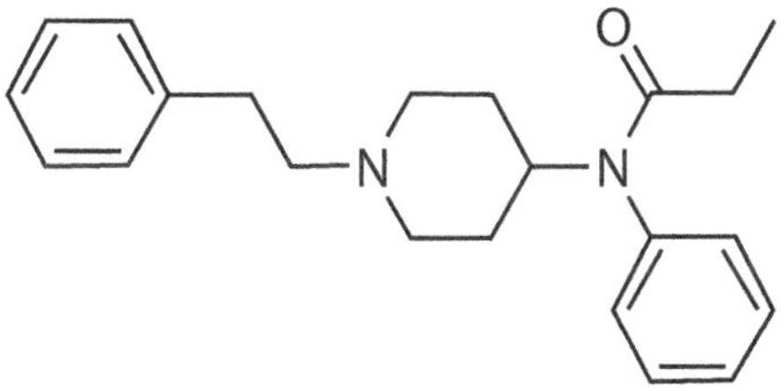

7.4 Butorphanol

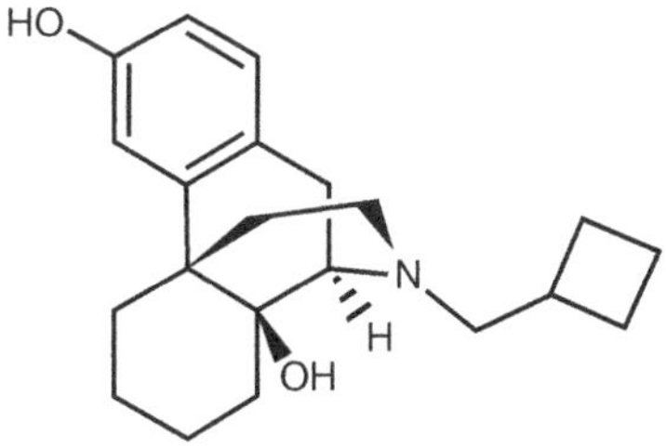

7.5 Nalbuphine

7.6 Buprenorphine

References

1. Mather LE. Pharmacokinetic and pharmacodynamic profiles of opioid analgesics: a sameness amongst equals? Pain. 1990;43:3–6.
2. Trescot AM, Datta S, Lee M, Hansen H. Opioid pharmacology. Pain Physician. 2008;11: s133–53.
3. Lebenow RL, Ivankovich AD, McCarthy RJ. Management of acute postoperative pain. In: Barash PG, editor. Clinical anesthesia. 4th ed. Philadelphia: Lippincott Williams & Wilkins; 2001.
4. Liu M, Wittbrodt E. Low-dose oral naloxone reverses opioid-induced constipation and analgesia. J Pain Symptom Manage. 2002;23(1):48.
5. Egan DE. Opioids. In: Miller RD, editor. Basics of Anesthesia. 6th ed. Philadelphia: Elsevier; 2011.
6. American Pain Society. Principles of analgesic use in the treatment of acute pain and cancer pain. 6th ed. Glenview: American Pain Society; 2008.
7. de Leon-Cassosla OA, Lema MJ. Postoperative epidural opioid analgesia: what are the best choices? Anesthesiol Analg. 1996;83:867–75.
8. Smith HS. Opioid metabolism. Mayo Clin Proc. 2009;84(7):613–24.

9. Sinatra R, deLeon-Cassola OA, Ginsberg B, et al. Acute pain management. New York: Cambridge University Press; 2009. p. 613.
10. Eckhardt K, Li S, Ammon S, et al. Same incidence of adverse drug events after codeine administration irrespective of the genetically determined differences in morphine formation. Pain. 1998;76(1–2):27–33.
11. Budd K. The role of tramadol in acute pain management. Acute Pain. 1999;2(4):189–96.
12. Sloan P. Review of oral oxymorphone in the management of pain. Ther Clin Risk Manag. 2008;4(4):777–87.
13. Bergams G, Vanacker B, Van Aken H, et al. Investigation of the pharmacokinetics and analgesic effects of an intramuscular injection of sustained-release sufentanil for postoperative pain: an open study. J Clin Anesthesiol. 1994;6:462–8.
14. Palmer PP, Miller RD. Current and developing methods of patient controlled analgesia. Anesthesiol Clin. 2010;28(4):587–99.
15. Egbert AM, Parks LH, Short LM, et al. Randomized trial of postoperative patient-controlled analgesia vs. intramuscular narcotics in frail elderly men. Arch Intern Med. 1990;150: 1897–903.
16. Hecker BR, Albert L. Patient-controlled analgesia: a randomized, prospective comparison between two commercially available PCA pumps and conventional analgesic therapy for postoperative pain. Pain. 1988;35:115–20.
17. Hug CC. Opioids: clinical use as anesthetic agents. J Pain Symptom Manage. 1992;7(6): 350–5.
18. Sussman G, Shurman J, Creed MR, Larsen LS, et al. Intravenous ondansetron for the control of opioid-induced nausea and vomiting. Clin Ther. 1994;6(6):462–8.
19. Philbin DM. Baillière Clin Anaesthesiol. 1989;3(1):205–16.
20. O'Conner AB, Lang VJ, Quill TE. Eliminating analgesic meperidine use with a supported formulary restriction. Am J Med. 2005;118:885–9.
21. Rosow CE. The clinical usefulness of agonist-antagonist analgesics in acute pain. Drug Alcohol Depend. 1987;20:329–37.
22. Land BL, Bruchas MR, et al. The dysphoric component of stress is encoded by activation of the dynorphin κ-opioid system. J Neurosci. 2008;28(2):407–14.
23. Miyoshi HR, Leckband SG. Systemic opioid analgesics. In: Loeser JD, Butler SH, Chapman CR, et al., editors. Bonica's management of pain. 3rd ed. Baltimore: Lippincott Williams & Wilkins; 2001. p. 1682–709.
24. Pasero C, Portenoy RK, McCaffery M. Opioid analgesics. Pain: a clinical manual. New York: Mosby; 1999. p. 161–99.
25. Power I. Fentanyl HCl iontophoretic transdermal system (ITS): clinical application of iontophoretic technology in the management of acute postoperative pain. Br J Anaesth. 2007;98(1):4–11 [http://bja.oxfordjournals.org/content/98/1/4.full.pdf+html].
26. Brose WG, Tanelian DL, Brodsky JB, Mark JB, Cousins MJ. CSF and blood pharmacokinetics of hydromorphone and morphine following lumbar epidural administration. Pain. 1991; 45:11–5.

Chapter 8
Analgesics: Opioids for Chronic Pain Management and Surgical Considerations

Roy Esaki and Alex Macario

Contents

R. Esaki, MD, MS (✉) • A. Macario, MD, MBA
Department of Anesthesiology, Perioperative and Pain Medicine,
Stanford University School of Medicine,
Stanford, CA, USA
e-mail: resaki@stanford.edu; amaca@stanford.edu

A.D. Kaye et al. (eds.), *Essentials of Pharmacology for Anesthesia,*
Pain Medicine, and Critical Care, DOI 10.1007/978-1-4614-8948-1_8,
© Springer Science+Business Media New York 2015

Overview

Opioids represent the third most commonly prescribed drug class in the United States in 2010, and the most prescribed medication, hydrocodone-acetaminophen, is an opioid [1]. Medicolegal issues continue to grow concerning misuse and diversion. The number of deaths from opioids in the United States quadrupled since 1999 and represents approximately three-quarters of all drug overdose deaths. In 2010, the amount of opioid analgesics sold was enough to "medicate every American adult with a typical dose of 5 mg of hydrocodone every four hours for one month" [2]. Simultaneously, with increasing emphasis on the recognition of pain as the "fifth vital sign" and per the second step of the WHO (World Health Organization) ladder, the proper management of chronic pain often requires judicious prescription of narcotics.

There are three major types of opioid receptors coupled to G-protein receptors which modulate synaptic transmission (Table 8.1). Although there is overlap in receptor location and function, many somatic side effects, such as respiratory depression and decreased GI mobility, are mediated through mu receptors, while kappa receptors play a role in sedation and dysphoria.

The various classes of opioids have varying ratios of receptor affinities or potency which result in characteristic clinical effects as well as differing analgesic responses to two different opioid classes despite an "equianalgesic" dose.

Table 8.1 Opioid receptors and their properties

Receptor	Location	Effect
Δ (delta)	Brain (pontine nuclei, amygdala, olfactory bulb, deep cortex), peripheral sensory neurons	Slight analgesia, physical dependence, antidepressant
K (kappa)	Brain (hypothalamus, periaqueductal gray), spinal cord (substantia gelatinosa)	Analgesia, sedation, miosis, dysphoria
μ (mu)	Brain (cortex, thalamus, periaqueductal gray), spinal cord (substantia gelatinosa), peripheral sensory neurons, intestine	Respiratory depression, miosis, euphoria, decreased GI mobility, physical dependence
	μ_1: peripherally located – central interpretation of pain	
	μ_2: CNS	
	μ_3: vascular tissue, leukocytes	

Across all opioid classes, side effects include drowsiness, changes in mood (which can include paradoxical excitation), miosis, respiratory depression, decreased gastrointestinal motility, nausea, vomiting, and autonomic dysregulation. Another side effect which may be beneficial in certain patients is depression of the medullary cough center.

A recent development is the FDA requirement of a formal risk evaluation and mitigation strategy (REMS) for commercializing and selling extended-release and long-acting opioid analgesics. This often entails REMS-compliant physician education programs and the patient counseling regarding the risks, safe use, storage, and disposal of opioids. Warnings common to all opioids include:

- Abuse potential: risk factors for opioid abuse, addiction, or diversion should be considered.
- Respiratory depression: life-threatening and fatal cases may occur even with recommended use, especially at the initiation of treatment or with dose increases.
- Accidental exposure: accidental ingestion, especially by children, can be fatal.
- Appropriate prescribing: opioids should be prescribed by health-care professionals knowledgeable in the use of potent opioids for chronic pain management.

The opioids in this chapter are generally classified as Schedule II controlled substances, which is the most restrictive classification that can be legally sold. Schedule II drugs have (1) a high potential for abuse, (2) a currently accept medical use, and (3) a potential for abuse with severe psychological or physical dependence. Some combination opioids (e.g., hydrocodone-acetaminophen) are Schedule III, which meet the first two criteria above but with a risk of "moderate to low physical dependence or high psychological dependence." Schedule III drugs have slightly less restrictive rules for prescribing. Generally, unlike Schedule II drugs, Schedule III prescriptions can be faxed or phoned in to a pharmacy. Of note, some states do allow e-prescribing of Schedule II drugs.

Drug Class: Morphine (Oral)

Introduction

Morphine is the prototypic opioid, with a multitude of immediate- and extended-release formulations available. The class effects common across all opioids are discussed below.

Mechanism of Action

Although at higher doses morphine can activate the kappa and delta receptors, morphine is relatively selective for the mu receptor. Morphine undergoes first-pass hepatic metabolism and is metabolized through Phase 2 conjugative reactions by uridine diphosphate glucuronosyltransferase (UGT) enzymes. Five to fifteen percent of morphine is conjugated to morphine 6-glucuronide, which has analgesic activity and may accumulate in patients with renal failure. Excretion is largely in the urine and bile as morphine 3-glucuronide and 6-glucuronide metabolites. Peak analgesia from immediate-release morphine formulations occurs in about 60 min and can last 3–7 h.

Indications/Clinical Pearls

Morphine is indicated "for the treatment of moderate to severe pain, when a continuous around-the clock opioid analgesic is needed for an extended period of time" [3]. Long-acting formulations such as MS Contin and Kadian are "not intended for use as a prn analgesic" or for acute pain, including postoperative pain. The exception to this is if the patient is already taking chronic opioids and the postoperative pain is expected to persist for an extended period.

In addition to highly variable bioavailability, there is greater inter-patient variability in minimum effective concentration, which is influenced by age, prior exposure to opioids, and comorbidities. This means that it is difficult to predict the optimal dose for a particular patient ahead of time without titrating to analgesia versus side effects.

The half-life of morphine can be prolonged in patients with cirrhosis or hepatic dysfunction. Renal impairment can result in accumulation of the morphine 3-glucuronide and 6-glucuronide. The dosage should be decreased by up to 50 % in severe renal failure.

Morphine crosses placental membranes and is Pregnancy Category C and can be transmitted to infants via breast milk.

Dosing Options

There are numerous morphine-containing oral preparations such as:

- Morphine sulfate is available in 15 and 30 mg tablets, to be taken every 3–4 h.
- MS Contin, a long-acting formulation, is available in 15, 30, 60, 100, and 200 mg pills to be taken every 8–12 h.
- Kadian is an extended-release capsule with morphine layered in an inert polymer that release morphine slowly. It is available in 10, 20, 30, 50, 60, 80, 100, and 200 mg capsules, to be taken daily.
- Avinza is an extended-release capsule available in 30, 60, 90, and 120 mg and contains both immediate- and extended-release beads of morphine sulfate and is meant for once daily administration. The daily dose of Avinza should be limited to 1,600 mg/day as the quantity of fumaric acid contained in the preparation poses a risk of renal toxicity.

Drug Interactions

There is an increased risk of hypotension, respiratory depression, or severe sedation when morphine formulations are consumed with CNS depressants including benzodiazepines, other opioids, tricyclic antidepressants, monoamine oxidase (MAO) inhibitors, and alcohol.

In particular, patients should be cautioned about concomitant alcohol consumption with extended-release preparations, as alcohol may cause the premature release of morphine.

Mixed agonist/antagonist analgesics (e.g., nalbuphine, butorphanol) can reduce the analgesic effect and may precipitate withdrawal symptoms in patients chronically taking morphine. Cimetidine may precipitate CNS toxicity, including apnea, confusion, muscle twitching, and seizures. MAO inhibitors may potentate the action of morphine; the FDA advises that morphine not be administered concomitantly or within 14 days of MAOI treatment [3].

Side Effects/Black Box Warnings

Morphine should be used in caution with acute abdominal conditions, such as proven or suspected paralytic ileus. In addition, given the risk of sphincter of Oddi spasm, morphine should be used with caution with biliary tract disease or pancreatitis.

Caution should also be used in administering morphine to patients with head injuries or increased intracranial pressure, as the vasodilation from morphine-induced carbon dioxide retention can elevate intracranial pressure.

Given the risk of respiratory depression, morphine should be given with caution to patients having conditions resulting in hypoxia or hypercapnia or decreased respiratory reserve. This includes asthma, chronic obstructive pulmonary disease or cor pulmonale, severe obesity, sleep apnea syndrome, or CNS depression.

Extended-release preparations such as Avinza, which contain microcapsules, should not be chewed, crushed, or dissolved given a risk of a rapid release of a potentially fatal dose of morphine. In the case of parenteral abuse, the talc content can also cause tissue necrosis, pulmonary granulomas, endocarditis, and valvular injury.

Morphine-containing formulations may contain black box warnings regarding *abuse potential, respiratory depression, and accidental ingestion.* MS Contin and Kadian both contain black box warnings: "*100 and 200 mg tablets are for use in opioid-tolerant patients only...these tablet strengths may cause fatal respiratory depression when administered to patients not previously exposed to opioids.*" Avinza uniquely carries a specific black box warning that co-ingestion of alcohol can "*result in the rapid release and absorption of a potentially fatal dose of morphine*" (www.fda.gov).

Summary

Morphine is the opioid prototype, with broadly representative indications and side effects of this class of analgesics. It has immediate and extended-release preparations. Dosing should be adjusted for age and hepatic and renal dysfunction, and prescribers should be mindful of the potential for abuse, appropriate patient selection and dosage, and respiratory depression.

Drug Class: Oxymorphone

Introduction

Oxymorphone is a potent semisynthetic mu-opioid agonist. Initially designed to decrease the side effects as well as euphoria of morphine and heroin, it is an alternative opioid indicated for the treatment of moderate to severe pain.

Mechanism of Action

Oxymorphone is an agonist relatively selective for the mu-opioid receptor. It is more lipid soluble than morphine or oxycodone, resulting in rapid transfer across the blood-brain barrier. This produces a faster onset of analgesia and peak plasma concentration [4]. Oral bioavailability of oxymorphone is approximately 15–30 %. Oxymorphone is principally metabolized through Phase 2 glucuronidation and is renally excreted. Immediate-release oxymorphone has an analgesic onset of 30 min, peak analgesia at 60 min, and analgesic duration of 4–6 h. Extended-release oxymorphone (Opana ER) has a 12 h dosing interval, as the drug is released over time via a hydrophilic matrix.

Indications/Clinical Pearls

Immediate-release oxymorphone is indicated for moderate to severe acute pain, often in the setting of postsurgical pain, or as a rescue analgesic for cancer and chronic nonmalignant pain. Extended-release oxymorphone is indicated for the long-term treatment of chronic pain. Ten milligrams of oral oxymorphone is roughly equianalgesic to 30 mg of oral morphine. Given the low bioavailability of oxymorphone, the conversion ratio of parenteral to oral oxymorphone has been reported as 10:1 [4].

The half-life of oxymorphone can be prolonged in patients with cirrhosis or hepatic dysfunction, and appropriate dose reductions should be made. Oxymorphone is contraindicated in severe liver failure. Severe renal failure increase oxymorphone bioavailability by 65 %.

The elimination half-life is approximately 8 h (twice that of morphine and oxycodone) and steady state concentrations require 3 days of dosing of immediate relief oxymorphone [5]. Dose escalation should thus be undertaken judiciously.

Oxymorphone crosses placental membranes and is Pregnancy Category C. It has also been found in breast milk.

Dosing Options

- Numorphan (suppository) is available in a 5 mg dose win a polyethylene glycol base to be taken every 4–6 h.
- Opana IR (immediate-release) 5 and 10 mg PO every 4–6 h.
- Opana ER (extended-release) 5, 7.5, 10, 15, 20, 30, 40 mg every12 h.

Drug Interactions

There is an increased risk of hypotension, respiratory depression, or severe sedation when oxymorphone formulations are consumed with CNS depressants including benzodiazepines, other opioids, tricyclic antidepressants, MAO inhibitors, and alcohol.

Patients should be cautioned about concomitant alcohol consumption with extended-release preparations such as Opana ER, as alcohol consumption may also cause the premature release of oxymorphone. Mixed agonist/antagonist analgesics (e.g., nalbuphine, butorphanol) can reduce the analgesic effect and may precipitate withdrawal symptoms in patients chronically taking oxymorphone.

In addition, oxymorphone use with anticholinergics may worsen urinary retention or severe constipation. Use with cimetidine may precipitate CNS toxicity, including apnea, confusion, muscle twitching, and seizures.

Side Effects/Black Box Warning

Oxymorphone side effects include those common to all opioids: CNS depression including sedation, confusion, and mood changes; GI effects including nausea, vomiting, and decreased motility; cardiovascular changes including orthostatic hypotension and increased pulmonary vascular resistance; respiratory depression; urinary retention; or itching.

Opana IR and Numorphan do not have any black box warnings. In addition to standard black box warnings about *appropriate use, abuse potential, respiratory depression, and accidental exposure,* Opana ER has a unique black box warning that alcohol *"may result in an increase of plasma levels and potentially fatal overdose of oxymorphone"* (www.fda.gov).

Summary

Oxymorphone is a potent semisynthetic mu-opioid agonist with typical opioid side effect for the treatment of moderate to severe pain. It has immediate as well as extended-release preparations. Dosing should be adjusted for age and hepatic and renal dysfunction, and alcohol use should be avoided with extended-release preparations.

Drug Class: Hydrocodone

Introduction

Hydrocodone is the most commonly prescribed drug in the United States, with almost 125 million prescriptions. It is most often sold as a combination, such as Vicodin which combines acetaminophen with hydrocodone. The potential for abuse, as well as the dangers of acetaminophen-induced hepatotoxicity of combination products, has lead to recent deliberations by the FDA regarding possibly reclassifying hydrocodone as Schedule II, rather than the current Schedule III [6].

Mechanism of Action

Hydrocodone is a mu-opiate receptor agonist. It is a metabolite of codeine, and Phase 1 hepatic metabolism occurs by cytochrome p450 2D6 (CYP2D6), to yield hydromorphone which is also biologically active. Hydrocodone and its metabolites undergo renal excretion. It has an analgesic onset of 15–60 min and duration of 4–6 h.

Clinical Pearls/Indications

Hydrocodone is indicated for the relief of moderate to moderately severe pain. Ten to fifteen milligrams of hydrocodone is approximately equianalgesic to 10 mg of oral morphine. It should be used with caution or in reduced dosage in elderly patients or those with hepatic or renal dysfunction.

Care must be given when combination drugs include an acetaminophen component because patients who take more medication than prescribed may have a risk not only of opioid-related side effects but of acetaminophen-induced hepatotoxicity as well. The most recent FDA recommendation is no greater than 3,250 mg of acetaminophen a day, although 3,000 mg is a commonly presented maximum daily dose by acetaminophen manufacturers [7].

The fact that hydrocodone is metabolized to hydromorphone by CYP2D6 has clinical implications with respect to inter-patient variability in enzymatic activity [8]. Approximately 10 % of Caucasians, and a greater percentage of African Americans, are "poor metabolizers." However, the decreased formation of hydromorphone formulation on analgesic effectiveness is not clear [9]. Conversely, ultra-rapid metabolizers, often found in North African and Middle Eastern populations, may have a greater effect than expected.

Hydrocodone crosses placental membranes and is Pregnancy Category C; in standard postpartum dosages, the amount of hydrocodone found in breast milk has been found to be minimal and safe for the infant [10].

Dosing Options

A plethora of products exist that combine hydrocodone with various dosages and combinations of adjunctive medications. These may be acetaminophen (e.g.,

Vicodin, Lortab, and Norco) or ibuprofen (Ibudone, Vicoprofen). Below, the use of Vicodin (5/300 mg) as a prototypic drug is reviewed. Initial dosing starts at 5–10 mg of the hydrocodone component every 4–6 h.

Drug Interactions

There is an increased risk of hypotension, respiratory depression, or severe sedation when morphine formulations are consumed with CNS depressants including benzodiazepines, other opioids, tricyclic antidepressants, monoamine oxidase (MAO) inhibitors, and alcohol.

Mixed agonist/antagonist analgesics can reduce the analgesic effect and may precipitate withdrawal symptoms in patients chronically taking hydrocodone. For hydrocodone-acetaminophen combination drugs, patients should be counseled to avoid taking acetaminophen or other acetaminophen-containing products and to keep the total daily dose under 3,000 mg to minimize the risk of hepatotoxicity.

Inhibitors of CYP2D6, such as selective serotonin reuptake inhibitors (SSRIs) such as fluoxetine, may reduce the metabolism of hydrocodone to hydromorphone, an active metabolite.

Side Effects/Black Box Warnings

Warnings of side effects include those common to all opioids, such as potential for misuse, abuse, and diversion and respiratory depression. In addition, acetaminophen-containing hydrocodone products such as Norco, Lortab, Lorcet, or Vicodin have a black box warning which describes the association between acetaminophen and cases of acute liver failure. The FDA has recently reduced the amount of acetaminophen allowed in opioid preparations to 325 mg and has reduced the daily amount guidelines from 4,000 to 3,000 mg/day (www.fda.gov).

Summary

Hydrocodone, often prescribed in the Vicodin formulation, is a commonly prescribed drug for the relief of moderate to moderately severe pain. The risk of hepatotoxicity from the acetaminophen component of combination drugs deserves attention.

Drug Class: Codeine

Introduction

Codeine is an opioid analgesic available as a single-component drug. However, due to its limited analgesic potency as a single agent, it is often combined with acetaminophen (e.g., Tylenol 3), aspirin (co-codaprin), or ibuprofen (Nurofen Plus). As such, it is often prescribed as a "milder" alternative to other opioids when non-opioid analgesia is insufficient.

Mechanism of Action

Codeine is a prodrug without inherent mu-agonist activity. This means that codeine must be metabolized to have analgesic benefit. About 5–10 % is metabolized to morphine by cytochrome CYP2D6; up to 80 % of codeine is metabolized by uridine diphosphate glucuronosyltransferase (UGT2B 7) to codeine-6-glucuronide (C6G). The analgesic effect of codeine is generally thought to be from the conversion of codeine to morphine. Codeine has a 90 % bioavailability, and approximately 90 % of the total codeine dose is renally excreted, 10 % of which is unchanged. It has an analgesic onset between 15 and 30 min, peaks within 30–60 min, and lasts for 4–6 h.

Clinical Pearls/Indications

Codeine is indicated for the treatment of mild to moderately severe pain where the use of an opioid analgesic is appropriate. Ten mg of codeine is approximately equianalgesic to 1.5 to 2 mg of oral morphine.

The fact that codeine is a prodrug that must be metabolized to morphine by CYP2D6 has important clinical implications with respect to inter-patient variability in enzymatic activity. Approximately 10 % of Caucasians are poor metabolizers, with a greater frequency of metabolizers in African Americans. These individuals would experience less analgesia than expected.

Notably, the properties of C6G in humans have not been fully elucidated; C6G has been shown in animal studies to have analgesic effect comparable to codeine, leading to suggestions that even poor CYP2D metabolizers who are unable to metabolize codeine to morphine would still experience analgesic benefit from the C6G metabolite [11].

Conversely, some patients are "ultrarapid" metabolizers, due to a specific CYP2D6 phenotype often carried by patients of North African or Middle Eastern descent. Sixteen to twenty-eight percent of such patients, compared to 1–10 % in Caucasians and 0.5–1 % in East Asian and Hispanic patients, are rapid metabolizers [12]. The rapid conversion into the active metabolite morphine results in increased opioid effects and possible overdose.

A common belief exists that there is a "ceiling effect," where dosages greater than 60 mg will not provide additional analgesia because saturation of CYP2D6 limits the usual metabolism of codeine to morphine. Some have questioned this assertion, citing the analgesic properties of the main metabolite, C6G [13]. The lack of conclusive evidence notwithstanding, in practice, there are other more potent opioids available for patients with high opioid requirements.

Codeine is often used as an antitussive as its weak agonism results in fewer opioid-related side effects when used in low doses.

Codeine crosses placental membranes and is Pregnancy Category C and also has been found in breast milk. Of note, the FDA has issued a warning that infants may be at risk of opioid overdose if their nursing mothers who take codeine are ultrarapid metabolizers.

Dosages

Codeine is available in 15, 30, and 60 mg tablets, as well as in combination products with varying compositions. When used for analgesia, a usual dose is 15–60 mg every 4–6 h.

If an acetaminophen-containing preparation is used, the acetaminophen component should be limited to 3,000 mg/day. Caution should be used in patients who are elderly or with renal dysfunction.

Drug Interactions

As with all opioids, there is an increased risk of hypotension, respiratory depression, or severe sedation when codeine formulations are consummated with CNS depressants including but not limited to other opioids, benzodiazepines, barbiturates, alcohol, and SSRIs. CYP2D6 inhibitors, such SSRIs, diphenhydramine, and bupropion, can reduce or eliminate the conversion of codeine to morphine, potentially reducing its effectiveness. Other medications such as rifampicin and dexamethasone can induce CYP450 isozymes and increase the conversion to morphine, resulting in increased effect or overdose.

Side Effects/Black Box Warnings

Warnings of side effects include those common to all opioids, such as the potential for misuse and respiratory depression. In addition, acetaminophen-containing products such as Tylenol #3 have a black box warning which describes the association between acetaminophen and cases of acute liver failure. The FDA has recently reduced the amount of acetaminophen allowed in opioid preparations to 325 mg and has reduced the daily amount guidelines from 4,000 to 3,000 mg/day (www.fda.gov).

Summary

Codeine is a weak opioid agonist, often used in combination with acetaminophen or as an antitussive. There is wide inter-patient variability in response to codeine, as genetic or drug-induced alterations in CYP2D6 function may experience either inadequate analgesia or unintentional opioid overdose.

Drug Class: Tramadol

Introduction

Tramadol is a central synthetic analgesic for the treatment of moderate to moderately severe pain. It is considered to have a relatively low risk of respiratory depression and abuse potential given its weak opioid activity. However, it has unique inhibition of norepinephrine and serotonin reuptake which have important clinical implications, such as mood alteration or serotonin syndrome.

Mechanism

Tramadol is a synthetic codeine analog, with weak but selective mu-opioid agonism. For instance, tramadol has one-tenth the mu-opioid agonism of codeine. Tramadol is about 70 % bioavailable and undergoes extensive first-pass hepatic metabolism, and its metabolites undergo renal excretion. The CYP2D6 pathway results in a metabolite, O-desmethyltramadol (M1), which has 4–200 times greater mu-opioid receptor affinity than the parent compound. In addition to its properties as a weak opioid, tramadol's weak inhibition of norepinephrine and serotonin reuptake also contributes to its analgesic effect. Analgesia begins within 1 h after oral administration and peaks in 2–3 h. The plasma half-life is about 6 h.

Indications/Clinical Pearls

Tramadol is indicated for the management of moderate to moderately severe pain in adults. The analgesic potency of tramadol is fairly limited. Ten milligrams of oral tramadol is roughly equianalgesic to 1 to 2 mg of oral morphine.

Tramadol is metabolized via CYP2D6 and CYP3A4 pathways. Poor CYP2D6 metabolizers can have a 20 % elevation of tramadol plasma concentration and 40 % lower M1 concentration [14]. The full analgesic and safety implications of reduced CYP2D6 activity is not fully elucidated, but there is suggestion that poor CYP2D6 metabolizers may have less intense but prolonged analgesia, while rapid metabolizers may have greater peak analgesic effect [15].

Tramadol is Pregnancy Category C and there is very low excretion into breast milk.

Dosing

Tramadol is available as a 50 mg immediate-release tablet (Ultram), 50 mg orally dissolving tablet (Rybix ODT), and various extended-release formulations. It is commonly dosed 50–100 mg every 4–6 h. The maximum daily oral dosage recommended is 400 mg.

Dose reductions are advisable in the elderly (maximum 300 mg/day for patients >75 years old) and those with hepatic impairment (maximum 100 mg/day in cirrhotic patients). This is because both conditions can increase bioavailability. Renal impairment can result in decreased excretion of tramadol and its active metabolites. If the creatinine clearance is <30, a maximum of 200 mg/day is recommended.

CYP2D6 inhibitors such as quinidine, fluoxetine, paroxetine, amitriptyline, diphenhydramine, and bupropion as well as CYP3A4 inhibitors such as ketoconazole and erythromycin can reduce metabolic clearance of tramadol, increasing the risk of both opioid side effects as well as serotonin effects such as seizures and serotonin syndrome. Signs of serotonin syndrome include mental status changes such as agitation, hallucinations, or coma, autonomic instability, hyperthermia, hyperreflexia, or gastrointestinal symptoms (e.g., nausea, vomiting, and diarrhea).

The risk of serotonin syndrome is also increased by the use of drugs affecting the serotonergic system, including SSRIs, MAO inhibitors (which impair serotonin metabolism), triptans, linezolid, lithium, or St John's wort.

Patients taking carbamazepine may have reduced analgesic effect of tramadol and may also increase seizure risk.

Side Effects/Black Box Warnings

Warnings of side effects include those common to all opioids, such as the potential for misuse, abuse, and diversion, and respiratory depression. There are no black box warnings associated with immediate-release tramadol. As noted above, patients should be monitored for signs of serotonin syndrome in addition to signs of opioid overdose. In addition, given the psychiatric effects of serotonin and norepinephrine reuptake inhibition, tramadol is contraindicated in patients at risk of suicide.

Summary

Tramadol is a weak opioid indicated for the treatment of moderate to moderately severe pain. Prescribers should be aware of interaction with CYP2D6 inhibitors, and appreciate the risk of serotonin syndrome, especially if co-administered with serotonergic agents.

Drug Class: Methadone (Oral)

Introduction

Methadone has many unique mechanistic and pharmacokinetic properties which make it a drug with unique indications but also has challenging clinical considerations. Methadone was involved in 30 % of the 15,500 deaths in 2009 from prescription opioid overdoses even though it represented only 2 % of the total prescriptions [16].

Oral methadone can be used in the treatment of chronic pain as well as for maintenance therapy for opioid dependence, for which the long duration of effect is useful in preventing withdrawal. In many countries, including the United States, the prescription of methadone for maintenance therapy (as opposed to the treatment of pain) is subject to additional regulatory requirements and restrictions.

Mechanism of Action

Methadone primarily binds to the mu-opioid receptor but also has activity at the kappa and delta opioid receptors. A unique feature of methadone is its inhibition of serotonin and norepinephrine reuptake, similar to tricyclic antidepressants. It also antagonizes N-methyl-D-aspartate receptors (NMDA) which helps prevent sensitization and promotes its effectiveness in opioid-tolerant patients.

The bioavailability of oral methadone is about 80 %. Its lipophilicity results in rapid distribution to organs and tissues, including the adipose, brain, kidney, liver, and muscle, which serve as tissue reservoirs. It has an analgesic onset of 30–60 min, peaks in 1–7.5 h, and has a biologic duration of 22–48 h with repeat dosing. The effective analgesic duration is shorter, often on the order of 4–12 h.

Indications/Clinical Pearls

Given that methadone has dose-dependent QT-prolonging effects, patients should be evaluated and advised regarding arrhythmia risks, and an EKG should be obtained prior to initiation of treatment. Periodic monitoring of QTc is indicated if there are risk factors for QTc prolongation or if methadone dosage exceeds 100 mg a day. A QTc interval between 450 and 500 ms should prompt careful examination of the risk/benefit ratio of therapy. A QTc exceeding 500 ms increases the risk of cardiac death 4-fold, and contraindicates further use of methadone [17].

The steady state plasma concentration can take 3 (and up to 10) days to achieve so titration should proceed slowly and patients monitored carefully after dose adjustments.

Dosing Options

Oral methadone is available in 5 mg, 10 mg, 40 mg, 5 mg/5 ml, 10 mg/5 ml, and 10 mg/ml solutions. The 40 mg tab is not approved for pain management and is restricted to authorized and DEA-registered opioid addiction detoxification and maintenance facilities and hospitals. When prescribed for analgesia, it is generally dosed every 8 h, starting with a very low dose and slow titration. In an outpatient setting, dosing increases should be made no more frequently than every 7 days, with appreciation of the fact that accumulation may occur. Since there is wide variation in half-lives among patients, peak respiratory depressant effects can be delayed [9].

Published morphine to methadone conversion ratios range from 4:1 to 12:1 [18]. A systematic review found a median ratio of 8.25:1 [19]. The conversion from morphine equivalent to methadone is generally considered nonlinear. This means that a larger morphine to methadone ratio (i.e., proportionately less methadone) should be used when converting from large morphine dosages.

Drug Interactions

As with all opioids, there is an increased risk of hypotension, respiratory depression, or severe sedation when methadone formulations are taken along with CNS depressants or other opioids.

Mixed agonist/antagonist analgesics can reduce the analgesic effect and may precipitate withdrawal symptoms in patients chronically taking methadone.

Methadone undergoes hepatic metabolism, largely by the CYP3A4 system. Substances such as protease inhibitors, ketoconazole, erythromycin, or grapefruit juice which inhibit CYP3A4 activity can increase the effect of methadone. Conversely, drugs such as carbamazepine, rifampicin, phenytoin, glucocorticoids, and St. John's wort can decrease the effect of methadone.

Medications which alkalinize urine (such as carbonic anhydrase inhibitors) can decrease clearance and thus increase the half-life of methadone to 42 h.

Methadone is classified as Pregnancy Category C. Although methadone can be transmitted to infants via breast milk, many studies have shown the safety of breast-feeding by women on methadone maintenance [20].

Side Effects/Black Box Warnings

The black box warning for methadone contains, like other opioids, reference to the potential for abuse of this medication. It also includes a strong warning against respiratory depression and the need for vigilant conversion, treatment initiation, and dose titration. This is particularly important in early stages of dosing, given that the peak respiratory effect of methadone occurs much later than its analgesic effects and considerably longer than typical analgesic preparations. Uniquely, methadone's black box warning states that it should be administered with the treatment standards cited in 42 CFR Section 8, including limitations on unsupervised administration. In addition, there is a warning that methadone can prolong the QT interval (www.fda.gov).

Methadone can cause serious and potential lethal arrhythmias (torsades de pointes) and most cases involve patients being treated for pain with large, multiple daily doses of the agent. Cases have also been reported in patients receiving doses commonly used for maintenance treatment of opioid addiction, and a baseline electrocardiogram should be obtained by the clinician to risk-stratify the patient. Patients with a baseline QTc interval greater than 450 to 480 milliseconds may be considered to be at increased risk.

Summary

Methadone is a very long-acting opioid used for both chronic pain and maintenance therapy that has agonist activity at opioid receptors and antagonist activity at NMDA receptors. Prescribers must appreciate its unique effects, including QT prolongation and a long half-life.

Perioperative Implications of Chronic Opioid Use

The management of patients with chronic opioid consumption presents many challenges in providing optimal analgesia in the perioperative period. Patients may require increased opioid secondary to the development of tolerance as well as opioid-induced hyperalgesia. Such patients would benefit from multimodal analgesia regimens, including adjunctive medications such as gabapentin, acetaminophen, intravenous lidocaine, ketamine, ketorolac, and neuraxial or regional nerve blockade, as appropriate. The utilization of patient-controlled analgesia (PCA) for postoperative pain may allow for effective dose titration, at least until the patient's postoperative opioid requirement is established.

Patients should be monitored for signs of opioid withdrawal, including anxiety or agitation, nausea, vomiting, or diaphoresis. Patients should also be instructed to continue their baseline opioids through the day of surgery. Their usual home regimen, or equivalent, should be administered intraoperatively in addition to what would be given for surgical analgesia.

Patients on chronic methadone should be monitored closely for signs of QTc prolongation, and a preoperative EKG should be obtained as appropriate. Many medications commonly administered intraoperatively can cause further QT prolongation, including ondansetron, dobutamine, dopamine, and clindamycin. Hypokalemia, hypomagnesemia, and hypocalcemia should be avoided, as these can exacerbate QT prolongation.

Patients using agonist-antagonists such as buprenorphine present additional challenges. Buprenorphine has partial mu-opioid agonist activity and is an antagonist of kappa-opioid receptors. The strong affinity of buprenorphine can block the binding of an opioid with stronger agonist activity at the mu receptor. Medications such as Suboxone which additionally contain naloxone may further impair effective analgesia.

There is no absolute guideline for whether buprenorphine should be discontinued preoperatively. While buprenorphine may facilitate analgesia intra- and postoperatively, patients who are relying on the drug for maintenance treatment of opioid dependence may be reluctant to discontinue its use out of concern for relapse. Intraoperatively, patients on buprenorphine may require higher doses of opioids to achieve analgesia, and multimodal analgesia should be provided. An opioid with a high binding affinity such as sufentanil has been suggested as an option for improved analgesia [21]. Postoperative approaches include continuing or increasing the buprenorphine dose for its analgesic effect (although there may be ceiling effect), converting buprenorphine to methadone and adding an additional opioid analgesic for breakthrough pain, or replacing the buprenorphine with another opioid [22]. If buprenorphine is discontinued, the patient will require re-induction with buprenorphine at a later time. Perioperative consultation with the prescribing physician and/or an addictionologist is advised for patients who are buprenorphine for maintenance of opioid addiction.

Chemical Structures

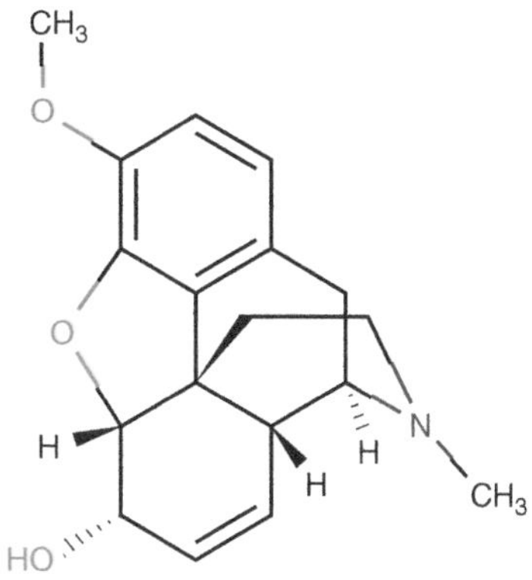

**Chemical Structure
8.1** Codeine

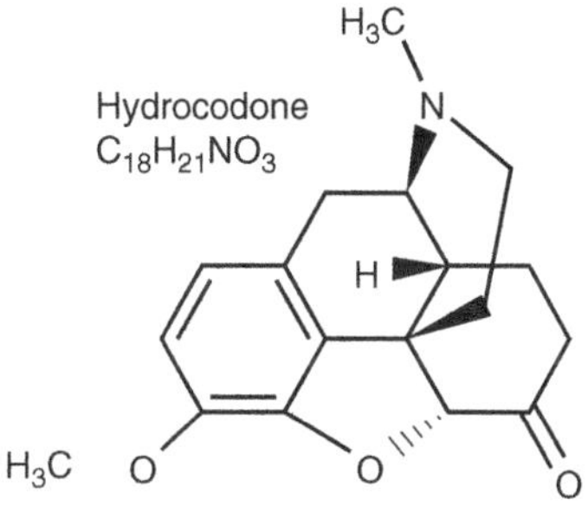

Hydrocodone
$C_{18}H_{21}NO_3$

**Chemical Structure
8.2** Hydrocodone

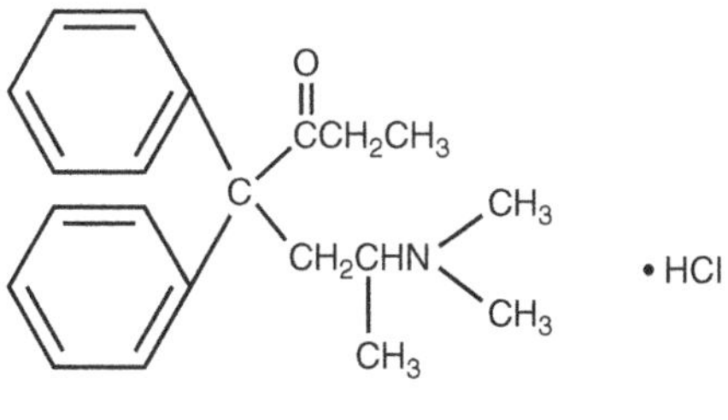

**Chemical Structure
8.3** Methadone
hydrochloride

Chemical Structure
8.4 Morphine sulfate

$\bullet\, H_2SO_4 \,\bullet\, 5H_2O$

Chemical Structure
8.5 Tramadol hydrochloride

$\bullet\, HCl$

References

1. The use of medicine in the United States: review of 2010. Parsippany: IMS Institute for Healthcare Informatics; 2011. http://www.imshealth.com/deployedfiles/imshealth/Global/Content/IMS%20Institute/Static%20File/IHII_UseOfMed_report.pdf. Accessed 6 Aug 2014.
2. Centers for Disease Control and Prevention. Vital signs: overdoses of prescription opioid pain relievers. Morb Mortal Wkly Rep. 2011;60(43):1487–92.
3. Morphine sulfate [package insert]. Columbus: Roxane Laboratories, Inc; 2012.
4. Sloan P. Review of oral oxymorphone in the management of pain. Ther Clin Risk Manag. 2008;4(4):777–87.
5. Adams MP, Ahdieh H. Single- and multiple-dose pharmacokinetic and dose-proportionality study of oxymorphone immediate-release tablets. Drugs RD. 2005;6:91–9.
6. Kuehn B. FDA Committee: more restrictions needed on hydrocodone combination products. JAMA. 2013;309(9):862.
7. Krenzelok EP, Royal MA. Confusion: acetaminophen dosing changes based on NO evidence in adults. Drugs RD. 2012;12(2):45–8.
8. Armstrong SC, Cozza KL. Pharmacokinetic drug interactions of morphine, codeine, and their derivatives: theory and clinical reality, Part II. Psychosomatics. 2003;44:515–20.
9. The Management of Opioid Therapy for Chronic Pain Working Group. VA/DoD clinical practice guideline for management of opioid therapy for chronic pain: guideline summary. [Internet]. Washington, DC: Department of Veterans Affairs; 2010 cited 3 March 2013. Available from: http://www.healthquality.va.gov/cot/cot_310_sum.pdf.
10. Sauberan JB, Anderson PO, Lane JR, Rafie S, Nguyen N, Rossi SS, Stellwagen LM. Breast milk hydrocodone and hydromorphone levels in mothers using hydrocodone for postpartum pain. Obstet Gynecol. 2011;117(3):611–7.
11. Srinivasan V, Wielbo D, Tebbett IR. Analgesic effects of codeine-6-glucuronide after intravenous administration. Eur J Pain. 1997;1(3):185–90.

12. Tylenol with codeine [package insert]. Titusville: Janssen Pharmaceuticals, Inc. 2012.
13. Vree TB, van Dongen RT, Koopman-Kimenai PM. Codeine analgesia is due to codeine-6-glucuronide, not morphine. Int J Clin Pract. 2000;54(6):395–8.
14. Ultram [package insert]. Raritan: Pricara; 2009.
15. Poulsen L, Arendt-Nielsen L, Brosen K, et al. The hypoalgesic effect of tramadol in relation to CYP2D6. Clin Pharmacol Ther. 1996;60:636–44.
16. Center for Disease Control and Prevention. Prescription Painkiller Overdoses [Internet]. Georgia: Center for Disease Control and Prevention; c2012 updated 3 July 2002; cited 20 March 2013. Office of the Associate Director for Communications; about 2 screens. Available http://www.cdc.gov/vitalsigns/MethadoneOverdoses/.
17. Christie J. Opioid prescribing: methadone risk mitigation [Internet]. Delaware; 2011 [cited 23 March 2013]. Available from: http://www.apsf.org/newsletters/html/2011/spring/01_opioid.htm.
18. Mercadante S. Conversion ratios for opioid switching in the treatment of cancer pain: a systematic review. Palliat Med. 2011;25(5):504–15.
19. Weschules D, Bain K. A systematic review of opioid conversion ratios used with methadone for the treatment of pain. Pain Med. 2008;9:595–612.
20. Jansson LM, Choo RE, Harrow C, Velez M, Schroeder JR, Lowe R, Huestis MA. Concentrations of methadone in breast milk and plasma in the immediate perinatal period. J Hum Lact. 2007;23(2):184–90.
21. Scholz J, Steinfath M, Schulz M. Clinical pharmacokinetics of alfentanil, fentanyl and sufentanil. An update. Clin Pharmacokinet. 1996;31(4):275–92.
22. Bryson EO, Lipson S, Gevirtz C. Anaesthesia for patients on buprenorphine. Anesthesiol Clin. 2010;28(4):611–7.

Chapter 9
Nonopioid Analgesic and Adjunct Drugs

Mary Bekhit, Kaveh Navab, Andrew Ghobrial, and Tod Aust

Contents

M. Bekhit, MD (✉)
Department of Anesthesiology, Ronald Reagan UCLA Medical Center,
Los Angeles, CA, USA
e-mail: mbekhit@mednet.ucla.edu

K. Navab, MD • A. Ghobrial, MD • T. Aust, MD
Department of Anesthesiology, David Geffen School of Medicine at UCLA,
Los Angeles, CA, USA

A.D. Kaye et al. (eds.), *Essentials of Pharmacology for Anesthesia,*
Pain Medicine, and Critical Care, DOI 10.1007/978-1-4614-8948-1_9,
© Springer Science+Business Media New York 2015

General Introduction

Nonopioid analgesics play an integral role in multimodal perioperative management of acute surgical pain. Multimodal analgesia involves the use of several different classes of drugs, each in smaller doses, to achieve better pain control than that achieved with the use of any one agent alone. This approach to perioperative pain control aims to reduce narcotic requirements, optimize early return to function, and improve the quality of patients' perioperative experience by maximizing analgesia while minimizing side effects. Some of the more commonly studied nonopioid analgesics include nonsteroidal anti-inflammatory drugs (NSAIDs), steroids, magnesium, alpha-2 agonists, dexmedetomidine, acetaminophen (IV and PO), and NMDA receptor antagonists. The following sections further elaborate some of the clinical literature supporting the benefit these agents offer as adjuncts to narcotics within a multimodal approach to perioperative pain control.

NSAIDs

Drug Class and Mechanism of Action

These pharmacologic agents employ a mechanism of anti-inflammation unique from steroids and opiates, and thus a different profile of adverse drug reactions (ADRs), so are a useful alternative or supplemental treatment. Using multimodal analgesic therapy, these drugs can be employed in concert with corticosteroid anti-inflammatory medications, thus reducing the cumulative effect of ADRs that would result from administering high doses of any one class.

The analgesic mechanisms of action for NSAIDs apply both centrally and peripherally [1]. Inhibition of prostaglandin synthesis has been the most long-standing established mechanism of their action. However, with the understanding that two distinct forms of cyclooxygenase exist (COX-1) and (COX-2), the role of NSAIDs has become further elucidated and their formulations more site specific [2]. COX-1 is a constitutive enzyme present in noninflammatory cells, whereas COX-2 is induced in inflammatory cells, upregulated by cytokines and growth factors. COX-2 is understood to work centrally, mediating hyperalgesia and allodynia [3]. NSAID-mediated analgesia in particular is presumably gained by the inhibition of COX-2, while the ratio of COX-1 to COX-2 inhibition accounts for the variability in ADRs associated with preferentially inhibiting one or the other. A considerable benefit of selective COX-2 inhibitors (e.g., celecoxib) over nonselective COX inhibitors (e.g., aspirin, ibuprofen, naproxen, Toradol) is low-to-absent risk of gastric perforation and bleeding associated with the former. The mechanism of this complication of nonselective COX inhibitors is embarrassment of prostaglandin synthesis in the gastric mucosa. COX-1 inhibition also interrupts platelet aggregation, furthering hemostatic instability. However, the ADRs of selective COX-2 inhibitors may be even more catastrophic, including significantly increased risk of cerebrovascular accidents (CVA) and myocardial infarction (MI) (Bing). COX-2 inhibition favors thrombotic events (CVA, MI) by increasing the production of thromboxane, a pro-thrombotic eicosanoid [4].

Indications/Clinical Pearls

Both classes of COX inhibitors have proven useful in multimodal perioperative analgesia. Used with caution and acknowledgment of their side effects, their administration can help control pain while reducing the reliance on opiates, minimizing their ADRs. NSAIDs have earned considerable standing in perioperative analgesia for dental procedures in particular [3], shown to be even superior to opiate analgesia.

Toradol (ketorolac) is a nonselective NSAID commonly utilized in the perioperative setting. De Oliveira et al. conducted a meta-analysis of 13 randomized trials, comprising 782 patients [5]. They determined that single-dose Toradol effectively improved pain control at the 2 h – but not the 24 h – mark, decreasing total opioid requirement and consequent nausea and vomiting. These benefits were only found at the 60 mg dose, not the 30 mg dose, and IM administration had greater opioid-sparing effects, as compared with IV administration.

Selective COX-2 inhibitors have enjoyed an increasing role in reducing perioperative opioid requirements in a wide variety of surgeries, including orthopedic [6], gynecologic [3], and general intra-abdominal surgery [7]. Despite their prothrombotic risk, their lack of a tendency to promote postop bleeding gives them a certain appeal. Lin et al. identified eight studies, comprising a total of 571 patients, in a systematic review and meta-analysis of selective COX-2 inhibitors in the perioperative setting of total knee arthroplasty (TKA) [6]. They found statistically significant outcome improvements including augmentation of pain control and active range of motion, as well as diminution of opioid consumption and its anticipated side effects of pruritus, nausea, and emesis. Viscusi et al. conducted their own trial of the COX-2 inhibitor etoricoxib, in the setting of total abdominal hysterectomy, and reported similarly encouraging results, in addition to more rapid bowel recovery than in the placebo group. Viscusi et al. demonstrated that both 90 and 120 mg of oral etoricoxib were equally effective at reducing perioperative opioid requirements and improving analgesia.

Sinatra et al. investigated the utility of oral rofecoxib, 25 and 50 mg, in the setting of lower abdominal surgery, with outcomes focused on effort-dependent pain and pulmonary function [7]. They found that in a dose-dependent fashion, rofecoxib tempered opiate requirements and led to improved pulmonary function and improved overall pain control. Sinatra et al. on the other hand found that there was a dose-dependent effect of rofecoxib on postop pain control and reduced opioid requirements, where 50 mg was superior to 25 mg. Whether this is a function of the drug itself, the type of surgery, or the study design is difficult to ascertain.

The only cyclooxygenase-2 selective nonsteroidal anti-inflammatory drug currently approved by the FDA is celecoxib. Merck voluntarily withdrew rofecoxib from the market because of concerns about increased risk of heart attack and stroke associated with long-term, high-dosage use. Etoricoxib is currently approved in more than 70 other countries worldwide – but not in the United States.

Dosing Options

Toradol's optimum dosing schedule has yet to be defined. A one-time perioperative 60 mg IM dose is implicitly recommended by the results of De Oliveira's meta-analysis, to effectively decrease opiate requirements. However, postoperative bleeding complications remains a concern as with all nonselective COX inhibitors, and a discussion of risks and benefits with the surgical team is advisable. Long-term oral use is strictly prohibited due to potential side effects associated with use over 5 days.

FDA black box warnings include the following:

There are four specific black box warnings involving Toradol ORAL (ketorolac tromethamine), a nonsteroidal anti-inflammatory drug (NSAID) (www.fda.gov):

- Indicated for short-term (up to 5 days in adults) management.
- Not indicated for the pediatric population.
- Not indicated for minor or chronic painful conditions.
- In adults increasing the dose beyond the maximum daily amount of 40 mg does not improve pain management but does increase the risk that serious adverse events will develop.

Drug Interactions

NSAIDs are relatively contraindicated in patients on anticoagulation (due to high risk of bleeding), as well as methotrexate (risk of bone marrow toxicity, renal failure, hepatic dysfunction). Lithium toxicity is a concern if coprescribed. Phenytoin and oral hypoglycemics should preclude the use of pyrazoles and salicylates. Naproxen should replace high-dose aspirin if prescribed with sodium valproate [8].

Side Effects/Black Box Warnings

Renal disease, papillary necrosis, and interstitial nephritis are complications of both categories of NSAIDs (Bing). Dilation of the afferent arteriole of the glomerulus requires prostaglandin, whereas NSAIDs effectively curtail this action and can lead to parenchymal hypoperfusion. Black box warnings are included on the COX-2 inhibitor Celebrex and nonselective COX inhibitor meloxicam for risk of thrombotic events and GI bleeding.

Steroids

Drug Class and Mechanism of Action

Glucocorticoids are a powerful group of drugs with numerous systemic effects, used therapeutically for many indications. Their role ranges from facilitating the autonomic sympathetic response to anti-inflammatory action and reducing postoperative nausea and vomiting (PONV). All of these properties of glucocorticoids are utilized in the perioperative setting. Their effects are systemic and profound, owing to the expression of glucocorticoid receptors on essentially all cells and the central role of the hypothalamic-pituitary-adrenal (HPA) axis in normal physiology [9]. Glucocorticoids, including the endogenous cortisol, act on cells in three ways. Two are so-called genomic, including non-DNA-dependent regulation of protein activity and even repression or activation of actual gene expression at the nucleic acid level through glucocorticoid-responsive DNA sequences. The third non-genomic pathway is glucocorticoid signaling through membrane-associated receptors and second messengers.

Indications and Clinical Pearls

Glucocorticoids are intimately associated with the pain and inflammation pathways in the body. Activation of peripheral pain receptors by inflammatory mediators leads to central nociceptive inputs and ultimately to HPA activation to quell the inflammatory response. Molecular mechanisms of glucocorticoid-associated analgesia include reduced release of neuropeptides, inhibition of nociceptive c-fibers and ectopic discharge from traumatized nerves, improved nerve recovery and regeneration, and a rapid inhibitory effect on voltage-dependent Ca channels in dorsal root ganglion neurons [10]. The modulation of the inflammatory and pain pathways by endogenous glucocorticoids can be augmented by exogenous varieties as well. Commonly employed glucocorticoids in the perioperative setting include dexamethasone and methylprednisolone.

The perioperative use of dexamethasone analgesia was thoroughly investigated by Waldron et al., who conducted a systematic review and meta-analysis [11] in 2013. They determined that a single IV dose of perioperative dexamethasone had small, but statistically significant, analgesic benefits. Their endpoints were pain scores and opioid requirements at 2 and 24 h, as well as length of PACU stays, all of which were reduced. However, the clinical utility of this effect is questionable, and endpoints such as reduced opioid side effects and accelerated time to bowel recovery were not evaluated. While postoperative glucose levels were increased in dexamethasone-treated patients compared to placebo-treated patients, wound healing time and incidence of infectious complications were not increased.

Other studies have also shown underwhelming effects of dexamethasone on perioperative analgesia. Tolver and colleagues examined its utility in laparoscopic inguinal hernia repair and only found that it improved PONV, not pain or discomfort [12].

Lunn et al. conducted trials evaluating the use of methylprednisolone (MP) in both total hip arthroplasty and total knee arthroplasty [13, 14]. They found that for THA, analgesia was improved in the first 24 h, but that time to functional discharge criteria was not decreased. Their study of MP administration before TKA revealed improved analgesia during walking, along with decreased serum CRP levels, although clinical evidence of inflammation, i.e., knee swelling, was unchanged between treatment and placebo groups.

Interestingly, Bauer et al. found that while ibuprofen vs. placebo showed no difference in postop pain scores s/p molar surgery, ibuprofen in conjunction with dexamethasone did show statistically significant improvement in postop pain. Unfortunately, this study did not include a dexamethasone-only branch, so the role of synergy vs. a simple cumulative effect cannot be ascertained [15].

Dosing Options

Effective doses of dexamethasone IV range from 4 to 10 mg, although higher doses on the order of 15 mg may be superior in reducing postoperative opioid requirements [16]. Methylprednisolone dosing ranges from 100 to 150 mg IV. 0.75 mg dexamethasone is equivalent to 4 mg methylprednisolone and 5 mg prednisolone.

Drug Interactions

One significant drug interaction to consider is that rifampicin treatment can reduce the efficacy of glucocorticoid therapy, so increasing the dosage of steroids may be indicated in this population to achieve comparable results [17].

Side Effects

Glucocorticoids play a role in the physiologic balance of inflammation and anti-inflammation, which can be deranged by diseases and iatrogenic processes. The extreme of HPA hyperactivity in Cushing's syndrome can lead to excessive anti-inflammation, i.e., immunosuppression and susceptibility to infection, whereas HPA quiescence in chronic corticosteroid therapy or Addison's disease, for example, leads to excessive inflammation and cytokine toxicity, requiring supplemental glucocorticoid administration [9]. While chronic steroid therapy can lead to such consequences, there is no strong evidence that single-dose perioperative glucocorticoid therapy has a negative impact on wound healing [15], immunocompetence, or long-term glucose control [14].

Magnesium

Introduction

Magnesium plays an important role in many enzymatic reactions including DNA and protein synthesis, energy metabolism, glycolysis, fatty acid breakdown and synthesis, as well as the regulation of calcium, potassium, and membrane excitability. Magnesium also affects the release of neurotransmitters and works to stabilize axonal membranes. In addition to its role in treating cardiac dysrhythmias, in the regimen against cerebral vasospasm, post-subarachnoid hemorrhage, preterm labor, and preeclampsia, magnesium has the potential to be used as an analgesic.

Mechanism of Action

The mechanism by which magnesium can function as an analgesic is thought to be secondary to its ability to block NMDA receptors and possibly its antagonistic effects on calcium release.

Indications and Dosing

A meta-analysis of 25 trials comparing magnesium to placebo revealed that magnesium infusions significantly decreased the amount of morphine required and overall pain scores in the first 24 h postoperatively [18]. In the analysis, the different studies used between 1.03 and 23.5 g total dose in the 24 h period. Despite this large range, there was no correlation between total magnesium dose and total morphine dose. The total dose of morphine required was decreased by 24 % regardless of the method of magnesium administration (bolus vs. infusion vs. bolus with infusion). Bradycardia was more common in the magnesium group, but hypotension was not. Given the lack of correlation between total dose and amount of morphine required and given the ease of administration, the authors suggest that a bolus dose may be the most reasonable approach. Bolus doses of 40–50 mg/kg were used in the various studies.

In a blinded randomized control trial, epidural magnesium added to a local anesthetic and opioid patient-controlled epidural infusion for 48 h did not lead to decreased incidence of chronic postoperative pain after VATS [19]. Magnesium infiltration in robotic-assisted laparoscopic prostatectomies led to decreased doses of remifentanil infusions required intraoperatively and also led to increased time to the first postoperative analgesic requirement [20]. The same investigators failed to find a benefit with an intravenous magnesium bolus and infusion in patients undergoing thyroidectomies under a remifentanil infusion [21]. Intravenous magnesium bolus and infusion intraoperatively (50 mg/kg over 15 min followed by 15 mg/kg/h) during spinal anesthesia for a total hip replacement led to decreased PCA requirements with an increase in serum magnesium concentrations without an increase in the adverse effects associated with hypermagnesemia [22]. In a study out of Cairo University, magnesium intrathecally (50 mg) and epidurally (100 mg/h) prolonged the anesthesia associated with a spinal anesthetic technique for lower-extremity surgery and decreased analgesic requirements in the postoperative period [23]. Epidural fentanyl plus magnesium compared to epidural fentanyl alone leads to decreased total fentanyl consumption in a 24 h period after hip surgery in patients using patient-controlled epidural analgesia [24].

In a study out of Turkey in a gynecologic population, the use of intravenous magnesium decreased the total propofol and atracurium required during the case and the amount of morphine required in the postoperative period. Furthermore, they showed that this was accomplished with a 40 mg/kg bolus upon induction and a

10 mg/kg/h infusion with no added benefit when a 20 mg/kg/h infusion was used. In fact, more hemodynamic side effects were seen [25]. Magnesium may have a role in the treatment of chronic pain as well. Patients with chronic low back pain benefited from a 2-week intravenous infusion of magnesium followed by 4 weeks of oral magnesium when added to a regimen of analgesics and physical therapy leading to decreased pain scores and increased range of motion [26].

Side Effects

Caution must be used especially in those with already high serum magnesium concentrations and those with impaired renal function. Hypermagnesemia greater than 2.5 mg/dL can lead to neuromuscular blockade and skeletal muscle weakness due to its antagonistic effect on the release of acetylcholine. Other symptoms of hypermagnesemia include lethargy, flushing, nausea, and vomiting, and at high concentrations (>7), one can also see hypotension and ECG changes leading to complete heart block and finally cardiac arrest.

Summary

In summary, it appears that magnesium whether given intravenously, intrathecally, epidurally, or through skin infiltration can be a safe and effective adjunct to pain control chronically, intraoperatively, and postoperatively.

Alpha-2 Agonists

Introduction

Clonidine and dexmedetomidine (Precedex) have been used as adjuncts to analgesia in the perioperative period.

Mechanism of Action

The mechanism of action is alpha-2 agonism leading to decreased release of norepinephrine in the locus coeruleus, substantia gelatinosa, and peripherally. Clonidine and dexmedetomidine also bind to alpha-1 receptors, but the alpha-2/alpha-1 binding affinity ratios for both are 220:1 and 1,620:1, respectively.

Indications

A meta-analysis showed that both clonidine and dexmedetomidine decreased opioid consumption in the perioperative period by 4.1 mg and 14.5 mg of morphine, respectively [27]. Furthermore, both decreased the incidence of early nausea. Clonidine did lead to more cases of hypotension, whereas dexmedetomidine led to more incidences of postoperative bradycardia. Recovery time was not increased in these patients. In children, premedication with oral clonidine at doses of 2 or 4 µg/kg led to improved sedation, mask acceptance, and postoperative analgesia when compared to oral midazolam [28]. Dexmedetomidine given intravenously (0.5 µg/kg) in patients undergoing carpal tunnel release under IVRA had improved analgesia and sedation intra- and postoperatively. This held true also when dexmedetomidine was added to the lidocaine solution used for the bier block [29]. In patients undergoing colorectal surgery, epidural clonidine given prior to surgery and then added to a local anesthetic and opioid PCEA led to decreased total opioid requirement postoperatively, faster return of bowel function, and decreased levels of inflammatory cytokines measured at 12 and 24 h after surgery [30]. A study in rat pups with intrathecal clonidine showed no damage at the cellular level of the spinal cord even when used at supra-analgesic doses [31]. In 6–8-year-old children undergoing orthopedic surgery, both intrathecal and intravenous clonidine (1 µg/kg) administered in addition to intrathecal bupivacaine led to decreased propofol required for intraoperative sedation, improved pain scores, higher sedation scores postoperatively, and increased time to first rescue analgesia without a change in adverse events. Motor and sensory blocks were prolonged with intrathecal clonidine [32]. In patients undergoing breast surgery for breast cancer, dexmedetomidine infusion intraoperatively not only had MAC and opioid-sparing effects perioperatively but also led to decreased incidence of chronic pain and better quality of life when assessed 3 months postsurgery [33].

Dosing

Clonidine is administered as a premedication orally in a dose of 5 µg/kg, as a transdermal patch (0.2 mg/24 h), intrathecally (15–45 µg), as part of a peripheral nerve block (0.5–1 µg/kg), or intra-articularly. Dexmedetomidine is usually given as an infusion (0.2–0.7 µg/kg/h) with or without a loading dose given over 10 min (1 µg/kg). It can also be given intranasally (1 µg/kg) or orally (3–4 µg/kg) especially in the pediatric population as a premedication.

Side Effects

Dexmedetomidine infusion, when compared to placebo or morphine, triples gastric emptying time and gastrointestinal transit in healthy volunteers [34]. The renal effects of dexmedetomidine were evaluated in a study of CABG patients, which found that markers of renal function were unchanged although urinary output did increase in the first 4 h after urinary catheter insertion [35].

Summary

In summary, alpha-2 agonists can be useful as safe adjuncts to multiple modes of anesthesia with benefits in both analgesia and sedation without significant adverse consequences although caution may be warranted in those patients who bradycardia and hypotension could have more significant impact on outcomes.

Acetaminophen

Introduction

Acetaminophen (Tylenol, APAP, paracetamol) is one of the most widely used analgesics. It is available in oral, rectal suppository and as an IV formulation. It is a common coanalgesic agent found in many frequently prescribed combination products. It is an effective pain reliever and antipyretic.

Drug Class and Mechanism of Action

Acetaminophen belongs to a class of drugs called the nonacidic antipyretic analgesics. The mechanism for analgesia is not completely understood, but it is believed to work through the inhibition of COX enzymes (similar to NSAIDs) with a preference for COX-2 over COX-1. These enzymes are responsible for catalyzing the production of prostaglandins from arachidonic acid. Circulating prostaglandins make nociceptors more sensitive to noxious stimuli resulting in increased pain. The inhibition of these enzymes by acetaminophen results in decreased prostaglandin synthesis and thus less sensitive nociceptors, increasing the pain threshold. Compared to NSAIDs, acetaminophen has little to no anti-inflammatory or antiplatelet effects [36].

Indications/Clinical Pearls

The FDA has approved acetaminophen for use in adults and children in the oral or IV form for the reduction of fever and the treatment of mild to moderate pain. It has also approved the IV form as an adjunct in the treatment of moderate to severe pain. Common off-label use includes acetaminophen for the treatment of osteoarthritis and as prophylaxis for potential adverse reactions to vaccines or infusions. Acetaminophen is also used as part of a multimodal analgesic approach in order to improve pain relief while minimizing side effects [37, 38]. Acetaminophen has been used in combination with NSAIDs in order to provide better pain relief than what is achieved with either drug alone [39, 40].

Dosing Options

For adults and children aged 13 and older with fever and/or mild to moderate pain: oral immediate release 650–1,000 mg orally every 4–6 h as needed with a maximum dose of 4,000 mg in 24 h, or oral extended-release 1,300 mg orally every 8 h as needed with a maximum dose of 3,900 mg in 24 h, or rectal, 650 mg per rectum every 4–6 h as needed with a maximum of six suppositories per day, or IV 650–1,000 mg IV every 4–6 h as needed with a maximum daily dose of 4,000 mg. If the patient is less than 50 kg, 12.5 every 4 h or 15 mg/kg IV every 6 h with a maximum daily dose of 75 mg/kg. The IV dose can also be given as an adjunct for moderate to severe pain. For infants and children, the oral dose is 10–15 mg orally every 4–6 h with a maximum of 75 mg/kg/day for infants and either 100 mg/kg/day or 4,000 mg/day, whichever is less, for children. The rectal dose is 10–20 mg/kg per rectum every 4–6 h as needed with a maximum of 75 mg/kg/day for infants and either 100 mg/kg/day or 4,000 mg/day, whichever is less, for children. The IV dose for children aged 2–12 is 12.5 mg every 4 h or 15 mg every 6 h with a maximum single dose of 15 mg/kg and a maximum daily dose of 75 mg/kg/day. The effect of IV acetaminophen has not been studied in children less than 2 years old.

Drug Interactions

Acetaminophen should be used cautiously with any drug which has an adverse effect on the liver. Special consideration should be taken with the combined use of acetaminophen with either methotrexate (MTX), propylthiouracil (PTU), or isoniazid (INH). The use of acetaminophen along with isoniazid may increase the potential for hepatotoxicity and, possibly, nephrotoxicity due to isoniazid's ability to induce cytochrome P450, resulting in a greater proportion of acetaminophen being converted to its toxic metabolite. It is important to remember that many combination analgesia preparations contain acetaminophen, so great care should be taken that the total amount of acetaminophen from all sources does not exceed the daily maximum recommended dose in order to avoid hepatic injury.

Side Effects/Black Box Warnings

Acetaminophen is hepatotoxic in doses exceeding the daily maximum. An overdose of acetaminophen can lead to acute liver failure or death. Liver dysfunction, hypovolemia, malnutrition, renal dysfunction, and chronic alcohol abuse can increase the risk of hepatotoxicity, and dose reductions should be considered.

Summary

When dosed appropriately, acetaminophen is a safe and extremely useful analgesic drug to be used alone or in combination with other drugs as part of a multimodal analgesic approach.

NMDA Receptor Antagonists

Introduction

Ketamine, in addition to being an effective agent for anesthesia and sedation, has an important place in both acute and chronic pain control. Ketamine has been in clinical use since 1970 and is still widely used in both the inpatient and outpatient setting. Ketamine provides effective analgesia as a single agent and is also highly effective as part of a multimodal analgesia approach [37].

Drug Class and Mechanism of Action

Ketamine belongs to a class of drugs called NMDA receptor antagonists. NMDA (N-methyl-D-aspartate) receptors are nonspecific cation channels that are highly permeable to calcium which play a critical role in learning and memory. Blockade of the NMDA receptors is also effective for anesthesia and sedation and has an important role in the management of both acute and chronic pain. Other NMDA receptor antagonists include inhaled anesthetics such as cyclopropane, nitrous oxide and xenon, other analgesic agents such as tramadol and methadone, and other drugs such as memantine (Namenda), amantadine, and dextromethorphan.

Ketamine acts on the CNS by depressing neuronal function in selective areas of the cortex and the thalamus, while simultaneously activating the hippocampus and other parts of the limbic system. This creates a dissociation between the thalamocortical and limbic system resulting in what is often referred to as dissociative anesthesia. Ketamine has an analgesic effect in the spinal cord by inhibiting neuronal activity in the dorsal horn, and it can help prevent the development of chronic pain by its effect on synaptic plasticity and by interfering with nociceptive central hypersensitization. Ketamine acts as a catecholamine reuptake inhibitor which increases circulating levels of epinephrine and norepinephrine. It is also active at norepinephrine, serotonin, and muscarinic acetylcholine receptors.

Indications/Clinical Pearls

NMDA receptor antagonists like ketamine can be used for the induction and maintenance of anesthesia, sedation, analgesia for acute pain, and prevention of chronic pain. Ketamine increases pain thresholds at plasma levels as low as 0.1 μg/mL, so ketamine given for anesthesia can continue to reduce pain in the immediate postoperative period [37, 39]. Small doses of ketamine can significantly reduce the amount of opiates used for acute pain control and can reduce the side effects of opiate use [39, 41, 42]. Ketamine also reduces acute tolerance to opiates [43]. Ketamine may also be effective in difficult to treat chronic pain states such as cancer pain, neuropathic pain, visceral pain, phantom limb pain, fibromyalgia, CRPS, and migraine. This is supported by multiple small studies and case reports [44].

Dosing Options

Ketamine readily crosses the blood-brain barrier and a bolus dose has a 30–60 s onset of action with maximal effect occurring in 1 min. It has a short half-life of around 3 h and a steady state can be reached in 12–15 h. Induction of general anesthesia can be achieved with a dose of 0.5–2 mg/kg IV or 4–6 mg/kg IM. Anesthesia can be maintained with a 30–90 μg/kg/min IV infusion. Sedation and acute analgesia can be achieved with 0.2–0.8 mg/kg IV or 2–4 mg/kg IM. Preemptive analgesia doses range from 0.15 to 0.25 mg/kg IV. Continuous infusions are often used with a wide range of dosing protocols. A good starting point for intermittent dosing is 0.25–0.5 mg/kg TID given orally, IM, or IV [43]. Children may require higher plasma levels to achieve the same effect. Ketamine is metabolized in the liver, so a reduction of the dose is advised in patients with impaired hepatic function [39, 45].

Drug Interactions

Ketamine has the potential to interact with several drugs. Concurrent use with opiates such as hydromorphone and oxycodone may result in an increase in CNS and respiratory depression. Concurrent use with tramadol may further increase this risk since tramadol is also an NMDA receptor antagonist. Its use with atracurium and tubocurarine may increase neuromuscular blockade. Its use with metrizamide may result in an increased risk of seizures and theophylline with ketamine can lower the seizure threshold. Ketamine with St. John's wort carries an increased risk for cardiovascular collapse and delayed emergence from anesthesia.

Side Effects/Black Box Warnings

Ketamine has multiple side effects. Dilated pupils, nystagmus, lacrimation, and increased muscle tone are common. Ketamine is also a bronchial smooth muscle relaxant and has been used to treat refractory bronchospasm and status asthmaticus. Ketamine can increase salivation which can lead to laryngospasm and airway obstruction. Ketamine increases intraocular pressure and intracerebral pressure, so it should be avoided in patients with intracranial mass effect or increased ICP. The increase of circulating catecholamines associated with ketamine results in the stimulation of the cardiovascular system causing elevations in blood pressure, heart rate, cardiac output, and myocardial oxygen consumption [43]. These cardiovascular effects are not related to dose. Caution should be used in patients with existing hypertension or ischemic heart disease. NMDA receptor antagonists can also cause unfavorable psychological reactions including vivid dreams, a sense of detachment from the body, illusions, and hallucinations. The visual disturbances may be accompanied by excitement, confusion, euphoria, or fear. Pediatric patients have lower incidence of psychological adverse reactions. Both the psychological and cardiovascular effects can be reduced by the use of benzodiazepines [43].

Summary

NMDA receptor antagonists such as ketamine provide an excellent adjunct to almost any analgesic regimen in addition to having predictable and manageable side effects.

Chemical Structures

Chemical Structure
9.1 Dexamethasone

Chemical Structure
9.2 Dexmedetomidine

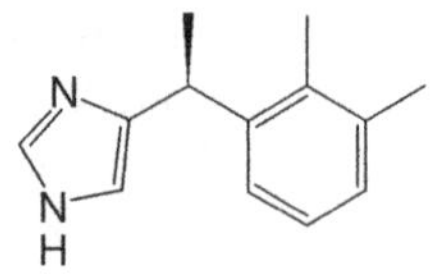

Chemical Structure
9.3 Acetaminophen/
paracetamol

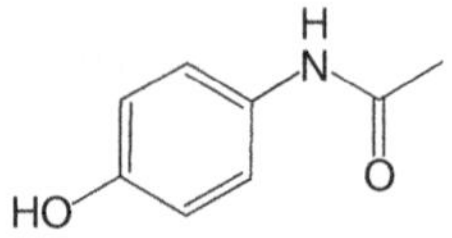

Chemical Structure
9.4 Ketamine

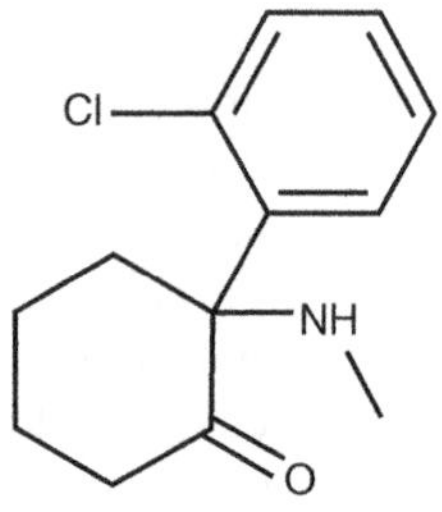

Chemical Structure
9.5 Ketorolac

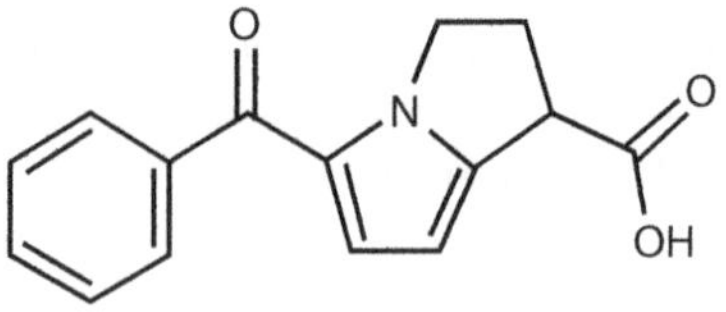

Chemical Structure
9.6 Celecoxib

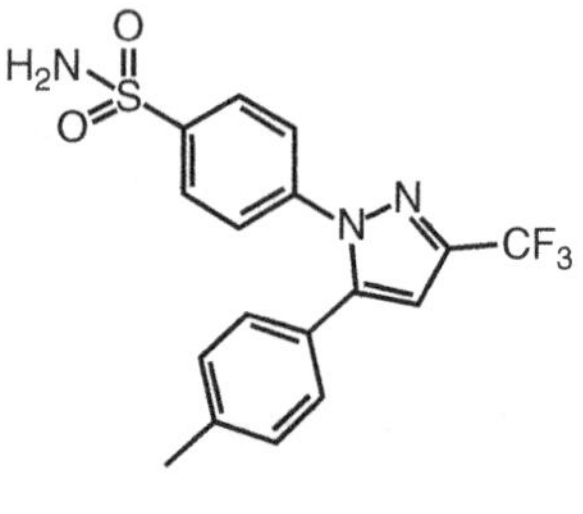

References

1. Cashman JN. The mechanisms of action of NSAIDs in analgesia. Drugs. 1996;52 Suppl 5: 13–23. Review.
2. Jackson LM, Hawkey CJ. COX-2 selective nonsteroidal anti-Inflammatory drugs: do they really offer any advantages? Drugs. 2000;59(6):1207–16. Review.
3. Viscusi ER, Frenkl TL, Hartrick CT, Rawal N, Kehlet H, Papanicolaou D, et al. Perioperative use of etoricoxib reduces pain and opioid side-effects after total abdominal hysterectomy: a double-blind, randomized, placebo-controlled phase III study. Curr Med Res Opin. 2012;28(8): 1323–35.

4. Bing RJ, Lomnicka M. Why do cyclo-oxygenase-2 inhibitors cause cardiovascular events? J Am Coll Cardiol. 2002;39(3):521–2.
5. De Oliveira GS, Jr AD, Benzon HT. Perioperative single dose ketorolac to prevent postoperative pain: a meta-analysis of randomized trials. Anesth Analg. 2012;114(2):424–33.
6. Lin J, Zhang L, Yang H. Perioperative administration of selective cyclooxygenase-2 inhibitors for postoperative pain management in patients after total knee arthroplasty. J Arthroplasty. 2013;28(2):207–13.
7. Sinatra RS, Shen QJ, Halaszynski T, Luther MA, Shaheen Y. Preoperative rofecoxib oral suspension as an analgesic adjunct after lower abdominal surgery: the effects on effort-dependent pain and pulmonary function. Anesth Analg. 2004;98(1):135–40.
8. Johnson AG, Seidemann P, Day RO. NSAID-related adverse drug interactions with clinical relevance. An update. Int J Clin Pharmacol Ther. 1994;32(10):509–32.
9. Rhen T, Cidlowski JA. Antiinflammatory action of glucocorticoids – new mechanisms for old drugs. N Engl J Med. 2005;353:1711–23.
10. Romundstad L, Stubhaug A. Glucocorticoids for acute and persistent postoperative neuropathic pain: what is the evidence? Anesthesiology. 2007;107(3):371–3.
11. Waldron NH, Jones CA, Gan TJ, Allen TK, Habib AS. Impact of perioperative dexamethasone on postoperative analgesia and side-effects: systematic review and meta-analysis. Br J Anaesth. 2013;110(2):191–200.
12. Tolver MA, Strandfelt P, Bryld EB, Rosenberg J, Bisgaard T. Randomized clinical trial of dexamethasone versus placebo in laparoscopic inguinal hernia repair. Br J Surg. 2012;99(10): 1374–80.
13. Lunn TH, Andersen L, Kristensen BB, Husted H, Gaarn-Larsen L, Bandholm T, et al. Effect of high-dose preoperative methylprednisolone on recovery after total hip arthroplasty: a randomized, double-blind, placebo-controlled trial. Br J Anaesth. 2013;110(1):66–73.
14. Lunn TH, Kristensen BB, Andersen L, Husted H, Otte KS, Gaarn-Larsen L. Effect of high-dose preoperative methylprednisolone on pain and recovery after total knee arthroplasty: a randomized, placebo-controlled trial. Br J Anaesth. 2011;106(2):230–8. doi:10.1093/bja/aeq333. Epub 2010 Dec 3.
15. Bauer HC, Duarte FL, Horliana AC, Tortamano IP, Perez FE, Simone JL. Assessment of preemptive analgesia with ibuprofen coadministered or not with dexamethasone in third molar surgery: a randomized double-blind controlled clinical trial. Oral Maxillofac Surg. 2013;17(3):165–71.
16. Schulze S, Andersen J, Overgaard H, Nørgard P, Nielsen HJ, Aasen A. Effect of prednisolone on the systemic response and wound healing after colonic surgery. Arch Surg. 1997;132(2):129–35.
17. Powell-Jackson PR, Gray BJ, Heaton RW, Costello JF, Williams R, English J. Adverse effect of rifampicin administration on steroid-dependent asthma. Am Rev Respir Dis. 1983;128(2): 307–10.
18. Albrecht E, Kirkham KR, Liu SS, Brull R. Peri-operative intravenous administration of magnesium sulphate and postoperative pain: a meta-analysis. Anaesthesia. 2013;68(1):79–90.
19. Lee JH, Yang WD, Han SY, Noh JI, Cho SH, Kim SH, Chae WS, Jin HC. Effect of epidural magnesium on the incidence of chronic postoperative pain after video-assisted thoracic surgery. J Cardiothorac Vasc Anesth. 2012;26(6):1055–9.
20. Lee C, Song YK, Jeong HM, Park SN. The effects of magnesium sulfate infiltration on perioperative opioid consumption and opioid-induced hyperalgesia in patients undergoing robot-assisted laparoscopic prostatectomy with remifentanil-based anesthesia. Korean J Anesthesiol. 2011;61(3):244–50.
21. Song JW, Lee YW, Yoon KB, Park SJ, Shim YH. Magnesium sulfate prevents remifentanil-induced postoperative hyperalgesia in patients undergoing thyroidectomy. Anesth Analg. 2011;113(2):390–7.
22. Hwang JY, Na HS, Jeon YT, Ro YJ, Kim CS, Do SH. I.V. infusion of magnesium sulphate during spinal anaesthesia improves postoperative analgesia. Br J Anaesth. 2010;104(1):89–93.
23. El-Kerdawy H. Analgesic requirements for patients undergoing lower extremity orthopedic surgery–the effect of combined spinal and epidural magnesium. Middle East J Anesthesiol. 2008;19(5):1013–25.

24. Bilir A, Gulec S, Erkan A, Ozcelik A. Epidural magnesium reduces postoperative analgesic requirement. Br J Anaesth. 2007;98(4):519–23.
25. Seyhan TO, Tugrul M, Sungur MO, Kayacan S, Telci L, Pembeci K, Akpir K. Effects of three different dose regimens of magnesium on propofol requirements, haemodynamic variables and postoperative pain relief in gynaecological surgery. Br J Anaesth. 2006;96(2):247–52.
26. Yousef AA, Al-Deeb AE. A double-blinded randomised controlled study of the value of sequential intravenous and oral magnesium therapy in patients with chronic low back pain with a neuropathic component. Anaesthesia. 2013;68(3):260–6.
27. Blaudszun G, Lysakowski C, Elia N, Tramèr MR. Effect of perioperative systemic α2 agonists on postoperative morphine consumption and pain intensity: systematic review and meta-analysis of randomized controlled trials. Anesthesiology. 2012;116(6):1312–22.
28. Cao J, Shi X, Miao X, Xu J. Effects of premedication of midazolam or clonidine on perioperative anxiety and pain in children. Biosci Trends. 2009;3(3):115–8.
29. Mizrak A, Gul R, Erkutlu I, Alptekin M, Oner U. Premedication with dexmedetomidine alone or together with 0.5 % lidocaine for IVRA. J Surg Res. 2010;164(2):242–7.
30. Wu CT, Jao SW, Borel CO, Yeh CC, Li CY, Lu CH, Wong CS. The effect of epidural clonidine on perioperative cytokine response, postoperative pain, and bowel function in patients undergoing colorectal surgery. Anesth Analg. 2004;99(2):502–9.
31. Walker SM, Grafe M, Yaksh TL. Intrathecal clonidine in the neonatal rat: dose-dependent analgesia and evaluation of spinal apoptosis and toxicity. Anesth Analg. 2012;115(2): 450–60.
32. Cao JP, Miao XY, Liu J, Shi XY. An evaluation of intrathecal bupivacaine combined with intrathecal or intravenous clonidine in children undergoing orthopedic surgery: a randomized double-blinded study. Paediatr Anaesth. 2011;21(4):399–405.
33. Jain G, Bansal P, Ahmad B, Singh DK, Yadav G. Effect of the perioperative infusion of dexmedetomidine on chronic pain after breast surgery. Indian J Palliat Care. 2012;18(1):45–51.
34. Iirola T, Vilo S, Aantaa R, Wendelin-Saarenhovi M, Neuvonen PJ, Scheinin M, Olkkola KT. Dexmedetomidine inhibits gastric emptying and oro-caecal transit in healthy volunteers. Br J Anaesth. 2011;106(4):522–7.
35. Leino K, Hynynen M, Jalonen J, Salmenperä M, Scheinin H, Aantaa R. Renal effects of dexmedetomidine during coronary artery bypass surgery: a randomized placebo-controlled study. Dexmedetomidine in Cardiac Surgery Study Group. BMC Anesthesiol. 2011;11:9.
36. Miller RD, Eriksson LI, Fleisher LA, Wiener-Kronish JP, Young WL, editors. Miller's anesthesia. 7th ed. Churchill Livingstone: An Imprint of Elsevier; 2009.
37. Reme'rand F, Le Tendre C, Baud A, Couvret C, Pourrat X, et al. The early and delayed analgesic effects of ketamine after total hip arthroplasty: a prospective, randomized, controlled, double-blind study. Anesth Analg. 2009;109:1963–71.
38. Maund CE, McDaid S, Rice K, Wright BJ, Woolacott N. Paracetamol and selective and non-selective non-steroidal anti-inflammatory drugs for the reduction in morphine-related side-effects after major surgery: a systematic review. Br J Anaesth. 2011;106(3):292–7.
39. Barash PG, Cullen BF, Stoelting RK, Cahalan MK, Stock MC, editors. Clinical anesthesia. 6th ed. Philadelphia: Wolters Kluwer Health/Lippincott Williams & Wilkins; 2009.
40. Ong CKS, Seymour RA, Lirk P, Merry Alan F. Combining paracetamol (acetaminophen) with nonsteroidal antiinflammatory drugs: a qualitative systematic review of analgesic efficacy for acute postoperative pain. Anesth Analg. 2010;110:4.
41. Yamauchi M, Asano M, Watanabe M, Iwasaki S, Furuse S, Namiki A. Continuous low-dose ketamine improves the analgesic effects of fentanyl patient-controlled analgesia after cervical spine surgery. Anesth Analg. 2008;107:1041–4.
42. Zakine J, Samarcq D, Lorne E, Moubarak M, Montravers P, Beloucif S, et al. Postoperative ketamine administration decreases morphine consumption in major abdominal surgery: a prospective, randomized, double-blind, controlled study. Anesth Analg. 2008;106: 1856–61.

43. Okon T. Ketamine: an introduction for the pain and palliative medicine physician. Pain Physician. 2007;10:493–500.
44. Nama S, Meenan DR, Fritz WT. The use of sub-anesthetic intravenous ketamine and adjuvant dexmedetomidine when treating acute pain from CRPS. Pain Physician. 2010;13:365–8.
45. Olofsen E, Noppers I, Niesters M, Kharasch E, Aarts L, Sarton E, et al. Estimation of the contribution of norketamine to ketamine-induced acute pain relief and neurocognitive impairment in healthy volunteers. Anesthesiology. 2012;117(2):353.

Chapter 10
Benzodiazepines and Muscle Relaxants

Joyce C. Lo and Alan David Kaye

Contents

J.C. Lo, MD (✉)
Department of Anesthesiology, Pain, and Perioperative Care,
Stanford University School of Medicine, Palo Alto, CA, USA
e-mail: joycelo@gmail.com

A.D. Kaye, MD, PhD
Department of Anesthesiology, Tulane Medical Center, New Orleans, LA, USA

Department of Anesthesiology, Louisiana State University Health Sciences Center,
New Orleans, LA, USA
e-mail: alankaye44@hotmail.com

A.D. Kaye et al. (eds.), *Essentials of Pharmacology for Anesthesia,*
Pain Medicine, and Critical Care, DOI 10.1007/978-1-4614-8948-1_10,
© Springer Science+Business Media New York 2015

Benzodiazepines

Introduction

The first benzodiazepines, chlordiazepoxide and valium, were introduced in the 1960s, and benzodiazepines are now among the most widely prescribed class of drugs and are used for a number of indications such as muscular spasm, spasticity, convulsive disorders, anxiety disorder, panic disorder, alcohol withdrawal, insomnia, jet lag, and muscle spasticity. Benzodiazepines can be classified by their elimination half-life as short acting (median elimination half-life of 1–12 h), intermediate acting (median elimination half-life of 12–40 h), and long acting (median elimination half-life of 40–250 h). They can also be classified based on their relative potency. The early benzodiazepines (e.g., chlordiazepoxide, oxazepam, temazepam) were low-potency agents with relatively low toxicity and were utilized to treat insomnia and anxiety. As benzodiazepines with higher potency (e.g., alprazolam, lorazepam, clonazepam) were developed, they became more widely prescribed for a number of new indications, including agitation and panic disorders, and were used as adjuncts to antipsychotics, selective serotonin reuptake inhibitors (SSRIs), and other neuropsychiatric drugs.

Drug Class and Mechanism of Action

Gamma-aminobutyric acid (GABA), an inhibitory neurotransmitter, is the most common neurotransmitter in the central nervous system (CNS) and decreases the excitability of neurons. Benzodiazepines act as positive allosteric modulators of the GABA-A receptor, a ligand-gated chloride-selective ion channel, and induce a conformational change that facilitates GABA binding [1]. GABA-A receptors have two α subunits, two β subunits, and one γ subunit.

Benzodiazepine receptors differ in terms of α subunit isoforms and the subsequent clinical effects from ligand binding. The BZ1 receptor contains the α1 isoform and is highly concentrated in the cortex, thalamus, and cerebellum [2]. It mediates sedative and anticonvulsive effects of benzodiazepines and also produces anterograde amnesia. BZ2 receptors contain the α2 isoform, which is responsible for the anxiolytic and myorelaxant effects of benzodiazepines. It is believed that BZ2 receptors mediating anxiolytic effects are found in the limbic system, whereas those mediating myorelaxant effects are located in motor neurons and the dorsal horn of the spinal cord. Sixty percent of GABA-A receptors contain the α1 isoform and, thus, amnesia as a common side effect of benzodiazepine use. Drugs across this class may interact with different affinities to each type of receptor and these differences correspond to the range of clinical manifestations seen with each drug. Benzodiazepines with higher lipid solubility have higher absorption rates and faster onset of clinical effects, as well as greater risk for amnesia. Drug titration should be incremental with consideration to the agent's pharmacodynamics and patient's preexisting comorbidities and condition [3].

Indications/Clinical Pearls

Benzodiazepines have been used in diverse clinical settings, including for the treatment of anxiety, seizures, alcohol withdrawal, insomnia, spasticity, and preoperative anterograde amnesia. Benzodiazepines and their metabolites are highly protein bound. Most undergo oxidative metabolism by cytochrome P450 (CYP450) enzymes and then are conjugated with glucuronide and excreted in urine. Many benzodiazepines have prolonged elimination half-lives and produce active metabolites, which may have additional clinical effects. Diazepam, for example, is a long-acting benzodiazepine with the active metabolites oxazepam, desmethyldiazepam, and temazepam, which further increase the duration of action. This potential needs to be considered in the selection and dosing of drugs to patients with impaired hepatic function or the elderly, particularly if multiple daily doses are prescribed. As an entire drug class, benzodiazepines are listed on the Beers Criteria by the American Geriatrics Society as a group of medications with strong evidence for avoidance in geriatric patients [4].

To reverse the sedative effects of benzodiazepines, flumazenil, a benzodiazepine receptor antagonist, can be given intravenously at a dose of 0.2 mg and repeated every minute if needed to a maximum dose of 1 mg. The dose may need to be repeated every 20 min if resedation occurs. In cases of benzodiazepine overdose, a large dose, 0.5 mg, may be required. Flumazenil administration needs to be carefully considered as there is a serious risk of seizures and withdrawal symptoms, and one should be prepared to treat these should they occur.

Benzodiazepine use is associated with tolerance and dependence and is limited by its addiction and abuse potential [5]. Abrupt discontinuation or rapid dose reduction of benzodiazepines may result in withdrawal symptoms including anxiety, dysphoria, insomnia, diaphoresis, vomiting, diarrhea, tremor, muscle spasms, seizure, and death. To avoid withdrawal symptoms, it is recommended that practitioners taper down drug dosage over weeks and consider transitioning to a low-potency long-acting benzodiazepine in dependent patients.

Dosing Options

Benzodiazepines can be administered via intravenous, intramuscular, oral, sublingual, intranasal, and rectal routes. Some commonly used benzodiazepines will be described below and in Table 10.1.

Alprazolam is a short-acting, high-potency benzodiazepine used in the treatment of anxiety and panic disorders. It may also be used for pre-procedural sedation. It is highly lipid soluble and has an increased risk of amnesia. While its shorter half-life makes it an appealing drug, patients can be at risk for rebound symptoms if abruptly discontinued.

Lorazepam is another short- to intermediate-acting benzodiazepine with high potency. In addition to having less affinity for GABA-A receptors than alprazolam, it is also less lipid soluble and may therefore carry a lower risk of causing amnesia.

Table 10.1 Commonly used oral benzodiazepines

Drug	Common dosing	Half-life (h)	Time to peak plasma concentration (h)	Elimination
Short- to intermediate-acting benzodiazepines				
Alprazolam (Xanax)	0.25–0.5 mg BID–TID for anxiety; *maximum 4 mg/day*	11.2 (6.3–26.9)	1–2	Renal
Clonazepam (Klonopin)	0.25–0.5 mg BID–TID for anxiety; 0.5–2 mg BID for panic disorder; *maximum 4 mg/day*	17–60	1–4	Renal
Lorazepam (Ativan)	2–6 mg/day divided BID–TID for anxiety; *maximum 10 mg/day*	10–20	2	Renal, fecal
Oxazepam (Serax)	10–30 mg TID–QID for anxiety	5–15	1–4	Renal
Temazepam (Restoril)	7.5–30 mg QHS for insomnia	9.5–12.5	2–3	Renal
Long-acting benzodiazepines				
Chlordiazepoxide (Librium)	5–25 mg TID–QID for anxiety; 50–100 mg PRN for alcohol withdrawal; *maximum 300 mg/day*	5–25	0.5–2	Renal
Clorazepate (Tranxene)	15–60 mg/day divided BID–TID for anxiety	40–50	0.5–2	Renal, fecal
Diazepam (Valium)	2–10 mg TID–QID for muscle spasm; 2–10 mg BID–QID for anxiety; 5 mg TID–QID PRN for alcohol withdrawal	20–50	0.25–2	Renal

Lorazepam is commonly used for the treatment of anxiety, agitation, and seizures. When administered intramuscularly, absorption is rapid and complete. Unlike most benzodiazepines which are metabolized by CYP450, lorazepam undergoes glucuronidation and elimination and is therefore less affected by the many drugs that may interact with CYP450.

Midazolam is a short-acting benzodiazepine with almost twice the potency of diazepam. It is commonly used preoperatively for anxiolysis and amnesia and can be administered via intravenous, intramuscular, oral, sublingual, intranasal, and rectal routes. It is highly lipophilic and therefore has a quick onset of action. Its elimination half-life is 2–6 h due to rapid reabsorption, making its effects shorter than lorazepam and suitable for use in a continuous infusion for sedation in the intensive care unit. The hypnotic effects of midazolam are due to its interference with GABA reuptake.

Clonazepam is an intermediate-acting, high-potency benzodiazepine. In addition to its effects at the GABA-A receptor, it also has some serotoninergic activity. It is used in the treatment of seizures, anxiety, panic disorder, and acute mania. It has lower lipid solubility than other benzodiazepines and tends to cause less anterograde amnesia.

Diazepam is a long-acting, medium-potency benzodiazepine prescribed for many indications, including anxiety, muscle spasms, seizures, and alcohol withdrawal. At low doses, diazepam binding to BZ2 receptors in the limbic system results in anxiolysis. At higher doses, diazepam binding to BZ2 receptors in the spinal cord and motor neurons provides muscle relaxation, but there are also increasing BZ1-mediated effects at these doses, such as sedation and anterograde amnesia. Diazepam has a number of active metabolites—oxazepam, temazepam, and desmethyldiazepam—which prolong the time in which a patient may experience sedation, amnesia, and other effects.

Drug Interactions

Most benzodiazepines are metabolized by CYP450 enzymes. A smaller group (e.g., lorazepam, oxazepam, temazepam) undergoes direct glucuronidation and is less affected by other drugs. Drugs that inhibit CYP450 enzymes (e.g., oral contraceptive pills, antifungals, some antibiotics) decrease the rate of benzodiazepine elimination and can worsen side effects or precipttate drug overdose. Drugs that induce CYP450 enzymes (e.g., carbamazepine, phenytoin, rifampin, St. John's wort) increase the metabolism of benzodiazepines and patients may thus require higher dosages.

Respiratory depression may occur if alcohol, opioids, or other psychotropic medications are co-administered, and consideration is needed before initiation in patients with pulmonary disease, neuromuscular weakness and obstructive sleep apnea. Similarly, cardiovascular effects from peripheral vasodilation and CNS depression may be more pronounced.

Side Effects/Black Box Warnings

The most common side effects include sedation, somnolence, memory and cognitive impairment, depression, anterograde amnesia, respiratory depression, changes in weight and appetite and decreased libido. Hypotension may result from peripheral vasodilation. Thrombophlebitis and venoirritation may be seen with intravenous administration of diazepam and lorazepam and Bdue to the diluent, propylene glycol. Intensive care unit patients who receive large doses of these drugs are at risk for propylene glycol toxicity. Paradoxical reactions, including agitation, irritability, aggression and impulsivity, rarely occur but may be seen more frequently in patients with psychiatric or cognitive disorders using higher dosages of high-potency benzodiazepines or in the setting of chronic benzodiazepine use. Drug clearance may be significantly delayed in elderly patients as hepatic and renal functions are commonly impaired and there is an inability to metabolize and eliminate the dose efficiently. As a result, elderly patients are highly sensitive to benzodiazepines and their administration may lead to significant adverse outcomes such as respiratory depression, altered mental status and oversedation, which could lead to injury via falls or motor vehicle accidents.

Muscle Relaxants

Introduction

Muscle relaxants alleviate pain caused by muscle spasms and spasticity of various origins. Both muscle spasms and spasticity involve involuntary muscular contraction that can be associated with significant pain. Many of these treatments, however, are limited by their side effect profile. The muscle relaxants described in this chapter are primarily centrally acting muscle relaxants and are distinct from agents that target the neuromuscular junction, such as succinylcholine and the non-depolarizing neuromuscular blocking agents.

Drug Class and Mechanism of Action

Muscle relaxants are a broad class of drugs that are not fully understood yet and do not generally share a common structure or mechanism of action. These drugs do not act directly at the neuromuscular junction and sedation likely plays a large role in the effectiveness of these centrally acting drugs as it is believed that sedation decreases the firing of painful nerve stimuli. Specific known mechanisms will be discussed below with each drug.

Indications/Clinical Pearls

This diverse group of drugs can be used in multiple settings, ranging from the treatment of muscle spasms and spasticity related to chronic CNS disorders such as spinal cord injury, stroke and multiple sclerosis to acute pain due to herniated intervertebral disks, muscle strains and postoperative pain. While the clinical effects of these centrally-acting muscle relaxants are in large part due to their sedative effects, sedation also becomes dose limiting. This class of drugs also carries a risk of addiction and abuse, and routine reevaluation and dose titration are indicated. Abrupt withdrawal or rapid downward dose titration may result in withdrawal symptoms.

Table 10.2 Commonly used oral muscle relaxants

Drug	Common dosing	Half-life (h)	Elimination
Cyclobenzaprine (Amrix, Flexeril)	5–10 mg QD–TID for muscle spasms; *maximum 40 mg/day*	18–24	Renal
Chlorzoxazone (Parafon Forte)	250–500 mg TID–QID for musculoskeletal pain and spasm; *maximum 750 mg/dose*	1–2	Renal
Carisoprodol (Soma)	350 mg QID or QHS for acute treatment of muscle spasms	10	Renal
Metaxalone (Skelaxin)	400–800 mg TID–QID for acute musculoskeletal pain	2–3	Renal
Methocarbamol (Robaxin)	1,500 mg QID for muscle spasm in first 72 h, then decrease; *maximum 8,000 mg/day initially, then 4,500 mg/day*	1–2	Renal
Orphenadrine citrate (Norflex)	100 mg BID for musculoskeletal pain	14	Renal, fecal
Tizanidine (Zanaflex)	2–8 mg TID–QID for spasticity; *maximum 12 mg/dose, 24 mg/day*	2.5	Renal, fecal
Dantrolene (Dantrium)	25 mg BID for spasticity; *maximum 400 mg/ day for 3 weeks*	4–8	Fecal, renal
Baclofen (Lioresal)	Start 5 mg TID for spasticity and increase every 3 days by 5 mg/dose; *maximum 80 mg/day*	2.5–4	Renal, fecal

Dosing Options

Some common muscle relaxants are described below and in Table 10.2.

Cyclobenzaprine is used in the treatment of muscle spasms. It is not used in the treatment of spasticity resulting from CNS pathology. Cyclobenzaprine acts on the descending pathways in the brainstem and ventral spinal cord where it blocks serotonergic receptors and interferes with signals from the raphe nuclei that travel to alpha-motor neurons [6]. These alpha-motor neurons interact directly with skeletal muscles and trigger muscle contraction. Cyclobenzaprine has a structure similar to tricyclic agents and has many similar side effects generally related to its anticholinergic properties, including dry mouth and dry eyes. Cyclobenzaprine should not be coadministered with monoamine oxidase inhibitors to prevent serotonin syndrome.

Carisoprodol is used in the acute treatment of muscle spasms but has little efficacy in the treatment of spasticity. The mechanism of action of carisoprodol is unknown but it is thought to disrupt neuronal communication. The drug and its metabolite, meprobamate, interact with GABA-A receptors in a manner similar to barbiturates. It is highly addictive with significant abuse potential. In discontinuation of the drug, the dose should be titrated slowly to avoid withdrawal symptoms.

Orphenadrine is not generally considered a first-line therapy for pain but rather is an adjuvant for myofascial pain, joint pain, neuropathic pain and spasms.

It is a mood-altering agent that can be useful in the treatment of depression. Its mechanism of action is thought to be due to its role as an N-methyl-D-aspartic acid (NMDA) receptor antagonist, possible sodium channel antagonist and, because it shares a similar structure to diphenhydramine, antihistamine and anti-cholinergic effects [6].

Chlorzoxazone has been used in the temporary treatment of muscle spasms but not in the treatment of spasticity resulting from CNS pathology. The exact mechanism of action of chlorzoxazone is unknown; however, it is thought to block reflexes in the spinal cord that affect muscle contraction [6]. Gastrointestinal symptoms, dizziness, and lethargy have been reported, but serious adverse reactions are uncommon. Hepatotoxicity is extremely rare.

Tizanidine is among the newer muscle relaxants used to treat spasticity and also may be an adjuvant agent in patients with insomnia. Unlike other drugs in this class, it stimulates alpha-2 adrenergic receptors thus decreasing the release of presynaptic excitatory neurotransmitters and also interferes with spinal reflex transmission resulting in decreased spasticity.

Baclofen has a structure similar to GABA and activates GABA-B receptors located within the CNS, which inhibits the release of excitatory neurotransmitters [7]. It is known to inhibit monosynaptic and polysynaptic spinal reflexes. It has been used in the treatment of spasticity associated with CNS pathology, such as multiple sclerosis or spinal cord injury, muscle spasms and trigeminal neuralgia. In addition to oral and parenteral routes, baclofen can also be administered intrathecally because it has low lipid solubility and otherwise poor CNS penetration. Intrathecal pumps allow for direct drug delivery with decreased systemic side effects. While less sedating than agents such as benzodiazepines, baclofen can also cause somnolence, as well as weakness, dizziness, gastrointestinal distress and hypotension.

Dantrolene may be best known for its role in the treatment of malignant hyperthermia, but it is also used as a peripheral-acting muscle relaxant. Dantrolene blocks the release of calcium from the sarcoplasmic reticulum interfering with excitation-contraction coupling and prevents muscle contraction [7]. As a result of its inhibition of muscle contraction, dantrolene may cause a significant decrease in muscle tone and is generally reserved for patients who are not ambulatory. In particular, it may be used to treat patients with spasticity associated with chronic disorders such as spinal cord injury, multiple sclerosis, cerebral palsy and cerebral vascular accident. One benefit of dantrolene is that it is less sedating than centrally-acting muscle relaxants. Dantrolene has also been used for the treatment of neuroleptic malignant syndrome.

Black Box Warnings
Dantrolene sodium has a potential for hepatotoxicity and should not be used in conditions other than those recommended. Symptomatic hepatitis (fatal and nonfatal) has been reported at various dose levels of the drug.

Drug Interactions

CNS depression and psychomotor impairment may occur when muscle relaxants are administered along with benzodiazepines, barbiturates or any other psychoactive drugs as their effects can be additive. Cyclobenzaprine should not be used within 14 days of recciving any monoamine oxidase inhibitor due to risk of serotonin syndrome. Methocarbamol should not be prescribed to a patient taking pyridostigmine as it prevents inhibition of acetylcholinesterase. Coadministration of agents that inhibit CYP450 may result in prolonged drug effect. Drug interactions are otherwise limited.

Side Effects/Black Box Warnings

Side effects of cyclobenzaprine include sedation, dry mouth, blurry vision, urinary retention, elevated intraocular pressure, constipation, dizziness and arrhythmias. Drug use may be limited by these anticholinergic effects worsening preexisting medical conditions, including benign prostatic hyperplasia, conduction abnormalities, glaucoma and congestive heart failure.

Carisoprodol's side effects include drowsiness, ataxia, tremor, irritability, insomnia, confusion, disorientation, tachycardia and postural hypotension. It is highly addictive and withdrawal symptoms similar to those seen with barbiturate withdrawal (e.g., restlessness, insomnia, anorexia, anxiety, seizures, death) may occur with abrupt discontinuation.

Metaxalone can cause hepatotoxicity and hemolytic anemia. Routine liver function monitoring is suggested.

Orphenadrine's side effects are generally mild and related to anticholinergic and antihistamine effects, such as dry mouth, blurry vision and urinary retention. Aplastic anemia is a rare severe adverse reaction. This drug was withdrawn from the Scandinavian market in 2005 because of lethal intoxications. If given intravenously, there is a risk for anaphylaxis.

Rapid intravenous infusion of *methocarbamol* can cause bradycardia, hypotension and syncope, as well as increase the risk of convulsions. As such, intravenous infusion is contraindicated in patients with a history of seizures. Other side effects include sedation, dizziness, nausea, thrombophlebitis, jaundice, leukopenia and metallic taste.

An alpha-2 agonist, *tizanidine* may cause hypotension although this is an uncommon side effect [8]. Nevertheless, it is generally recommended to avoid concomitant use of other alpha-2 agonist agents. Other side effects include headache, weakness, sedation, dry mouth, hallucinations and gastrointestinal symptoms. Hepatocellular injury may also occur and routine monitoring of liver function is recommended within the first 6 months of therapy and periodically afterward. Consideration should be taken prior to initiating this drug in a patient with liver dysfunction or who is on drugs that inhibit CYP450 as it will result in prolonged drug effect.

Side effects of *dantrolene* include drowsiness, dizziness, muscle weakness, malaise, diarrhea and hepatotoxicity, which is more commonly seen in women over the age of 40. Muscle weakness may be significant and dantrolene may be more appropriate for use in non-ambulatory patients.

Summary

Benzodiazepines are commonly prescribed drugs that have been effective in the treatment of a wide range of disorders, including anxiety, muscle spasms, insomnia and seizures. Muscle relaxants, which have been used to treat muscle spasms and spasticity, generally act via central mechanisms. While both classes of drugs are generally safe to use, these drugs can produce significant adverse effects, particularly when used in combination with alcohol, opioids and other drugs that may affect respiratory or central nervous system function. In addition to the potential side effects, these drugs are also associated with an abuse and addiction potential. Careful consideration must be taken when prescribing these drugs.

Chemical Structures

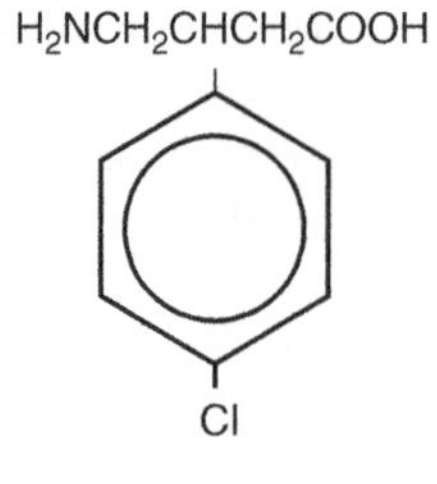

$H_2NCH_2CHCH_2COOH$

Cl

Chemical Structure
10.1 Baclofen

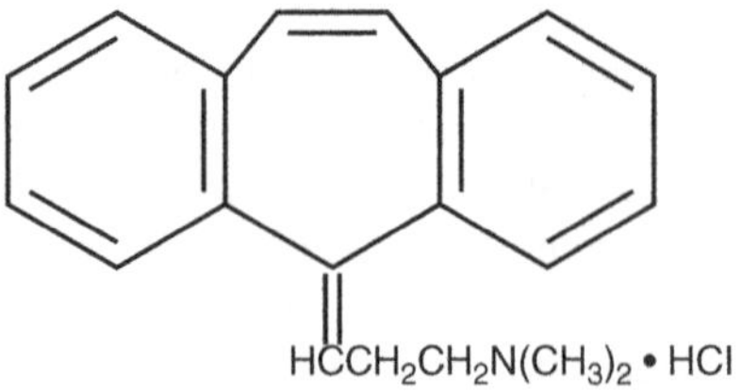

$HCCH_2CH_2N(CH_3)_2 \bullet HCl$

Chemical Structure
10.2 Cyclobenzaprine
hydrochloride

Chemical Structure 10.3 Dantrolene sodium

**Chemical Structure
10.4** Tizanidine

Chemical Structure 10.5 Orphenadrine citrate

References

1. Griffin CE, Kaye AM, Bueno FR, Kaye AD. Benzodiazepine pharmacology and central nervous system-mediated effects. Oschner Clin J. 2013;13(2):214–23.
2. Sieghart W. Pharmacology of benzodiazepine receptors: an update. J Psychiatry Neurosci. 1994;19(1):24–9.

3. Kaye AD, Gayle K, Kaye AM. Pharmacological agents in moderate and deep sedation. In: Kaye AD, Urman R, editors. Moderate and deep sedation. New York: Cambridge Press; 2011. p. 8–32.
4. American Geriatrics Society. Beers criteria update expert panel. American geriatrics society updated beers criteria for potentially inappropriate medication use in older adults. J Am Geriatr Soc. 2012;60:616–31.
5. World Health Organization. Programme on substance abuse: rational use of benzodiazepines. World Health Organization. 1996.
6. Stout T, Kaye AD, Kaye AM. Muscle relaxants and antispasticity drugs. In: Manchikanti L, editor. In: Foundations of interventional pain management and pain medicine ASIPP publishing. Paducah, KY. Chapter VI–10, 607–14.
7. Zafonte R, Lombard L, Elovic E. Antispasticity medications: uses and limitations of enteral therapy. Am J Phys Med Rehabil. 2004;83:S50–8.
8. Onur M, Benzon HT. Muscle relaxants. In: Essentials of pain medicine and regional anesthesia. New York: Churchill Livingstone; 1999. p. 78–82.

Chapter 11
Pharmacology of Local Anesthetics

Neesa Patel and Alireza Sadoughi

Contents

N. Patel, MD (✉)
Department of Anesthesiology,
UCLA- Santa Monica Medical Center and Orthopedic Hospital,
Santa Monica, CA, USA

Department of Anesthesiology, Ronald Reagan UCLA Medical Center,
Los Angeles, CA, USA

Department of Anesthesiology, David Geffen School of Medicine, University of California,
Los Angeles, CA, USA
e-mail: nnpatel@mednet.ucla.edu

A. Sadoughi, MD
Department of Anesthesiology, UCLA- Santa Monica Medical Center and Orthopedic
Hospital, Santa Monica, CA, USA

Department of Anesthesiology, David Geffen School of Medicine, University of California,
Los Angeles, CA, USA
e-mail: asadoughi@mednet.ucla.edu

A.D. Kaye et al. (eds.), *Essentials of Pharmacology for Anesthesia,*   179
Pain Medicine, and Critical Care, DOI 10.1007/978-1-4614-8948-1_11,
© Springer Science+Business Media New York 2015

Introduction

The development of local anesthetics dates to the first use by the Incas of Peru, using cocaine for its medicinal properties. They treated headaches with trepanation or by burrowing holes in the skull with chewed cocaine as the local anesthetic [1]. Today, the use of local anesthetics by anesthesia providers has gained increasing popularity, traditionally in both obstetric and regional anesthesia. This chapter will focus on the types of local anesthetics, dosing and mechanism of action, indications with clinical pearls, and drug interactions/toxicity profile.

Drug Classes

The majority of injectable local anesthetics are tertiary amines. Only a few (e.g., prilocaine and hexylcaine) are secondary amines. All local anesthetics are amphipathic and possess both lipophilic and hydrophilic parts. The lipophilic part is the largest portion derived from benzoic acid, aniline, or thiophene. The hydrophilic part is an amino derivative of ethyl alcohol or acetic acid. Local anesthetics that lack a hydrophilic part are mostly used as topical anesthetics (e.g., benzocaine). The structure is completed by an intermediate hydrocarbon chain link which contains either an ester or an amide linkage. Variations in this intermediate chain portion of the basic local anesthetic molecule have resulted in the development of two basic classes of local anesthetics, the esters and the amides.

The ester-type local anesthetics are less stable in solution, are rapidly metabolized by plasma pseudocholinesterase, and appear to be associated with rare true allergic reactions. The amide-type local anesthetics are very stable in solution, are

Table 11.1 Anesthetic agents and their common uses

Agent	Commonly used for	Agent	Commonly used for
Cocaine	Topical	Mepivacaine	Infiltration, PNB, spinal (not FDA approved), epidural
Benzocaine	Topical	Prilocaine	Infiltration, PNB, epidural
Procaine	Infiltration	Bupivacaine	PNB, epidural, spinal, infiltration
Dibucaine	Spinal	Ropivacaine	Infiltration, PNB, epidural
Tetracaine	Spinal	Lidocaine	PNB, spinal, epidural, topical, infiltration
Chloroprocaine	PNB, epidural, infiltration		

PNB peripheral nerve block

Covino B, Vassallo H. Local anesthetics: mechanisms of action and clinical use. Orlando: Grune & Stratton; 1976.

metabolized in the liver by cytochrome P450 enzymes, and are almost never associated with true allergic reactions.

Commonly used amino amides include lidocaine, mepivacaine, prilocaine, bupivacaine, etidocaine, and ropivacaine (Table 11.1). Commonly used amino esters include cocaine, procaine, tetracaine, chloroprocaine, and benzocaine. An easy way to remember which drug belongs in which category is that all of the amino amides contain the letter "i" twice, as does the term "amino amides."

Local Anesthetic Properties

Activity of local anesthetics may be affected by their lipid solubility, percent ionization at physiologic pH, affinity for protein binding, and vasodilatation effect.

Lipid Solubility

Lipid solubility appears to be the most significant property of local anesthetic molecules in determining anesthetic potency. Local anesthetic molecules which are highly lipophilic easily penetrate nerve cell membranes and become intracellular, resulting in more blockades. For example, bupivacaine is considerably more lipid soluble and more potent than lidocaine.

Ionization

Local anesthetics exist in ionized and nonionized forms, the proportions changed by pH of the environment. The nonionized portion is the form that is capable of diffusing across nerve membranes and blocking sodium channels. The nonionized form also has a faster onset of action due to fast diffusion. Local anesthetics differ in respect to the pH at which the ionized and nonionized forms are present at equilibrium (7.6–8.9). The more closely the equilibrium pH for a given anesthetic approximates the physiologic pH of tissues (i.e., 7.35–7.45), the more rapid the onset of action.

A decrease in pH shifts equilibrium toward the ionized form, delaying onset of action. This explains why local anesthetics are slower in onset of action and less effective in the presence of inflammation, which creates a more acidic environment with lower pH. By addition of sodium bicarbonate to certain local anesthetics, we may enhance the onset of action. Overalkalinization, however, can cause local anesthetic molecules to precipitate from solution [2].

Protein Binding

Protein binding is related to the duration of action. The more firmly the local anesthetic binds to the protein of the sodium channel, the longer the duration of action. Poorly protein-bound agents, such as procaine, are readily washed out in in vitro experiments, and duration of local anesthetic blockade can be extremely short, whereas those which are highly protein bound, such as bupivacaine, are less easily washed out in in vitro experiments, and conduction blockade is interrupted for a longer period of time. The clinical activity of the agents which are more protein bound such as bupivacaine and etidocaine are associated with a longer duration of clinical anesthesia. The less well protein-bound agents such as procaine and chloroprocaine are associated with short duration of clinical activity.

Vasodilatation

Most local anesthetics, with the exception of cocaine, have a biphasic effect on vascular smooth muscle. At low doses, they cause vasoconstriction, and at high doses, they cause vasodilation via direct relaxation of peripheral arteriolar smooth muscle fibers. The more vasodilatory property the local anesthetic has, the faster the absorption and thus the shorter the duration of action of the local anesthetic. To counteract this vasodilatation, epinephrine is often included in local anesthetic solutions [3].

Mechanism of Action

Once the local anesthetic reaches the neuron, it reversibly binds to voltage-gated sodium channels, blocking Na+ movement through the channels and thus blocking the action potential and neural conduction. At adequate dosage, these drugs should reversibly inhibit conduction of all neurons.

Na+ (Sodium) Channels

Na+ channels are heterotrimeric transmembrane proteins, consisting of α (Mr~260 kDa), β1 (36 kDa), and β2 (33 kDa) subunits. The α subunit contains four homologous domains (I–IV); each domain contains 6 α-helical transmembrane segments (S1–S6). The voltage sensor is located in the fourth transmembrane segment of each domain which is rich in positively charged residues. The loop between domains III and IV serves as an inactivation gate which folds to block the pore shortly after opening of the channel. The binding site for local anesthetics is located in the S6 transmembrane domain of segment IV close to the intracellular side of the membrane [4].

Function of Na+ (Sodium) Channels

Na+ (sodium) channels can be found in three states. First, there is the closed state at potentials below –70 mV. The pore in the channel is occluded so that Na$^+$ ions cannot pass from one side to the other. Second, the open state of the channel is initiated by depolarization of the transmembrane potential to the threshold potential (usually above –40 mV). In response to depolarization, the channel opens within a millisecond and allows Na$^+$ ions to diffuse down their concentration gradient through the pore, causing an inward current and depolarizing the transmembrane potential even further, which continues a self-driven depolarization [5].

This process underlies the upstroke of the action potential of most excitable cells. During channel opening the S4 segment twists back, driven by both the changed potential difference and intrinsic charge changes, which allow the outer pore mouth to expand, resulting in a 20° twist of the α-helix. The third state follows activation during prolonged depolarization and is termed the inactivated state. The inactivated state was shown to be a nonconducting mode of the channel. The order of affinity of local anesthestics for different sodium channel states is open, inactivated, and lastly, resting. Thus, the open state of the sodium channel is the primary target of local anesthetic molecules. The blocking of propagated action potentials is therefore a function of the frequency of depolarization.

Mechanism of Differential Blockade

After administration of local anesthetics, molecules diffuse from the extraneural site toward the nerves. The rate of diffusion depends on several factors; the most significant of which is the concentration gradient. The greater the initial concentration of the local anesthetic, the faster is the diffusion of its molecules and the more rapid its

Table 11.2 Short- and long-acting anesthetic agents

Short-acting agents	Long-acting agents
Procaine, lidocaine, mepivacaine, prilocaine, chloroprocaine	Tetracaine, bupivacaine, etidocaine, ropivacaine

onset of action. It is important to note that the fasciculi that are located near the surface of the nerve are termed mantle bundles and are reached by the local anesthetic first and blocked completely. The fasciculi found closer to the center of the nerve are called core bundles and are exposed to less concentrated anesthetic solution and delayed response [6].

Thus, small unmyelinated C fibers (pain) and small myelinated Aδ fibers (pain and temperature) are blocked before larger myelinated Aγ, Aβ, and Aα fibers (postural, touch, pressure, and motor signals). In large nerve trunks, motor nerves are usually located circumferentially and may be affected before the sensory fibers. In the extremities, proximal sensory fibers are located more circumferentially than distal sensory fibers. Thus, loss of sense may spread from proximal to distal part of the limb.

It is important to understand that nerves with higher firing frequency and more positive membrane potential are more sensitive to local anesthetic block because the charged (active form) local anesthetic molecules are more likely to access to the binding sites in the open Na+ channel and less likely to dissociate from its binding sites in the open or inactivated channels in comparison with the resting Na+ channels. Sensory fibers, especially pain fibers, have a high firing rate and relatively longer action potential duration than motor fibers and thus are more sensitive to lower concentrations of local anesthetics.

Indications/Clinical Pearls

Local anesthetics are commonly used for the blockade of nerve impulses to abolish a specific sensorimotor function. Specifically, local anesthetics bind to voltage-gated Na+ channels, blocking electrical impulses propagated by neuronal action potentials.

There are many uses of local anesthetics. These include topical applications, injection around nerve endings via peripheral nerve blockade, intrathecal or epidural injections, or intravascular injections for arrhythmia management (see Table 11.2).

In our practice, local anesthetics are most commonly used for peripheral nerve blocks; intravenous regional anesthesia, i.e., Bier blocks; topical and infiltration anesthesia; and neuroaxial blocks. In addition, lidocaine is used as a ventricular antiarrhythmic. In plastic surgeon offices, local anesthesia is also used as tumescent anesthesia. The type and quantity of local anesthetic depends on the type of nerve block, surgical procedure, and physical status of the patient.

Table 11.3 Anesthetic drugs and their suggested max dose

Drug (per 70 kg patient)	Concentration %	Volume CC	Suggested max dose (mg)
Lidocaine	1–2	30–50	500
Mepivacaine	1–1.5	30–50	500
Prilocaine	1–2	30–50	600
Bupivacaine	0.25–0.5	30–50	225
Levobupivacaine	0.25–0.5	30–50	225
Ropivacaine	0.2–0.5	30–50	250

Peripheral Nerve Blocks

A significant difference exists between the onset times of various agents when blocks are done for peripheral nerves. In general, agents of intermediate potency have a more rapid onset than the more potent compounds do. Onset times of approximately 14 min for lidocaine and mepivacaine have been reported versus approximately 23 min for bupivacaine. Epinephrine will increase the duration of most local anesthetics for peripheral nerve blocks, but should not be used for ankle or digit blocks for risk of ischemia (Table 11.3).

When combining two local anesthetics for a given block, usually a short-acting local anesthetic for surgical anesthesia is used, with the combination of a long-acting agent for postoperative pain control. It is recommended to not use the maximum doses for two local anesthetics in combination, because the toxicities are additive [7].

Topical and Infiltrative Local Anesthesia

Infiltrative
All local anesthetics have an immediate onset of action and any local anesthetic may be used for infiltration anesthesia. Duration of action varies and depends on the type of local anesthetic used. Epinephrine can be used to prolong the duration, and it is more pronounced when added to lidocaine. Dilute concentrations will provide equal analgesia.

Topical
Lidocaine, cocaine, dibucaine, tetracaine, and benzocaine are most commonly used for short duration of topical analgesia. EMLA cream, which is a combination of lidocaine and prilocaine, can be used for IV placements. Tetracaine and lidocaine sprays are available for endotracheal intubation, bronchoscopies, and endoscopies.

Intravenous
Bier block is a technique for intravenous regional anesthesia. It traditionally requires 3 mg/kg of low-concentration short-acting agents such as 0.5 % prilocaine or lidocaine without epinephrine. It is not recommended to use bupivacaine for intravenous regional

anesthesia as it is associated with local anesthetic toxicity and death [8]. Dilute solutions of long-acting amide and adjuvants such as tramadol, ketorolac, or clonidine have been used to prolong sensory blockade and analgesia after deflation of the tourniquets [9]. Bier blocks can be used for both upper- and lower-extremity surgeries.

Central Neuroaxial Block

Epidural
Any of the local anesthetic drugs may be used for epidural anesthesia. Potency affects duration of action, with the long-acting agents producing analgesia for 3–4 h and intermediate agents for about 1–2 h. Procaine and tetracaine are rarely used because of their long onset times. Interestingly, the duration of short- and intermediate-acting drugs is significantly prolonged by the addition of epinephrine (1:200,000), but the duration of long-acting drugs is minimally prolonged.

Clinical Pearl
Local anesthetics can be used for differential inhibition of sensory and motor activity. They have a unique property of having a motor-sparing effect; low concentrations will allow for a motor-sparing sensory blockade. Bupivacaine is widely used in obstetrics and for postoperative pain management for its ability of differential inhibition at varying concentrations. Low concentrations will have a motor-sparing effect while providing adequate sensory analgesia.

Increasing the dosage of the local anesthetic can increase the duration of satisfactory anesthesia. This is done by administering either a larger volume or a more concentrated solution. Increasing the concentration of epidurally administered local anesthetic while maintaining the same volume of injectate results in shorter latency, an improved incidence of satisfactory analgesia, and a longer duration of sensory analgesia [10].

Clinical Pearl
Caution should be taken in pregnant patients, as nerve tissue is particularly sensitive to local anesthetics. Lower doses or local anesthetics should be used (Table 11.4).

Spinal
Most of the local anesthetics can be used intrathecally. Caution must be taken with the intermediate local anesthetics such as mepivacaine or lidocaine, as they have an increased incidence of limited transient neurologic symptoms (back pain, paresthesias, radicular pain, or hypoesthesia) [11, 12]. Long-acting agents like bupivacaine are less likely to do so.

Clinical Pearl
The spread of the local anesthetic in the intrathecal space is determined by the baricity of the solution, positioning of the patient immediately after placement, and dose of the injectate.

Table 11.4 Anesthetic drugs and their concentrations for pregnant patients

Drug	Concentration (%)	Volume (cc)
Procaine	10.0	1–2
Lidocaine	1.5, 5.0	1–2
Mepivacaine	4	1–2
Tetracaine	0.25–1.0	1–4
	0.25	2–6
	1.0	1–2
Bupivacaine	0.5	3–4
	0.75	2–3
Levobupivacaine	0.5	3–4
	0.75	2–3
Ropivacaine	0.5	3–4
	0.75	2–3

Tumescent Anesthesia

This is a new technique in the use of local anesthetics for plastic surgery use. During liposuction procedures, surgeons will inject subcutaneously large volumes of dilute local anesthetic in combination with epinephrine. Caution must be taken to prevent adverse outcomes, because very large doses are typically used, typically of lidocaine 35–55 mg/kg [13].

Dosing Options

Absorption of local anesthetics is affected by the following factors: dosage, site of injection, speed of administration, local tissue vascularity, drug-tissue binding, pH, and presence of vasoconstricting drugs.

The maximum dose of each local anesthetic varies as seen in Table 11.2. As seen there is variability in the maximum dosage with and without addition of epinephrine. Since local anesthetics are vasodilators, they tend to be absorbed into the bloodstream from the operative field because of vasodilatation of peripheral arterioles especially in vey vascular tissues. Epinephrine induces vasoconstriction, delaying absorption of the local anesthetic for longer duration of action at the site of injection. By delaying absorption, epinephrine also increases the safe dose of local anesthetic that may be administered.

Each patient situation must be taken into account given that protein binding is an important factor in dosing of local anesthetics. Decreasing protein binding allows more free drugs to be available. For example, in parturient patients, the local anesthetics are more potent and there is a higher level of free drugs, therefore toxicity, in blood due to decreased protein binding.

Bicarbonate is another drug that is commonly added to local anesthetic solutions, particularly when the patient is awake. Because the pH of local anesthetic solutions is generally 4–5 to prolong shelf life, patients often experience burning on injection. Bicarbonate also helps in onset of medication by increasing the nonionic form of the local anesthetic and allowing faster diffusion through tissue. Addition of sodium bicarbonate decreases the latency of onset and increases potency of local anesthetics.

Speed of administration is also important because toxicity develops as a result of peak serum concentration. When multiple areas are to be anesthetized with local anesthetic, inject each site sequentially rather than all at once at the beginning of the procedure. If an area will not be operated on at the beginning of the procedure, wait to inject it until ready to extend the procedure to that site. This spreads the total dose of local anesthetic over a longer period, leading to lower peak serum levels.

Drug Interactions

Ester local anesthetics are rapidly metabolized in the blood via pseudocholinesterases [14]. Amide-type local anesthetics are metabolized by the liver. Anything that reduces hepatic blood flow, i.e., liver or heart failure or certain classes of medications, will increase the likelihood of local anesthetic toxicity. Drugs such as B-blockers and H2 receptor blockers may inhibit cytochrome CYP2D6, responsible for the local anesthetic metabolism [14]. Itraconazole inhibits CYP3A4 and may decrease bupivacaine elimination by 20–25 % [15].

Local Anesthetic Side Effects

Allergic Reactions

These are usually more common with esters, which are infrequently used, since they are derivatives of para-aminobenzoic acid which is a well-recognized allergen. They usually contain methylparaben as a preservative, which is a neurotoxin. Allergy to amides though extremely rare can occur. The reactions range from hypersensitivity to anaphylaxis [16].

Methemoglobinemia

A side effect unique to prilocaine is methemoglobinemia at doses of at least 600 mg. The liver metabolizes prilocaine to o-toluidine which oxidizes hemoglobin to methemoglobin. It is clinically insignificant in healthy adults with normal oxygen-carrying capacity but can cause hypoxemia in infants. Methemoglobinemia is readily treated with methylene blue [17].

Myotoxicity

Skeletal muscle toxicity is a rare and uncommon side effect of local anesthetic drugs. Intramuscular injections of these agents regularly result in reversible myonecrosis. The extent of muscle damage is dose dependent and worsens with serial or continuous administration. All local anesthetic agents that have been examined are myotoxic, whereby procaine produces the least and bupivacaine the most severe muscle injury [18].

Neurotoxicity

In the late 1970s and early 1980s, prolonged sensory and motor deficits were reported in some patients after the epidural or subarachnoid injection of large doses of chloroprocaine. Some studies suggest that the combination of low pH, sodium bisulfite, and inadvertent intrathecal dosing is responsible in part for the neurotoxic reactions observed after the use of large amounts of chloroprocaine solution; other studies have disputed this claim and note that chloroprocaine itself at high concentrations can also be neurotoxic, but these concentrations are probably rarely achieved during properly positioned epidural anesthesia, as opposed to inadvertent spinal anesthesia [19].

Transient Neurologic Syndrome

Single-shot spinal anesthesia with commonly recommended doses and concentrations of many different local anesthetics can produce more limited and transient neurologic symptoms (back pain, paresthesia, radicular pain, or hypoesthesia). The addition of vasoconstrictors to local anesthetic solutions may also increase the risk [20]. Intraoperative positioning also appears to be a risk factor. Patients undergoing surgery in the lithotomy position appear to be at increased risk for neurologic symptoms after either spinal or epidural anesthesia.

Systemic Toxicity

A major cause of adverse reactions to these drugs is high plasma concentration of free unbound medication which may be due to excessive dose, rapid absorption from injection site, diminished tolerance, inadvertent intravascular injection, reduced elimination, or slow metabolic degradation.

The most common toxicities that require immediate countermeasures are related to the central nervous system and the cardiovascular system.

Central Nervous System Effects

Central nervous system toxicity often starts with a change in mentation, followed by perioral paresthesia, a feeling that the subject's whole body is flushing, tinnitus, and generalized seizure as excitation phase followed by depression phase—coma and respiratory and cardiac arrest.

The effects on the CNS may be affected by hypercarbia given that decreased arterial CO_2 pressure also lowers seizure threshold with local anesthetic administration. There is a concomitant increase in cerebral blood flow which allows more local anesthetic to be delivered to the CNS. An increase in intracellular pH leads to ion trapping of the local anesthetic. The acidosis caused by hypercarbia decreases the protein binding of local anesthetics making more drugs available to the CNS. On the other hand, patients receiving CNS depressant drugs such as benzodiazepines or anesthetic drugs will have higher seizure threshold and may not manifest seizure activity before complete CNS depression results.

Cardiovascular System

Toxicity with low doses of local anesthetics may cause hypertension due to vaso-constriction, whereas moderate or high doses result in vasodilatation and decreased SVR.

Local anesthetics have direct effects on the heart and peripheral blood vessels. They block the fast sodium channels in the fast-conducting tissue of Purkinje fibers and ventricles resulting in a decrease rate of depolarization. The effective refractory period and action potential duration are also reduced by local anesthetics. High concentrations can decrease conduction times leading to prolonged PR intervals and widened QRS complexes and even sinus bradycardia/arrest. Ventricular arrhythmias, including fibrillation, are more likely to occur with bupivacaine than lidocaine. Local anesthetics have a dose-dependent negative inotropic effect. This depressant effect is directly proportional to the drugs' relative potency. Patients with acidosis and/or hypoxia are at a greater risk for the cardiac depressant effects of local anesthetics. Cardiotoxicity of local anesthetics can be compared using the CC/CNS dose ratio that is the ratio of the dose causing cardiac collapse (CC) to the dose causing seizure/convulsions. The cardiotoxicity of bupivacaine is unique in that the ratio of the dose required for irreversible cardiovascular collapse (CC) and the dose that will produce CNS toxicity is lower for bupivacaine than other agents. Cardiac resuscitation is more difficult after bupivacaine-induced cardiac arrest. It is important to note that patients under general anesthesia will typically present with cardiotoxicity as the first sign of local anesthetic toxicity given that patients are usually not alert [21]. The very slow reversal of Na^+ channel blockade after a cardiac action potential, which is a hallmark of bupivacaine, is considerably faster with ropivacaine. In addition to these electrical differences, the negative inotropic potency of ropivacaine on isolated cardiac tissue appears to be considerably less than that of bupivacaine. Both electrical and mechanical differences in the toxic profiles may arise from the selective inhibition of Ca^{2+} currents by bupivacaine [22].

Location of Block

With the same amount of local anesthetic, serum levels can differ depending on location and vascularity of the site. For example, serum levels are highest following intercostals blocks followed by epidural/caudal blocks, followed by brachial plexus and femoral/sciatic nerve blocks, followed by subcutaneous injections. This order parallels the vascular supply of each tissue.

Pregnancy

Bupivacaine has been shown to have increased cardiotoxicity in pregnant women resulting in a decreased CC/CNS dose ratio. The FDA discourages the use of 0.75 % concentration of bupivacaine for obstetrical anesthesia. There have been reports of cardiac arrest with difficult resuscitation or death despite the correct management and treatment [23].

Management of Local Anesthetic Toxicity

The treatment of local anesthetic systemic toxicity (LAST) has unique resuscitative measures. Calling for help early, airway management which includes ventilating with 100 % oxygen, seizure treatment with benzodiazepines, and avoiding propofol in cardiovascular instability are important. In cardiopulmonary instability, basic and advanced cardiac life support (ACLS) is necessary but with prolonged effort and avoiding vasopressin, calcium channel blockers, beta-blockers, or local anesthetics. Most importantly, the patients must be treated with lipid emulsion (20 %) with dosing of 1.5 ml/Kg (lean body mass) bolus over 1 min with continuous infusion of 0.25 mL/kg/min. Bolus may be repeated for persistent cardiovascular collapse and the infusion may be doubled [24].

New Vistas

Exparel™ is a novel long-acting liposomal bupivacaine injectable suspension, which was approved by the FDA in Oct. 2011. The technology involves DepoFoam, tiny lipid-based particles containing small discrete water-filled chambers dispersed through the lipid matrix. The particles are 10–30 μm in diameter and the suspension can be injected through a fine needle. Levels persist for approximately 96 h. Thus, this agent could prove quite beneficial clinically as an ultra long-acting local anesthetic.

Summary

Many local anesthetics are available commercially and provide a unique option for analgesia and anesthesia for health-care providers. With the onset of ultrasound technology and improvements in pain management, regional anesthetics will continue to rise. Caution must be taken in administering the local anesthetics as both cardiovascular and central nervous system toxicities are a known risk.

Chemical Structures

Chemical Structure
11.1 Bupivacaine

Chemical Structure
11.2 Benzocaine

Chemical Structure
11.3 Prilocaine

References

1. Vandam LD. Some Aspects of the history of local anesthesia. Local anesthetics: handbook of experimental pharmacology. Heidelberg: Springer; 1987. p. 1–19
2. Wong K, Strichartz GR, Raymond SA. On the mechanisms of potentiation of local anesthetics by bicarbonate buffer: drug structure-activity studies on isolated peripheral nerve. Anesth Analg. 1993;76:131–43.
3. Johns RA, DiFazio CA, Longnecker DE. Lidocaine constricts or dilates rat arterioles in a dose-dependent manner. Anesthesiology. 1985;62:141–4.
4. Arcisio-Miranda M, Muroi Y, Chowdhury S, Chanda B. Molecular mechanism of allosteric modification of voltage-dependent sodium channels by local anesthetics. Physiology. 2010;136(5):541–54.
5. Scholz A. Mechanisms of (local) anaesthetics on voltage-gated sodium and other ion channels. Br J Anaesth. 2002;89:52–61.
6. Zahedi S. Retrospective review of dental local anesthetic induced paresthesia in the United Kingdom. Thesis for masters degree. University of Toronto; 2012. https://tspace.library.uto-ronto.ca/bitstream/1807/33617/1/Zahedi_Sepehr_201211_MSc_thesis.pdf.
7. Badgwell JM, Heavner JE, Kyttä J, Rosenberg PH. Cardiovascular and central nervous system effects of co-administered lidocaine and bupivacaine in piglets. Reg Anesth. 1991; 16:89–94.
8. Davies JAH, Wilkey AD, Hall ID. Bupivacaine leak past inflated tourniquets during intravenous regional analgesia. Anaesthesia. 1984;39:996.
9. Atanassoff PG, Aouad R, Hartmannsgruber MW, Halaszynski T. Levobupivacaine 0.125% and lidocaine 0.5% for intravenous regional anesthesia in volunteers. Anesthesiology. 2002; 97:325.
10. Littlewood DG, Scott DB, Wilson J, Covino B. Comparative anaesthetic properties of various local anaesthetic agents in extradural block for labour. Br J Anaesth. 1979;49:75–9.
11. Freedman JM, Li DK, Drasner K, et al. Transient neurologic symptoms after spinal anesthesia: an epidemiologic study of 1,863 patients. Anesthesiology. 1998;89:633–41 [erratum appears in Anesthesiology 1998 Dec;89(6):1614].
12. Eberhart LH, Morin AM, Kranke P, et al. Transient neurologic symptoms after spinal anesthesia. A quantitative systematic overview (meta-analysis) of randomized controlled studies. Anaesthesist. 2002;51:539–46.
13. Nordström H, Stånge K. Plasma lidocaine levels and risks after liposuction with tumescent anaesthesia. Acta Anaesthesiol Scand. 2005;49:1487–90.
14. Tetzlaff J. Clinical pharmacology of local anesthetics. Woburn: Butterworth-Heinemann; 2000.
15. Palkama VJ, Neuvonen PJ, Olkkola KT. Effect of itraconazole on the pharmacokinetics of bupivacaine enantiomers in healthy volunteers. Br J Anaesth. 1999;83:659–61.
16. Boren E, Teuber SS, Naguwa SM, Gershwin ME. A critical review of local anesthetic sensitivity. Clin Rev Allergy Immunol. 2007;32(1):119–28.
17. Lund P, Cwik J. Propitocaine (Citanest) and methemoglobinemia. Anesthesiology. 1980; 53:259.
18. Zink W, Graf BM. Local anesthetic myotoxicity. Reg Anesth Pain Med. 2004;29(4):333–40.
19. Reisner LS, Hochman BN, Plumer MH. Persistent neurologic deficit and adhesive arachnoiditis following intrathecal 2-chloroprocaine injection. Anesth Analg. 1980;59:452–4.
20. Pollock JE. Transient neurologic symptoms: etiology, risk factors, and management. Reg Anesth Pain Med. 2002;27(6):581–6.
21. De Jong RH, Ronfeld RA, DeRosa RA. Cardiovascular effects of convulsant and supraconvulsant doses of amide local anesthetics. Anesth Analg. 1982;61(1):3–9.
22. Clarkson CW, Hondeghem LM. Mechanism for bupivacaine depression of cardiac conduction: fast block of sodium channels during the action potential with slow recovery from block during diastole. Anesthesiology. 1985;62:396–405.

23. Tsen LC, Tarshis J, Denson DD, Osanthanondh R. Measurements of maternal protein binding of bupivacaine throughout pregnancy. Anesth Analg. 1999;89(4):965–8.
24. Neal JM, Bernards CM, Butterworth JF, Di Gregorio G, Drasner K, Hejtmanck MR, Mulroy MF, Rosenquist RW, Weinberg GL. Checklist for treatment of local anesthetic systemic toxicity. Reg Anesth Pain Med. 2010;35:152–61.

Chapter 12
Neuromuscular Blockers

Gabriel Goodwin and Vilma Joseph

Contents

Introduction

Muscle relaxants were first used on poisonous darts by South American Indians during hunting, according to accounts found in the court of King Ferdinand and Queen Isabella. It took several hundred years until their therapeutic potential was realized in the medical setting [1]. Tubocurarine, the first muscle relaxant used clinically, often produced hypotension and tachycardia through histamine release.

G. Goodwin (✉) • V. Joseph
Department of Anesthesiology, Montefiore Medical Center,
Albert Einstein College of Medicine, Bronx, NY, USA
e-mail: gabrielvangoodwin@gmail.com; vjoseph@montefiore.org

A.D. Kaye et al. (eds.), *Essentials of Pharmacology for Anesthesia,*
Pain Medicine, and Critical Care, DOI 10.1007/978-1-4614-8948-1_12,
© Springer Science+Business Media New York 2015

Today, we have sophisticated neuromuscular blockers (NMBs) that keep the patient paralyzed providing ideal surgical conditions, facilitating intubation and artificial ventilation, with minimal changes to vital signs [2].

Drug Class and Mechanism of Action

Biochemistry of Receptor and Ach

NMBs are classified by their action on the nicotinic acetylcholine receptor (nACHR), as either depolarizing or non-depolarizing. The nACHR has five sub-units. Attachment of acetylcholine to the two alpha subunits causes a conformational change in the receptor. The receptor is opened by this change, allowing depolarization and subsequent muscle twitch. NMBs are quaternary ammonium compounds and thus structurally related to Ach. Due to this similarity, NMBs are able to mimic Ach by attaching to the nACHR, preventing attachment of Ach and subsequent depolarization [3]. Both alpha subunits must be activated by Ach to cause depolarization. Thus, blockade is accomplished even if only one alpha unit is blocked [2].

Categories and Examples

The only clinically relevant depolarizing NMB is succinylcholine (SUX). Biochemically, it consists of two Ach molecules attached by acetate methyl groups. This structure (see figures in "Chemical structures" section at the end of the chapter) explains why succinylcholine acts as an agonist at the nACHR during phase I.

Non-depolarizing NMBs are categorized by their class and by their duration of action. The clinically relevant NMBs are either benzylisoquinolone compounds (long duration of action, d-tubocurarine, metocurarine, doxacurium; intermediate duration of action, atracurium, cisatracurium; short duration of action, mivacurium) or steroids (long duration of action, pancuronium, pipecuronium; intermediate acting, vecuronium, rocuronium).

Depolarizers vs. Non-depolarizers (Mechanism)

The action of a depolarizing NMB is divided into two phases. In the first phase, a depolarizing NMB attaches to the alpha receptor, causing depolarization of the receptor, muscle twitch, and a rise in extracellular potassium levels. In the second phase, the NMB remains attached to the alpha subunit. As a result of its prolonged attachment, it blocks the attachment of Ach molecules, preventing further depolarization. This is considered noncompetitive antagonism since no amount of Ach administered can reverse this blockade.

The action of a non-depolarizing NMB is similar to phase II of a depolarizing NMB. It attaches to the alpha subunit, without causing depolarization, thus preventing the attachment of Ach. This type of blockade is considered competitive, since increasing the concentration of Ach can overcome the blockade and cause depolarization [3].

Chronic disease states associated with decreased release of Ach result in upregulation of extrajunctional receptors, which leads to an increased response to depolarizing NMBs and an increased release of potassium. Contrastingly, these same diseases will cause a decreased response to non-depolarizing NMBs, because more receptors need to be blocked [2].

Indications/Clinical Pearls

NMBs are primarily used to cause paralysis of the vocal cords to facilitate tracheal intubation and to provide surgical relaxation when needed (i.e., laparoscopy). In order to choose the appropriate NMB, the practitioner must consider the type of surgery and patient characteristics.

Rapid sequence induction is a method of inducing and intubating the patient when aspiration of gastric content is of concern. Succinylcholine and rocuronium are the NMBs most commonly chosen. Succinylcholine is the relaxant of choice for rapid sequence induction due to its fast action (60–90 s). A small dose of non-depolarizing muscle relaxation can be used before the use of succinylcholine in order to prevent fasciculations (pre-curarization). If a non-depolarizer must be used for rapid sequence, rocuronium when used at a higher dose is chosen for its short onset of activation. For example, succinylcholine-induced increases in intraocular pressure would be detrimental during an open-globe case. Thus, if the case necessitates the use of succinylcholine, pre-curarization could be used to prevent depolarization, therefore preventing an increase in intraocular pressure.

Organ dysfunction often dictates which NMB is chosen. Atracurium and cisatracurium are spontaneously degraded in the plasma by the Hofmann reaction, making them good choices for muscle relaxation in patients with hepatic or renal dysfunction. Atracurium is also degraded by ester hydrolysis. Mivacurium, like succinylcholine, is degraded by pseudocholinesterase, making it another good choice for patients with hepatic or renal dysfunction [3]. In 2006, mivacurium was discontinued by the manufacturer and is no longer available in the United States [7]. Pancuronium and dTC (d-tubocurarine) are largely degraded by the kidney. Vecuronium is degraded by both the kidney and liver in fairly equal proportions. Rocuronium is largely degraded by the liver [3].

Table 12.1 Relationship between receptor occupancy, T1, T4, T4/T1 ratio, and tetanus during non-depolarizing block [9]

Percentage blocked receptors	T1 (% normal)	T4 (% normal)	T4/T1 (% normal)	Tetanus
100				
95				
	0		T1 lost	
90	10		T2 lost	
	20		T3 lost	
80	25	0	T4 lost	Onset of fade at 30 Hz
	80–90	55–65	0.6–0.7	
	95	70	0.7–0.75	
75	100	75–100	0.75–1	
	100		0.9–1	Onset of fade at 50 Hz
50				Onset of fade at 100 Hz
30				Onset of fade at 200 Hz

Recovery

Recovery from NMB is necessary during emergence from anesthesia, prior to extubation. Incomplete recovery may lead to respiratory depression, necessitating positive-pressure ventilation and/or reintubation. Recovery should be assessed clinically and with a twitch monitor.

The twitch monitor stimulates a nerve (i.e., ulnar nerve), allowing the clinician to assess the patient's level of relaxation. For example, if the patient is completely paralyzed, no amount of stimulation will cause thumb adduction during ulnar nerve stimulation. During "train of four," or TOF, the nerve is stimulated four consecutive times over 2 s. The clinician assesses the strength of each corresponding contraction. If the patient adducts their thumb four times equally, they have 4/4 twitches. However, if the patient only has two strong twitches, the patient has 2/4 twitches. Unfortunately, assessment of twitch is subjective and is thus subject to error. When the patient has 0/4 twitches, >95 % of the receptors are blocked. With four strong twitches (T4/T1 = 1), there could still be blockade of 75 % (see Table 12.1). Therefore, the patient may not be strong enough to maintain spontaneous breathing despite four strong twitches. The four twitches will be weak but equal after administration of a depolarizer. If a non-depolarizer is administered, however, each subsequent twitch will be weaker than the last [4].

Other types of stimulation include tetanus and double burst. During tetanus the patient is stimulated for 5 s at 30–100 Hz. Fade will occur during tetanus during phase II of a depolarizing block and with the use of a non-depolarizer. Phase I will not demonstrate any fade. During double burst stimulation, the nerve is stimulated by two 50 Hz stimuli, separated by 750 msec. In a patient with partial paralysis, the second twitch will be weaker than the first.

Recovery is facilitated with the use of acetylcholinesterases. Acetylcholinesterases antagonize NMBs by increasing Ach. The three most commonly used acetylcholinesterases are neostigmine, pyridostigmine, and edrophonium. An antimuscarinic must be used along with one of the three aforementioned acetylcholinesterases to prevent undesirable cholinergic effects. Glycopyrrolate is administered with neostigmine and atropine is administered with edrophonium because of similarities in onset of activation [2].

Abductor pollicis is a better indicator of recovery of the muscles of the upper airway for reversal than orbicularis oculi or corrugator supercilii. Thus, train of four should be assessed at the abductor pollicis before reversal is administered [5]. Head lift for 5 s correlates with a train of four of 0.6 or less [10].

Neuromuscular blockers are agonized or antagonized by a variety of medications. Most antibiotics can cause blockade even without the use of a NMB. Magnesium enhances non-depolarizing NMBs but most likely antagonizes succinylcholine blockade. Calcium antagonizes muscle relaxation, whereas dantrolene enhances NMB by preventing release of calcium (recall that depolarization at the neuromuscular junction causes a surge of calcium release, leading to muscle contraction). Lithium can both enhance and antagonize NMBs secondary to its structural relationship to sodium and potassium. Local anesthetics enhance NMBs. Acute furosemide usage enhances dTC and succinylcholine. Acetazolamide antagonizes acetylcholinesterase. Steroids antagonize non-depolarizing NMBs. Antiestrogen medication potentiates non-depolarizing NMBs [3]. By decreasing the level of pseudocholinesterase, pregnancy, as well as hepatic and renal failure, prolongs the action of succinylcholine. This can lead to dangerous elevations of potassium levels secondary to the depolarization succinylcholine causes during phase I blockade. Acidosis, hypokalemia, and hypothermia prolong the effects of NMBs.

Dosing Options (Table 12.2)

The intubation dose is twice the ED95 (95 % depression of twitch). Less blockade is needed for surgical relaxation post-intubation. Maintenance is achieved by redosing the NMB at slightly less than ED95. When considering dosages, it is important to remember that drug interactions might increase or decrease the amount of NMB that is required [3].

Drug Interactions

Concomitant usage of medications can alter the duration of action and dosages of NMBs. Other drug interactions can cause hemodynamic effects.

Table 12.2 Drugs and their dosing options [2]

Drug	ED95 for adductor pollicis during N_2/O_2 anesthesia (mg/kg)	Intubation dose (mg/kg)	Onset of action for intubating dose (min)	Duration of intubating dose (min)	Maintenance dosing by boluses (mg/kg)	Maintenance dosing by infusion (mcg/kg/min)
Succinylcholine	0.5	1.0	0.5	5–10	0.15	2–15 mg/min
Rocuronium	0.3	0.8	1.5	35–75	0.15	9–12
Mivacurium	0.08	0.2	2.5–3.0	15–20	0.05	4–15
Atracurium	0.2	0.5	2.5–3.0	30–45	0.1	5–12
Cisatracurium	0.05	0.2	2.0–3.0	40–75	0.02	1–2
Vecuronium	0.05	0.12	2.0–3.0	45–90	0.01	1–2
Pancuronium	0.07	0.12	2.0–3.0	60–120	0.01	–
Pipecuronium	0.05	0.1	2.0–3.0	80–120	0.01	–
Doxacurium	0.025	0.07	4.0–5.0	90–150	0.05	–

Duration

Prolonged depolarization after administration of succinylcholine occurs if administered after neostigmine and pyridostigmine secondary to inhibition of pseudocholinesterase. Pancuronium can also prolong the effects of succinylcholine by inhibiting pseudocholinesterase.

Mivacurium-rocuronium combinations have a faster onset of activation and shorter duration of activation than either relaxant used in isolation.

Hemodynamics

Vecuronium, atracurium, and cisatracurium cause bradycardia with concomitant opioid usage.

Requirements

Inhaled anesthetics decrease requirements by 30–50 % in order from greatest to least: desflurane>sevoflurane>isoflurane>halothane>NO_2-barbiturate-opioid or propofol. NMBs of the same class have additive effects. NMBs of differing classes have synergistic effects.

Side Effects/Black Box Warnings

After phase II blockade, succinylcholine diffuses away from the end plate to be degraded by plasma cholinesterase/pseudocholinesterase. Since this enzyme is made in the liver, patients with advanced liver disease may be predisposed to prolonged blockade by succinylcholine. Similarly, pregnancy prolongs the duration of succinylcholine by decreasing pseudocholinesterase levels. Patients with genetic pseudocholinesterase deficiency are also susceptible to prolonged blockade by succinylcholine. The amount of deficiency can be quantified by the dibucaine number. Dibucaine is a local anesthetic that inhibits normal pseudocholinesterase to a greater extent than abnormal pseudocholinesterase. The dibucaine number is the percentage of enzyme that is inhibited. A patient with a dibucaine number of 70–80 is considered normal, 50–60 is considered to have a heterozygous atypical enzyme, and 20–30 is considered to have a homozygous atypical enzyme.

Succinylcholine can cause cardiac arrhythmias from two separate mechanisms. As it is structurally related to Ach, it can cause bradycardia through vagal stimulation. Alternately, as a result of depolarization in phase I, potassium is transferred out of the cells. Succinylcholine typically elevates the potassium level by 0.5 meq/l. Hyperkalemia can cause arrhythmias or asystole. Patients with immobility greater than 24 h or disorders that result in increased levels of extrajunctional Ach receptors, such as stroke, muscular dystrophies, Guillain-Barre, trauma, and burn patients, should not receive succinylcholine due to the risk or hyperkalemia. Of note, succinylcholine can be administered safely within the first 24 h after a burn has occurred since extrajunctional Ach receptors have not proliferated yet. Other miscellaneous side effects of succinylcholine include increased intraocular pressure, gastric pressure, and intracranial pressure; masseter spasm; and myalgias due to the diffuse fasciculations during phase I blockade and tachycardia.

Laudanosine is a metabolite of atracurium. This metabolite can cause central nervous system stimulation and cardiovascular depression. As opposed to atracurium's spontaneous degradation in the plasma, laudanosine's degradation is largely dependent on the liver [3].

Long-term administration of vecuronium to patients in intensive care units has resulted in prolonged neuromuscular blockade (up to several days), possibly from accumulation of its active 3-hydroxy metabolite, changing drug clearance, or the development of a polyneuropathy [2]. Further prolongation may occur with hepatic and/or renal failure, as vecuronium is degraded by the two aforementioned organ systems.

Pancuronium has become less clinically relevant due to its ability to cause tachycardia. These cardiovascular effects are a combination of vagolytic activity and sympathetic stimulation of ganglions. Since pancuronium is almost exclusively degraded in the kidney, renal failure can cause increased duration of action, with pronounced vagolytic action [3].

Several NMBs cause the release of histamine. These include succinylcholine, mivacurium, atracurium, and dTC. The release of histamine can result in tachycardia and hypotension.

NMB can alter the pulmonary tree. Depending on which muscarinic receptor is stimulated, NMBs can cause either bronchoconstriction or bronchorelaxation. Stimulation of the muscarinic receptor M3 causes bronchoconstriction. This effect is enhanced if M2 is simultaneously stimulated. Contrastingly, the stimulation of M1 results in bronchorelaxation [8]. Rapacuronium, a short-acting non-depolarizer, was removed from clinical practice because of its association with bronchospasm secondary to its action on the M2 receptor [11].

NMB administration causes the most allergic reactions out of all medications administered by the anesthesiologist. This is a result of the ammonium ion in the NMB. The NMBs that are most commonly implicated for allergic reactions were rocuronium followed by atracurium [3].

Succinylcholine, as well as volatile anesthetics can cause the patient to develop malignant hyperthermia (MH). This is an autosomal dominant genetic disorder, characterized by a hypermetabolic state, increased sympathetic drive, and rhabdomyolysis secondary to skeletal muscle activation. The first signs include hypercarbia and tachycardia. Afterwards, hypertension, masseter muscle rigidity, and hyperthermia may develop. Ironically, hyperthermia is often a late sign. MH is thought to occur due to an abnormal ryanodine receptor, leading to increased calcium release from the sarcoplasmic reticulum, thus causing increased muscle depolarization. This is a true medical emergency which must be addressed promptly [6].

Summary

What was once used to hunt game (neuromuscular blockade) is now commonplace in the operating room. When administered properly, it can allow the anesthesiologist to intubate with ease and facilitate the job of the surgeon. For safe administration, however, the practitioner must be familiar with its dosage, interactions, and side effects.

Chemical Structures

Chemical Structures
12.1 Tubocurarine chloride

Chemical Structures
12.2 Pancuronium

Chemical Structures 12.3 Succinylcholine

Chemical Structures
12.4 Succinylcholine

Succinylcholine modecule

Chemical Structures
12.5 Rocuronium bromide

References

1. Thandla R. Neuromuscular blocking drugs: discovery and development. J R Soc Med. 2002;95(7):363–7.
2. Morgan GE, Mikhail MS, Murray MJ. Clinical Anesthesiology. 4th ed. New York: McGraw-Hill Companies, Inc; 2006.
3. Miller R, Eriksson L, Fleisher L, Wiener-Kronish J, Young W. Miller's Anesthesia. 7th ed. Churchill Livingstone: Elsevier; 2009.
4. Waud BE, Waud DR. The relation between the response to "train-of-four" stimulation and receptor occlusion during competitive neuromuscular block. Anesthesiology. 1972;37(4):413–6.

 5. Thilen SR, Hansen BE, Ramaiah R, Kent CD, Treggiari MM, Bhananker SM. Intraoperative neuromuscular monitoring site and residual paralysis. Anesthesiology. 2012;117(5):964–72.
 6. Kim DC. Malignant hyperthermia. Kor J Anesthesiol. 2012;63(5):391–401.
 7. FDA (last updated 1/24/2013). Drugs to be discontinued. http://www.fda.gov/drugs/drug-safety/drugshortages/ucm050794.htm.
 8. Stuckmann N, Schwering S, Wiegand S, Gschnell A, Yamada M, Kummer W, Wess J, Haberberger R. Role of muscarinic receptor subtypes in the constriction of peripheral airways: studies on receptor-deficient mice. Mol Pharmacol. 2003;64(6):1444–51.
 9. Padmaja D, Mantha S. Monitoring of neuromuscular junction. Indian J Anaesth. 2002;46(4):279–88.
10. Barash P, Cullen B, Stoelting R, Cahalan M, Stock C, Ortega R. Clinical anesthesia. 7th ed. Philadelphia: Lippincott; 2013.
11. Jooste E, Klafter F, Hirshman CA, Emala CW. A mechanism for rapacuronium-induced bronchospasm: M2 muscarinic receptor antagonism. Anesthesiology. 2003;98(4):906–11.

Chapter 13
Reversal Agents

Andrew Sim and Angela Vick

Contents

A. Sim, MD (✉) • A. Vick
Department of Anesthesiology, Montefiore Medical Center, Albert Einstein
College of Medicine, Bronx, NY, USA
e-mail: ansim@montefiore.org; avick@montefiore.org

A.D. Kaye et al. (eds.), *Essentials of Pharmacology for Anesthesia,*
Pain Medicine, and Critical Care, DOI 10.1007/978-1-4614-8948-1_13,
© Springer Science+Business Media New York 2015

Introduction

One of the clinical indications for administering cholinesterase inhibitors, or anticholinesterases, is to reverse the effect of muscle relaxation by non-depolarizing neuromuscular blocking agents at the conclusion of surgery. The purpose of administering antimuscarinic drugs concomitantly with anticholinesterases is to minimize the muscarinic side effects associated with increased acetylcholine transmission at muscarinic receptors. Besides their routine uses in the operating room, anticholinesterases and antimuscarinic drugs have a host of other important clinical uses. This chapter will review cholinergic pharmacology, the indications for using anticholinesterases and anticholinergic agents, and the mechanisms of action as well as adverse effects of anticholinesterases and anticholinergic agents.

Drug Class and Mechanism of Action

In the peripheral nervous system, acetylcholine is the neurotransmitter at the neuromuscular junction between the motor nerve and skeletal muscle. In the autonomic nervous system, acetylcholine is the neurotransmitter in the preganglionic sympathetic and parasympathetic neurons. Acetylcholine also serves as the neurotransmitter at the adrenal medulla and serves as the neurotransmitter in all parasympathetic innervated organs [1].

Acetylcholine is synthesized from two precursors: choline and acetyl coenzyme A by the enzyme choline O-acetyltransferase in the nerve terminal [2]. It is released into the synapse where it then binds to acetylcholine receptors and is then rapidly hydrolyzed in the synapse by acetylcholinesterase into acetate and choline. Acetylcholinesterase is a type B carboxylesterase in the neuromuscular junction that can catalyze 4,000 molecules of acetylcholine per active site per second [3]. The active surface of acetylcholinesterase has two sites: the anionic site, which binds and orients the substrate molecule, and the esteratic site, which is responsible for hydrolysis.

The primary acetylcholine receptor subtypes were named after the alkaloids originally used in their identification: muscarine and nicotine. Muscarine, a chemical isolated from mushroom, causes effects similar to those produced by activation of the parasympathetic nervous system. The muscarinic receptor is a G protein-coupled receptor. Drugs that mimic the effects of muscarine on parasympathetically innervated organs, such as the heart, smooth muscles, and glands, have been called muscarinic drugs. In the early 1900s, nicotine was found to act on autonomic ganglia and skeletal muscle receptors [1]. These receptors were known as nicotinic. The nicotinic receptor acts as an ion channel, and drugs that act on these receptors system are called nicotinic drugs. While nicotinic and muscarinic receptors differ in their response to nicotine and muscarine, they both respond to acetylcholine and were thus both recognized as cholinoceptor subtypes.

Neuromuscular transmission is dependent on acetylcholine binding to nicotinic receptors on the motor end plate. Non-depolarizing muscle relaxants act via competitive antagonism by competing with acetylcholine for receptor binding sites, thus blocking neuromuscular transmission. Depolarizing muscle relaxants such as succinylcholine act as receptor agonists. Succinylcholine binds to acetylcholine receptors, generating a muscle action potential. However, succinylcholine is not metabolized by acetylcholinesterase, so its continued presence in the synaptic cleft leads to prolonged depolarization of the muscle end plate.

Since depolarizing muscle relaxants are not metabolized by acetylcholinesterase, they diffuse away from the neuromuscular junction and are hydrolyzed in plasma and the liver by pseudocholinesterase. However, the recovery from non-depolarizing neuromuscular blockade is dependent on an increase in the acetylcholine concentration in the neuromuscular junction relative to the concentration of muscle relaxant. The relative increase of acetylcholine must occur in order to overcome competitive blockade. This relative increase depends on redistribution, metabolism, and excretion of the drug, as well as the administration of reversal agents [4].

Anticholinesterases

After acetylcholine is released from autonomic and somatic motor nerves, its action is terminated by the rapid hydrolysis of the molecule by acetylcholinesterase. The anticholinesterase drugs (cholinesterase inhibitors) are indirect-acting cholinomimetics; that is, they exert their primary effect at the active site of the enzyme, rendering it inactive. By inhibiting enzyme function, they prevent the hydrolysis of acetylcholine, indirectly increasing the concentration of endogenous acetylcholine in the neuromuscular junction. This allows for more acetylcholine molecules to bind to postsynaptic receptors, "overcoming" the non-depolarizing blockade.

The commonly used anticholinesterases fall into three chemical groups: (1) simple alcohols bearing a quaternary ammonium group (e.g., edrophonium), (2) carbamic acid esters of alcohols bearing quaternary or tertiary ammonium groups (the carbamates, e.g., neostigmine), and (3) organic derivatives of phosphoric acid (organophosphates, e.g., echothiophate) [5].

Neostigmine, edrophonium, and pyridostigmine are all clinically used anticholinesterases. They are lipid insoluble, quaternary ammonium compounds that do not cross the blood-brain barrier, and thus have no effect on cholinergic function in the central nervous system. Physostigmine is a lipid soluble, tertiary ammonium compound that crosses the blood-brain barrier, and thus is not used clinically to reverse neuromuscular blockade.

Before further discussion of the anticholinesterases, an understanding of the mechanism of action of acetylcholinesterase is required. The enzymatic action of acetylcholinesterase is a two-step process. In the first step, acetylcholinesterase binds acetylcholine at the enzyme's active site. Acetylcholine is hydrolyzed to free choline and acetylated enzyme. In the second step, the covalent acetyl-enzyme bond is split by the addition of water.

Neostigmine and pyridostigmine are oxydiaphoretic (acid-transferring) anticholinesterases. They transfer a carbamate group to acetylcholinesterase and form a covalent bond at the esteratic site. The covalent bond of the carbamoylated enzyme resists breakdown by hydration and lasts on the order of 30 min to 6 h. Edrophonium is a prosthetic inhibitor; it reversibly binds to the anionic site on the enzyme by electrostatic attraction and to the esteratic site by hydrogen bonding. The enzyme-inhibitor complex does not involve a covalent bond and is correspondingly short-lived (2–10 min). The organophosphates undergo initial binding and hydrolysis by acetylcholinesterase, but the result is a phosphorylated active site. The covalent phosphorylated enzyme bond is extremely stable and hydrolyzes water at a slow rate [5].

The inhibition of acetylcholinesterase by anticholinesterases occurs at every cholinergic synapse in the peripheral nervous system, including at muscarinic receptors. Thus, when attempting to reverse non-depolarizing neuromuscular blockade, the resulting activation of muscarinic receptors causes several undesired side effects, depending on the organ involved. Therefore, the goal of reversing neuromuscular blockade with anticholinesterases is to maximize nicotinic transmission while minimizing untoward muscarinic effects.

Sugammadex

Although not yet available for clinical use in the United States (as of this writing), sugammadex is an important new drug in neuromuscular pharmacology. Sugammadex is the first selective relaxant binding agent, meaning that it acts by forming a complex with steroidal neuromuscular blocking agents (rocuronium > vecuronium >> pancuronium). For example, the intravenous administration of sugammadex during rocuronium-induced neuromuscular blockade causes rapid removal of free rocuronium molecules from plasma. This causes a concentration gradient of rocuronium molecules between the neuromuscular junction and plasma, favoring movement away from the junction into circulating plasma. There, they continue to form complexes with free sugammadex molecules, terminating the neuromuscular blockade of rocuronium. Sugammadex has no effect on acetylcholinesterase or any receptor system of the body, thus eliminating the need for anticholinergic drugs and their side effects [3].

The implications of sugammadex-induced reversal neuromuscular blockade are that the combination of rocuronium and sugammadex can possibly replace succinylcholine for rapid-sequence induction as well as completely eliminate residual paralysis in the postanesthesia recovery room [3].

Antimuscarinics

Muscarinic receptors are present in end-organ effector cells in smooth muscle, the sinoatrial node and atrioventricular node, and the lacrimal and salivary glands. Anticholinesterases will act on muscarinic receptors in the sinoatrial and atrioventricular node by causing bradycardia, which can progress to sinus arrest. In bronchial smooth muscle, muscarinic receptor activation can lead to bronchospasm and increased respiratory tract secretions. Gastrointestinal receptors respond to increased acetylcholine with increased glandular secretions and peristaltic activity. These undesired side effects of anticholinesterase administration are attenuated by prior or concomitant administration of antimuscarinic medications.

Antimuscarinics are often called parasympatholytic because they block the effects of parasympathetic autonomic discharge. Naturally occurring antimuscarinic compounds have been known and used for centuries as medicines, poisons, and cosmetics [5].

Atropine, the prototypical antimuscarinic, is a tertiary amine alkaloid ester of tropic acid. It is highly selective for muscarinic receptors, causing reversible blockade of cholinomimetic actions. When atropine binds to the muscarinic receptor, it prevents the release of inositol triphosphate and the inhibition of adenylyl cyclase caused by muscarinic agonists [5].

Indications

The major therapeutic uses of the anticholinesterases are for reversal of neuromuscular blockade following surgery, diseases of the eye, the gastrointestinal and urinary tracts, the neuromuscular junction, and the heart.

Surgery

One of the most common indications for administering anticholinesterases is to reverse residual neuromuscular blockade at the end of surgery. In the United States, anticholinesterases are the only compounds currently used clinically to reverse neuromuscular blockade [2]. Anticholinesterases are indicated only for patients who have received non-depolarizing muscle relaxants. Complete reversal, or return of neuromuscular function, should be achieved at the end of surgery unless continued mechanical ventilation is planned. Three anticholinesterases are used to antagonize residual neuromuscular blockade – neostigmine, pyridostigmine, and edrophonium.

Myasthenia Gravis

Myasthenia gravis is a disease affecting the neuromuscular junction. It is an autoimmune process that causes antibodies to nicotinic receptors on motor end plates. Clinical signs include ptosis and diplopia, and symptoms include difficulty speaking and swallowing and extremity weakness that classically worsens with repetition. Severe disease may affect the muscles of respiration.

Anticholinesterases are valuable therapeutic agents for myasthenia gravis. Edrophonium is used as a diagnostic test for myasthenia. A dose is administered intravenously after baseline muscle strength has been established. If the patient has myasthenia, a temporary improvement in muscle strength will be observed.

Neostigmine and pyridostigmine are used for long-term therapy. Since these agents are relatively short acting, they require frequent dosing (every 4 h for neostigmine and every 6 h for pyridostigmine) [5].

Gastrointestinal and Urinary Tracts

For disease states that depress smooth muscle activity without obstruction, such as postoperative ileus, congenital megacolon, urinary retention, or neurogenic bladder, anticholinesterases may be helpful. Of the anticholinesterases, neostigmine is the most widely used [5].

Alzheimer's Disease

Alzheimer's disease is a neurodegenerative disorder with a poorly understood etiology and limited effective therapy. The cholinergic system has been recognized as being affected by the pathological processes of the disease, and a lack of acetylcholine has been identified in the early phases of degradation. Donepezil, galantamine, and rivastigmine are anticholinesterases used in the treatment of Alzheimer's disease.

The Eye

Glaucoma is a disease of the eye characterized by increased intraocular pressure. Physostigmine has been used in the past to cause contraction of the ciliary body, which increases the outflow of aqueous humor and thus reduces intraocular pressure.

Antimuscarinic Drug Intoxication

Severe muscarinic receptor blockade, produced by antimuscarinics such as atropine, or drugs with antimuscarinic properties such as the tricyclic antidepressants, can cause severe behavioral disturbances and fatal arrhythmias. The receptor blockade caused by these drugs can be overcome by increasing the amount of endogenous acetylcholine reaching the muscarinic receptor, and physostigmine has been used clinically because of its ability to cross the blood-brain barrier. Since it is able to enter the central nervous system, it can reverse the central as well as the peripheral signs of muscarinic blockade.

Antimuscarinics

Antimuscarinics are routinely administered prior to or concomitantly with the administration of anticholinesterases when reversing non-depolarizing neuromuscular blockade. This is done to prevent the untoward side effects of muscarinic activity following an increase in acetylcholine concentration. Antimuscarinic agents have a host of therapeutic uses based on their site of action.

Central Nervous System

Centrally acting antimuscarinic drugs were among the first drugs used to treat the tremor of Parkinson's disease. Since Parkinsonian tremor and rigidity are the result of a relative excess of cholinergic activity due to a deficiency of dopaminergic activity in the basal ganglia-striatum system, antimuscarinics are sometimes used with dopamine agonists for therapy.

Motion sickness and other vestibular disorders respond to antimuscarinics, as well as antihistamine agents with antimuscarinic effects. Scopolamine is one of the oldest and most effective treatments for seasickness.

Eye

Pupillary constrictor muscle activation is blocked by antimuscarinic drugs. The result is unopposed sympathetic dilation and mydriasis. Ciliary muscle contraction is also weakened by antimuscarinic drugs, causing the loss of accommodation. Both mydriasis and cycloplegia are useful for ophthalmology when performing a complete eye exam. Antimuscarinics also act to decrease lacrimal gland secretion, which can produce the sensation of dry, sandy eyes.

Respiratory

Antimuscarinics relax the bronchial smooth musculature, decrease respiratory tract secretions, and thus reduce airway resistance. For these reasons, atropine was routinely used preoperatively when older volatile anesthetics such as ether were used, because these anesthetics were associated with increased airway secretions and laryngospasm. Today's volatile anesthetics are less irritating, but premedication with glycopyrrolate or atropine is useful for reducing airway secretions for awake endotracheal intubation or fiberoptic bronchoscopy. Patients with reactive airways such as asthmatics have found therapeutic benefit with the inhalational antimuscarinics ipratropium and tiotropium. Patients with COPD also benefit from the use of these inhaled agents.

Cardiovascular

Blockade of M2 receptors in the sinoatrial node results in tachycardia. The SA node is sensitive to antimuscarinics, and they are particularly useful in reversing bradycardia secondary to vagal discharge.

Gastrointestinal

As mentioned above, airway secretions are reduced by antimuscarinics. Salivary and gastric secretions are also reduced by these agents. Antimuscarinics also decrease intestinal motility and peristalsis, prolonging gastric emptying time. For these reasons, antimuscarinic agents can be used to provide symptomatic relief in traveler's diarrhea and other conditions of hypermotility.

Urinary

Antimuscarinics decrease ureter and bladder tone as a result of smooth muscle relaxation. They have been used to provide some relief in the treatment of urinary urgency, incontinence, bladder spasm, and ureteral smooth muscle spasm.

Dosing Options

This section will focus on dosing options for reversal of residual neuromuscular blockade at the conclusion of surgery. The time required to recover from neuromuscular blockade caused by non-depolarizing muscle relaxants is dependent on several factors, including the choice and dose of cholinesterase inhibitor administered, the muscle relaxant being antagonized, and the extent of blockade before reversal [6]. Recovery of muscle strength is dependent primarily on an increase in the acetylcholine concentration relative to that of muscle relaxant in the neuromuscular junction to overcome the competitive blockade. This increase in acetylcholine is first dependent on the ongoing movement of muscle relaxant from the motor end plate into the central circulation, followed by its elimination from the circulating blood volume [1]. Generally, more time is needed to antagonize profound levels of blockade than lesser levels [7].

Dosage requirements of anticholinesterases depend on degree of block, which can be partially determined by response to peripheral nerve stimulation. Peripheral nerve stimulators should be used to monitor progress and confirm adequacy of reversal; however, peripheral nerve stimulation is both unreliable by visual measurement (train-of-four) and uncomfortable in awake patients, so end points of recovery can be sustained tetanus for 5 s in response to 100 Hz stimulus in anesthetized patients or sustained head lift in awake patients [6].

Some spontaneous recovery must be present before reversal can be attempted, and reversal takes longer when deep blockade (no twitch or one twitch present to train-of-four stimulation) than if four twitches are present. Under the conditions of moderate depth of blockade, the speed of antagonism of residual blockade by anticholinesterases is edrophonium > neostigmine > pyridostigmine. In general, larger doses of anticholinesterases should antagonize neuromuscular blockade more rapidly than smaller doses. However, this relationship only holds true to the point of the maximum effective dose, beyond which additional amounts of anticholinesterase will not produce any further antagonism (60–80 μg/kg neostigmine, 70 μg/kg pyridostigmine, 1–1.5 mg/kg edrophonium) [1]. It is actually not advisable to administer additional anticholinesterase if these doses fail to antagonize residual blockade, as they may actually render patients weaker [8].

Neostigmine

The maximum recommended dose of neostigmine is 80 μg/kg. The maximum antagonistic effect of neostigmine occurs in 10 min or less; if adequate recovery does not occur within this amount of time, then recovery requires further elimination of the muscle relaxant from circulating plasma [1]. Pediatric and elderly patients experience a more rapid onset and require a smaller dose than adults, as they appear to be more sensitive to its effects [6]. As discussed earlier in this chapter, an antimuscarinic is administered prior to or concomitantly with an anticholinesterase in order to minimize muscarinic side effects. Glycopyrrolate is often administered with neostigmine (0.2 mg glycopyrrolate per 1 mg neostigmine) because of a similar onset of action.

Pyridostigmine

The maximum recommended dose of pyridostigmine is 0.4 mg/kg. It has a slower onset than that of neostigmine, and its duration is slightly longer (>2 h). It is administered with either glycopyrrolate or atropine, with glycopyrrolate being preferred due to its slower onset of action [6].

Edrophonium

Edrophonium has the most rapid onset of action (1–2 min) and the shortest duration of effect of the anticholinesterases used to reverse non-depolarizing neuromuscular blockade. This is due to the electrostatic and hydrogen bonds formed by the enzyme and the anticholinesterase. The recommended dosage is 0.5–1 mg/kg, and its rapid onset is best paired with atropine (0.014 mg atropine per 1 mg edrophonium) [6]. Unlike with neostigmine, pediatric patients and elderly patients are not more sensitive to edrophonium reversal. Edrophonium does not produce the same degree of muscarinic side effects at equipotent doses as neostigmine and pyridostigmine. Glycopyrrolate can also be paired with edrophonium, but because of a slower onset, it should be administered several minutes prior to edrophonium to avoid bradycardia.

Drug Interactions

Many drugs have been shown to interact with neuromuscular blocking drugs and anticholinesterases, affecting duration of block and time for recovery. Drugs that potentiate neuromuscular blockade can slow reversal if given after anticholinesterase administration. We will review some of the more important drug interactions in this section.

Inhaled Anesthetics

Inhaled anesthetics enhance the neuromuscular blocking effects of non-depolarizing neuromuscular blocking drugs. They decrease the dose of drug required for paralysis, as well as prolong both the duration of block and recovery from block [9]. Withdrawal of the inhaled anesthetic at the end of surgery will speed anticholinesterase reversal [10].

Antibiotics

Antagonism of neuromuscular blockade has been reported to be more difficult after the administration of certain antibiotics, particularly aminoglycosides [11]. Aminoglycosides, polymyxins, and clindamycin will inhibit the prejunctional release of acetylcholine and also depress postjunctional nicotinic acetylcholine receptor sensitivity to acetylcholine. When combined with neuromuscular blocking drugs, these antibiotics can potentiate neuromuscular blockade.

Magnesium

Magnesium potentiates the neuromuscular blockade induced by non-depolarizing neuromuscular blocking drugs, and neostigmine-induced recovery is also attenuated in patients treated with magnesium [12]. This potentiation may be due to magnesium's inhibitory effect both on calcium channels at presynaptic nerve terminals responsible for release of acetylcholine and on postjunctional potentials, causing decreased excitability of muscle fiber membranes.

Local Anesthetics

Local anesthetics act on presynaptic, postsynaptic, and muscle membranes. In small doses, they enhance the neuromuscular blockade produced by both depolarizing and non-depolarizing neuromuscular blocking drugs; in large doses, they block neuromuscular transmission [13].

Side Effects

Anticholinesterases

Many of the side effects of anticholinesterases are actually direct extensions of their pharmacologic actions. The dominant initial signs are those of muscarinic excess: miosis, salivation, bronchospasm, increased respiratory secretions, vomiting, increased peristalsis, fecal incontinence, and bradyarrhythmias. CNS signs follow, accompanied by peripheral nicotinic effects, especially depolarizing neuromuscular blockade causing weakness [5]. When reversing non-depolarizing neuromuscular blockade with anticholinesterases, the muscarinic effects are prevented or attenuated with concomitant antimuscarinic treatment with atropine or glycopyrrolate. If acute toxicity is from organophosphate exposure or accidental anticholinesterase overdose, the therapy includes maintenance of vital signs and atropine and pralidoxime in organophosphate exposure.

Neostigmine has been reported to cross the placenta, resulting in fetal bradycardia. Thus, atropine may be a better choice of anticholinergic agent than glycopyrrolate in pregnant patients receiving neostigmine [6].

Anticholinesterases are excreted via the kidneys by active secretion into the tubular lumen so that clearance is reduced (and duration of action increased) in renal failure.

Antimuscarinics

Side effects of antimuscarinics are related to their effects on each organ system. Tachycardia, dry mouth/throat, xerostomia, ataxia and drowsiness, ileus, urinary retention, mydriasis, cycloplegia, diplopia, and increased intraocular pressure are all consequence of organ systems discussed. In addition, inhibition of sweat glands can cause impaired thermoregulation and an increase in body temperature, and dilation of cutaneous blood vessels can cause a red, flushed appearance.

At higher concentrations, atropine causes block of all parasympathetic functions. Children, especially infants, are very sensitive to the hyperthermic effects of atropine, with deaths following doses as low as 2 mg. Antimuscarinic overdose is generally treated symptomatically, requiring temperature control with cooling blankets and seizure control with benzodiazepines [5].

Summary

While anticholinesterases and antimuscarinics are fundamental agents in the operating room, they also have a huge host of other clinical applications. Although neuromuscular blockade is an essential component of a balanced anesthetic and airway management, residual neuromuscular blockade can lead to airway obstruction, inadequate ventilation, and hypoxia. As clinicians, our knowledge of anticholinesterases and antimuscarinics is paramount in both providing safety to our patients from extubation to postoperative recovery and caring for our patients outside of the surgical setting.

Chemical Structures

Chemical Structure
13.1 Neostigmine

Chemical Structure
13.2 Physostigmine

Chemical Structure
13.3 Pyridostigmine

Chemical Structure   Acetlcholine
13.4 Acetylcholine

Succinylcholine (diacetylcholine)

References

1. Glick DB. The autonomic nervous system. In: Miller RD, editor. Miller's anesthesia. 7th ed. Orlando: Churchill Livingstone; 2009.
2. Pohanka M. Acetylcholinesterase inhibitors; a patent review (2008-present). Expert Opin Ther Pat. 2012;22:871–86. doi:10.1517/13543776.2012.701620.

3. Naguib M, Lien CA. Pharmacology of muscle relaxants and their antagonists. In: Miller RD, editor. Miller's anesthesia. 7th ed. Orlando: Churchill Livingstone; 2009.

4. Donati F, Bevan DR. Neuromuscular blocking agents. In: Barash PG, editor. Clinical anesthesia. 6th ed. Philadelphia: Lippincott Williams & Wilkins; 2009.

5. Katzung BG. Cholinoceptor-blocking drugs. In: Basic and clinical pharmacology. 12th ed. New York: McGraw-Hill; 2011.

6. Morgan GE, Mikhail MS. Cholinesterase inhibitors. In: Clinical anesthesiology. 4th ed. New York: McGraw-Hill; 2006.

7. Bevan JC, Collins L, Fowler C, et al. Early and late reversal of rocuronium and vecuronium with neostigmine in adults and children. Anesth Analg. 1999;89:333–9.

8. Caldwell JE. Reversal of residual neuromuscular block with neostigmine at one to four hours after a single intubating dose of vecuronium. Anesth Analg. 1995;80:1168–74.

9. Saitoh Y, Toyooka H, Amaha K. Recoveries of post-tetanic twitch and train-of-four responses after administration of vecuronium with different inhalation anaesthetics and neuroleptanaesthesia. Br J Anaesth. 1993;70:402–4.

10. Baurain MJ, D'Hollander AA, Melot C, et al. Effects of residual concentrations of isoflurane on the reversal of vecuronium-induced neuromuscular blockade. Anesthesiology. 1991;74:474–8.

11. Burkett L, Bikhazi GZB, Thomas Jr KC, et al. Mutual potentiation of the neuromuscular effects of antibiotics and relaxants. Anesth Analg. 1979;58:107–15.

12. Sinatra RS, Philip BK, Naulty JS, Ostheimer GW. Prolonged neuromuscular blockade with vecuronium in a patient treated with magnesium sulfate. Anesth Analg. 1985;64:1220–2.

13. Usubiaga JE, Wikinski JA, Morales RL. Interaction of intravenously administered procaine, lidocaine and succinylcholine in anesthetized subjects. Anesth Analg. 1967;46:39–45.

Chapter 14
Drugs Acting on the Autonomic Nervous System

John Pawlowski

Contents

Introduction

The autonomic nervous system is a coordinated motor system that consists of inner-vated cardiac muscle, smooth muscle, and glands. The ANS maintains homeostasis and provides a coordinated response to external stimulation. Much of homeostasis

J. Pawlowski
Division of Thoracic Anesthesia, Beth Israel Deaconess Medical Center, Boston, MA, USA
e-mail: jpawlows@bidmc.harvard.edu

A.D. Kaye et al. (eds.), *Essentials of Pharmacology for Anesthesia,*
Pain Medicine, and Critical Care, DOI 10.1007/978-1-4614-8948-1_14,
© Springer Science+Business Media New York 2015

occurs involuntarily, but some autonomic processes have a degree of voluntary control (urination, sexual activity). The major components are the sympathetic and parasympathetic nervous systems. This review will focus on those aspects of the autonomic nervous system that are most crucial in the clinical assessment and treatment of disease. Many elements of the ANS, thermoregulation and the emotional component to sympathetic stimulation, for example, will be omitted.

The sympathetic nervous system is mainly located in the thoracolumbar area of the body. Sensory afferents send nerve fibers to the central nervous system. The motor sympathetic pathway starts in the intermediolateral cell column of the spinal cord. These cells send mostly myelinated axons via the white ramus to the adjacent sympathetic ganglion. In the ganglion, the axon synapses with postganglionic cells that send axons via the unmyelinated gray ramus to the effector organ, smooth muscle, or gland.

A coordinated activation of the sympathetic nervous system results in the "fight or flight" response [1]. Pupils dilate, the heart rate increases and contracts more forcefully, bronchioles dilate, and glucose is released. Blood flow is diverted away from the skin and gut and toward the skeletal muscles. All of these actions can prepare the individual for a rapid expenditure of energy. A similar coordinated response of the parasympathetic nervous system does not exist. In fact, the widespread activation of the parasympathetic nervous system, as evidenced by nerve agents such as sarin, can be incapacitating and fatal.

A number of autonomic reflexes exist, but the most important clinically is the baroreceptor reflex. The neural pathway for the baroreceptor reflex begins with stretch sensory nerves located in the carotid sinus and the aortic arch. These axons travel from the carotid sinus via the nerve of Hering to the glossopharyngeal nerve (IX), which projects to the nucleus of the tractus solitaries in the medulla. Efferent sympathetic fibers exit the CNS via the intermediolateral cell column as described and innervate arteriolar blood vessels, which cause vasodilation and a decrease in blood pressure. Vagal efferents also are inactivated, which causes a slowing of the heart rate. A decrease in carotid stretch can also elicit a baroreceptor response – this decrease in stretch causes an increase in heart rate as well as the sympathetic stimulation of the adrenal gland to secrete epinephrine and norepinephrine into the blood stream, with a resultant increase in blood pressure. Therefore, profound drops in blood pressure often are accompanied by a reflex increase in the heart rate via the baroreceptor pathway [2].

Parasympathetic ganglia are located in the cranial and sacral areas of the body. Preganglionic parasympathetic neurons are located near the cranial nerves (III, VII, IX, X), and postganglionic parasympathetic cells are located near their effector organs.

All preganglionic autonomic fibers contain acetylcholine as the neurotransmitter. The only exception is in the enteric system at the level of the myenteric and submucosal plexuses, where other neuropeptides also exist.

All sympathetic postganglionic fibers contain the neurotransmitter norepinephrine, with the exception of the apocrine sweat glands that contain acetylcholine. Postganglionic parasympathetic fibers contain acetylcholine.

The different types of sympathetic receptors (alpha-1, alpha-2, beta-1, beta-2, beta-3) exist in the neural endings in the eye, lung, heart, blood vessels, GI tract, bladder, sex organs, skin, fat, and adrenal medulla [3]. The different types of parasympathetic receptors (M1, M2, M3, M4, M5) exist in the neural connections of the same organs although with different effects and to a different degree than the sympathetic. For example, there are very few parasympathetic (muscarinic) receptors in the blood vessels. The response to activation of the receptor subtypes can depend on the location of the receptor, either pre- or postsynaptic, and to the receptor coupling mechanism.

Excitatory neurotransmitters can cause a local depolarization called an excitatory post synaptic potential (EPSP), through an increase in cation permeability (usually Na^+). With enough excitatory potential change, an action potential can propagate down the postsynaptic axon. Inhibitory neurotransmitters, in contrast, can create a local hyperpolarization of the postsynaptic membrane or inhibitory postsynaptic potential (IPSP), usually through K^+ or Cl^- channels.

Activity at the postsynaptic level can also be altered by the rate of degradation of the neurotransmitters, the rate of reuptake of the neurotransmitters into the presynaptic nerve ending, or by diffusion away from the synapse. Other regulatory steps that can influence neural activity are neurotransmitter synthesis, transmitter sequestration into vesicles, and receptor degradation and downregulation. All of these mechanisms will be discussed with clinical examples.

Certain organs have dual control from the sympathetic and parasympathetic nervous system. The neural pathways that control pupillary dilation, bronchodilation, cardiac activation, micturition, and autonomic reflexes contain both sympathetic and parasympathetic elements.

With knowledge of the anatomy of the autonomic nervous system, we should be able to predict where sympathomimetic drugs and parasympathomimetic drugs might offer a therapeutic effect for patients with bronchospasm, symptomatic bradycardia, and neurogenic bladder conditions.

Sympathetic Stimulation

Sympathetic or adrenergic stimulation usually involves the neurotransmitter norepinephrine at the level of the postganglionic fiber. Norepinephrine, as well as the other catecholamines dopamine and epinephrine, is synthesized in the body from the precursor tyramine. In adrenergic neurons, NE is packaged into vesicles. In the adrenal medulla, most of the norepinephrine is methylated to form epinephrine and packaged into vesicles. NE also finds its way back to the presynaptic axon terminal across the axoplasmic membrane through the action of the norepinephrine transporter (NET). Both cocaine and the tricyclic antidepressants block the NET and can lead to supranormal concentrations of norepinephrine in the synaptic cleft. Other sympathomimetic drugs such as tyramine and ephedrine act as indirect agonists.

Ephedrine displaces NE from the presynaptic nerve terminal and into the extracellular space by competing with NE for vesicle incorporation and by hastening outward transport of NE by facilitated exchange diffusion using the norepinephrine transporter. The increased concentration of NE in the synapse causes increased activation of postsynaptic receptors. These indirect-acting sympathomimetic agents, however, are prone to exhibit tachyphylaxis. Repeated doses of ephedrine, for instance, result in rapidly diminishing efficacy.

The metabolism of catecholamines involves the enzymatic activity of monoamine oxidase (MAO) and catechol-O-methyltransferase (COMT). Inhibitors of MAO, for example, can produce therapeutic increases in the catecholamine concentrations of NE, dopamine, and serotonin in the CNS and improve the symptoms of depression. Inhibitors of COMT can be useful in the therapy of Parkinson's disease.

Catecholamines can have variable and sometimes opposite effects on the same organs due to a diversity of adrenergic receptors. For example, sympathetic stimulation of smooth muscle can produce both contraction and relaxation. The identification of multiple adrenergic receptors as well as an understanding of the receptor coupling mechanisms can explain this phenomenon. The characterization of alpha and beta receptors led to the development of selective alpha antagonists such as phenoxybenzamine and of selective beta-blockers such as propranolol. Further discovery of alpha and beta subtypes has enabled the development of increasingly more selective adrenergic agents. The beta-3 receptor, mostly present in adipose tissue, will be ignored here. Beta-3 agonists produce lipolysis and an active thermogenic response. The most potent adrenergic agonist for beta receptors is isoproterenol. The most potent catecholamine agonist for alpha receptors is epinephrine. Beta-1 receptors were described in the myocardium, while beta-2 receptors were characterized in smooth muscle.

Alpha receptors vary in their effects based on the intracellular G protein-mediated second messenger activity. The G protein can be either stimulatory or inhibitory. For example, alpha-1 subtypes involve the action of the stimulatory G protein Gq, which increases the enzymatic activity of phospholipase C and results in vasoconstriction. Alpha-2 subtypes are coupled to an inhibitory G protein, Gi, which inhibits hormone release from the adrenal medulla. The beta-1 and beta-2 receptors are both coupled to a stimulatory G protein, Gs, which in the heart causes cyclic AMP-mediated activation of calcium channels and positive inotropic and chronotropic effects, whereas in smooth muscle, an elevated cAMP results in vasodilatation from enhanced activity of the myosin light-chain phosphatase.

Long-term exposure to catecholamines has been known to cause a decrease in the ability of these adrenergic target cells to respond to repeated sympathetic stimulation. This behavior is alternatively called tachyphylaxis, refractoriness, or desensitization and may actually represent multiple consequences of long-term adrenergic exposure. The mechanisms may include receptor phosphorylation by G protein receptor kinases (GRKs) with an effect on beta-arrestin binding and by signaling kinases such as PKA and PKC [4]. Other mechanisms may be receptor sequestration, uncoupling from G proteins, and activation of cyclic nucleotide phosphodiesterases. Slower phenomena may also occur such as receptor endocytosis. Thus, a complex series of events occur with long-term catecholamine stimulation, which may help explain the deleterious consequences of such chronic diseases like congestive heart failure, which is associated with overstimulation of the sympathetic nervous system [5].

Parasympathetic Stimulation

Parasympathetic or vagal stimulation involves the release of acetylcholine from a nerve terminal. In contrast to the acetylcholine-mediated activation of the skeletal muscle, the activation of postganglionic parasympathetic nerves involves Ach binding to the muscarinic receptor. The presynaptic synthesis of acetylcholine occurs from the association of the mitochondrial product acetyl coenzyme A and dietary choline. Once synthesized, Ach is packaged into vesicles. Calcium activation causes the vesicles to fuse with the cell membrane, assisted by a vesicle-associated membrane protein (VAMP) and a synaptosome-associated protein (SNAP), which promotes exocytosis and release of Ach into the synapse. This action of the SNAPs is blocked by botulinum toxin or Botox. The Ach binds to muscarinic receptors on the postganglionic cell and works through a G protein-coupled reaction. As with adrenergic receptor families, muscarinic activity depends on the muscarinic receptor subtype and its G protein type. There are at least five muscarinic subtypes, M1, M2, M3, M4, and M5. All subtypes are present in the CNS. M2 is also in the heart and vasculature. M3 is in the bladder and salivary glands. The stimulatory subtypes are M1, M3, and M5. The inhibitory subtypes are M2 and M4. As might be expected, the stimulatory effects involve the Gq and the inhibitory effects involve either Gi or Go. The pharmacodynamics action of a particular muscarinic agonist, therefore, will depend not only on the specific muscarinic subtype that is activated but also on the location of the specific effector tissue that possesses that receptor subtype.

Knowledge of the anatomy, motor function, and control elements of the autonomic nervous system is essential to the description of the therapeutic manipulation of autonomic responses. In practice, much of the autonomic nervous system is manipulated pharmacologically to reduce autonomic side effects from other medications. For example, the antimuscarinic drugs are used to reduce side effects from the administration of neostigmine, an anticholinesterase inhibitor. The following review will not discuss the parasympathomimetic or parasympatholytic (vagolytic) drugs nor will ganglionic blocking drugs be mentioned. Instead, the following discussion will focus on adrenergic agonists and antagonists, their clinical uses, dosage strategies, interactions, and potential side effects.

Drug Class and Mechanism of Action

Sympathomimetics

The sympathomimetics represent a broad class of pharmacologic agents that act to enhance sympathetic nervous activity. In contrast, the catecholamines consist of drugs that resemble epinephrine and norepinephrine in structure and that may have similar or more selective actions in patients. *Epinephrine* stimulates both alpha and beta receptors, with specific binding to alpha-1, beta-1, and beta-2. The indirect-acting agent *ephedrine* has similar effects on alpha and beta receptors as does epinephrine, although to a lesser efficacy. *Norepinephrine* activates both alpha-1 and beta-1 and a similar action can be produced with *metaraminol. Isoproterenol* stimulates both beta-1 and beta-2. *Dopamine* stimulates alpha-1, beta-1, and dopaminergic receptors. *Dobutamine* stimulates beta-1 more than beta-2 and alpha-1. Thus, both synthetic and naturally occurring adrenergic agonists can be employed for their specific activation of adrenergic receptor subtypes.

Several sympathomimetics possess more selective binding to individual classes of adrenergic subtypes. For instance, *methoxamine* and *phenylephrine* can be used as a selective alpha-1 agonist. These two agents are potent vasoconstrictors and can be used to treat low blood pressure, especially that caused by low systemic vascular resistance. Methoxamine tends to act on the arterial side, whereas phenylephrine vasoconstricts both arteries and veins. Therefore, treatment with phenylephrine often results in an increase in preload due to venoconstriction and a reduction in venous capacitance. The increase in preload can increase the stroke volume and cardiac output when phenylephrine is used.

Selective alpha-2 agonists include *clonidine* and *dexmedetomidine*, which have vasodilatory effects on the vasculature and potentiate central effects of anesthetics and sedatives. The vasodilatory response is best explained by a predominance of presynaptic location of the alpha-2 receptor, thus reducing the presynaptic release of norepinephrine into the synapse.

The beta-agonists have effects on multiple organs and tissues in the body. Beta-1 agonists have both chronotropic and inotropic effects on the heart. *Dobutamine* is the most selective and the most widely used of the beta-1 agonists [6]. Beta-2 agonists act by dilating smooth muscle in the vasculature, airways, and uterus. Thus, *terbutaline* and *albuterol* are potent bronchodilators and terbutaline and *ritodrine* are effective tocolytics.

Several nonadrenergic agents are sympathomimetics through a mechanism of inhibiting phosphodiesterase (PDE) and causing an increase in the intracellular concentrations of cAMP. *Aminophylline, theophylline*, and *amrinone* inhibit PDE-3 and act as inodilators and bronchodilators [7]. Other inotropic agents exist, such as thyroxine, glucagon, and digoxin, but will not be addressed in this chapter.

Sympatholytics

Several compounds exist that can block the activity of adrenergic receptors in the sympathetic nervous system. *Prazosin* is a selective postsynaptic alpha-1 antagonist that produces orthostatic hypotension and is often accompanied by a reflex tachycardia, due to a compensatory baroreceptor response. In contrast, the drug *phentolamine* is a nonselective and competitive antagonist of both alpha-1 and alpha-2 receptors. In addition to tachycardia, both prazosin and phentolamine are associated with miosis and nasal stuffiness. The mixed antagonist, *labetalol*, blocks alpha-1 and beta receptors. Therefore, labetalol has the action of simultaneously lowering both heart rate and blood pressure. The nonselective antagonism of beta-1 and beta-2 receptors makes labetalol susceptible to cause a worsening of bronchospasm and congestive heart failure.

Among a long list of beta-blockers, several stand out as useful to anesthesiologists. The selective beta-1 blocker, *esmolol*, is an ultrashort-acting medication with a plasma half-life of 9 min [8]. Esmolol can rapidly lower both heart rate and blood pressure in an immediate fashion and as an emergency measure. Another selective beta-1 beta-blocker is *metoprolol*, which has a more gradual onset when compared with esmolol and a more prolonged half-life [9]. These two beta-blockers are both available as intravenous preparations and should be proximate to any anesthetic where treatment of tachycardia, ischemia, or hypertension is anticipated.

Indications/Clinical Pearls

Sympathomimetics

The indications for alpha and beta receptor agonists are in the treatment of abnormal vital signs such as symptomatic hypotension and bradycardia, as well as the treatment of local organ conditions, such as nasal congestion and bronchospasm. In specific instances, beta-agonists can be employed to reveal an abnormal arrhythmia. In the setting of anaphylaxis, the effects of epinephrine are useful to both restore the hemodynamic condition and modulate the immune response. For this complex therapy of anaphylaxis, it is not possible to substitute other medications in place of epinephrine. Adding an alpha-1 agonist to a beta-1 agonist plus a beta-2 agonist does not equal the effects of epinephrine. In the setting of severe, uncompensated congestive heart failure, it is possible to substitute inotropes in place of epinephrine. Dopamine, in high doses, has similar effects to epinephrine. Dobutamine can produce a significant increase in the cardiac output with little elevation of the heart rate. Results on the cardiac function are similar to that of dobutamine when dopexamine is used. Isoproterenol should be avoided in this circumstance, due to an exaggerated action in raising the heart rate as well as a beta-2 mediated effect on the vasculature to lower blood pressure.

Another indication for the use of alpha- and beta-agonists is the restoration of normal vital signs after the administration of anesthetic agents. To counter the vasodilatory and cardiodepressive effects of anesthesia, both alpha- and beta-agonists can be given. Neuraxial anesthesia, such as spinal and epidural, inhalational anesthesia, and total intravenous anesthesia are all associated with the side effects of lower blood pressure and lower systemic vascular resistance [10]. To counter a low systemic vascular resistance, a selective alpha-1 agonist, such as *methoxamine* or *phenylephrine*, can be used. Phenylephrine is also useful as a continuous infusion. These agents, however, can produce a reflex bradycardia and a decrease in cardiac output. For this reason, drugs with mixed alpha- and beta-agonist activity are often utilized. *Mephentermine, metaraminol,* and *ephedrine* act on both alpha and beta receptors to raise blood pressure and improve cardiac output. Ephedrine is a derivative of the active ingredient in ephedra tea, an herbal supplement. The action of ephedrine is as an indirect agonist and repeated doses of ephedrine are less effective, a phenomenon known as tachyphylaxis. Thus, ephedrine is not appropriate as a continuous infusion. The efficacious use of ephedrine in reversing the blood pressure drop following the administration of a spinal anesthetic has been well described.

The most common indication for the use of a selective beta-2 agonist is the relief of bronchospasm. In reactive airways disease, such as asthma, the resistance airways can be in a state of continuous muscular tension. Beta-2-mediated activity causes the airway smooth muscle to relax and the bronchioles to dilate and to facilitate exhalation. Classes of selective beta-2 agonists can be separated as short acting and long acting. Among the short-acting beta-2 agonists are *albuterol, metaproterenol,* and *terbutaline.* Albuterol either can be administered as an inhalant or can be taken orally to counteract the symptoms of bronchospasm. When inhaled, albuterol produces bronchodilation within 15 min and has a therapeutic half-life of 2–3 h. In the United States, the metered dose inhaler contains hydrofluoroalkane as a propellant, which does not disrupt the ozone layer. Less selective than albuterol is metaproterenol, which is rapidly acting in the parenteral preparation but is more resistant than albuterol to methylation by the enzyme COMT and subsequent excretion. Therefore, the half-life is longer for metaproterenol than for albuterol. Terbutaline is approved for the long-term treatment of COPD. Even longer acting is the agonist *salmeterol,* which has a duration of action greater than 12 h. Salmeterol is approved for the chronic treatment of asthma only in those patients where the chronic treatment with corticosteroids alone has failed to achieve good control.

The demonstration of long-term improvement of symptoms and relief of disease progression with beta-agonists suggests that these agents are doing more than dilating airways. Beta-2 agonists have been shown to lower levels of leukotrienes, inhibit phospholipase A2, decrease the release of histamine from mast cells, decrease capillary permeability, and augment mucociliary function. Thus, beta-2 agonists have been shown to be more effective in improving symptoms, lung function, and quality of life in patients with COPD than other bronchodilators such as theophylline and the parasympatholytic agent ipratropium.

Sympatholytics

The use of sympatholytics is to control the vital signs and to protect the body from effects of overstimulation of the sympathetic nervous system (SNS). The need to block the SNS becomes more critical in patients who cannot tolerate increases in the heart rate and the blood pressure. Patients with critical aortic stenosis or mitral stenosis, for example, do not tolerate tachycardias well. Patients with ischemic heart disease may not tolerate exaggerated increases in blood pressure without the development of angina. Therefore, medications to modulate and lower the heart rate and blood pressure can be useful therapeutic agents [11]. The beta-1 selective beta-blockers such as *metoprolol* can be used to control the heart rate and blood pressure.

All other beta-blockers are only interesting as to their reason for being used as a chronic medication. Beta-blockers are chosen for their long-term effects on hypertension and for their specific side effects and metabolism. For example, selectivity is desirable in many patients, but nonselective beta-blockers are often cheaper. Generic forms of these beta-blockers may also be less expensive. Certain beta-blockers have been shown to be effective in the long-term treatment of hypertension, congestive heart failure, postinfarction, and ischemic heart disease. Other agents are chosen for their relative lipid insolubility or their lack of hepatic metabolism. Beta-blockers with intrinsic sympathetic activity are selected to reduce the risk of symptomatic bradycardia. Other beta-blockers have vasodilatory properties or more antiarrhythmic effects. Therefore, the types and combinations of beta-blockers may be varied, depending on the desirable side effects and metabolisms of these agents in the treatment of chronic conditions.

Dosing Options

Sympathomimetics

In a clinical setting of low blood pressure, a bolus of a sympathomimetic agent can temporarily restore normal hemodynamics. In a single bolus, both direct- and indirect-acting adrenergic agonists can be used. For example, *phenylephrine* 100 mcg, *methoxamine* 10 mg, *metaraminol* 5 mg, *mephentermine* 30 mg, or *ephedrine* 10 mg can be used to restore the vital signs. In cases of extremely low blood pressures, where end organ perfusion is in jeopardy, boluses of catecholamines such as *epinephrine* 8 mcg, *norepinephrine* 16 mcg, or *dopamine* 200 mcg can be administered as an intravenous bolus, usually through a central venous line. After administration of these vasopressors, the clinician should rule out other causes of low blood pressure, such as hypovolemia, hemorrhage, drug overdose, and myocardial infarction. These causes need other treatments besides sympathomimetic agents to reverse their underlying pathology.

Table 14.1 Doses of commonly used sympathomimetic agents. These doses are intended for adult patients via an intravenous route. See text for details

Drug	Bolus dose	Infusion rate
Phenylephrine	100 mcg	1 mcg/kg/min
Methoxamine	10 mg	NA
Norepinephrine	16 mcg	0.1 mcg/kg/min
Epinephrine	8 mcg	0.05 mcg/kg/min
Metaraminol	5 mg	NA
Ephedrine	10 mg	NA
Mephentermine	30 mg	NA
Dopamine	200 mcg	10 mcg/kg/min
Dobutamine	NA	10 mcg/kg/min
Vasopressin	40 Units	0.6 Units/min

If several boluses of the sympathomimetic drugs do not restore normal vital signs, an infusion may become necessary. Not all the sympathomimetic agents are amenable to prolonged infusion, usually due to issues of tachyphylaxis as an indirect-acting agent or from protracted effects due to the context sensitive half-lives. Table 14.1 shows typical intravenous bolus doses as well as typical intravenous infusion rates of several commonly used sympathomimetic agents. As with most medications used to restore the vital signs, it is useful to titrate to effect and to attempt to correct the underlying disorder that is responsible for the lowered blood pressure. In extreme cases of hypotension, such as pulseless electrical activity, it may be necessary to administer vasopressin. *Vasopressin* does not work by activating adrenergic receptors, but rather, vasopressin binds to vasopressin receptors in the vasculature and causes intense and efficacious vasoconstriction. A usual bolus dose of 40 Units of vasopressin and an infusion rate of 0.6 Units per minute can restore a perfusing blood pressure in many patients who are resistant to catecholamine stimulation.

Sympatholytics

For both acute and chronic treatment of hypertension, beta-blockers have been a valuable clinical tool. The role of beta-blockers in anesthesia relates to both pre-anesthetic conditions and perioperative situations. In general, chronic beta-blocker therapy should be continued throughout the perioperative period. Perioperatively, abnormally high blood pressures can be treated with beta-blockers or with *labetalol*, an alpha- and beta-blocking agent. Both nonselective and selective beta-1-blocking agents can also be employed to lower high blood pressures. *Esmolol* is an ultrashort-acting beta-1 selective beta-blocker with an extremely short half-life of 9 min. *Metoprolol*, while selective, is longer acting than esmolol. The utility of metoprolol

Table 14.2 Doses of commonly used sympatholytic agents for the perioperative period. These doses are intended for adult patients via an intravenous route. See text for details

Drug	Bolus dose	Infusion rate
Labetalol	5 mg	NA
Esmolol	30 mg	100 mcg/kg/min
Metoprolol	5 mg	100 mcg/kg/min
Nitroprusside	100 mcg	5 mcg/kg/min

is for more sustained treatment of hypertension, such as when the patient has failed to take his or her daily beta-blocker. Other drugs, such as alpha-methyldopa, clonidine, and trimethaphan, no longer have practical clinical utility in controlling perioperative hypertension. Table 14.2 demonstrates several of the clinically useful beta-blocking agents in the prevention and treatment of perioperative hypertension. Included in the table are labetalol, a mixed alpha- and beta-blocker, and *nitroprusside*, a nitrovasodilator. Both these drugs are useful when conventional beta-blockade has not produced the desired reduction in blood pressure.

Drug Interactions

Sympathomimetics

In general, serious drug interactions can arise when sympathomimetics are combined with agents that accentuate all or a portion of the actions of these adrenergic agonists. For example, classes of *tricyclic antidepressants* (TCAs) and *monoamine oxidase inhibitors* (MAOIs) potentiate the sympathetic effects of adrenergic agonists by causing higher synaptic levels of the neurotransmitter norepinephrine. In some cases, this combination of sympathomimetic and MAOI can cause a fatal hypertensive crisis. In other drug combinations, only a part of the sympathetic action is seen. One of the side effects of the use of *droperidol* or *haloperidol* is a profound alpha-blockade. In combination with epinephrine, the effect of droperidol can be to cause further decreases in blood pressure: not only from the alpha-blockade but also from the unopposed beta-2 stimulation by epinephrine on the peripheral vasculature. When epinephrine is given to patients who are taking a nonselective beta-blocker, there can be an exaggerated increase in blood pressure due to unopposed alpha activity with no activation of beta-2 in the vasculature. Note that the *nonselective beta-blocker* can be the antiarrhythmic agent propranolol (taken orally) or the anti-glaucoma medication timolol (given as eye drops). In both cases, there can be enough systemic absorption to cause these cardiovascular drug interactions. Sympathomimetic agents can also interact with *volatile anesthetic agents* to promote arrhythmias.

Sympatholytics

Drug interactions with sympatholytic agents can arise whenever there is an effect on the clinical action or the metabolism or excretion of the drug. Sympatholytic drugs tend to lower blood pressure and reduce contractility and they often have additive effects with other antihypertensive drugs and in clinical conditions such as congestive heart failure. *Calcium channel blockers* must be given cautiously to patients already on beta-blockers. Beta-blockers may decrease the effectiveness of *oral hypoglycemic* agents in the treatment of diabetes. Beta-blockers can reduce the effectiveness of *theophylline* in the treatment of asthma, as theophylline can reduce the effectiveness of beta-blockers in treating hypertension. *Aspirin and NSAIDs* can counteract the antihypertensive effects of beta-blockers, probably through their inhibition of prostaglandins. The combination of beta-blockers and *MAO inhibitors* can lead to increased blood pressure, through an unopposed beta-2 blockade in the resistance arterioles. Cold remedies that contain *caffeine, pseudo-ephedrine, or ephedrine* can counteract the effects of beta-blockers with their sympathomimetic effects.

Many drugs can influence the effects of sympatholytic medications by altering their metabolism. The antituberculin drug *rifampicin* and the barbiturate *phenobarbital* both induce the activity of liver enzymes that metabolize beta-blockers (such as propranolol and metoprolol). Thus, rifampicin and phenobarbital make these beta-blockers less effective. The antimalarial drug *mefloquine* decreases liver enzyme activity and therefore increases the effective concentration of a given dose of propranolol, for example. Many other drugs merely share the same cytochrome P450 enzyme as do these beta-blockers and, thus, compete for metabolism. These drugs include the *statins, antiulcer drugs, warfarin, and oral hypoglycemic drugs. Thioridazine and chlorpromazine* can lead to hypotension by interfering with the elimination of propranolol and pindolol. For a variety of pharmacodynamic actions or the influences on metabolism and excretion, the sympatholytics can demonstrate important side effects with a host of other medications.

Side Effects/Black Box Warnings

Sympathomimetics

Any sympathomimetics will have side effects from the activation of the undesirable consequences of the sympathetic nervous system. Sympathomimetics can worsen narrow-angle glaucoma, neurogenic bladder, or chronic constipation. Used as a diet drug, sympathomimetics act to suppress the appetite, but in other situations, this is an unwanted side effect. Other signs of sympathetic activation are restlessness, headache, anxiety, dry mouth, dizziness, shaking, sweats, palpitations, and insomnia. Excess sympathetic stimulation can lead to hypertension, tachycardia, tachyarrhythmias, palpitations, chest pain, congestive heart failure, myocardial infarction, stroke, and death. Intravenous administration of catecholamines has been associated with extravasation, skin sloughing, and loss of digits. Administration of isoproterenol has produced tachycardia and chest pain. Included in the sympathomimetics are several recreational drugs of abuse, such as cocaine and methamphetamine. Both of these drugs have added problems. In addition to the signs and symptoms of sympathetic activation are the signs of intoxication and effects of withdrawal. There can be damage to the nasal septum, bleeding, confusion, paranoid hallucinations, cold sweats, nausea, and vomiting. Therefore, sympathomimetic agents can activate any target organ of the sympathetic nervous system as well as any other area of the body that is reached by the circulation.

Sympatholytics

The obvious side effects from sympatholytics are the exaggerated declines in blood pressure and the phenomenon of orthostatic hypotension. Orthostatic hypotension in the extreme can result in syncope. In addition, more selective blockers have more selective side effects. Phenoxybenzamine can cause reflex tachycardia and can interfere with ejaculation. Beta-blockers are associated with sexual dysfunction in the form of erectile dysfunction as well as the symptoms of fatigue and clinical depression [12]. In patients with uncompensated congestive heart failure, beta-blockers can have synergistic negative inotropic effects in combination with calcium channel blockers and can lead to low cardiac output and cardiogenic shock [13].

Summary

The autonomic nervous system is a coordinated system that allows both voluntary and vegetative control of a variety of organs and bodily functions. The sympathetic and parasympathetic nervous systems provide the architecture of the central nervous system control of these functions. Many of the specific organs are regulated by dual control: by both sympathetic and parasympathetic input. Usually, this input is opposing in nature. A level of intrinsic tone provides a baseline homeostasis that can be perturbed by a variety of external stimuli and by a variety of pharmacologic agents. Various drugs have been described which act as sympathomimetics and sympatholytics. The clinical usefulness and the relevant side effects of these agents were described.

Chemical Structures

Chemical Structure
14.1 (*R*)-(–)-L-Epinephrine
or (*R*)-(–)-L-adrenaline

Chemical Structure
14.2 Dobutamine

Chemical Structure 14.3 Phenylephrine hydrochloride

Chemical Structure
14.4 Theophylline

Chemical Structure
14.5 Albuterol

References

1. Opie LH, Gersh BJ, editors. Drugs for the heart. 8th ed. Philadelphia: Elsevier Saunders; 2013.
2. Brunton LL, Chabner BA, Knollmann BC, editors. Goodman and Gilman's the pharmacological basis of therapeutics. 12th ed. New York: McGraw-Hill Companies, Inc; 2011.
3. Drazen JM, O'Byrne PM. Risks of long acting beta-agonists in achieving asthma control. N Engl J Med. 2009;360:1671–2.
4. Lefkowitz RJ, et al. Transduction of receptor signals by beta-arrestins. Science. 2005;308:512–7.
5. Felker GM, et al. Clinical Trials of pharmacological therapies in acute heart failure syndromes: lessons learned and directions forward. Circ Heart Fail. 2010;3:314–25.
6. Andrus MR, Loyed JV. Use of beta-adrenoceptor antagonists in older patients with chronic obstructive pulmonary disease and cardiovascular co-morbidity. Drugs Aging. 2008;25:131–44.
7. Hasenfuss G, et al. Cardiac inotropes: current agents and future directions. Eur Heart J. 2011;32:1838–45.
8. Webers C, Beckers H, Nuijts R, Schouten J. Pharmacological management of primary open-angle glaucoma: second line options and beyond. Drugs Aging. 2008;25:729–59.
9. Bangalore S, et al. Cardiovascular protection using beta blockers. J Am Coll Cardiol. 2007;50:563–72.
10. Miller RD, Eriksson LI, Fleisher LA, Wiener-Kronish JP, Young WL, editors. Miller's anesthesia. 7th ed. Philadelphia: Churchill Livingstone; 2010.
11. Varon J. Treatment of acute severe hypertension: current and newer agents. Drugs. 2008;68:283–97.
12. Williams B. Beta-blockers and the treatment of hypertension. J Hypertens. 2007;25:1351–3.
13. RESOLVD Investigators. Effects of metoprolol CR in patients with ischemic and dilated cardiomyopathy. The randomized evaluation of strategies for left ventricular dysfunction pilot study. Circulation. 2000;101:378–84.

Chapter 15
Antihypertensives, Diuretics, and Antidysrhythmics

Ryan Field

Contents

R. Field, MD
Department of Anesthesiology and Perioperative Care, School of Medicine,
University of California–Irvine, Irvine, CA, USA
e-mail: zkain@uci.edu, fieldr@uci.edu

A.D. Kaye et al. (eds.), *Essentials of Pharmacology for Anesthesia,*
Pain Medicine, and Critical Care, DOI 10.1007/978-1-4614-8948-1_15,
© Springer Science+Business Media New York 2015

Introduction

Anesthesiology, pain medicine, and critical care all experience heavy exposure to antihypertensives, diuretics, and antidysrhythmics. Whether patients require new therapy acutely or have used therapies for a long time, whether requiring titration or merely knowledge of how they affect medical decision making, and whether using them to improve patient outcomes or in an emergency situation, these therapies represent great advances in healthcare as well as potentially very dangerous pitfalls. Thorough knowledge of classification, mechanism of action, medical indication, dosing options, drug-drug interactions, and side effects help the clinician wisely choose and titrate therapy while minimizing patient harm.

Drug Class and Mechanism of Action

Alpha-Blockers

Alpha-blockers include phentolamine, prazosin, and phenoxybenzamine. They directly act on alpha adrenergic receptors. At alpha adrenergic receptors, they collectively reduce or prevent the action of endogenous and exogenous catecholamines. Removing adrenergic tone causes smooth muscle within vessels to relax, lowering systemic vascular resistance. Phentolamine and prazosin reversibly bind alpha adrenergic receptors and competitively antagonize circulating catecholamine action. Phenoxybenzamine irreversibly binds alpha adrenergic receptors and inhibits circulating catecholamine action. Although all three pharmaceuticals exhibit nonselective properties, phenoxybenzamine acts on alpha-1 postsynaptic receptors 100 times more potently than alpha-2. Prazosin too exhibits large preference for alpha-1 potency and is considered alpha-1 selective. Phentolamine, on the other hand, affects alpha-1 and alpha-2 postsynaptic receptors with much more equality.

Beta-Blockers

Beta-blockers treat cardiovascular disease and hypertension. Receptor activity largely defines function between beta-1 blockers and nonselective beta-blockers. Beta-1 blockers, such as esmolol, atenolol, and metoprolol, selectively bind beta-1 receptors making the heart their primary site of action, while nonselective beta-blockers, such as propranolol, nadolol, and sotalol, also affect the vascular, metabolic, and bronchial smooth muscle systems through their beta-2 blockade. No beta-blocker is completely selective. Labetalol and carvedilol, mixed antagonists, selectively block alpha-1 receptors and nonselectively block beta-1 and beta-2 receptors.

Calcium Channel Blockers

Calcium channel blockers act at the cellular membrane to alter calcium concentration. This change in calcium concentration produces vasodilation, decreased myocardial contractility, decreased heart rate, and slow cardiac conduction. Commonly used calcium channel blockers include nicardipine, nifedipine, nimodipine, diltiazem, and verapamil. Importantly, calcium channel blockers vary in relative strength of site effect, including cardiac and vascular action.

Angiotensin Antagonists

All angiotensin antagonists act upon the renin-angiotensin-aldosterone system. Lisinopril, captopril, and enalapril all prevent the conversion of angiotensin I to angiotensin II. Angiotensin II receptor blockers prevent the successful action of active angiotensin II. Losartan and valsartan most commonly represent this class. In either case, the angiotensin II receptor is unable to be stimulated such that aldosterone, norepinephrine, and ADH levels are reduced.

Other Vasodilators

Hydralazine, nitroglycerin, and sodium nitroprusside largely comprise this functional class. Hydralazine directly relaxes vascular smooth muscle through an unknown mechanism. Nitroglycerin, a predominantly venodilator, decreases cardiac preload. Sodium nitroprusside works indiscriminately on both venous and arterial systems, reducing both preload and afterload.

Loop Diuretics

Loop diuretics, such as furosemide and bumetanide, work by inhibiting sodium and chloride resorption at the loop of Henle, the distal convoluted tubule, and the proximal convoluted tubule. Loop diuretics obtain their name from their primary site of action.

Thiazide Diuretics

Thiazide diuretics act at the distal convoluted tubule to inhibit sodium and chloride resorption. They act similarly to loop diuretics but narrow their site of action. Hydrochlorothiazide is the most frequently prescribed thiazide. It is seen alone and in combination with other medications in many oral formulations.

Osmotic Diuretics

Mannitol is a commonly used osmotic diuretic in perioperative and critical care environments. Osmotics are normally filtered by glomeruli but abnormally reabsorbed. This abnormality creates an osmotic gradient in the tubular fluid limiting water resorption. As an intravenous medication, similarly to its effect in the tubules, the osmotic gradient liberates fluid from the cellular space and mobilizes it to the vascular space enhancing renal blood flow.

Carbonic Anhydrase Inhibitors

Carbonic anhydrase inhibitors prevent bicarbonate reformation from carbonic acid and re-accumulation of hydrogen ions available for counter transport with sodium into the proximal tubule. Without this co- and counter transport, sodium and bicarbonate remain in the proximal tubule, creating a favorable gradient for diuresis. Acetazolamide is most commonly used.

Antidysrhythmics

Lidocaine is a class Ib antidysrhythmic interacting with sodium channels to shorten cardiac action potentials and is commonly thought of as a sodium channel blocker. Amiodarone is a class III antidysrhythmic that prolongs repolarization by blocking potassium channels. It also acts as a sodium, beta, and calcium channel blocker. Sotalol also represents class III antidysrhythmics but also functions as a beta-blocker. Adenosine represents class V antidysrhythmics directly acting at the AV node or functioning by an unknown mechanism.

Digoxin and magnesium also belong in this class most commonly. Digoxin most likely binds the sodium and potassium ATPase channels, thereby preventing the counter transport of intracellular calcium. This increase in intracellular calcium lengthens phases 0 and 4 of the cardiac action potential, which decreases overall rate. There may be some synergy or additive effects with vagal and possibly even direct AV nodal effects of digoxin. Intracellular calcium rises and the calcium levels in the sarcoplasmic reticulum elevate and increase inotropy. Magnesium acts as a calcium channel blocker, slows SA nodal activity, and prolongs conduction.

Indications and Clinical Pearls

Alpha-Blockers

Alpha-blockers largely find use in refractory hypertensive patients, such as those with end-stage renal disease and concomitant secondary hypertension, as well as those with pheochromocytoma both perioperatively and intraoperatively. Oral alpha-1 blockers, such as prazosin, doxazosin, and tamsulosin, are often encountered in the preoperative assessment and intensive care arenas and may be used for the improvement of urinary tract function in patients with benign prostatic hypertrophy. Tamsulosin typically is not prescribed for hypertension.

Preloading patients with intravenous crystalloid solutions prior to general anesthesia may very well avoid the typical induction hypotension patients experience due to masked hypovolemia in the preoperative unit. Direct-acting alpha adrenergic agonists, such as phenylephrine, may increase systemic vascular resistance and alpha adrenergic tone as well. Phenylephrine should almost never be used in lieu of appropriate volume resuscitation.

Alpha-blockers should be continued perioperatively without obvious contraindication. Abdominal cramping and diarrhea, typical of phentolamine administration, may improve with concomitant administration of atropine. Interestingly, phenoxybenzamine administration is thought not to affect coronary or cerebral vascular resistance. Prazosin, being considered alpha-1 selective, commonly does not exhibit the reflex tachycardia of other alpha-blockers because inhibitory alpha-2 receptors are left with intact function. Prazosin acts on both arteries and veins which often requires diuretic therapy for preload optimization in hypertensive patients.

Beta-Blockers

Beta-blockers are widely used for the treatment of many pathologies including hypertension and congestive heart failure and provide rate control for tachydysrhythmias, such as atrial fibrillation. They are useful in myocardial recovery from infarction and likely provide cardiac protection during the perioperative period in patients who already follow a beta-blocker regimen. Beta-1 selective blockade allows use in patients with obstructive pulmonary disease, peripheral vascular disease, and hyperglycemia with caution. Immediate preoperative initiation of beta-blockade therapy prior to presentation for elective surgery may 1 day be suggested for subpopulations; however, it is currently too controversial to suggest as routine practice.

Indications for propranolol include the treatment of hypertension, angina pectoris, post-MI cardiovascular event prophylaxis, atrial fibrillation and flutter, supraventricular tachydysrhythmia, migraine headache prophylaxis, essential tremor therapy, adjunct preoperative pheochromocytoma therapy, portal hypertension, and idiopathic hypertrophic subaortic stenosis. It is important to appreciate that therapeutic dosing ranges vary greatly with the intended use.

Labetalol, used in early postoperative hypertensive therapy, may display a time to peak effect of 20–30 min, making titration of labetalol challenging in this setting and sometimes leading to unintended hypotension and bradycardia. Interestingly, labetalol additionally exhibits partial beta-2 agonism and may increase glycogenolysis, increasing glycemic state. Where hyperglycemia may worsen outcomes, such as neurologic injury, this aspect of labetalol may warrant more frequent glucose monitoring and may increase need for antihyperglycemic therapies. Conversely, partial agonism may foster an improved safety profile in patients with reactive airway disease. Carvedilol, commonly used in patients with congestive heart failure, exhibits no partial agonism and should be continued in the perioperative period. Carvedilol may also be used in the treatment of hypertension and post-MI prophylaxis.

Calcium Channel Blockers

Nicardipine serves well as a titratable drip for control of hypertensive crisis. It predominantly affects vascular smooth muscle. Nifedipine acts at cardiac and vascular sites with equipotency; however, in vivo, increased cardiac output and increased heart rate are frequently seen with afterload reduction. Nifedipine is frequently prescribed for use in Prinzmetal's angina, unstable angina, and myocardial infarction. Nimodipine uniquely dilates the cerebral vasculature secondary to its extreme lipophilic nature, and therefore it is often used orally, intravenously, or by catheter-directed administration to dilate vasospastic cerebral arteries. Diltiazem acts more effectively on myocardium and coronary arteries than on peripheral smooth muscle. It prolongs AV nodal conduction, effectively treating supraventricular tachydysrhythmias. Verapamil too prolongs AV nodal conduction; however it acts more strongly on peripheral vasculature and may therefore be less desirable in patients who cannot tolerate afterload reduction.

Angiotensin Antagonists

ACE inhibitors and ARBs are frequently used in conjunction with benign essential hypertension; malignant, renal, and other secondary hypertensions; as well as congestive heart failure. These drugs improve potassium by reducing aldosterone levels, do not typically increase vasomotor tone or sympathetic reflexive nervous system activity, and reduce cardiac afterload without effecting left ventricular filling pressure. Their use may be beneficial in patients with nephropathy, diabetes at risk for development of clinical nephropathy, and acute myocardial infarction as well. Losartan carries an indication for cerebrovascular accident prophylaxis. Valsartan also is approved for use in post-MI patients with left ventricular dysfunction.

Other Vasodilators

Hydralazine is often used in acute hypertension and as an as-needed parenteral therapy. Nitroglycerin enjoys wide use to reduce blood pressure and myocardial ischemia. Sodium nitroprusside is used to decrease acutely increased blood pressure by parenteral means.

Loop Diuretics

Loop diuretics are used to treat cardiopulmonary overload in the ICU and the OR, as well as to treat congestive heart failure, both acute and chronic decompensation.

They find use in neurosurgery, as a second-line diuretic, for improvement of brain relaxation and surgical exposure enhancement. They also help patients with chronic kidney injury and may achieve a desired end result in acute on chronic kidney injury under the guidance of the skilled clinician. Potassium stores can easily become depleted with the use of a loop diuretic. It is important to monitor these stores and supplementation with oral potassium in chronic therapy, or more intensive potassium replacement may become important in the acute setting. Pairing a potassium-sparing diuretic with a loop diuretic may help limit this with effective titration and combination.

Thiazide Diuretics

Thiazide diuretics see wide use in the treatment of benign essential hypertension, control of peripheral edema, as well as control of edema in pregnancy. They see little to no use in the operative or critical care environment, but remain important factors in preoperative assessment of the patient for surgery and as factors for home medication.

Osmotic Diuretics

Because osmotic diuretics quickly and effectively mobilize fluid from cells to vascular space and vascular space to urinary output, osmotic diuretics most commonly find use in acute or worsening chronic cerebral edema, particularly with threatened intracranial hypertension and herniation. Furthermore, in cases of desired increased renal blood flow, such as acute therapy after renal transplantation, osmotic diuretics can provide acute renal failure prophylaxis and therapy. It likely does not help with prophylaxis before contrast loads and does not act as a substitute for intravenous fluid therapy in these circumstances or for other mild injury. Mannitol is frequently employed in craniotomy to improve surgical exposure.

Carbonic Anhydrase Inhibitors

Carbonic anhydrase inhibitors enjoy particular advantages in the treatment of altitude sickness, urinary alkalization, drug-induced edema, and glaucoma and can be used in both absence and generalized seizure disorder and pseudotumor cerebri. Acetazolamide may be helpful in diuresing the patient with metabolic alkalosis. It is imperative to consider that the source of metabolic alkalosis may be fluid contraction, which may be a sign of over-diuresis.

Antidysrhythmics

Lidocaine is approved for use in ventricular dysrhythmia, ACLS with ventricular fibrillation or pulseless ventricular tachycardia. It also acts as a drug for status epilepticus and enjoys wide use as a local anesthetic. Amiodarone is approved for malignant ventricular dysrhythmia, as well as ACLS with ventricular fibrillation or pulseless ventricular tachycardia. Additionally, amiodarone is used in ACLS for wide complex tachycardia, atrial fibrillation, supraventricular tachycardia, and hypertrophic cardiomyopathy. As an antidysrhythmic, sotalol is used in ventricular dysrhythmia for a 1–2-week course. Adenosine may convert paroxysmal supraventricular tachycardia. It is indicated in narrow complex tachycardia in ACLS. It may be used in SVT with aberrancy, which may appear wide. Digoxin is used in CHF therapy and atrial fibrillation and flutter and may convert paroxysmal supraventricular tachycardia. Magnesium is largely used in electrolyte replacement and ventricular dysrhythmia and treats both seizures and preeclampsia. It may induce labor arrest and treats torsades de pointes.

Dosing Options

Alpha-Blockers

Parenterally administered phentolamine may be used as a bolus dose medication or titratable drip. Typical onset time is 2 min with a typical duration of action approaching 10–15 min by most sources. A bolus dose range of 30–70 mcg/kg/dose will produce reliable and short-lived decreases in blood pressure. Phenoxybenzamine is generally orally dosed 10 mg twice daily and requires up to 24 h for conversion into active drug, while prazosin is typically orally dosed 1 mg twice daily.

Beta-Blockers

Esmolol typically has a short duration of action of only 10–20 min, dosed at 0.25–0.5 mg/kg/bolus. For use as a titratable drip, a loading dose of 0.5 mg/kg over 2 min follows with a titratable rate from 0.05 to 0.2 mg/kg/min. Atenolol begins with an intravenous 5 mg bolus over 5 min and may follow with single daily dosing of 25–50 mg/day orally. Parenteral metoprolol effectively reduces myocardial strain and blood pressure at doses of 1.25–5 mg, every 6–12 h. Post-myocardial infarction therapy can include progressive dosing of 2–5 mg every 2 min for up to three doses followed by oral therapy of 50 mg every 6 h, thereafter.

Propranolol, frequently used for indications other than hypertension, has many oral dosing regimens tailored to the condition intended for treatment. Uncommonly, propranolol may be dosed parenterally 0.5–1 mg up to a ceiling of 5 mg total bolus dose. Labetalol may be given either orally or parenterally; however, the beta to alpha antagonism ratio is different for each. The ratio with which there is beta-blockade preference over alpha-blockade activity by labetalol in parenteral and oral therapy is 1:7 to 1:3, respectively. This difference makes oral to parenteral and parenteral to oral conversion potentially challenging. An initial intravenous dose can start as low as 2.5 mg and range as high as 10 mg. Common cardiac dosing in patients with congestive heart failure includes a range of 3.125–25 mg orally, twice daily.

Calcium Channel Blockers

Nicardipine is often initially infused at 5 mg/h with an increase of approximately 2.5 mg/h every 15 min until control is achieved. Peak effects are achieved within 15 min after 3–4 min onset and bolus dose effects last at least 25 min on average. It is suggested to reduce the drip rate to 3 mg/h after goal blood pressure is reached. Nifedipine is dosed orally 10–20 mg three times daily. An extended action formulation can be dosed 30–90 mg once daily. Nimodipine in cerebral vasospasm after subarachnoid hemorrhage, most commonly from ruptured cerebral aneurysm, can be orally dosed 60 mg very 4 h for up to 3 weeks. Alternatively, selective intra-arterial injection by invasive neurovascular catheter placement can relax cerebral vasospasm at the effect site.

Oral diltiazem, 60–90 mg three times daily, provides effective relief from angina. Two extended release formulations exist: 120–180 mg twice daily provides effective therapy for hypertension, while a 24 h formulation ranges from 180 to 480 mg once daily and provides effective relief from angina, as well as treatment for hypertension. Intravenous dosing of 0.25 mg/kg as a bolus may convert supraventricular tachydysrhythmia, and repeat bolus dosing may occur 15 min thereafter with a dose of 0.35 mg/kg. A successful chemical conversion may be supported with a variable infusion rate of 5–15 mg/h thereafter for up to 24 h.

Verapamil may be used orally 80 mg three times daily for migraine prophylaxis. It may also be used for rate control, 80–120 mg three to four times daily, with a maximum 24 h dose of 480 mg. Hypertensive patients benefit from 80 to 120 mg orally, three times daily. A 12 h extended release formula of 120–480 mg/day, divided into daily or twice daily dosing, a 24 h AM extended release formulation of 120–480 mg orally started at 240 mg every morning, and a 24 h PM extended release formulation of 100–400 mg orally started at 200 mg at bedtime. Initial dosing should be halved in the elderly. For supraventricular tachydysrhythmia abortive therapy, 2.5–10 mg IV may be used with a repeat dose not earlier than 15 min later and not to exceed a total dose of 20 mg.

Angiotensin Antagonists

Enalapril, normal converted by liver esterase to active enalaprilat, is available directly in parenteral form as enalaprilat. Enalaprilat may be dosed 0.625–1.25 mg every 6 h with a maximum dose of 5 mg every 6 h. 1.25 mg is considered equivalent to 5 mg by mouth, a typical oral starting dose daily of enalapril. Enalapril may be increased gradually to a maximum dose of 40 mg daily for hypertensive patients and is divided twice daily for congestive heart failure patients. Lisinopril may be dosed 10–40 mg daily and offers a very long duration of action. Captopril is typically dosed 25–50 mg two to three times daily and is divided secondary to a shorter duration of action. Losartan sees a therapeutic range of 25–100 mg daily or divided to twice daily.

Other Vasodilators

Hydralazine is typically bolus dosed 5–10 mg every 15–20 min. Intramuscular dosing of 10–40 mg is reported, but less often used. Nitroglycerin works well as a titratable drip at 1–3 mcg/kg/min. Nitroglycerin response is rapid and effects terminate rapidly after drip cessation as well. Sodium nitroprusside, similarly to nitroglycerin, has rapid onset and offset times, works well as a titratable drip, and is typically started at 0.25–0.5 mcg/kg/min and may increase to as much as 2 mcg/kg/min with little fear for cyanide toxicity.

Loop Diuretics

Furosemide is largely a parenteral and oral medication; although it may be dosed IM, this is rarely done. Orally, 40–120 mg/day divided by the most effective interval, once to twice daily is typical, generally produces a desired result. The dosing of loop diuretics exhibits an all or none effect and does not exhibit a dose-dependent relationship with diuresis. It has been suggested not to exceed 600 mg/day of oral furosemide. Furosemide is twice as potent IV and, as such, should be dosed at 50 % of the previously successful oral dose. Forty milligram parenterally may be a good starting dose for evacuating pulmonary edema. Bumetanide is dosed equally between oral and parenteral forms. As with any oral to parenteral conversion, and the reverse, it is important to understand the conversion may not be purely generalizable to all patients in all situations. Some trial and error will likely be required. Similarly to furosemide, bumetanide is largely orally and parenterally dosed, yet may also find use as an IM therapy. A typical oral dose may range from 0.5 to 10 mg/day divided up to twice daily. IV recommendations are identical. Initially, bumetanide administration may be repeated every 4–5 h until a response is measured.

Thiazide Diuretics

Thiazide diuretics are available as oral tablet and liquid suspension mainly as hydrochlorothiazide but also as metolazone. Hydrochlorothiazide is typically dosed 12.5–50 mg daily for control of hypertension and 25–200 mg daily for peripheral edema. Dosing need not be daily in those intolerant of daily dosing. Every other day dosing or three to five doses per week have also found success.

Osmotic Diuretics

Mannitol is only available in a parenteral form. It is dosed 0.2 g/kg for renal prophylaxis in kidney transplantation and 0.25 g/kg in non-threatening cases of cerebral edema. For intracranial hypertension and threatened herniation, a dose of 0.25–2 g/kg may be needed to achieve acute lowering of intracranial pressure. For surgical exposure during craniotomy, a dose of 0.5–1 g/kg is typically employed.

Carbonic Anhydrase Inhibitors

Acetazolamide is available in both oral and parenteral forms. For glaucoma, a dose of 125–250 mg orally every 4–12 h is typical. Twenty-four to forty-eight hours prior to altitude elevation, patients may begin 250 mg twice to four times daily. Dosing continues until up to 48 h after symptoms resolve or peak altitude is reached. Congestive heart failure sees increased dosing, usually 250–375 mg daily to every other day. Seizure disorders may require as much as 1,000 mg daily, which may be divided up to four times daily. Pseudotumor cerebri patients may require 1–2 g daily. This dose may be divided up to four times daily.

Antidysrhythmics

Lidocaine for ventricular dysrhythmia may be dosed 1–4 mg/min parenterally. An initial dose of 1–1.5 mg/kg intravenously may be appropriate. Lidocaine toxicity generally occurs at a dose of 4.5 mg/kg with a total maximal hourly dose of 300 mg. Importantly, the blood concentration of lidocaine is much more important than the dose delivered, and as such, toxicity may be encountered at doses significantly lower, or higher. ACLS dosing for ventricular fibrillation and pulseless ventricular tachycardia is 1–1.5 mg/kg intravenous or intraosseous, with a maximum limit of 3 mg/kg. The dose for status epilepticus is 1 mg/kg intravenous bolus.

Amiodarone may be given 200–600 mg orally, loading 800–1,600 mg daily until response, with reduction thereafter. Intravenous dosing may start at 1 mg/min after a 150 mg load over 10 min. After conversion, therapy may be titrated to 0.5 mg/min, typically after 6 h. This is generally converted to oral dosing after an additional 18 h. ACLS use has different methodologies for different conditions. If the patient is pulseless, then 300 mg amiodarone may be pushed intravenously. However, if the patient retains a pulse, it is preferred to administer this dose over a 10 min time period. One hundred fifty milligrams intravenous dosing may be repeated every 10 min as needed until conversion. Maintenance dosing for oral amiodarone is typically 200–600 mg daily.

Sotalol may be dosed 80–160 mg every 12 h orally. The dose may be titrated every 3 days. A suggested maximum daily dose is 480 mg, 640 mg/day in refractory cases. Adenosine ACLS paroxysmal and persistent supraventricular tachycardia treatment is 6 mg intravenously followed by a flush volume to clear the intravenous tubing. Twelve milligrams may be used after the 6 mg dose and may be repeated 1–2 min later up to two times.

Digoxin use in congestive heart failure, atrial fibrillation or flutter, and conversion of paroxysmal supraventricular tachycardia is typically dosed orally 0.125–0.5 mg; however, a fasting patient may receive 0.1–0.4 mg intravenously. Digoxin is typically loaded and may be loaded orally 0.75–1.25 mg orally in three doses: 50 % total, 25 % total, and 25 % total every 4–8 h as tolerated. Parenteral load is administered identically with a total dose range of 0.5–1 mg. Patients with renal impairment should have reduced dosing.

Magnesium sulfate may be administered for ventricular dysrhythmia 3–20 mg/min for 5–48 h. It may be loaded 2–6 g over several minutes. For torsades de pointes, magnesium may be given 1–2 g intravenous or intraosseously. After conversion, it may be appropriate to administer 0.5–1 g/h intravenously. Magnesium may still be used in the renally impaired patient, but it should be limited to 20 g over a 48 h period when impairment is severe.

Drug Interactions

Alpha-Blockers

Patients administered alpha-blockers chronically will not exhibit a traditional compensatory response to further methods of autonomic challenge, such as regional blockade, volatile anesthesia, and surgical stress. Without alpha adrenergic response, unopposed beta-agonism may decrease, rather than reflexively increase systemic vascular resistance. The use of alpha adrenergic blockers may be inadvisable or require increased diligence in patients on chronic niacin therapy. Any vasodilating medications affect largely additive results and may increase the risks for either hypotension or orthostatic hypotension.

Beta-Blockers

Drug interactions may include insulin and NSAIDs, due to reduced renal prostaglandin production in patients on chronic NSAID therapy. Hepatically metabolized beta blockade may interact with histamine blockers, such as cimetidine, or antidysrhythmics such as amiodarone. Any drugs that increase hepatic metabolism reduce efficacy, and any drug that decreases hepatic function may increase beta-blocker efficacy. Atenolol is minimally hepatically metabolized.

Bupropion may augment beta-blockade efficacy. Caution is advised with pseudoephedrine containing products due to alpha adrenergic stimulation. Therapy may increase digoxin levels. Combination with metformin and sulfonylureas may mask hypoglycemia and prolong it. Combination with octreotide may result in unintended bradycardia.

Calcium Channel Blockers

Calcium channel blockers may interact with beta-blockers and increase levels of statins. They should not be combined with amiodarone due to a risk of progression of sick sinus syndrome or AV nodal block.

Angiotensin Antagonists

Angiotensin antagonists are often used in conjunction with thiazide and loop diuretics secondary to their ability to help maintain normal potassium stores; however, they may work too effectively in combination with potassium-sparing diuretics. All NSAIDs, including aspirin, may also inadvertently increase potassium stores.

Other Vasodilators

NSAIDS may decrease hydralazine efficacy. Beta-blocker levels may be increased. Use of vasodilators with niacin therapy may increase orthostatic hypotension tendency. Nitroprusside with dobutamine may increase cardiac output in a synergistic fashion. Use of nitroprusside with acetaminophen may increase the risk of methemoglobinemia. Nitroglycerin should not be used in patients on sildenafil. Use of alcohol may increase the effects of nitroglycerin. For unknown reasons, nitroglycerin may create heparin resistance. Alteplase and other thrombolytics may have reduced efficacy in patients receiving nitroglycerin. Sublingual formulations may be poorly absorbed in patients with recent administration of anticholinergics and tricyclic antidepressants secondary to reduced salivation.

Loop Diuretics

Combination of loop diuretics with other nephro- and ototoxic pharmacotherapies may have additive effects. Loop diuretics synergize with ACE inhibitors as well as angiotensin receptor blockers. Aspirin should be used sparingly with loop diuretics. Loop diuretics should be used cautiously in those on other potassium-wasting medications, such as amphotericin and beta-2 agonists. Similarly beta-blocker use may increase the need for potassium store monitoring. Hypokalemia associated with loop diuretics may increase the risk of digoxin toxicity or sensitivity to QT prolongation. Diabetics may require increased insulin dosing with use of loop diuretics. Use with NSAIDS may both decrease efficacy of diuresis and increase nephrotoxic effects. Use with common PPI such as omeprazole may increase the risk of hypomagnesemia. SIADH in combination with SSRI use has been reported.

Thiazide Diuretics

Thiazides may elevate triglyceride levels and are not recommended for those on fibrate therapy. The use of fluoroquinolone antibiotics with thiazides may increase phototoxicity. Thiazide diuretics may increase the lithium serum level of patients under treatment. NSAID and aspirin therapy may have increased nephrotoxic effects with use of thiazides. Patients requiring amiodarone may have increased QT prolongation with the use of thiazides; other QT-prolonging medications may be inadvisable in patients on thiazide therapy. Potassium-wasting medications may have additive effects with thiazides. Proton pump inhibitors may increase the risk for hypomagnesemia.

Osmotic Diuretics

Mannitol should not be avoided for fear of drug interaction in patients with threatened herniation. Proton pump inhibitors may combine with mannitol to worsen hypomagnesemia. Through increased renal blood flow, lithium levels may decrease. Use with octreotide may create undesirable electrolyte shifts, and a decreased dose of mannitol may be appropriate in this case. SSRI use with mannitol can create an increased likelihood of SIADH and hyponatremia.

Carbonic Anhydrase Inhibitors

Acetaminophen and aspirin may increase carbonic anhydrase inhibitor levels. CNS toxicity with increased metabolic acidosis may result. Caution should be used in patients abusing methamphetamine or with prescribed amphetamines for other disorders. Combination with topiramate may increase the risk of nephrolithiasis, worsen metabolic acidosis, and create hyperthermic conditions. Carbonic anhydrase inhibitors should be used thoughtfully in combination with other serum potassium-lowering medications. Use of QT-prolonging medications with carbonic anhydrase inhibitor therapy should be limited. Digoxin toxicity may be increased. Similar to other diuretics, lithium levels may be decreased secondary to increased renal excretion. Hypomagnesemia may be enhanced in patients also on proton pump inhibitors. Acetazolamide may increase the toxicity of anticonvulsants and may increase the chance of osteomalacia with increased use.

Antidysrhythmics

Lidocaine use with scheduled acetaminophen, barbiturates, and nitrates may increase methemoglobinemia. All medications, such as ciprofloxacin and amiodarone, that inhibit hepatic metabolism may increase lidocaine levels. Propranolol may decrease the clearance of lidocaine. Patients on hepatic enzyme-inducing medications, such as cimetidine and TNF-blocking agents, may see decreased lidocaine levels through increased hepatic metabolism. Additive sedating effects with opiates and other sedating medications have been observed. Lidocaine is best not combined with sotalol until two to three half-lives as increased cardiac dysrhythmia may be observed. Lidocaine prolongs the duration of action of depolarizing neuromuscular blockade agents.

Similarly to lidocaine, any medication that inhibits hepatic metabolism may increase amiodarone levels. Any medication that induces hepatic metabolism may decrease amiodarone levels. Concomitant use of statins with either antidysrhythmic therapy should be thoughtfully dosed and considered. Amiodarone may have additive effects with all QT-prolonging medications and should also be thoughtfully and carefully dosed in duality. QT prolongation may be observed with ephedrine use. Some pharmaceuticals, such as methadone, trazodone, tricyclic antidepressants, serotonin-epinephrine reuptake inhibitors, and ondansetron, exhibit both additive QT prolongation and hepatic metabolism inhibition. Electrolytes should be carefully monitored in patients on amiodarone and diuretic therapy.

Calcium channel blockers may reduce hepatic metabolism and have additive effects, resulting in unexpected bradycardia and hypotension. Beta-agonists may increase QT prolongation and dysrhythmia, while beta-blockers may increase bradycardia. Colchicine gout therapy should be carefully weighed and reduced in dose when patients have no renal or hepatic impairment. Otherwise, concomitant therapy is contraindicated. Cyclosporine and amiodarone may increase each other's levels to toxicity through glycoprotein-mediated transport and hepatic metabolism inhibition mechanisms. Digoxin use with amiodarone should be decreased by 50–70 % and digoxin levels should be monitored carefully. Use with corticosteroids may increase QT prolongation, alter electrolyte levels, and induce cardiac dysrhythmia. Lastly, amiodarone may induce an elevated INR in patients on warfarin. Warfarin dosing should be decreased by one-third to one-half in anticipation of hepatic metabolism inhibition. INR levels should be monitored more frequently than usual.

Sotalol should be used with caution in patients also on beta-agonist therapy secondary to the beta-blockade mechanism of sotalol. QT-prolonging medications may add to sotalol's effects. Phenylephrine may combine dangerously with sotalol to cause excess alpha adrenergic stimulation with severe vasoconstriction, hypertension, and induction of dysrhythmia. This has been observed in nasal decongestant phenylephrine as well, but less so than intravenous administration. Advanced AV block has been reported with use of verapamil.

Side Effects and Black Box Warnings

Alpha-Blockers

Alpha-blockers do not act equally at all sites. Those vessels with increased nascent alpha adrenergic tone will experience a higher degree of smooth muscle relaxation than other sites. This may result in side effects such as orthostatic hypotension, near syncope, syncope, hypotension, reflex tachycardia, diarrhea, miosis, nasal congestion, and ejaculatory sexual dysfunction. Phentolamine may exhibit antihistaminic and cholinomimetic effects. Cardiac dysrhythmia and myocardial ischemia with angina pectoris may ensue.

Beta-Blockers

Controversially, patients with asthma may not be candidates for even the most selective beta-1 blockade therapy as these drugs are not purely beta-1 selective. Increased symptoms secondary to decreased sympathetic tone in the bronchial smooth muscle can worsen a patient's quality of life, morbidity, or even mortality. Furthermore, diabetics may experience decreased gluconeogenesis, leading to hypoglycemia or difficult recovery from hypoglycemia. Cold-turkey removal of chronic beta-blockade therapy can contribute to hemodynamic withdrawal with increased tachydysrhythmia. Consequently, the metabolic rate for oxygen in myocardial tissue may increase above its oxygen supply, resulting in unintended myocardial ischemia in the acute perioperative period.

Importantly, patients experiencing significant blood loss in the perioperative period may reduce end-organ perfusion by combining reduced cardiac output with reduced blood volume. Mortality and morbidity may increase from their use in these patient populations. Bradycardia, increased or new heart block, cardiogenic shock, angina on withdrawal, myocardial infarction on withdrawal, ventricular arrhythmia on withdrawal, hepatitis, photosensitivity, lupus erythematosus, agranulocytosis, fatigue, dizziness, diarrhea, pruritus, depression, and dermal rash may all result from beta-blocker pharmacotherapy. Most beta-blockers carry a black box warning against abrupt cessation due to withdrawals mentioned above. Notably, atenolol, labetalol, esmolol, and carvedilol do not carry this warning.

Calcium Channel Blockers

Nicardipine may produce or worsen flushing or headache with its use. Verapamil may increase AV nodal conduction delay to the point of cardiac arrest. Those with sick sinus syndrome or other conduction delay or block may best avoid its use. This effect is exacerbated in combination with propranolol. In general, calcium channel blockers delay recovery from both depolarizing and non-depolarizing neuromuscular blockade. Calcium channel blockers, verapamil in particular, may be best avoided in those with Duchenne's muscular dystrophy. Calcium channel overdose can lead to constipation and unintended myocardial ischemia.

Angiotensin Antagonists

All angiotensin antagonists carry a black box warning regarding use during pregnancy. Affecting the renin-angiotensin-aldosterone system during pregnancy has evidence to support an increase in both fetal and neonatal morbidity and mortality. Bradykinin-mediated angioedema is an uncommon but terrifying and threatening side effect possible with the use of this drug class. Angiotensin antagonists may worsen a patient's condition in acute kidney injury by reducing GFR and elevating potassium levels; thus it is recommended to stop angiotensin antagonism during acute kidney injury or acute on chronic kidney injury. Use of angiotensin antagonists may create refractory hypotension in the anesthetized patient. Somewhat controversially, it is recommended to stop angiotensin antagonists just prior to surgery. Both cough and rash have similarly been reported.

Other Vasodilators

This functional class is not without its side effects. Hydralazine may produce a reflex tachycardia due to the decrease in cardiac afterload that can be undesirable. Lupus-like syndromes, rashes, neuropathy, fever, and pancytopenia have all been associated with its use. Nitroglycerine has few side effects of note and importantly carries no risk of cyanide toxicity. Sodium nitroprusside does carry a risk of cyanide toxicity, which is worsened by increased dose and duration of infusion. It may be avoided in obstetric patients for this very reason and fetal intolerance of even low cyanide level increases. Sodium nitroprusside carries black box warnings for warning to dilute in 5 % dextrose, causing precipitous decreases in blood pressure and cyanide toxicity when used for long durations or at a dose greater than 2 mcg/kg/min.

Loop Diuretics

Loop diuretics carry a black box warning for their potency as both diuretics and their potential to disturb electrolyte balance. Loop diuretics should only be managed under medical supervision. Loop diuretics may contribute to a contraction alkalosis in excess. They are potently oto- and nephrotoxic. Thrombocytopenia has been reported with their use. Bone marrow suppression similarly has been identified. Both anaphylaxis and Stevens-Johnson syndrome have been described with loop diuretic therapy. Loop diuretics may exacerbate connective tissue disease, such as lupus. Rarely, eosinophilia may become laboratory evident upon investigation. More commonly, rash, dizziness, nausea and vomiting, weakness, muscle cramps, transaminitis, tinnitus, and paresthesia are traditionally seen. Cholesterol and triglyceride levels may increase. Patients should reduce their sun exposure.

Thiazide Diuretics

Thiazide therapy has been associated with cholestatic jaundice, interstitial nephritis, Stevens-Johnson syndrome, photosensitivity, bone marrow suppression, hemolytic anemia, severe hypokalemia, lupus exacerbation, and, rarely, angle-closure glaucoma. Orthostatic hypotension, dizziness, diarrhea, anorexia, headache, weakness, sexual dysfunction, abdominal pain and cramping, and hyperglycemia have all been reported. Thiazide diuretics carry no black box warnings.

Osmotic Diuretics

Patients may experience seizures with mannitol use, possibly due to electrolyte perturbation. Congestive heart failure, pulmonary edema, coma, and extravasation necrosis are serious reactions. More commonly, headache, nausea, vomiting, dizziness, and blurred vision may be confused with CNS symptoms. Rash and large derangement of electrolytes, particularly in the young, may cause unwanted side effects. Mannitol administration is directly irritating to the vascular space and can cause thrombophlebitis. Osmotic diuretics carry no black box warnings.

Carbonic Anhydrase Inhibitors

Carbonic anhydrase inhibitors may induce Stevens-Johnson syndrome. Hepatic impairment, even necrosis, is possible. Bone marrow suppression has been reported. Nephrolithiasis and seizures may ensue. More commonly, patients may express fatigue, anorexia, GI upset, tinnitus and hearing impairment, rash, photosensitivity, and melena.

Antidysrhythmics

After lidocaine administration, seizures, respiratory arrest or status asthmaticus, heart block or other bradycardia, coma, anaphylaxis, and methemoglobinemia have all been reported. Confusion, hypotension, anxiety, tinnitus, blurred vision, sedation, and nausea with or without vomiting occur more commonly. Amiodarone carries a black box warning for potential pulmonary and hepatic toxicity, as well as for prodysrhythmic effects in 2–5 % of patients. Amiodarone may cause severe bradycardia, QT prolongation, torsades de pointes, congestive heart failure, cardiogenic shock, acute respiratory distress syndrome, skin rash, altered thyroid function, rhabdomyolysis, pancreatitis, blood dyscrasia, and peripheral neuropathy with prolonged use. More commonly corneal deposits with prolonged therapy, malaise, ataxia, tremor, hyperkinesia, nausea with or without vomiting, constipation, anorexia, hypotension, photosensitivity, and visual disturbance occur. Over long-term use, skin may change color to a bluish or gray tone.

Sotalol carries black box warnings to guide use to minimize the induction of a new arrhythmia, as well as to only use the atrial fibrillation and flutter formulations for those arrhythmias. Sotalol may induce congestive heart failure, severe bradycardia, a withdrawal reaction of angina pectoris or even myocardial infarction, QT prolongation, torsades de pointes, bronchospasm, and lupus erythematosus. More commonly, dyspnea, hypotension, headache, nausea with or without vomiting, edema, sleep disturbance, diarrhea, diaphoresis, and dyspepsia have been reported. Adenosine carries no black box warnings, ventricular fibrillation or tachycardia, atrial fibrillation, and even cardiac arrest. Bronchospasm, flushing, dyspnea, nausea, headache, and lightheadedness may also occur.

Digoxin may cause total AV block, severe bradycardia, new ventricular dysrhythmia, thrombocytopenia, delirium, and intestinal necrosis or ischemia. Dizziness, headache, diarrhea, abdominal pain, anorexia, weakness, visual disturbance, confusion, mood change, gynecomastia, and rash may occur more frequently. Magnesium may cause cardiovascular collapse, respiratory paralysis, hypothermia, pulmonary edema, depressed deep tendon reflexes, hypotension, flushing, drowsiness, diaphoresis, hypocalcemia, hypophosphatemia, hyperkalemia, and vision changes.

Closing Comments

Each antihypertensive, diuretic, and antidysrhythmic carries a dizzying array of uses, dosing options, adverse reactions, and side effects. Most of the negative outcomes associated with a therapy occur during regular and prudent use. Some occur due to rare drug-drug interactions. To further complicate matters, many of these medications enjoy many off-label uses outside the scope of this text. What remains important is developing a strong and organized working knowledge of the most common and most dangerous aspects of each medication and/or drug class and maintaining a low threshold to consult a reference whenever doubt remains.

Chemical Structures

**Chemical Structure
15.1** Amiodarone

**Chemical Structure
15.2** Atenolol

**Chemical Structure
15.3** Esmolol

Chemical Structure
15.4 Lidocaine

Chemical Structure
15.5 Acetazolamide

Further Reading

1. Barash PG, et al. Clinical anesthesia. 5th ed. Philadelphia: Lippincott, Williams and Wilkins; 2013.
2. Epocrates Rx. Version 5.1.2. San Mateo: Epocrates, Inc. Copyright 2009. [Updated 21 Dec 2012]. http://www.epocrates.com.
3. Micromedex Healthcare Series [Internet Database]. Greenwood Village: Thomson Healthcare. Updated periodically.
4. Morgan GE, Mikhail MS, et al. Clinical anesthesiology. 4th ed. New York: Lange; 2013. ISBN 0-071-42358-3.
5. Rang HP. Pharmacology. Edinburgh: Churchill Livingstone; 2003. ISBN 0-443-07145-4.
6. Rosenfeld GC, et al. Board review series pharmacology. 5th ed. Philadelphia: Lippincott, Williams & Wilkins; 2013.

Chapter 16
Peripheral Vasodilators

Ratan K. Banik and Jay S. Berger

Contents

> We were looking for a drug that would dilate coronary arteries. More blood, more oxygen, less angina—better lifestyle. …..we were doing clinical tests in V.A. hospital…….And we found we couldn't get the pills back from the vets. Then doctors started finding pills missing from the hospital cabinets. Very quickly we learned the reason. The drug is now known as Viagra, or "the little blue pill," and is prescribed for impotence. -James R. Gardner, Ph.D., Vice President, Pfizer Inc. [1]

Vasodilators, as their name imply, treat hypertension by causing the smooth muscle walls of blood vessels to relax, thus dilating the vessel. The systemic peripheral vascular resistance (afterload) is reduced by dilating on the arterial side of the

R.K. Banik, MD, PhD • J.S. Berger, MD, PhD (✉)
Department of Anesthesiology, Montefiore Medical Center, Albert Einstein College of
Medicine, Bronx, NY, USA
e-mail: rbanik@montefiore.org; jberger@montefiore.org

A.D. Kaye et al. (eds.), *Essentials of Pharmacology for Anesthesia,*
Pain Medicine, and Critical Care, DOI 10.1007/978-1-4614-8948-1_16,
© Springer Science+Business Media New York 2015

Table 16.1 Principles of vasodilator therapy

Preload reduction	Afterload reduction
Decreased pulmonary venous congestion	Reduction in ventricular wall stress
Decreased ventricular wall stress	Increased coronary blood flow
Increased coronary blood flow	Enhanced oxygen delivery
Improved myocardial oxygen delivery	Improved systolic contractile function
	Reduction in mitral regurgitation

Vasodilators work by reducing preload, afterload, or both preload and afterload. Preload reduction results in decreased intraventricular pressures and improved myocardial oxygen delivery. Afterload reduction results in decreased work for the heart which improves hemodynamics in patients with heart failure

Table 16.2 Classification of systemic vasodilators

Therapeutic objective	Medication
Arterial vasodilation	Hydralazine
(Decreased afterload)	Fenoldopam
Venous vasodilation	Nitroglycerin
(Decreased preload)	
Mixed	Nitroprusside
(Decreased afterload and preload)	ARBs (e.g., losartan)
	ACEI (e.g., enalapril)

ARB angiotensin receptor blocker, *ACEI* angiotensin-converting enzyme inhibitors

vascular system. The peripheral venous return (preload) is reduced by dilating the veins. The overall effect is a decrease in arterial blood pressure, an increase in ventricular output, and a decrease in end-diastolic volume (Table 16.1). In hypovolemic states, vasodilators must be used with caution because they can worsen perfusion to vital organs. Most vasodilating medications to some degree work on both the arterial side and the venous side of the vascular system. However, some vasodilators work more specifically on one side or the other (Table 16.2). These medications are used in a wide variety of disease states, such as coronary artery disease, heart failure, and hypertension. The effectiveness of vasodilator treatment for patients with chronic congestive heart failure has been demonstrated in large multicenter clinical trials (Vasodilator-Heart Failure Trial I and II) [2–4]. The combination of different vasodilators has been shown to significantly improve symptoms, exercise tolerance, and survival of heart failure patients.

Nitroglycerin

Class: Antianginal Agent, Nitrate, Vasodilator

Nitroglycerin is originally discovered in 1847 by Swedish Scientist Dr. Sobrero by interacting glycerol, nitric acid, and sulfuric acid. Originally discovered as an explosive, nitroglycerin was quickly shown to relieve the chest pain associated with

Fig. 16.1 Mechanism of action of nitric oxide (*NO*) induced vasodilation. NO activates the cytosolic guanylate cyclase, to form cyclic guanosine monophosphate, which in turn activates protein kinases. These kinases block calcium entry inside the cell and enhance migration of calcium to intracellular stores resulting in vasodilation. *NO* nitric oxide, *GC* guanylyl cyclase, *cGMP* cyclic GMP

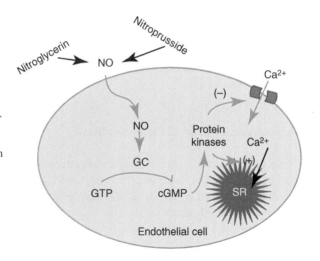

angina pectoris. The exact mechanism for the pain relief remained a mystery for greater than 100 years. It is now known that nitroglycerin releases nitric oxide from vascular smooth muscle cells, which initiates a cascade of events that results in venous relaxation. The investigator Ferid Murad won the Nobel Prize in 1998 for his discovery (along with Robert F. Furchgott, Louis J. Ignarro) [5].

Mechanism of Action

Nitroglycerin binds to the surface of endothelial cells and acts as substrate for formation of nitric oxide (NO). The nitric oxide then moves out of the endothelial cells and binds with its receptor on smooth muscle cell (Fig. 16.1). Once inside the smooth muscle cells, NO converts guanosine triphosphate (GTP) to cyclic guanosine monophosphate (cGMP). The cGMP reduces cytosolic calcium levels by two mechanisms: First, cGMP-dependent protein kinase G is activated which prevents calcium entry into the cell. Second, mitochondrial uptake of calcium is simulated. The overall effect is decreased intracellular calcium levels resulting in smooth muscle cell relaxation [5].

Indications

The primary indication of nitroglycerin is the treatment and prevention of acute chest pain associated with angina pectoris. Acute onset of chest pain can be treated with quickly dissolving sublingual tablets (0.3–0.6 mg) or oral spray (0.4–0.8 mg) administered every 5 min until pain is relieved up to three doses within 15 min [6]. Prevention of pain can be achieved with quickly acting sublingual tablets (0.3–0.6 mg) or oral spray (0.4–0.8 mg) just prior to activity, or extended release tablets (isosorbide-5-mononitrate). The IV form of nitroglycerin is indicated for persistent unstable angina that is poorly responsive to oral form, congestive heart failure with acute MI, hypertensive emergency with acute pulmonary edema, and induction of intraoperative hypotension. Start 10–20 mcg/min and titrate up by 5–10 mcg/min every 5–10 min until desired effect. The maximum dose is 500 mcg/min [7]. Not recommended in pediatrics. Pregnancy safety: Category C, not known if it is secreted in breast milk.

Drug Interactions and Contraindications

Nitroglycerin decreases the anticoagulation effect of heparin, increases the paralytic effect of pancuronium, and potentiates the vasodilatory effect of phosphodiesterase inhibitors which can result in vasodilatory shock. Patients taking ASA >500 mg may have decreased metabolism of nitroglycerin. Nitroglycerin is contraindicated in hypersensitivity to nitrates, glaucoma and hypovolemia, head trauma, constrictive pericarditis, and cardiac tamponade.

Side Effects

The most common side effect is headache, which can be persistent and severe due to dilation of cerebral blood vessels. Other side effects include postural hypotension, tachycardia, syncope, palpitation, anxiety, dizziness, vertigo, anxiety, and weakness. Most of these side effects are related to excessive vasodilation.

Clinical Pearls

  I. Nitroglycerine is the first-line treatment of acute chest pain.
 II. Must use nonabsorbable infusion set because of absorption of the nitroglycerine by standard PVC tubing.
III. Warn patients about the most common side effects of nitroglycerine: headache, orthostatic hypotension, and dry mouth.
 IV. Administration of IV nitroglycerine requires continuous hemodynamic monitoring.
  V. Administration of nitroglycerine with other vasodilators can precipitate a shock state.

Nitroprusside (SNP)

Class: Antihypertensive, Nitrate, Vasodilator

The first recorded use of sodium nitroprusside (SNP) in humans was in 1928; however, FDA approval was delayed until 1974, because of safety concern over cyanide toxicity. SNP is a rapidly acting (<30 s) powerful vasodilator, which affects both arterial and venous smooth muscle cells. In addition to its quick onset, the vasodilatory effect of SNP ceases within 1–3 min of discontinuing the infusion.

Mechanism of Action

Sodium nitroprusside is comprised of five cyanide moieties and one nitrosyl group. Once infused, it converts oxyhemoglobin (Fe^{++}) to methemoglobin (Fe^{+++}) and releases cyanide and NO moieties. Unlike nitroglycerin, SNP directly generates NO, which relaxes vascular smooth muscle by a similar mechanism described above. The cyanide moiety is converted to thiocyanate by thiosulfate sulfurtransferase within the liver. The conversion of cyanide to thiocyanate utilizes sulfur stores. Depletion of sulfur stores by malnutrition or in postoperative patients facilitates accumulation of cyanides and increases the risk of developing cyanide toxicity. The metabolite thiocyanate is excreted in the urine [8].

Indications

The rapid onset of action makes SNP ideal for the treatment of hypertensive crisis. The short duration of action allows SNP to be utilized for deliberate hypotension in a variety of surgical procedures, such as major spinal surgery.

Dosing Options

The only route of administration of SNP is via an intravenous infusion. The dosing for pediatrics and adults is the same. The initial infusion rate is started low at 0.3 g/kg/min and is titrated up every few minutes to a maximum does of 10 g/kg/min [9]. It is not indicated in patients with renal impairment (creatinine clearance <10 ml/min). The use of higher doses limited to a maximum duration of 10 min. Nitroprusside should not be given to pregnant women. It is not known if SNP and its metabolites are excreted in human milk [6].

Drug Interactions and Contraindications

The most common side effects are hypotension, palpitations, restlessness, retching, retrosternal discomfort, and muscle twitching which are related to rapid reduction of blood pressure and disappear once infusion is discontinued. Less commonly seen are the following: significant methemoglobinemia whose incidence increases when the maximum recommended dose of 10 g/kg/min is infused for more than 16 h and when medications such as benzocaine and lidocaine that cause methemoglobinemia are concurrently administered. The administration of >2 mcg/kg/min in patients with renal insufficiency or administration at the maximum dose for greater than 24 h can increase the risk of cyanide toxicity [9]. The signs and symptoms of cyanide toxicity (>5 mg/dl) include metabolic acidosis, nausea, mental confusion, and muscle weakness. The degree of pulmonary shunting can also increase due to SNP attenuating the normal physiologic response of pulmonary artery constriction to hypoxia.

Clinical Pearls

I. Methemoglobinemia should be suspected in patients exhibiting low oxygen saturation (~85 %) despite adequate cardiac output and PO_2. Pay attention at chocolate color blood while taking ABG sample [8].

II. Cyanide toxicity is a clinical diagnosis because cyanide level assay is technically difficult to perform and metabolic acidosis is a lagging indicator. In an awake, spontaneously breathing patient, their breath will smell like almonds and the patient will suddenly become confused. Suspicion should be high when the drug's hypotensive effect is gone despite increased infusion rates. Treatment should include stopping the infusion, mechanical ventilation with 100 % oxygen, and administering sodium thiosulfate (150 mg/kg over 15 min) or 3 % sodium nitrate (5 mg/kg over 5 min) [10].

III. If blood pressure is not controlled by the maximum rate after 10 min, check acid-base balance and venous oxygen concentration for evidence of cyanide toxicity; however, these indicators are not reliable.

IV. Nitroprusside administration is contraindicated in patients with glucose-6-phosphate dehydrogenase deficiency because these patients are unable to clear methemoglobin [11].

Hydralazine

Class: Antihypertensive, Arterial Vasodilator

Hydralazine is a direct arteriolar vasodilator with almost no effect on the venous circulation. It was discovered in 1950 by Franz Gross. The increase in renal blood flow despite the fall in blood pressure has been considered a unique feature of this drug [12].

Mechanism of Action

Hydralazine reduces afterload by causing arterial vasodilation. The decrease in diastolic blood pressure is greater than the decrease in the systolic blood pressure. Some studies suggest that potassium channels are opened for prolonged period causing hyperpolarization of the smooth muscle cells. Another proposed mechanism involves the production of NO stimulating cGMP as described previously [13]. Lastly, hydralazine has been shown to interfere with the release of calcium from the endoplasmic reticulum which inhibits vasoconstriction.

Indications

Hydralazine specifically dilates arteries which minimizes orthostatic hypotension that is associated with other vasodilators. Renal flow is usually maintained or slightly increased by hydralazine making it an ideal medication to use in patients with renal disease; however, clearance is dependent on renal function. Similarly, hydralazine is a first-line medication for the treatment of preeclampsia because it slightly increases uteroplacental blood flow. The reduction of afterload by this drug is beneficial for treatment of congestive heart failure when conventional therapy fails.

Dosing Options

The oral dose is 10–50 mg every 6 h. The IV/IM dose is 5–20 mg every 4 h. Blood pressure starts to decrease within 10–30 min of administration. Pediatric dose is 0.2–0.5 mg/kg IV every 4–6 h [6].

Drug Interactions and Contraindications

The arterial vasodilation causes an increase in cerebral blood flow which contraindicates its use in patients with increased intracranial pressure. It is also contraindicated in the treatment of aortic dissection because the reflex tachycardia may propagate the dissection. Similarly, the reflex tachycardia increases the work of the heart and contraindicates its use in patients with underlying coronary artery disease.

Side Effects

Arterial vasodilation by hydralazine causes stimulation of the sympathetic nervous system which causes tachycardia, myocardial contractility, and increase plasma renin activity. Increased plasma renin stimulates aldosterone resulting in fluid and water retention. Side effects include fluid retention, tachycardia, palpitations, headache, lupus-like syndrome, and neonatal thrombocytopenia.

Clinical Pearls

I. The reflex tachycardia can be prevented by the administration of a low-dose beta-blocker.
II. Genetic variations in the liver enzyme N-acetyltransferase expression determine the hypotensive effect of hydralazine. High levels of enzyme expression result in less vasodilatory effect [14].

III. Lupus can occur in as many as 10 % of patients and presents as joint pain, fever, and anemia. Seventy-three percent of patients experiencing hydralazine-induced lupus are HLA-DRw4 positive [14].

IV. Chronic (>3 months) use of hydralazine can cause peripheral neuropathy by inhibiting the enzymes involved in pyridoxine metabolism. Prophylactic treatment with pyridoxine with oral hydralazine [15].

Calcium Channel Blockers (CCB)

Class: Antihypertensive, Antiarrhythmic, Calcium Channel Blocker, Vasodilator

Calcium channel blockers inhibit the influx of calcium into vascular smooth muscles and cardiac cells. This class of medications is a heterogeneous group with dissimilar structures and function. Dihydropyridines (drug with suffix "dipine," e.g., nifedipine, amlodipine, and nicardipine) cause arterial vasodilation, and non-dihydropyridines (e.g., verapamil and diltiazem) decrease myocardial contractility and heart rate. Further discussion of non-dihydropyridines is outside the scope of this chapter.

Mechanism of Action

Dihydropyridines inhibit voltage-sensitive L-type calcium channels preventing calcium entry into the smooth muscle cells and thus contraction of these cells.

Indications

The patient's comorbidities play a large role in choices of which calcium channel blocker is administered. Nifedipine and nicardipine are used for isolated hypertension in patients with asthma, diabetes mellitus, or renal dysfunction and in the elderly and African American patients. Nifedipine is useful for the treatment of Prinzmetal's angina. In addition to coronary artery vasodilation, the reduced afterload and left ventricular volume results in decrease in myocardial oxygen demand. Nifedipine has minimal negative inotropic activity, minimal effect on nodal activity, and no antiarrhythmic activity, which therefore causes no electrocardiographic changes. Nimodipine has greater effect on cerebral arteries and is indicated for cerebral spasms after subarachnoid hemorrhage or ruptured intracranial aneurysm [16].

Dosing Options

Nifedipine is available as both a short-acting and an extended release form, which are not FDA approved for pediatric use. The short-acting form is used to treat acute coronary spasm titrating from low doses of 20–30 mg 3–4 times per day to a maximum dose of 180 mg per day [6]. The extended release form is used to treat chronic coronary spasm and hypertension by starting at 30–60 mg once per day to a maximum of 120 mg per day [6]. Nicardipine is available in an oral form as are all calcium channel blockers; however, it is the only one available in intravenous form. Thus, nicardipine is the only calcium channel blocker that can be utilized to tightly modulate blood pressure. Start the infusion at 2.5 mg/h titrating up every 15 min to a maximum dose of 15 mg/h [6]. Nimodipine is prophylactically administered to prevent cerebral artery spasm after subarachnoid hemorrhage at a dose of 60 mg every 4 h for 21 days [17].

Drug Interactions and Contraindications

The dihydropyridines are potent vasodilators; therefore, they should not be given to patients with aortic stenosis, cardiomyopathy, heart failure, or recent MI.

Side Effects

Short-acting dihydropyridines (e.g., nifedipine) cause rapid onset of vasodilation which is associated with flushing, tachycardia, palpitation, and headache. These side effects are negligible with the extended release preparations. Peripheral edema has an incidence of 7–30 % of patients taking a calcium channel blocker regardless of the preparation used.

Clinical Pearls

I. Calcium entry blockers may augment the effects of both depolarizing and non-depolarizing muscle relaxants [11].
II. Hypotension induced by calcium channel blocker administration is often not responsive to the administration of intravenous calcium; however, it usually responds to direct vasoconstrictors such as phenylephrine.

Angiotensin-Converting Enzyme (ACE) Inhibitors

Class: Antihypertensive, Vasodilator

In the late 1960s, the Nobel Prize winning scientist Sir John Vance observed that the effects of Brazilian viper venom was due to sudden decrease in blood pressure. A potent inhibitor of the angiotensin-converting enzyme (ACE) was isolated in the venom. This inhibitor was used to develop the first synthetic

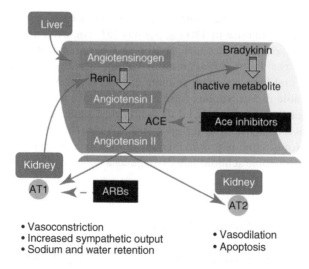

Fig. 16.2 Mechanism of action of angiotensin-converting enzyme (*ACE*) inhibitors and angiotensin receptor blockade. Angiotensinogen is converted to angiotensin I by renin secreted from juxtaglomerular apparatus in the kidney. Angiotensin I is further converted to angiotensin II by ACEIs, which are released in the lungs and also responsible for breakdown of bradykinin, a potent vasodilator. Angiotensin II acts on AT1 receptor in the kidney, which is blocked by ARBs. The role of AT2 receptor in adults remains poorly understood. Note that the production of bradykinin is enhanced by ACE inhibitors (not by ARBs) which is largely responsible for major side effects of these drugs (e.g., dry cough, angioedema)

ACE inhibitor, captopril, for treatment of hypertension. This class of medication is now a mainstay in the treatment of hypertension, heart failure, and chronic kidney disease.

Mechanisms of Action

ACE inhibitors attenuate effects of the renin-angiotensin system (Fig. 16.2). The juxtaglomerular apparatus of the renal cortex secretes renin, which acts on plasma angiotensinogen to form angiotensin I. ACE is then converts angiotensin I to angiotensin II in the lung. Angiotensin II directly constricts vascular smooth muscle cells and stimulates the adrenal gland to release aldosterone and epinephrine. By interfering with the formation of angiotensin II, ACE inhibitors inhibit vasoconstriction [13]. In addition, ACE inhibitors slow the degradation of kinins, which directly cause vasodilation. An elevated level of bradykinin results in an increased conversion of arachidonic acid to prostaglandins, which are also potent vasodilators [13].

Indications

In hypertensive diabetic patients, ACE inhibitors have been shown to delay the progression of diabetic nephropathy. Vasodilation of the afferent arteriole leads to an increase in the renal blood flow; however, vasodilation of the efferent arteriole causes a decrease in the glomerular filtration rate. In heart failure patients, the administration of an ACE inhibitor has been shown in multiple trials to significantly reduce morbidity and mortality. Often an ACE inhibitor is administered in conjunction with a diuretic. The hypovolemia induced by the diuretic triggers vasoconstriction via the angiotensin II system, which is prevented by the ACE inhibitor.

Dosing Options

To avoid hypotension and other adverse side effects, start with a low dose and gradually titrate the dose to the targeted response. Captopril: The starting dose is 6.25–12.5 mg TID and can be titrated up to a maximum dose of 50 mg TID. In pediatrics, the starting dose is 0.15–0.3 mg/kg/day in 3 divided doses and can be titrated up to a maximum dose of 6 mg/kg/day in 3 divided doses. Lisinopril: The starting dose is 2.5 mg per day and may be titrated up to a maximum dose of 40 mg per day. In pediatrics (age >6 years old), the starting dose is 0.07 mg/kg per day and can be titrated up to a maximum dose of 5 mg per day [6].

Contraindications and Drug Interactions

The development of side effects such as a cough or angioedema as described below should prompt the discontinuation of therapy. Bilateral renal artery stenosis is a contraindication to ACE inhibitor administration. Angiotensin II causes vasoconstriction of the efferent arterioles in the glomerulus, increasing the relative glomerular filtration rate. This vasoconstriction is prevented by an ACE inhibitor. The glomerular filtration rate is maintained by vasodilation of the afferent arterioles; however, if bilateral renal artery stenosis exists, the decrease in glomerular filtration rate cannot be compensated for. Pregnancy is also a contraindication to ACE inhibitor administration, which may in the second or third trimester cause pulmonary hypoplasia, intrauterine growth retardation, and oligohydramnios secondary to fetal hypotension [18].

Side Effects

In general, ACE inhibitors are well tolerated and have a low incidence of side effects. Like all vasodilators, ACE inhibitors can cause hypotensive related symptoms such as dizziness and headache. Roughly 20 % of patients will complain of a dry cough. The etiology of the cough is unclear but may be related to the increased kinin level. Symptoms typically cease after the discontinuation of therapy. Less frequently, patients on ACE inhibitors develop angioedema which depending on severity may necessitate endotracheal intubation. Fortunately most cases resolve spontaneously after discontinuation of the medication. In patients with renal insufficiency, the incidence of hyperkalemia increased by the administration of an ACE inhibitor [11].

Clinical Pearls

I. Patients undergoing general anesthesia are likely to experience post-induction hypotension, which must be anticipated and aggressively treated [19].
II. Angioedema is an infrequent life-threatening complication of ACE inhibitors (incidence approximately 0.1 %). Patients typically present with lip and tongue swelling and possibly laryngeal edema. These patients require close monitoring, and if the airway appears to be at risk, early endotracheal intubation is prudent [19].

Angiotensin Receptor Blockers (ARBs)

Class: Antihypertensive, AT1 Receptor Antagonists, Vasodilator

The disruption of the renin-angiotensin system by ACE inhibitors is an effective means to treat hypertension; however, as mentioned previously ACE inhibitors are associated with some unwanted side effects. ACE inhibitors prevent the formation of angiotensin II. The interaction of angiotensin II with the smooth muscle cells is prohibited by ARBs (Fig. 16.2). In circumstances where the side effects of ACE inhibitors cannot be tolerated, ARBs have been shown to effectively control blood pressure.

Mechanism of Action

The conversion of angiotensin I to angiotensin II is catalyzed by angiotensin-converting enzyme in the lung. Angiotensin II then interacts with the AT1 receptor on smooth muscle cells causing vasoconstriction. This interaction is prevented by ARBs. Unlike ACE inhibitors, ARBs do not interfere with kinin degradation and consequently bradykinin levels do not increase. The difference in mechanism of action may explain the significantly lower incidence of cough associated with ARBs versus ACE inhibitors [13].

Dosing Options

The typical starting dose of losartan is 50 mg per day, but the dose can be reduced to 25 mg per day in hypovolemic patients. The maximum dose is 100 mg per day. Losartan is also marketed as a combination medication with hydrochlorothiazide (HCTZ) that comes in the following concentrations: losartan/HCTZ 50 mg/12.5 mg, 100 mg/12.5 mg, and 100 mg/25 mg. The pediatric dose of losartan is 0.7 mg/kg per day to a maximum dose of 50 mg/ day [6].

Indications

ACE inhibitors are superior to ARBs in the treatment of hypertension in patients with heart failure. The difference in their mechanism of action of these two classes of medication may explain the difference in their efficacy. ACE inhibitors result in reduced levels of angiotensin II, which downregulates the activity at both AT1 and AT2 receptors. ARBs only interfere with the interaction between angiotensin II and the AT1 receptor (Fig. 16.2). There is limited evidence regarding the beneficial effects of administering both and ARB and an ACE inhibitor. The combination is, however, contraindicated in post-MI patients. Losartan has been shown to increase uric acid levels, questioning its benefit in patients with hypertension and gout.

Contraindications and Drug Interactions

Fluconazole inhibits metabolism of ARBs, causing an increased antihypertensive effect. Indomethacin, phenobarbital, and rifampin decrease their effectiveness of ARBs. Telmisartan enhances insulin sensitivity, which may help in blood sugar control in diabetic patients. ARBs may increase lithium levels out of the therapeutic levels and into toxic levels. ARBs should be used with caution in patients who have difficulty regulating potassium levels. ARBs are contraindicated in pregnancy and in patients who have angioedema with ACE inhibitors.

Side Effects

ARBs are well tolerated and relatively have a low incidence of side effects. Cough and angioedema may occur; however, the incidence is much less than compared for ACE inhibitors. ARBs are associated with a significantly higher rate of symptomatic hypotension than are ACE inhibitors.

Clinical Pearls

I. The risk of post-induction hypotension is greater in patients who continue to take ARBs up to the day of surgery; nevertheless, studies show that the benefits of blood pressure control outweigh this risk of perioperative hypotension [20].

II. The patients with poorly controlled hypertension should be medically optimized before proceeding to elective surgery. In general, it is recommended that elective surgery should be canceled for patients with blood pressure >170/110 in multiple measurements [20].

Fenoldopam

Class: Antihypertensive, Dopamine Agonist, Vasodilator

Fenoldopam is a selective dopamine-1 receptor agonist which lowers blood pressure by decreasing peripheral vascular resistance, diuresis, and renal vasodilation. The drug is 6–10 times more potent than dopamine in producing renal vasodilatation and has no adrenergic effects.

Mechanism of Action

Stimulation of dopamine DA1 receptor causes systemic arterial vasodilation, specifically in renal, coronary, cerebral, and mesenteric arteries. Generalized arterial vasodilation rapidly reduces peripheral vascular resistance and blood pressure. In the kidney, both the afferent and efferent arterioles are dilated, which results in a large increase in renal blood flow with little effect on the glomerular filtration rate. In addition, it inhibits the Na-K-ATPase pump in the proximal tubular cells and sodium reabsorption in the collecting tubules. The net effect is natriuresis and diuresis.

Indications

The drug is indicated for treatment of severe hypertension and short-term (<4 h) blood pressure reduction in pediatric patients. It may be useful in patients with acute renal failure, as it selectively activates renal dopamine DA1 receptor without affecting additional receptors, lowers renal vascular resistance, and increases urinary output [21].

Dosing Options

Oral bioavailability is poor, limiting administration to continuous intravenous infusion. The initial infusion rate is 0.03–0.1 mcg/kg/min and increased in increments of 0.05–0.1 mcg/kg/min every 15 min until targeted response is reached. The maximal infusion rate is 1.6 mcg/kg/min. In children under the age of 12 years, the initial infusion rate is 0.2–0.3 mcg/kg/min and is titrated up to a maximum dose, 0.8 mcg/kg/min. The onset of action is 5 min and the peak effect is reached within 20 min. The medication is rapidly metabolized by the liver and excreted in the urine [6].

Drug Interaction and Contraindications

No drug interaction is reported. There are no contraindications.

Side Effects

The drug increases intraocular pressure and decreases serum potassium levels. The other side effects are related to vasodilation, which included hypotension, dizziness, headache, flushing, and tachycardia.

Clinical Pearls

I. Fenoldopam contains sulfite and is therefore contraindicated in patients with a sulfur allergy.
II. Fenoldopam may increase intraocular pressure. Monitor patients for any changes in vision during and after the treatment [21].
III. Monitoring of potassium levels is required to prevent dangerous hypokalemia [21].

Chemical Structures

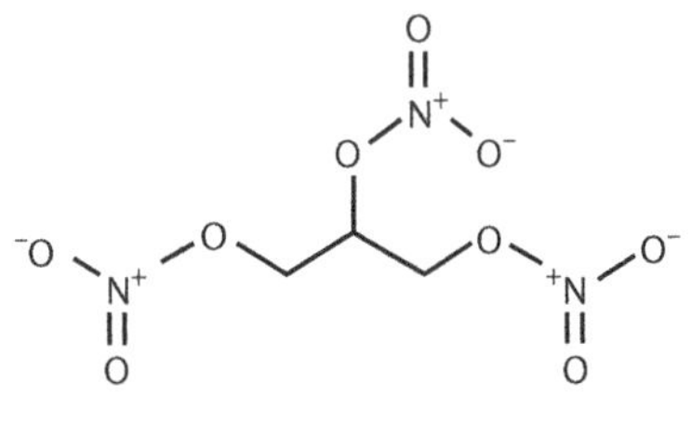

Chemical Structure 16.1 Nitroglycerin

Chemical Structure 16.2 Hydralazine

Chemical Structure 16.3 Nifedipine

Chemical Structure 16.4 Captopril

Chemical Structure 16.5 Losartan

References

1. Studies PSUOotVPfRaG, School PSUOotVPfRaDotG. Research/Penn State: Pennsylvania State University, Office of the Vice President for Research and Graduate Studies. 1998.
2. Cohn JN, Johnson G, Ziesche S, Cobb F, Francis G, Tristani F, Smith R, Dunkman WB, Loeb H, Wong M. A comparison of enalapril with hydralazine-isosorbide dinitrate in the treatment of chronic congestive heart failure. N Engl J Med. 1991;325:303–10.
3. Loeb HS, Johnson G, Henrick A, Smith R, Wilson J, Cremo R, Cohn JN. Effect of enalapril, hydralazine plus isosorbide dinitrate, and prazosin on hospitalization in patients with chronic congestive heart failure. The V-HeFT VA Cooperative Studies Group. Circulation. 1993;87:VI78–87.
4. Rector TS, Johnson G, Dunkman WB, Daniels G, Farrell L, Henrick A, Smith B, Cohn JN. Evaluation by patients with heart failure of the effects of enalapril compared with hydralazine plus isosorbide dinitrate on quality of life. V-HeFT II. The V-HeFT VA Cooperative Studies Group. Circulation. 1993;87:VI71–7.
5. Meinertz T. Nitroglycerin 9: nitrates and mobility. Berlin: Walter de Gruyter; 2000.
6. In: Lexi-Drugs Online [Internet Database]. Hudson OL-C, Inc. Accessed 26 Mar 2014.
7. Kannam JP, Gersh BJ. Nitrates in the management of stable angina pectoris. In: Biller J, Wilterdink JL, GM, editors. Uptodate Inc. Retrieved from http://www.uptodatecom/home/indexhtml. Accessed 25 Mar 2014.
8. Irwin RS, Rippe JM. Irwin and Rippe's intensive care medicine. Philadelphia: Wolters Kluwer Health/Lippincott Williams & Wilkins; 2008.
9. Kaplan NM. Drug treatment of hypertensive emergencies. In: Aronson MD, Holt NF, Sokol HN, editors. Uptodate Inc. Retrieved from http://www.uptodatecom/home/indexhtml. Accessed 25 Mar 2014.
10. Hensley FA, Gravlee GP, Martin DE. A practical approach to cardiac anesthesia. 4th ed. Philadelphia: Wolters Kluwer Health; 2008.
11. Barash PG, Cullen BF, Stoelting RK, Cahalan M, Stock C. Clinical anesthesia. 6th ed. Philadelphia: Wolters Kluwer Health; 2009.
12. Feldman AM. Heart failure: pharmacologic management. Hoboken: Wiley; 2008.
13. Agasti TK. Textbook of anaesthesia for postgraduates. New Delhi: Jaypee Brothers, Medical Publishers; 2011.
14. Izzo JL, Black HR, Goodfriend TL, Research CHBP. Hypertension primer: the essentials of high blood pressure. Philadelphia: Lippincott Williams & Wilkins; 2003.
15. Goljan EF. Rapid review pathology: with student consult online access. Elsevier – Health Sciences Division.
16. Modak RK. Anesthesiology Keywords Review. 2nd ed. Philadelphia: Wolters Kluwer Health; 2013.
17. Singer RJ, Ogilvy CS, Rordof G. Treatment of aneurysmal subarachnoid hemorrhage. In: Kaski JC, Shaperia GM, editors. Uptodate Inc. Retrieved from http://www.uptodatecom/home/indexhtml. Accessed 25 Mar 2014.
18. Schaefer C, Peters PWJ, Miller RK. Drugs during pregnancy and lactation: treatment options and risk assessment. 2nd ed. London: Elsevier Science; 2007.
19. Hines RL, Marschall K. Stoelting's anesthesia and co-existing disease. 5th ed. Philadelphia: Churchill Livingstone; 2008.
20. Lovich-Sapola JA. Anesthesia oral board review: knocking out the boards. New York: Cambridge University Press; 2009.
21. Frishman WH, Sica DA. Cardiovascular pharmacotherapeutics. 3rd ed. Minnesota: Cardiotext Publishing; 2011.

Chapter 17
Nitric Oxide and Pulmonary Vasodilators

Michelle Schlunt

Contents

Pulmonary vasodilators are predominantly used as target-directed therapy for patients diagnosed with pulmonary arterial hypertension, which has an annual mortality of approximately 10 %. Pulmonary arterial hypertension is defined as a mean pulmonary artery pressure of >25 mmHg at rest, a pulmonary wedge pressure ≤15 mmHg and pulmonary vascular resistance >3 Wood units [1]. In pediatric patients, pulmonary hypertension is commonly defined as a systolic

M. Schlunt, MD
Department of Anesthesiology, Children's Hospital Los Angeles, Los Angeles, CA, USA
e-mail: mschlunt@chla.usc.edu

A.D. Kaye et al. (eds.), *Essentials of Pharmacology for Anesthesia,*
Pain Medicine, and Critical Care, DOI 10.1007/978-1-4614-8948-1_17,
© Springer Science+Business Media New York 2015

Table 17.1 Updated clinical classification of pulmonary hypertension [3]

I. Pulmonary arterial hypertension
Idiopathic
Heritable
Drug and toxin induced
Associated with:
Connective tissue diseases
HIV infection
Portal hypertension
Congenital heart diseases
Schistosomiasis
Chronic hemolytic anemia
Persistent pulmonary hypertension of the newborn
I′. Pulmonary venoocclusive disease and/or pulmonary capillary hemangiomatosis
II. Pulmonary hypertension owing to left heart disease
III. Pulmonary hypertension owing to lung disease and/or hypoxia
IV. Chronic thromboembolic pulmonary hypertension
V. Pulmonary hypertension with unclear multifactorial mechanisms

pulmonary arterial pressure > half systemic arterial pressure [2]. Pulmonary arterial hypertension may be idiopathic or related to other causes such as left heart disease or lung disease. The classifications of pulmonary arterial hypertension were most recently updated at the fourth World Symposium in 2008 [3] (Table 17.1). The majority of clinical studies involving pulmonary vasodilator therapy involve patients in classification group 1. Pulmonary vasodilators are also utilized in the setting of acute increases in pulmonary vascular resistance, which can occur following cardiac or thoracic surgery, in the setting of adult respiratory distress syndrome (ARDS) or acute pulmonary embolism [4]. Three major neurohumoral signaling pathways modulate pulmonary vascular tone, and it appears to be an imbalance between these pathways resulting in the disorder of pulmonary arterial hypertension [5]. Each pathway will be discussed, as well as the agents, which influence each particular pathway.

Nitric Oxide

Class: Inhaled Selective Pulmonary Vasodilator

Nitric oxide (NO), previously termed endothelium-derived relaxing factor, is a potent endogenous vasodilator, as well as a valuable signaling molecule [6]. Originally described for its use in the treatment of persistent pulmonary hypertension of the newborn (PPHN) [7], inhaled nitric oxide (iNO) therapy has been extended to usage for right ventricular dysfunction with increased pulmonary

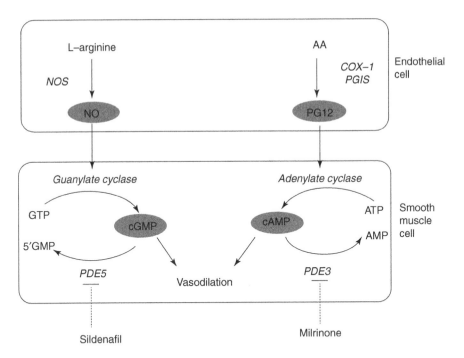

Fig. 17.1 Nitric oxide (*NO*) and prostacyclin (*PGI₂*) signaling pathways in the regulation of pulmonary vascular tone. NO is synthesized by NO synthase (*NOS*) from the terminal nitrogen of L-arginine. NO stimulates soluble guanylate cyclase (*sGC*) to increase intracellular cGMP. PGI₂ is an arachidonic acid (*AA*) metabolite formed by cyclooxygenase (*COX-1*) and prostacyclin synthase (*PGIS*) in the vascular endothelium. PGI₂ stimulates adenylate cyclase in vascular smooth muscle cells, which increase intracellular cAMP. Both cGMP and cAMP indirectly decrease free cytosolic calcium, resulting in smooth muscle relaxation. Specific phosphodiesterases (*PDE*) hydrolyze cGMP and cAMP, thus regulating the intensity and duration of their vascular effects. Inhibition of these PDE with such agents as sildenafil and milrinone may enhance pulmonary vasodilation (From Steinhorn [27] and Porta and Steinhorn [12]; with permission)

vascular resistance following left ventricular assist device placement [8], orthotopic heart [9], lung and liver transplantation [10], and surgery for congenital heart disease [11].

Mechanism of Action

Nitric oxide is synthesized by nitric oxide synthase (NOS) from L-arginine to citrulline in pulmonary endothelial cells. Nitric oxide generated in the endothelium diffuses into adjacent vascular smooth muscle cells. The generation of NO influences guanylate cyclase to increase production of cyclic-guanine monophosphate (cGMP). cGMP decreases free intracellular calcium thereby causing vascular smooth muscle relaxation [12] (Fig. 17.1). Nitric oxide is absorbed into the blood where it binds to oxyhemoglobin forming methemoglobin or it combines with deoxyhemoglobin forming nitrosyl-hemoglobin, which is oxidized to methemoglobin with the release of nitrates [13]. Because of its rapid degradation and inhalational delivery, administration of NO has virtually no systemic vasodilatory effects.

Indications

Nitric oxide is used in the setting of acute increases in pulmonary vasoreactivity with associated right ventricular dysfunction, as well as therapy to decrease intrapulmonary shunt. It is usually administered with mechanical ventilation but can also be administered with continuous positive airway pressure (CPAP) or nasal cannula apparatus. The initial recommended starting dose is 20 parts per million (ppm). A higher dose of 40 ppm may be utilized if no response is readily noted within 20 min of initiating therapy; however, it should be noted that failure to respond at 20 ppm is rarely associated with a favorable response at a higher dose [7]. Due to its inhalational delivery, nitric oxide is delivered only to ventilated lung units thereby increasing perfusion to those selective areas decreasing intrapulmonary shunt. Inhaled NO therapy for PPHN has reduced the need for extracorporeal membrane oxygenation (ECMO) in infants >35 weeks' estimated gestational age, yet it has not demonstrated a change in overall mortality [7]. Nitric oxide may also have a protective role in the inflammatory response as it has been shown to inhibit platelet aggregation, block monocyte adherence/migration, and inhibit vascular smooth muscle cell proliferation [6].

Inhaled NO is also used during diagnostic right heart catheterization to assess a patient's response to acute vasodilator therapy. Those patients with pulmonary arterial hypertension who meet the defined criteria of a decrease in mean pulmonary artery pressure ≥ 10 mmHg to a value of ≤ 40 mmHg with an increase or unchanged cardiac output are termed "responders" and are initially treated with calcium-channel blockers for their disease [4]. However, the proportion of patients with a favorable response is <10 % [14]. Additional agents which may be used in this type of provocative testing are intravenous epoprostenol and adenosine [4].

Drug Interactions and Contraindications

The administration of high doses of nitric oxide and prolonged usage can result in high levels of nitric oxide, which can compete with oxygen. The use of iNO treatment requires monitoring for the formation of nitrogen dioxide (NO_2) [6]. Cytotoxicity related to the formation of free oxygen radicals may worsen existing lung injury and interfere with mitochondrial respiration [6].

Prolonged administration and higher doses of nitric oxide increases the risk of developing significant methemoglobinemia. Methemoglobin levels should be measured frequently and kept <2.5 % [2]. The use of additional nitrate compounds such as nitroglycerin or sodium nitroprusside may have additive effects increasing the risk of developing methemoglobinemia.

Side Effects

Abrupt cessation in inhaled nitric oxide therapy may be followed by a severe rebound in pulmonary hypertension secondary to the downregulation of endogenous nitric oxide production. If deterioration occurs during weaning or after treatment has been discontinued, the dose should be increased to the previous level or inhaled NO therapy restarted [2]. The use of sildenafil prior to discontinuation of inhaled NO therapy has been shown to prevent rebound pulmonary hypertension [12].

Clinical Pearls

I. Initial dose is 20 ppm.
II. Requires specialized delivery system with monitoring for NO_2.
III. If difficulty is encountered with weaning, consider the addition of sildenafil and/or bosentan prior to reinitiating the weaning process.

Prostanoids

Prostacyclin is derived from the action of cyclooxygenase on arachidonic acid. Prostacyclin generated in pulmonary endothelial cells binds to the smooth muscle cell membrane-bound receptor stimulating adenylate cyclase to increase levels of cyclic adenosine monophosphate (cAMP) [12]. cAMP works to decrease intracellular calcium levels thereby causing vasodilatation [12] (Fig. 17.1). Prostacyclin is also a strong inhibitor of platelet aggregation, as well as an inhibitor of smooth muscle proliferation. Patients with pulmonary arterial hypertension are known to have decreased levels of prostacyclin causing an imbalance which favors vasoconstriction and pulmonary vascular remodeling [5].

Epoprostenol (Flolan®)

Class: Intravenous Synthetic Prostacyclin Analogue

Epoprostenol was approved by the FDA in 1995 for the treatment of pulmonary arterial hypertension. It is the only agent to date which has demonstrated survival benefit in this particular patient population [5].

Mechanism of Action

Epoprostenol functions like endogenous prostacyclin to increase cAMP levels which in turn decrease intracellular calcium levels thereby promoting pulmonary

Table 17.2 World Health Organization functional classifications of patients with pulmonary hypertension [26]

I.	No limitation of usual physical activity; ordinary physical activity does not cause increased symptoms
II.	Mild limitation of usual physical activity; no discomfort at rest, but normal physical activity causes symptoms
III.	Marked limitation of physical activity; no discomfort at rest, although less than normal activity causes symptoms
IV.	Unable to perform any physical activity and may have signs of right ventricular failure; dyspnea and/or fatigue present at rest, and any physical activity causes symptoms

smooth muscle cell vasodilatation. Due to its short half-life of 3 min, epoprostenol must be administered as a continuous intravenous infusion requiring a dedicated central venous catheter [15]. The drug must be reconstituted in an alkaline solution, kept in a cool pack during administration, and be protected from light [16]. Once reconstituted, the solution is only good for 24 h. Initial dosing is started at 2 nanograms per kilogram per minute (ng/kg/min) and increased by increments of 2 ng/kg/min every 15 min based on response and any noted side effects. The maximum recommended dose is 40 ng/kg/min. Epoprostenol is rapidly hydrolyzed at neutral pH in the blood with its metabolites excreted in the urine.

Indications

Epoprostenol is considered worldwide to be the first line of therapy in patients with advanced disease (World Health Organization [WHO] functional classes III–IV) or those who are unresponsive to oral pulmonary vasodilator therapies [14] (Table 17.2).

Drug Interactions and Contraindications

Epoprostenol has both systemic and pulmonary vasodilatory effects. If used in combination with other antihypertensives, there is an increased risk for exaggerated decreases in systemic blood pressure. Epoprostenol also has antiplatelet aggregation properties, and if used concurrently with other antiplatelet agents or anticoagulants, the risk for bleeding is increased. It has also been shown to decrease the clearance of digoxin, which is important as digoxin is commonly used as part of conventional treatment for pulmonary arterial hypertension.

Side Effects

The most concerning side effect is systemic vasodilatation. A drop in systemic blood pressure may compromise coronary blood flow particularly to the right ventricle leading to worsening of its function [17]. Other reported systemic side effects which usually limit further epoprostenol dosage increases are headache, flushing, jaw pain, bone pain, nausea, diarrhea, and dizziness. Because epoprostenol does increase pulmonary perfusion, the presence of underventilated lung areas may lead to worsening of ventilation/perfusion mismatch in patients with existing lung disease.

Clinical Pearls

   I. Tachyphylaxis is quite common.
  II. The interruption of the continuous infusion can lead to severe rebound pulmonary hypertension; therefore, patients should always have a backup infusion pump as well as a spare drug cartridge readily available.
 III. Risk of central line catheter infection.
 IV. At higher doses, it may cause high-output cardiac failure.

Treprostinil (Remodulin®, Tyvaso®)

Class: Subcutaneous/Intravenous/Inhalational Synthetic Prostacyclin Analogue

Mechanism of Action

Being a prostacyclin analogue, treprostinil stimulates increased production of cAMP which decreases intracellular calcium in pulmonary vascular smooth muscle cells causing vasodilatation. Treprostinil has a longer half-life of 3–4 h in comparison to epoprostenol. This longer half-life allows treprostinil to be administered via a continuous subcutaneous route. Its neutral pH solution is stable at room temperature, making it much more convenient for patient care administration compared to epoprostenol [15]. For those patients who cannot tolerate the subcutaneous route, intravenous administration is an alternative option. However, intravenous administration requires central venous access with its attendant risks of infection and thrombosis. Initial dosing for both continuous subcutaneous and intravenous administration begins at 0.625–1.25 ng/kg/min with incremental increases of 1.25 ng/kg/min weekly for the first month. Afterward, further incremental increases are done at 2.5 ng/kg/min with a maximum recommended dosage of 40 ng/kg/min. Inhalational delivery dosage starts at three breaths which is equal to 18 micrograms (mcg) per treatment which is done four times daily while awake. Dosing is increased by three breaths every 1–2 weeks up to nine breaths per treatment (54 mcg) [15].

Indications

Treprostinil was initially approved by the FDA in 2002 for the treatment of patients with pulmonary arterial hypertension in WHO functional classes II–IV. The approval for intravenous administration followed in 2004 and subsequent approval for inhalation delivery in 2009.

Drug Interactions and Contraindications

Subcutaneous and intravenous administration of treprostinil during concurrent administration of antihypertensives may result in exaggerated decreases in systemic blood pressure. As with other prostanoids, treprostinil inhibits platelet aggregation and may increase the risk of bleeding in the presence of other antiplatelet agents and anticoagulants. Treprostinil is metabolized in the liver by cytochrome P450 (CYP) 2C8. CYP inhibitors like gemfibrozil decrease the clearance of treprostinil, while CYP inducers such as rifampin increase its clearance. Treprostinil itself however does not induce or inhibit CYP enzymes.

Side Effects

With the subcutaneous route of administration, the most common reported side effect is pain and erythema at the injection site. As with other prostanoids, systemic vasodilatation occurs with its associated symptomatology of headache, flushing, jaw pain, bone pain, nausea, and diarrhea and dizziness.

Clinical Pearls

I. It is suggested with subcutaneous administration to change sites every 72 h.

Iloprost (Ventavis)

Class: Inhaled Synthetic Prostacyclin Analogue

Mechanism of Action

Being a prostacyclin analogue, iloprost stimulates increased production of cAMP which decreases intracellular calcium in pulmonary vascular smooth muscle cells causing vasodilatation. Initial dosing is 2.5–5 mcg/dose with six to nine doses daily while awake [15]. Recommended delivery is via an ultrasonic nebulizer, but each dose administration usually takes 10–15 min to complete. The maximum dosage is 45 mcg/day. The half-life of iloprost is 20–30 min, and it undergoes beta-oxidation to an inactive metabolite.

Indications

Iloprost was the first inhaled prostanoid approved by the FDA for the treatment of pulmonary arterial hypertension. It is recommended as a fourth-line agent for long-term treatment in WHO functional class III patients or as an optional agent with epoprostenol in WHO functional class IV patients [14].

Drug Interactions and Contraindications

Iloprost has both systemic and pulmonary vasodilatory effects. If used in combination with other antihypertensives, there is an increased risk for exaggerated decreases in systemic blood pressure. Iloprost also has antiplatelet aggregation properties, and if used concurrently with other antiplatelet agents or anticoagulants, the risk for bleeding is increased. Iloprost, unlike epoprostenol, has no effect on digoxin levels.

Side Effects

Common reported side effects associated with inhaled iloprost therapy include cough, headache, flushing, jaw pain, nausea, and dizziness.

Phosphodiesterase Inhibitors

Phosphodiesterases are enzymes involved in the degradation of both cGMP and cAMP attenuating their effects on pulmonary vasodilatation. It is the inhibition of these enzymes that is targeted by this particular class of pulmonary vasodilators.

Sildenafil

Class: Selective Phosphodiesterase-5 Inhibitor

Mechanism of Action

Nitric oxide signaling from pulmonary endothelial cells triggers guanylate cyclase to increase production of cGMP, which in turn decreases intracellular calcium leading to vasodilatation. Phosphodiesterase-5 breaks down cGMP. In pulmonary arterial hypertensive patients, increased levels of phosphodiesterase-5 which would cause an imbalance toward pulmonary vasoconstriction have been noted. Selective inhibition of this enzyme would therefore prohibit the breakdown of cGMP increasing its levels to promote pulmonary vasodilatation (Fig. 17.1). Dosing recommendation is 20 milligrams (mg) orally three times a day, with prior studies having reported doses up to 80 mg orally three times daily. Oral pediatric doses range from 1 to 5 mg/kg three times daily. An intravenous formulation was approved in 2009 to be used as a temporizing measure for those unable to take the oral formulation. The parenteral dose is 10 mg three times daily. Sildenafil is metabolized in the liver by the CYP system, mainly CYP3A4 and CYP2C9. Its estimated half-life is approximately 3–4 h with onset of effect within 15 min of administration.

Indications

In 2005, sildenafil became the first phosphodiesterase-5 inhibitor to receive FDA approval for the treatment of pulmonary arterial hypertension in WHO functional class II–III patients. Its use for erectile dysfunction preceded this. Sildenafil, although not approved in the pediatric population, has been used extensively off-label in the settings of PPHN [18] and pulmonary hypertension secondary to congenital heart disease.

Drug Interactions and Contraindications

Being metabolized by CYP3A4 and CYP2C9, sildenafil levels are affected by CYP inhibitors such as cimetidine and ketoconazole which would increase levels, whereas CYP inducers such as rifampin would decrease levels. Sildenafil potentiates the action of antihypertensives and is contraindicated in patients receiving concurrent nitrate therapy in any form.

Side Effects

Common side effects reported with sildenafil administration include headache, flushing, nasal congestion, nausea, diarrhea, and abdominal pain. In 2005, the FDA updated its labeling for phosphodiesterase-5 inhibitors due to reported cases of sudden vision loss (non-arteritic ischemic optic neuropathy) possibly associated with their use [15]. Other vision changes may include color perception changes (inability to distinguish between green and blue), blurry vision, and photosensitivity. There have also been unsettling reports of sudden hearing loss as well [15]. A recent 2012 FDA warning states that the off-label use of sildenafil in the pediatric population for the treatment of pulmonary arterial hypertension is not recommended, nor has it even been approved for such use. The warning was due to recent findings in a pediatric clinical trial which noted an increased risk of mortality in the children receiving higher dosages of sildenafil compared with the lower-dosage groups over a three-year period of treatment [19].

Clinical Pearls

I. Has been demonstrated to be useful in facilitating weaning of iNO therapy to prevent rebound pulmonary hypertension
II. Should not be substituted with the formulation used for erectile dysfunction (Viagra®)
III. Should not be combined for use with other phospodiesterase-5 inhibitors

Tadalafil (Adcirca®)

Class: Selective Phosphodiesterase-5 Inhibitor

Mechanism of Action

Tadalafil is a selective phosphodiesterase-5 inhibitor which has the same mechanism of action as described for sildenafil. It has a significantly longer half-life of 35 h allowing for once daily dosing of 40 mg orally. The dose should be decreased to 20 mg daily in those with decreased creatinine clearance or moderate liver dysfunction [15]. The pediatric dose is 1 mg/kg orally once a day.

Indications

Tadalafil is the second oral phosphodiesterase-5 inhibitor to be approved for the treatment of pulmonary arterial hypertension WHO functional class II–III patients.

Drug Interactions and Contraindications

Tadalafil is metabolized in the liver by the CYP system, mainly CYP3A4. As such its metabolism is affected by concurrent administration of CYP inhibitors and inducers. As with sildenafil, the use of tadalafil with concurrent administration of nitrate therapy in any form is contraindicated. Tadalafil is also contraindicated in patients with a creatinine clearance <30 ml/min and in those patients with severe liver dysfunction [15].

Side Effects

Common side effects reported with tadalafil administration include headache, flushing, nausea, diarrhea, abdominal pain, and extremity pain. Practitioners must also be aware of the possibility of associated sudden vision or hearing loss [15].

Clinical Pearls

I. The half-life of tadalafil is shortened to approximately 17 h with concurrent administration of bosentan [20].
II. Should not be combined with other phosphodiesterase-5 inhibitors.

Milrinone (Primacor®)

Class: Selective Phosphodiesterase-3 Inhibitor

Mechanism of Action

Milrinone is a selective phosphodiesterase-3 inhibitor which works to prevent the degradation of cAMP in pulmonary vascular smooth cells decreasing intracellular calcium levels thereby promoting pulmonary vasodilatation. Milrinone has both inotropic and vasodilatory effects, distinguishing it as an "inodilator." In cardiac myocytes, increased levels of cAMP enhance contractility, chronotropy, and dromotropy. Cardiac output is augmented with an accompanying decrease in afterload. It also improves left ventricular diastolic relaxation. Its intravenous dosing is 0.25–0.75 mcg/kg/min with an intravenous loading dose of 50 mcg/kg administered over 10 min. Its use has also been described via inhalational delivery at a dose of 2–5 mg [21].

Indications

Milrinone is used in the setting of acute decompensated heart failure, to facilitate weaning from cardiopulmonary bypass, and pulmonary hypertension with right ventricular dysfunction.

Drug Interactions and Contraindications

The use of furosemide and milrinone in the same intravenous line for infusion will cause precipitation to form.

Side Effects

The use of a continuous milrinone infusion is inevitably associated with a systemic arterial hypotension and may be accompanied by the appearance of ventricular arrhythmias.

Clinical Pearls

I. The initial loading dose is frequently not necessary to achieve response.
II. The use of pressor agents such as norepinephrine or vasopressin may be necessary to counteract the decrease in systemic vascular resistance [22].

Endothelin-Receptor Antagonists

Endothelins are a family of peptides that play a key role in the regulation of pulmonary vascular tone. Pulmonary vascular endothelial cells are a major source of endothelins. Endothelin-1 is a potent vasoconstrictor, as well as a potent stimulant inducing cell proliferation of vascular smooth muscle cells. Endothelins interact with two distinct receptors: endothelin receptor A (ET-A) and endothelin receptor B (ET-B). These receptors belong to the family of receptors connected to guanine nucleotide-binding G proteins which induce phospholipase C activation and consequent release of intracellular calcium. Endothelin-A receptors are located on pulmonary vascular smooth muscle cells. The activation of ET-A receptors mediates vasoconstriction. Endothelin B receptors are located on both pulmonary vascular endothelial cells and vascular smooth muscle cells. Activation of ET-B receptors mediates vasodilation via increased levels of NO and prostacyclin and also increases clearance of circulating ET-1 [12] (See Fig. 17.2).

There are currently two endothelin-receptor antagonists approved for the treatment of primary pulmonary hypertension.

Bosentan (Tracleer®)

Class: Oral Dual Endothelin-Receptor Antagonist

Indications

In 2001, bosentan became the first oral agent to receive FDA approval in the treatment of group I primary pulmonary hypertension patients in WHO functional classes III–IV. It is the only endothelin-receptor antagonist recommended for use in patients with Eisenmenger's syndrome [23].

Mechanism of Action

Bosentan is a dual endothelin-receptor antagonist with a higher affinity for ET-A receptors. By blocking the action of endothelin-1 on its receptors, vasodilatation of

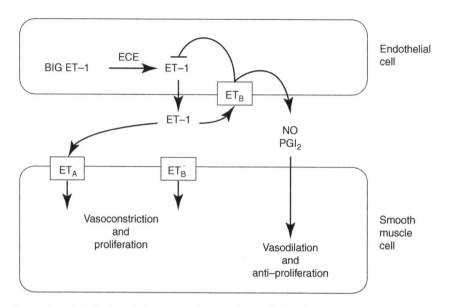

Fig. 17.2 Endothelin (*ET*)-1 signaling pathway in the regulation of pulmonary vascular tone. Big ET-1 is cleaved to ET-1 by endothelin-converting enzyme (*ECE*) in endothelial cells. ET-1 binds its specific receptors ET-A and ET-B with differential effects. Binding of ET-1 to ET-A or ET-B on smooth muscle cells leads to vasoconstrictive and proliferative effects. ET-B are transiently expressed on endothelial cells after birth; binding of ET-1 to ET-B on endothelial cells leads to downregulation of ECE activity and increased production of nitric oxide (*NO*) prostacyclin (*PGI₂*), which led to vasodilation and antiproliferation (Porta and Steinhorn [12]; with permission)

pulmonary vascular smooth muscle cells via NO and prostacyclin is favored. The initial dosing recommendations are 62.5 mg orally twice daily for 4 weeks, followed by an increase to 125–250 mg orally twice daily [15]. Pediatric dosing is 2 or 4 mg/kg orally twice daily.

Drug Interactions and Contraindications

The half-life of bosentan is 5 h. Bosentan is metabolized in the liver by CYP2C9 and CYP3A4 and eliminated through biliary excretion [24]. It also induces the action of these CYP enzymes with an associated decrease in the concentration of simvastatin, warfarin, and sildenafil. It is not recommended in patients receiving glyburide (increased risk of developing liver dysfunction), cyclosporine (decreases bosentan clearance), or tacrolimus (decreases bosentan clearance). Other drugs such as ketoconazole known to inhibit CYP2C9 and CYP3A4 should be avoided. The administration of bosentan is contraindicated in pregnant patients as it is teratogenic (category X). Women of childbearing age being treated with bosentan are recommended to practice two reliable methods of birth control and undergo monthly pregnancy testing. Bosentan is also contraindicated in patients with moderate to severe liver dysfunction.

Side Effects

Bosentan has been associated with dose-dependent increases in liver enzymes during treatment. The levels of alanine aminotransferase (ALT) and aspartate aminotransferase (AST) may reach over eight times above normal. Discontinuation of the drug usually results in return to normal levels of the liver enzymes. Due to the risk of hepatotoxicity, current mandates include baseline and monthly monitoring of liver function tests [25]. Bosentan is also associated with a drop in hemoglobin which usually manifests in the first 2 weeks following initiation of treatment and stabilizes by 1–3 months afterward. Other side effects noted are related to vasodilatory effects and include flushing, edema, headache, nasal congestion, and extremity pain. In men, bosentan may cause testicular atrophy and decrease sperm count [15].

Clinical Pearls

I. No need for dose adjustment in patients with renal dysfunction, even those on dialysis
II. Often used in conjunction with sildenafil as combination therapy in patients with primary pulmonary hypertension

Ambrisentan (Letairis®)

Class: Oral Selective Endothelin-A Receptor Antagonist

Mechanism of Action

Ambrisentan is a specific ET-A receptor antagonist. Theoretically, it preferentially inhibits activation of ET-A receptors thereby preventing vasoconstriction without inhibiting the vasodilatory actions mediated via activation of ET-B receptors.

Indications

Ambrisentan received FDA approval for treatment of patients with primary pulmonary hypertension in WHO functional classes II–III in 2007. The dosage recommendation is 5–10 mg orally once a day. Its longer half-life of 15 h compared to bosentan allows for once daily administration [25].

Drug Interactions and Contraindications

Ambrisentan is metabolized in liver by several CYP enzymes. It is currently contraindicated for usage in patients with moderate to severe liver dysfunction.

Ambrisentan is teratogenic (category X) and contraindicated in pregnant patients. Women of childbearing age should practice two reliable methods of birth control and undergo monthly pregnancy testing.

Side Effects

Ambrisentan administration has a much lower risk of inducing hepatotoxicity in comparison to bosentan; hence the mandate for monthly monitoring of liver function tests was lifted by the FDA after its release [25]. As seen with bosentan, anemia, peripheral edema, and lower sperm counts have been associated with ambrisentan treatment.

Pulmonary arterial hypertension is a chronic progressive condition with essentially no curative treatment. Pulmonary vasodilators serve mainly to decrease right ventricular afterload, improve exercise tolerance, improve quality of life, and lengthen time to clinical worsening [14]. Treatment with pulmonary vasodilators is usually in conjunction with background or conventional therapy consisting of supplemental oxygen, diuretics, digoxin, and anticoagulants, as well as calcium-channel blockers in the small minority of "responders." None of the pulmonary vasodilators discussed are approved by the FDA for the treatment of pulmonary arterial hypertension in the pediatric population. New pulmonary vasodilating agents are still being developed. Pulmonary vasodilating agents from different classes have been strategized in combination therapy for additive and beneficial effects; however, the actual cure all for pulmonary arterial hypertension remains elusive.

Chemical Structures

Chemical Structure
17.1 Prostacyclin

**Chemical Structure
17.2** Tadalafil

**Chemical Structure
17.3** Treprostinil

**Chemical Structure
17.4** Milrinone

**Chemical Structure
17.5** Sildenafil

References

1. McLaughlin VV, Archer SL, Badesch DB, Barst RJ, Farber HW, Lindner JR, et al. ACCF/ AHA 2009 expert consensus document on pulmonary hypertension: a report of the American College of Cardiology Foundation Task Force on expert consensus documents and the American Heart Association: developed in collaboration with the American College of Chest Physicians, American Thoracic society, Inc., and the Pulmonary Hypertension Association. Circulation. 2009;119:2250–94.
2. Checchia PA, Bronicki RA, Goldstein B. Review of inhaled nitric oxide in the pediatric cardiac surgery setting. Pediatr Cardiol. 2012;33:493–505.
3. Simonneau G, Robbins IM, Beghetti M, Channick RN, Delcroix M, Denton CP, et al. Updated clinical classification of pulmonary hypertension. J Am Coll Cardiol. 2009;54:S43–54.
4. Zamanian RT, Haddad F, Doyle RL, Weinacker AB. Management strategies for patients with pulmonary hypertension in the intensive care unit. Crit Care Med. 2007;35(9):2037–50.
5. Benedict N, Seybert A, Mathier MA. Evidence-based pharmacologic management of pulmonary arterial hypertension. Clin Ther. 2007;29(10):2134–53.
6. Levine AB, Punihaole D, Levine TB. Characterization of the role of nitric oxide and its clinical applications. Cardiology. 2012;122:55–68.
7. Peliowski A. Inhaled nitric oxide use in newborns. Paediatr Child Health. 2012;17(2):95–7.
8. Antoniou T, Prokakis C, Athanasopoulos G, Thanopoulos A, Rellia P, Zarkalis D, et al. Inhaled nitric oxide plus iloprost in the setting of post-left assist device right heart dysfunction. Ann Thorac Surg. 2012;94:792–9.
9. Gazit AZ, Canter CE. Impact of pulmonary vascular resistances in heart transplantation for congenital heart disease. Curr Cardiol Rev. 2011;7:59–66.
10. Granton J, Moric J. Pulmonary vasodilators – treating the right ventricle. Anesth Clin. 2008;26:337–53.
11. Caojin Z, Yigao H, Tao H, Wenhui H, Chunli X, Xinsheng H. Comparison of acute hemodynamic effects of aerosolized iloprost and inhaled nitric oxide in adult congenital heart disease with severe pulmonary arterial hypertension. Intern Med. 2012;51:2857–62.
12. Porta NF, Steinhorn RH. Pulmonary vasodilator therapy in the NICU: inhaled nitric oxide, sildenafil, and other pulmonary vasodilating agents. Clin Perinatol. 2012;39:149–64.
13. Iacovidou N, Syggelou A, Fanos V, Xanthos T. The use of sildenafil in the treatment of persistent pulmonary hypertension of the newborn: a review of the literature. Curr Pharm Des. 2012;18:3034–45.
14. Ventetuolo CE, Klinger JR. WHO group 1 pulmonary arterial hypertension: current and investigative therapies. Prog Cardiovasc Dis. 2012;55:89–103.
15. Bishop BM, Mauro VF, Khouri SJ. Practical considerations for the pharmacotherapy of pulmonary arterial hypertension. Pharmacotherapy. 2012;32(9):838–55.
16. Yao A. Recent advances and future perspectives in therapeutic strategies for pulmonary arterial hypertension. J Cardiol. 2012;60:344–9.
17. Greyson CR. Pathophysiology of right ventricular failure. Crit Care Med. 2008;36:S57–65.
18. Shah PS, Ohlsson A. Sildenafil for pulmonary hypertension in neonates (review). Cochrane Database of Systematic Reviews. 2011;8.
19. Barst RJ, Ivy DD, Gaitan G, Szatmari A, Rudzinski A, Garcia AE, et al. A randomized, double-blind, placebo-controlled, dose-ranging study of oral sildenafil citrate in treatment-naïve children with pulmonary arterial hypertension. Circulation. 2012;125:324–33.
20. Wardle AJ, Tulloh RM. Evolving management pediatric pulmonary arterial hypertension: impact of phosphodiesterase inhibitors. Pediatr Cardiol. 2013;34:213–9.
21. Gille J, Seyfarth HJ, Gerlach S, Malcharek M, Czeslick E, Sablotzki A. Perioperative anesthesiological management of patients with pulmonary hypertension. Anesthesiol Res Pract. 2012;2012:1–16.

22. Forrest P. Anaesthesia and right ventricular failure. Anaesth Intensive Care. 2009;37:370–85.
23. Monfredi O, Griffiths L, Clarke B, Mahadevan VS. Efficacy and safety of bosentan for pulmonary arterial hypertension in adults with congenital heart disease. Am J Cardiol. 2011;108:1483–8.
24. Carter NJ, Keating GM. Bosentan in pediatric patients with pulmonary arterial hypertension. Pediatr Drugs. 2010;12:63–73.
25. Rubin LJ. Endothelin receptor antagonists for the treatment of pulmonary artery hypertension. Life Sci. 2012;91:517–21.
26. Rich S. Primary pulmonary hypertension: executive summary from the world symposium on primary pulmonary hypertension. Evian: World Health Organization; 1998. p. 6–10.
27. Steinhorn RL. Lamb models of pulmonary hypertension. Drug Discov Today Dis Model. 2010;7:99–105.

Chapter 18
Asthma and COPD Agents

Alexis Appelstein and Mabel Chung

Contents

A. Appelstein, DO • M. Chung, MD (✉)
Department of Anesthesiology, Montefiore Medical Center,
Albert Einstein College of Medicine, Bronx, NY, USA
e-mail: aapplest@montefiore.org; mchung4621@gmail.com

A.D. Kaye et al. (eds.), *Essentials of Pharmacology for Anesthesia,*
Pain Medicine, and Critical Care, DOI 10.1007/978-1-4614-8948-1_18,
© Springer Science+Business Media New York 2015

Introduction

Chronic obstructive pulmonary disease (COPD) is a respiratory disorder characterized by inflammation leading to airflow obstruction. Its two main subtypes – chronic bronchitis and emphysema – can exist alone or in tandem. Asthma, another major disease characterized by airflow obstruction, differs greatly from COPD in the pathophysiology of its inflammation but commonly coexists with one or more of the subtypes of COPD (Fig. 18.1).

COPD affects approximately 5 % of the population according to the Centers for Disease Control and Prevention [2] with a mortality of over 120,000 individuals per year [3]. Chronic bronchitis is defined as a chronic productive cough for 3 months over two successive years and emphysema occurs as a result of destruction to alveolar walls causing permanent airspace dilation distal to the terminal bronchioles. The inflammation leading to these two processes is characterized by the infiltration of neutrophils, macrophages, and CD 8+ T lymphocytes [4]. Cigarette use is the most

Table 18.1 Management of asthma

Severity	Characteristics	Therapies
Intermittent – mild	Daytime symptoms ≤2×/week Nocturnal awakenings ≤2×/month Use SABA ≤2×/week FEV_1 or PEF ≥80 % predicted Asymptomatic between exacerbations 0–1 exacerbations/year requiring steroids	Short-acting β2 agonist
Persistent – mild	Daytime symptoms >2×/week but <1×/day Nocturnal awakenings 3–4×/month Use SABA >2×/week but not daily FEV_1 or PEF ≥80 % predicted	Inhaled glucocorticoid *Alternate* Leukotriene receptor antagonist Methylxanthines Mast cell stabilizer
Persistent – moderate	Normal FEV_1 between exacerbations ≥2 exacerbations/year requiring steroids Daily symptoms Nocturnal awakenings >1×/week Use SABA daily Some limitation in normal activity FEV_1 or PEF 60–80 % predicted	Inhaled glucocorticoid plus long-acting β2 agonist *Alternate* Leukotriene receptor antagonist or lipoxygenase inhibitor Methylxanthines
Persistent severe	≥2 exacerbations/year requiring steroids Symptoms throughout the day Frequent nocturnal awakenings Use SABA multiple times/day Extreme limitation in normal activity FEV_1 or PEF ≤60 predicted ≥2 exacerbations/year requiring steroids	Oral glucocorticoids (acutely) Immunomodulators

SABA short-acting β2 agonist, *PEF* peak expiratory flow

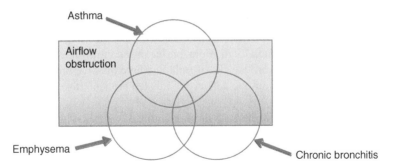

Fig. 18.1 A Venn diagram depicting the three entities of obstructive airway disease and the ways in which they can coexist. Asthma can exist as its own entity or as a bronchospastic component to COPD (chronic bronchitis and emphysema). Alternatively, COPD can exist purely without a reversible bronchospastic/asthmatic component. In addition, each subtype may also contain an element of the other. Asthma and COPD can exist as milder entities without significant airflow obstruction (*outside blue box*) or with significant obstruction (*within blue box*) (Modified from Ref. [1])

common cause of this inflammation, although inhalational exposures and α-1 antitrypsin deficiency can contribute as well. The diagnosis of COPD is suggested by symptoms of dyspnea with or without exertion, by chronic cough and sputum production, and by spirometric evidence of irreversible airflow limitation during forced expiration, i.e., an FEV_1/FVC <70 % and FEV_1 <80 % of the predicted value not reversible with bronchodilators.

According to the National Institutes of Health National Asthma Education and Prevention Program, asthma affects approximately 22 million people of all ages in the United States [5]. The inflammation associated with asthma is distinct from that of COPD and involves eosinophils, mast cells, and CD4+ T lymphocytes [4]. This inflammation leads to the destruction of epithelium, the remodeling and thickening of airway walls, airway edema, mucous plugging, and bronchial hyperresponsiveness, all of which can lead to airflow obstruction characterized by wheezing, cough, dyspnea, and chest tightness. The diagnosis of asthma is suggested by episodic symptoms, by triggers such as exercise, cold air, and allergens, and by the presence of a family history of atopy. In contrast to COPD, patients with asthma demonstrate reversibility of their airflow obstruction. Spirometric data suggestive of asthma includes an FEV_1/FVC <70 % and an FEV_1 <80 % of the predicted value with a post-bronchodilator response demonstrating an increase in FEV_1 >12 % from baseline with at least a 200 mL increase in FEV_1 [6].

The pharmacologic management of COPD and asthma is very similar with some exceptions. An asthma attack may be acutely managed with short-acting bronchodilators (β2 agonists and anticholinergics) and systemic glucocorticoids. COPD exacerbations, in addition to bronchodilators and systemic glucocorticoids, may also be treated with antibiotics, as approximately 50 % of exacerbations are precipitated by bacterial infections [7]. Depending on the severity, chronic asthma can be controlled with a combination of multiple agents including short- or long-acting β agonists, inhaled corticosteroids, mast cell stabilizers, methylxanthines, leukotriene modifiers (receptor antagonists or lipoxygenase inhibitors), systemic corticosteroids, or immunomodulators. Table 18.1 delineates the recommended therapies according to severity of asthma [5, 8]. Epinephrine, as an intravenous bronchodilator, may be of benefit in severe attacks of asthma where massive bronchoconstriction and restrictive airflow limit the delivery of inhaled bronchodilators to the lungs [9, 10].

COPD may be managed with short- or long-acting β2 agonists, long-acting anticholinergics, and inhaled glucocorticoids (sometimes combined as triple-inhaler therapy), methylxanthines, and PDE-4 inhibitors [11].

Drug Class and Mechanism of Action [5, 8, 12–14]

Short-Acting β2 Agonists (SABA)

Albuterol, Levalbuterol, Terbutaline, Bitolterol, Pirbuterol, and Metaproterenol

MOA

Binds to the β2 G-protein-coupled adrenergic receptor causing activation of adenyl cyclase, production of cAMP, stimulation of protein kinase A, and inactivation of myosin light-chain kinase leading to smooth muscle relaxation and bronchodilation.

Indications

Relief of acute bronchospasm in asthma and COPD. Prophylaxis against exercise-induced asthma.

Dosing

Albuterol: For use in patients >4 years: 1–2 puffs q4–6 h as needed. Two puffs 15 min before exercise to prevent exercise-induced asthma. Maximum: 12 inhalations/day.

Levalbuterol: Available in three different 3 mL dose vials: 0.31, 0.63, 1.25 mg. For ages 6–11 years: 0.31 mg three times/day q6–8 h by nebulizer. For patients >12 years: 0.63–1.25 mg three times/day q6–8 h by nebulizer.

Terbutaline: May be administered subcutaneously, PO, or inhaled. Subcutaneous dosing has a quick onset of action due to high lipid solubility: Inject 0.25 mg into the lateral deltoid area; additional 0.25 mg dose can be repeated every 15–30 min for a total of three doses. 2.5–5 mg PO q6 h, maximum 15 mg/24 h. 1–2 inhalations q4–6 h.

Bitolterol: Two inhalations q8 h. Maximum: Three inhalations q6 h or two inhalations q4 h.

Pirbuterol: For use in patients >12 years: Two puffs q4–6 h.

Metaproterenol: 2–3 inhalations q3–4 h. Maximum: 12 inhalations/day. Not recommended for children <12 years and in those with cardiac arrhythmias associated with tachycardia.

Side Effects/Drug Interactions

Tachycardia, skeletal muscle tremor, hypokalemia, increased lactic acid, headache, and hyperglycemia. Inhaled route usually causes few systemic side effects. Caution with use in patients with cardiovascular disease.

Anticholinergics

Ipratropium Bromide, Tiotropium Bromide

MOA

Blocks the action of acetylcholine on postsynaptic muscarinic receptors in the lung, thus inhibiting the influx of calcium and reversing vagally mediated bronchoconstriction. Decreases mucus gland secretion.

Indications

Ipratropium: Relief of acute bronchospasm in asthma and COPD in conjunction with a β2 agonist. Tiotropium: Long-term maintenance treatment of bronchospasm associated with COPD.

Dosing

Ipratropium bromide: For patients >12 years: Two inhalations q6 h. Maximum: 12 inhalations/day.

Tiotropium bromide: Two inhalations of powder contents of one capsule once daily.

Side Effects/Drug Interactions

Increased wheezing, drying of respiratory secretions and mouth, blurred vision if contact with eyes. If used as nebulizer treatment, usually produces less cardiac stimulation compared to SABAs. Reverses only cholinergic-induced bronchospasm, not antigenic or exercise-induced asthma. Treatment of choice for β-blocker-induced bronchospasm. Not proven to be adequate for long-term control method for asthma.

Inhaled Corticosteroids

Beclomethasone Dipropionate, Budesonide, Flunisolide, Fluticasone Propionate, Mometasone Furoate, Triamcinolone Acetonide

MOA

Anti-inflammatory. Decreases airway hyperresponsiveness, blocks release of cytokines, and inhibits inflammatory cell migration and activation. Reversal of $\beta2$ receptor downregulation.

Indications

Long-term prevention of symptoms and reversal of inflammation in asthma and COPD.

Dosing

Beclomethasone dipropionate: Available as a 40 mcg or 80 mcg puff. For children 5–11 years: 40–80 mcg twice daily. For adults: 40–320 mcg twice daily.

Budesonide: Available as a 90 mcg or 180 mcg inhaler. For children 6–17 years: 180 mcg twice daily with a maximum dose of 360 mcg twice daily. For patients >18 years: 360 mcg twice daily with a maximum of 720 mcg twice daily. Available as a budesonide/formoterol combination inhaler (80/4.5 and 160/4.5; for patients >12 years – two inhalations twice daily).

Flunisolide: 250 mcg/puff. For children >6 years: two inhalations twice daily. For adults: 2–4 inhalations twice daily.

Fluticasone propionate: Available as a 44, 110, or 220 mcg inhaler. Dosing varies and must be individualized to patient. Also available as a 50, 100, or 250 mcg Diskus delivery system – 1–2 puffs twice daily. Available as a fluticasone/salmeterol combination inhaler (45/21, 115/21, and 230/21; for patients >12 years – two inhalations twice daily) or Diskus (100/50, 250/50, or 500/50; Diskus with the 100/50 dose for children 4–11 years – one inhalation twice daily for all doses.)

Mometasone furoate: Available in 110 and 220 mcg preparations. For children 4–11 years, use of 110 mcg inhaler in the evening recommended. For patients >12 years, 220–880 mcg recommended. Available as a mometasone/formoterol combination in doses of 100/5 and 200/5; in patients >12 years – two puffs twice daily.

Triamcinolone acetonide: Available as a 75 mcg inhaler. For children 6–12 years: 2–8 puffs/day in divided doses. For adults: 4–16 puffs/day in divided doses.

Side Effects/Drug Interactions

Oral thrush (candidiasis), dysphonia, cough. In high doses, systemic side effects such as skin thinning, osteoporosis, easy bruising, and adrenal suppression may occur. In low to medium doses, possible suppression of growth velocity observed in children. Spacer/holding chambers and non-breath-activated MDIs with mouth washing after use decrease local side effects. Dexamethasone is not included for long-term inhalation use due to high absorption and suppressive side effects.

Long-Acting Beta Agonists (LABAs)

Formoterol Fumarate, Salmeterol Xinafoate

MOA

Binds to the $\beta2$ G-protein-coupled adrenergic receptor causing activation of adenyl cyclase, production of cAMP, stimulation of protein kinase A, and inactivation of myosin light-chain kinase leading to smooth muscle relaxation and bronchodilation. Compared to SABAs, formoterol has a similar onset of action (<5 min), while salmeterol has a longer onset (15–30 min). Both salmeterol and formoterol have longer durations of actions of at least 12 h.

Indications

Prevention of exercise-induced asthma and maintenance treatment of asthma and COPD. Not indicated for acute exacerbations. The FDA has recommended that LABAs be used only in conjunction with inhaled corticosteroids (see Black Box Warning below).

Dosing

Formoterol fumarate: For patients >5 years, inhalation of one 12 mcg capsule q12 h.
    Available as a combination product with budesonide and mometasone (see above).
Salmeterol xinafoate: For patients >4 years, inhalation of 50 mcg via Diskus q12 h.
    Available as a combination product with fluticasone (see above).

Side Effects/Drug Interactions

Tachycardia, skeletal muscle tremor, and prolongation of QT_c interval in overdose. A diminished bronchoprotective effect may occur with 1 week of use, with lack of evidence for clinical significance. Not for use as monotherapy or treatment of acute symptoms.

> **Black Box Warning**
> The SMART trial [15], which compared daily treatment with salmeterol versus placebo, showed a small but statistically significant increase in the risk of asthma-related deaths in the salmeterol group; as a result, the use of salmeterol as monotherapy without the use of a long-term asthma control medication such as an inhaled corticosteroid is contraindicated. This recommendation extends to formoterol on the basis of being in the same class of medication as salmeterol. The use of combination LABA/steroid inhalers is encouraged to ensure adherence to the use of the corticosteroid. Studies have suggested a higher incidence of severe asthma exacerbations with formoterol. It is unknown whether the rate of death is affected in patients with COPD who use LABAs.

Mast Cell Stabilizers

Cromolyn Sodium, Nedocromil

MOA

Anti-inflammatory. Stabilizes mast cells by inhibiting their ability to degranulate and release mediators. Response usually seen within 2 weeks from the start of treatment but may take up to 4–6 weeks to get maximum efficacy. Nebulizer delivery of cromolyn may be more effective in some patients.

Indications

Prophylactic, long-term prevention of symptoms in mild persistent asthma. Prevention of exercise- and allergen-induced asthma exacerbations.

Dosing

Cromolyn sodium: For patients >2 years, nebulizer – one 20 mg vial four times daily; metered dose inhaler – two inhalations four times daily.
Nedocromil: For patients >6 years, two inhalations four times daily (total 14 mg daily).

Side Effects/Drug Interactions

Main side effects: cough and throat irritation. 15–20 % of patients complain of the unpalatable taste of nedocromil.

Leukotriene Receptor Antagonists

Montelukast, Zafirlukast

MOA

Antagonizes leukotriene receptors thus decreasing bronchoconstriction and inflammation.

Indications

Long-term control and prevention of symptoms in mild persistent asthma for patients >1 year with montelukast and >7 years with zafirlukast. Prevention of exercise-induced asthma and relief of symptoms of allergic rhinitis. May be used in combination with inhaled corticosteroids in moderate persistent asthma.

Dosing

Montelukast: For children 12–23 months: One packet of 4 mg oral granules daily. For children 2–5 years: One 4 mg tablet once a day. For children 6–14 years: One 5 mg tablet once a day. For patients >15 years: One 10 mg tablet once a day.
Zafirlukast: For children 5–11 years: 10 mg tablet twice daily. For patients >12 years: 20 mg tablet twice daily.

Side Effects/Drug Interactions

No specific adverse effects identified. Rare cases of Churg-Strauss syndrome have occurred (uncertain relationship). Post-marketing surveillance of zafirlukast has uncovered cases of reversible hepatitis and rare irreversible hepatic failure leading to death and need for liver transplantation. Liver function should be monitored and patients should be advised to discontinue use of this medication with any signs/symptoms of liver dysfunction. Zafirlukast is a CYP 450 enzyme inhibitor that can inhibit the metabolism of warfarin; thus, INR should be monitored closely in affected patients. Zafirlukast does not appear to affect plasma levels of theophylline.

5-Lipoxygenase Inhibitor

Zileuton

MOA

Decreases the production of leukotrienes from arachidonic acid by inhibiting the 5-lipoxygenase enzyme.

Indications

Long-term control and prevention of symptoms of asthma in patients >12 years. May be used with inhaled corticosteroids in patients >12 years in moderate persistent asthma.

Dosing

For patients >12 years, two 600 mg tablets twice daily within 1 h of meals.

Side Effects/Drug Interactions

Elevation of liver enzymes has been reported with limited reporting of hyperbilirubinemia and reversible hepatitis. ALT levels should be monitored. Inhibits the CYP 450 enzyme and the metabolism of both warfarin and theophylline. Doses of these two medications should be carefully monitored.

Methylxanthines

Theophylline

MOA

Purported mechanism is the inhibition of PDE III and IV leading to an increase in cAMP, activation of protein kinase A, and relaxation of smooth muscle causing bronchodilation. May decrease eosinophil infiltration into bronchial mucosa and T lymphocyte migration in the epithelium. Found to improve diaphragm contractility and mucociliary clearance.

Indications

Long-term control and prevention of symptoms in mild persistent asthma and in combination with inhaled corticosteroids in moderate persistent asthma. Can be used as an adjunctive bronchodilator in stable COPD.

Dosing

Weight-based (use ideal body weight). Individualized to achieve steady states of 5–15 mcg/mL. Routine serum concentration monitoring is essential due to the narrow therapeutic range. Patients should discontinue theophylline if signs of toxicity develop. Not recommended for acute exacerbations.

Loading dose: If no theophylline received in the last 24 h: 5 mg/kg PO. Goal to achieve serum level of 10 mcg/mL.

Maintenance dose: Immediate release: For patients 16–60 years and weighing >45 kg, 300–600 mg/day divided q6–8 h; doses >600 mg/day should be titrated to serum level. For patients >60 years or with risk factors for decreased theophylline clearance (such as liver disease, hypothyroidism, congestive heart failure), final theophylline dose should not exceed 16 mg/kg/day to a maximum of 400 mg/day. Extended release: Same guidelines but with once daily dosing. Alternate dosing strategy: For patients >16 years (healthy, nonsmoking), 3 mg/kg q8 h; older patients and patients with cor pulmonale, 2 mg/kg q8 h; patients with congestive heart failure, 1–2 mg/kg q12 h. Check serum levels every 24 h for acute dosing and at 6–12-month intervals for chronic dosing. If serum levels are greater than 15 mcg/ml, decrease dose by 10 % to decrease risk of toxicities.

Side Effects/Drug Interactions

Dose-related acute toxicities include tachycardia, nausea and vomiting, tachyarrhythmias, headache, CNS stimulation, seizures, hematemesis, hyperglycemia, and hypokalemia. Adverse effects at usual doses include insomnia, gastric intolerance, aggravation of ulcer reflux, and increase in hyperactivity in children; elderly men with prostatism may experience difficulty with urination.

Systemic Corticosteroids

Prednisone, Methylprednisolone, Hydrocortisone

MOA

Anti-inflammatory. Decreases airway hyperresponsiveness; inhibits cytokine production, adhesion protein activation, and inflammatory cell migration. Reversal of $\beta2$ receptor downregulation.

Indications

For moderate to severe exacerbations of asthma and COPD with the goal of preventing progression, reversing inflammation, and facilitating recovery. Slow onset of action – clinical benefit may not be appreciated for up to 6 h.

Dosing

Typical doses include prednisone 40–60 mg/day PO in single or divided doses; continue until symptoms resolve or PEF reaches 70 % predicted or personal best, usually over 3–10 days. For patients with impending respiratory failure, methylprednisolone 60–125 mg IV. Alternatives include hydrocortisone 150–200 mg IV and dexamethasone 6–10 mg IV [5, 16]. Tapering of doses not typically necessary in duration less than 3 weeks.

Side Effects/Drug Interactions

With short-term use: Increased appetite, fluid retention, weight gain, facial flushing, mood alteration, reversible glucose metabolism abnormalities, hypertension, peptic ulcer, and rarely, aseptic necrosis. Caution when used in herpes virus, varicella, tuberculosis, and strongyloides infections, hypertension, peptic ulcer disease, diabetes, and osteoporosis as it can worsen these preexisting conditions.

PDE-4 Inhibitor

Roflumilast

MOA

PDE IV inhibitor leading to an increase in cAMP. May promote bronchodilation and decreased inflammation.

Indications

For the reduction of exacerbations in patients with COPD associated with chronic bronchitis and a history of exacerbations. Not for use in acute bronchospasm.

Dosing

500 mcg PO/day.

Side Effects/Drug Interactions

Diarrhea, weight loss, nausea, headache, and back pain. Should be used with caution when used in conjunction with strong cytochrome P450 inducers or inhibitors or with oral contraceptives containing gestodene and ethinyl estradiol.

Immunomodulators

Omalizumab

MOA

Binds to circulating IgE and prevents it from binding to high affinity receptors on mast cells or basophils. Decreases mast cell mediator release. Downregulates IgE receptors on basophils and submucosal cells.

Indications

Long-term control and prevention of symptoms in patients >12 years who have moderate to severe persistent allergic asthma that is ineffectively controlled with inhaled corticosteroids.

Dosing

Ranges from 150 to 375 mg subcutaneous every 2–4 weeks [17]. Dose determined by body weight and total IgE level before treatment (Tables 18.2 and 18.3). Maximum dose of 150 mg with each injection site.

Side Effects/Drug Interactions

Anaphylaxis (reported in 0.2 % of patients – monitor patient after injection), pain and bruising at injection site, upper respiratory tract infections, sinusitis, headache, pharyngitis, and the possibility of development of malignant neoplasms (found in 0.5 % of cases compared to 0.2 % of placebo – unclear association with drug).

Table 18.2 Omalizumab dosing in milligrams with administration every 4 weeks

Pretreatment serum IgE (IU/ml)	Body weight (kg)			
	30–60	>60–70	>70–90	>90–150
>30–100	150	150	150	300
>100–200	300	300	300	a
>200–300	300	a	a	a

a See Table 18.3

Table 18.3 Omalizumab dosing in milligrams with administration every 2 weeks

Pretreatment serum IgE (IU/ml)	Body weight (kg)			
	30–60	>60–70	>70–90	>90–150
>100–200	a	a	a	225
>200–300	a	225	225	300
>300–400	225	225	300	b
>400–500	300	300	375	b
>500–600	300	375	b	b
>600–700	375	b	b	b

[a]See Table 18.2
[b]Do not dose drug

Epinephrine

MOA

Binds to the β2 G-protein-coupled adrenergic receptor causing activation of adenyl cyclase, production of cAMP, stimulation of protein kinase A, and inactivation of myosin light-chain kinase leading to smooth muscle relaxation and bronchodilation. Also stimulates β1 receptors (increasing myocardial contractility and heart rate), and α1 receptors (increasing blood pressure).

Indications

Acute bronchospasm

Dosing

10 mcg IV titrated to response. Can also be administered IM and SC (0.3–0.5 mg IM/SC) [9, 11, 16].

Side Effects/Drug Interactions

Include coronary ischemia, ventricular dysrhythmias, and cerebral hemorrhage. Epinephrine should be reserved for patients who experience severe, life-threatening bronchospasm not responsive to inhaled β2 agonists and anticholinergic agents.

Asthma and Anesthetic Agents [9, 11, 16, 18]

In the absence of certain considerations (e.g. difficult airway, full stomach), a deep plane of anesthesia should be achieved prior to intubation in the patient with significant asthma due to the potential for inducing bronchospasm with instrumentation of the airway. Intravenous induction with propofol may decrease respiratory resistance and the incidence of wheezing after tracheal intubation [19, 20]. In addition, ketamine, through the release of catecholamines, has excellent bronchodilating properties and is especially beneficial in the setting of hemodynamic instability. Those agents with histamine-releasing properties should be avoided, including thiopental, atracurium, mivacurium, morphine, and meperidine. Ketorolac should be administered with caution, especially in patients with sensitivity to aspirin; inhibition of the cyclooxygenase enzyme can shunt arachidonic acid into the lipoxygenase pathway, increase the production of leukotrienes, and induce bronchospasm in susceptible individuals. With the possible exception of desflurane, the volatile agents have potent bronchodilating properties and are an important adjunct in balanced anesthesia for an asthmatic patient. Desflurane was originally shown to have direct smooth muscle relaxant effects on the bronchial segments of dogs [21], but a subsequent study in intubated humans showed that it caused an increase in airway resistance in smokers (with no effect on nonsmokers) [22].

Cholinesterase inhibitors such as neostigmine and anticholinergic agents such as glycopyrrolate have competing effects on the airway. Neostigmine increases parasympathetic tone and bronchoconstricts, but glycopyrrolate can counter this effect, especially if given prior to neostigmine. Intravenous lidocaine may prevent reflexive bronchospasm. If without contraindications (e.g., difficult airway, full stomach), a deep extubation may decrease the risk of bronchospasm on emergence.

The use of bronchodilating anesthetics in COPD only improves the reversible component of airflow obstruction, and thus expiratory airflow obstruction will still be observed despite a deep plane of anesthesia. Nitrous oxide should be avoided in patients with bullae to decrease the risk of pneumothorax. In both asthma and COPD, small to moderate tidal volumes with low respiratory rates may prevent air trapping, especially if combined with a generous I/E ratio (i.e., 1:3).

If there is no contraindication, a regional technique (e.g., epidural or spinal anesthesia or peripheral nerve blockade) or the use of the laryngeal mask airway may obviate the need for an endotracheal tube and may decrease the risk of bronchospasm that can occur with invasive airway manipulation.

Bronchospasm typically manifests with an increase in peak airway pressure, decrease in $EtCO_2$, and wheezing. Initial maneuvers should include an increase in the FiO_2 to 100 % and hand ventilation of the patient. The lungs should be auscultated and other causes of increased peak airway pressure such as endotracheal tube kinking, secretions, and main stem intubation should be sought. If bronchospasm is suspected as the cause of difficulty in ventilation, an inhaled $\beta2$ agonist such as albuterol can be administered directly into the endotracheal tube. Surgical stimulation should be stopped and the anesthetic should be deepened by increasing the concentration of volatile agent; if severe airflow obstruction prevents the delivery of an adequate amount of anesthetic, a bolus dose of an intravenous agent such as propofol or ketamine can be given. Terbutaline can be administered subcutaneously and should produce improvement 5–15 min after administration with maximal effect after 30–60 min. While not immediately effective, systemic glucocorticoids should be administered for an anti-inflammatory effect that may aid in longer-term stabilization of an acute asthma exacerbation. Refractory bronchospasm, especially that which results in minimal air movement and a decrease in

SpO_2, can be treated with epinephrine; 10 mcg IV titrated to response may be administered. Magnesium sulfate 2 g IV may augment bronchodilation in such cases of severe bronchospasm.

Clinical Pearls

- Terbutaline, a potent and rapidly acting bronchodilator, is underutilized intraoperatively.
- An old anecdotal technique for the treatment of bronchospasm and increased secretions includes injecting atropine, in a dose of 0.4 mg, directly into the endotracheal tube.
- Lidocaine 1 or 2 % via an endotracheal tube can be utilized as an adjuvant for certain types of bronchospasm though the mechanism is unclear at present.

Summary

Asthma and COPD are common in the operating room and postoperatively. Knowledge of the pathophysiology of these disease states as well as the myriad of agents available and how they intervene in the disease process is essential to safe and successful delivery of an anesthetic regimen and in effective postoperative management.

Chemical Structures

Chemical Structure 18.1 Formoterol

Chemical Structure
18.2 Cromolyn Sodium

Chemical Structure 18.3 Theophylline

Chemical Structure
18.4 Prednisone

Chemical Structure
18.5 Roflumilast

Chemical Structure
18.6 Montelukast

Chemical Structure
18.7 Terbutaline

References

1. Rennard I. Chronic obstructive pulmonary disease: definition, clinical manifestations, diagnosis, and staging. UptoDate Online. 2013.
2. Centers for Disease Control and Prevention. Chronic obstructive pulmonary disease among adults – United States, 2011. MMWR Morb Mortal Wkly Rep 2012;61:938.
3. Miniño AM, Murphy SL, Xu J, Kochanek KD. Deaths: final data for 2008. Natl Vital Stat Rep. 2011;59:1.
4. Sutherland ER, Martin RJ. Airway inflammation in chronic obstructive pulmonary disease: comparisons with asthma. J Allergy Clin Immunol. 2003;112(5):819.
5. National Asthma Education and Prevention Program: Clinical Practice Guidelines. Expert Panel Report 3. "Guidelines for the Diagnosis and Management of Asthma." National Institutes of Health: National Heart, Lung, and Blood Institute. August 2007.
6. Barreiro TJ, Perillo I. An approach to interpreting spirometry. Am Fam Physician. 2004;69(5):1107–15. http://www.aafp.org/afp/2004/0301/p1107.html.

7. Sethi S, Murphy TF. Infection in the pathogenesis and course of chronic obstructive pulmonary disease. N Engl J Med. 2008;359:2355.
8. Tucker J, Fanta CH. Integrative inflammation pharmacology: asthma. In: Golan DE, Tashjian AH, Armstrong E, Galanter JM, Armstrong AW, Arnaout RA, Rose HS, editors. Principles of pharmacology: the pathophysiologic basis of drug therapy. Philadelphia: Lippincott Williams & Wilkins; 2004. p. 699–711.
9. Woods BD, Sladen RN. Perioperative considerations for the patient with asthma and bronchospasm. Br J Anaesth. 2009;103 Suppl 1:i57–65.
10. Looseley A. Management of bronchospasm during general anaesthesia. Clinical Overview Articles. Update in Anaesthesia. 2011. p. 17–21. http://update.anaesthesiologists.org/.../ Bronchospasm_during_anaesthesia_Update_2011.pdf.
11. Global strategy for the diagnosis, management, and prevention of chronic obstructive pulmonary disease: Revised 2011. Global Initiative for Chronic Obstructive Lung Disease (GOLD). www.goldcopd.org.
12. American Academy of Allergy and Immunology. http://www.aaaai.org/conditions-and-treatments/ treatments/drug-guide. 1 Dec 2012.
13. Ogbru O, et al. RxList: The Internet Drug Index."WebMD. Accessed July 22, 2013. www. rxlist.com.
14. Fanta CH. Asthma. N Engl J Med. 2009;360:1002–14.
15. Nelson HS, Weiss ST, Bleecker ER, Yancey SW, Dorinsky PM, Smart Study Group. The salmeterol multicenter asthma research trial: a comparison of usual pharmacotherapy for asthma or usual pharmacotherapy plus salmeterol. Chest. 2006;129(1):15–26.
16. Fanta CH. Treatment of acute exacerbations of asthma in adults. Table 1. UpToDate Online. 2012.
17. Xolair® Omalizumab. http://www.accessdata.fda.gov/drugsatfda_docs/label/2003/omalgen062003LB.pdf. 23 Mar 2013.
18. Yao FF. Asthma and chronic obstructive pulmonary disease. In: Yao FF, Malhotra V, Fontes ML, editors. Yao & Artusio's anesthesiology: problem-oriented patient management. 6th edn. Philadelphia: Lippincott Williams & Wilkins; 2008. p 1–28.
19. Eames WO, Rooke GA, Wu RS, Bishop MJ. Comparison of the effects of etomidate, propofol, and thiopental on respiratory resistance following tracheal intubation. Anesthesiology. 1996;84:1307–11.
20. Pizov R, Brown RH, Weiss YS, Baranov D, Hennes H, Baker S, Hirshman CA. Wheezing during induction of general anesthesia in patients with and without asthma. A randomized, blind trial. Anesthesiology. 1995;82:1111–6.
21. Mazzeo AJ, Chen EY, Bosnjak ZJ, Coon RL, Kampine JP. Differential effects of desflurane and halothane on peripheral airway smooth muscle. Br J Anaes. 1996;76:841–6.
22. Goff MJ, Arain SR, Ficke DJ, Uhrich TD, Ebert TJ. Absence of bronchodilation during desflurane anesthesia. Anesthesiology. 2000;93:404–8.

Chapter 19
Hormones, Part 1: Thyroid and Corticosteroid Hormones

Joe C. Hong

Contents

J.C. Hong, MD
UCLA Department of Anesthesiology,
Ronald Reagan UCLA Medical Center,
Los Angeles, CA, USA
e-mail: jhong@mednet.ucla.edu

A.D. Kaye et al. (eds.), *Essentials of Pharmacology for Anesthesia,*
Pain Medicine, and Critical Care, DOI 10.1007/978-1-4614-8948-1_19,
© Springer Science+Business Media New York 2015

Thyroid Hormones

Introduction

The thyroid gland is responsible for the production, storage, and release of thyroid hormones. Adequate levels of these vital hormones are needed throughout life. Starting as a neonate, thyroid hormones are needed for the proper development of the central nervous system. During childhood, skeletal growth and maturation is dictated by thyroid hormones [1]. In adulthood, metabolism and the normal function of multiple organ systems are guided by proper thyroid hormone levels. Because thyroid hormones play such an integral part in normal physiology, it should come as no surprise that thyroid dysfunction is one of the most common endocrinopathies seen in clinical practice.

The two major thyroid hormones are L-thyroxine (T_4, Chemical Structure 19.1) and L-3,5,3'-triiodothyronine (T_3, Chemical Structure 19.2). Follicular cells within the thyroid gland produce and secrete T_4 and T_3 in a classic negative feedback loop. Thyroid-releasing hormone (TRH) secreted from the hypothalamus stimulates the release of thyroid-stimulating hormone (TSH) from the anterior pituitary gland. This in turn stimulates T_3 and T_4 production and release from the thyroid gland. T_3 and T_4 feedback to inhibit the synthesis and secretion of both TRH and TSH.

Hypothyroidism is the most common disorder of thyroid function. It is a clinical state resulting from insufficient circulating levels of T_4 and T_3. Primary hypothyroidism (~95 % of hypothyroidism) is defined by the inability of the thyroid gland to produce thyroid hormones. Secondary hypothyroidism is defined as a functional thyroid deprived of TSH stimulation due to pituitary failure. Tertiary hypothyroidism is due to hypothalamic failure. All etiologies of hypothyroidism can be treated with thyroid hormone replacement therapy either as synthetic or desiccated thyroid preparations.

Myxedema is a medical emergency and represents the clinical state of severe, long-standing hypothyroidism. Clinical features of myxedema include depression of the cardiovascular, respiratory, gastrointestinal, and central nervous systems. Impaired diuresis leads to profound hyponatremia and acidosis [2].

Drug Class and Mechanism of Action

Once released by the follicular cells of the thyroid gland, the thyroid hormones are transported in the plasma by thyroxine-binding globulins (TBG). Protein binding by TBG (>99 % of circulating hormones are protein bound) markedly increases the half-lives of thyroid hormones by protecting the hormones from metabolism and excretion [3]. However, it is only the unbound hormone that is metabolically active. Unbound T_3 and T_4 enter effector cells by either passive diffusion or via specific transporter proteins present on the cell membrane [4]. Once within the cell cytoplasm, T_4 is converted by deiodination to the much more biologically active T_3.

At the cellular level, the mechanism of action of thyroid hormone is mediated by the binding of T_3 to thyroid hormone receptors (TRs) within the nucleus of the effector cell. This complex of T_3 and TRs promotes DNA transcription and ultimately results in protein synthesis that mediates the clinical effects of the thyroid hormone [5]. Some of these clinical effects include thermogenesis, carbohydrate metabolism, and the regulation of myocardial gene expression which play a critical role cardiac inotropy and chronotropy [6]. As alluded to in the introduction, the lack of thyroid hormone during critical period of neurogenesis can lead to cretinism which is characterized by mental retardation from deranged axonal projections and decreased synaptogenesis.

Thyroid hormone preparations are available either as synthetic preparations or desiccated porcine thyroid gland preparations. The synthetic preparations are available as pure T_4, T_3, or as a mixture. The desiccated porcine preparations contain a 4:1 ratio of T_4 to T_3, although human thyroid secrets a roughly 11:1 ratio of T_4 to T_3.

Indications/Clinical Pearls

The major indication for the therapeutic use of thyroid hormones is for hormone replacement therapy in patients with clinical manifestations of hypothyroidism. Signs and symptoms include mental slowing, depression, periorbital edema, cold extremities, brittle hair, bradycardia, narrow pulse pressure, pericardial effusion, ascites, and edema. The goal of all etiologies of hypothyroidism is to render the patient clinically euthyroid. In primary hypothyroidism, serum TSH can be used as a marker to follow the effectiveness of therapy. In secondary and tertiary hypothyroidism, adequacy of therapy should be assessed by measuring serum free T_4 levels. Despite these serum markers to measure the adequacy of therapy, most experts believe mild hypothyroidism poses no increased surgical risk. The choice of using a pure T_4 or mixed thyroid hormones replacement is likely one of personal preference. Randomized blinded controlled trials have found no difference in the effectiveness of T_4 monotherapy versus T_4 and T_3 combination therapy [7].

As the biologically active form of thyroid hormone and thus a rapid onset of action, T_3 is indicated for the treatment of myxedema. Compared to T_4, T_3 is less protein bound resulting in a shorter plasma half-life. Thus, T_3 requires more frequent dosing but allows for a more rapid achievement of steady state. Careful cardiac monitoring is needed in conjunction with the use of T_3 to monitor the precarious state of the patient and also to prevent over titration and the precipitation of a hyperthyroid state. Patients with severe hypothyroidism or myxedema must be medically optimized prior to surgery.

Dosing Options

Levothyroxine is a synthetic T_4. Levothyroxine sodium is marketed under multiple brand names including Synthroid, Levoxyl, Levothroid, Tirosint, and Unithroid. Despite multiple brands of levothyroxine, the potency standards are all reported to be within 95–105 % of the standard set by the USP used to establish bioequivalence. In patients with clinical hypothyroidism, levothyroxine is typically started orally at 1.7 mcg/kg once daily. Due to its long half-life of roughly 7 days, steady state is achieved at 6–8 weeks, and upward dose adjustments of 25 mcg/day can be titrated every 4–6 weeks until euthyroid. Due to the slow onset of levothyroxine, it is not recommended for the treatment of myxedema.

Liothyronine is a synthetic T_3. Liothyronine sodium is marketed as an oral preparation under the brand names Cytomel and as an injectable form, Triostat. Because T_3 is the biologically active form of thyroid hormone, it has a faster onset as it does not require peripheral conversion of T_4 to T_3. Cytomel's onset of activity occurs within a few hours of administration with maximum pharmacologic response occurring within 2–3 days. The biological half-life is about 2.5 days. The recommended starting dosage is 25 mcg daily. Dosage can be increased by up to 25 mcg every 1 or 2 weeks until clinically euthyroid. The usual maintenance dose is 25–75 mcg daily. Cytomel may be preferred when impairment of peripheral conversion of T_4 to T_3 is suspected. While Cytomel has a faster onset of action compared to levothyroxine, the manufacturer recommends using intravenous Triostat for the management of myxedema.

Triostat is a synthetic intravenous formulation of T_3. It is indicated for the treatment of myxedema although the mainstay of therapy should include supportive care with ventilator support, inotropes, rewarming, and correction of electrolyte and acid/base derangements. Although there are no randomized controlled clinical trials to evaluate the optimal therapy in myxedema, recommendations for dosing come from collective case reports from scientific literature. An initial dose of Triostat ranging from 25 to 50 mcg is recommended in the emergency treatment of myxedema. Based on continuous monitoring of the patient's clinical condition and response, additional doses may be titrated. Administration of at least 65 mcg/day of T_3 in the initial days of therapy was associated with lower mortality. Doses in excess of 100 mcg/day have been shown to increase mortality. In patients with cardiovascular disease, the initial dose should be decreased and upward titration moderated to prevent precipitating myocardial ischemia. An addition concern with rapid upward titration of T_3 is the precipitation of adrenal crisis due to increased cortisol metabolism. Glucocorticoids should be coadministered with rapid thyroid hormone replacement therapy [8].

Desiccated preparations of porcine thyroid glands are marketed as Armour Thyroid and Nature-Throid. The starting dose for both of these preparations is 30 mg/day with increments of 15 mg every 2–3 weeks. A maintenance dosage of 60–120 mg/day is usually required to achieve euthyroidism.

Drug Interactions

Oral anticoagulants – Thyroid hormones increase the catabolism of vitamin K-dependent clotting factors. Patients on oral anticoagulants should have their INR followed carefully during initiation of thyroid hormone replacement therapy. Dosages of anticoagulants may need to be reduced.

Insulin or oral hypoglycemics – Thyroid replacement may cause increases in insulin or oral hypoglycemic requirements. The effects are poorly understood.

Estrogen, oral contraceptives – Estrogen and estrogen-containing contraceptives increases serum TBG concentration, resulting in decreased T_4. Thyroid replacement therapy may need to be increased.

Digitalis – Thyroid hormones may increase the metabolism and clearance of digitalis. Monitoring of digitalis levels is recommended when starting thyroid replacement therapy.

Cytochrome P450 inducers – Strong inducers of hepatic cytochrome P450 3A4 (including but not limited to phenytoin, carbamazepine, rifampin, and amiodarone) may increase hepatic metabolism and thereby thyroid hormone clearance.

Side Effect

Therapeutic overdose of thyroid hormone replacement accounts for the vast majority of side effects. In general, these side effects include heat intolerance, excessive sweating, nervousness, anxiety, and insomnia. Cardiovascular wise, patient may experience palpitations, angina, and myocardial infarction especially in patients with known coronary disease. Gastrointestinal symptoms of diarrhea and abdominal cramps may also occur. Little awareness exists in most of the medical community regarding the toxicity of excessive thyroid hormone and related bone loss. Suppressed thyroid-stimulating hormone (TSH) accelerates bone resorption due to modulation of TSH receptors on osteoclastic and osteoblastic cells. In situations of prolonged elevation of thyroid consumption, osteoporosis and increased fracture risk have been reported. Women may experience menstrual irregularities and impaired fertility. FDA warnings (www.fda.gov) regarding preparation of thyroid replacement therapy articulate:

- Not using thyroid hormones such as levothyroxine, alone or with other therapeutic agents, for the treatment of obesity or for weight loss.
- In euthyroid patients, doses within the range of daily hormonal requirements are largely ineffective for weight reduction.
- Increasing doses might produce serious or even life-threatening effects, especially when administered with sympathomimetic amines.

Summary

Hypothyroidism is typically treated by thyroid replacement therapy by using levothyroxine given once daily. Other forms of thyroid preparation are available but there is no clinical evidence that one particular preparation is superior to the others. The goal of the therapy is to relieve the signs and symptoms of hypothyroidism. Serum markers with the goal of normalizing TSH and serum free-T_4 can be used to track the progress of therapy. Because of the long half-life of oral thyroid hormone preparations, steady state requires 6–8 weeks after initiation of therapy. In patients with coronary artery disease, care must be taken during upward titration of therapy to reduce the risk of angina or myocardial infarction. Severe hypothyroidism or myxedema is a medical emergency. The management is supportive with intravenous T_3 titration.

Mild hypothyroidism poses no increased surgical risk and patients may be able to proceed for surgery. Patients with severe hypothyroidism or myxedema must be medically optimized prior to surgery. Should myxedematous patients require emergent surgery, appropriate invasive monitoring and inotropic support should be anticipated. Careful titration of short-acting opioid or the use of nonopioid analgesics may help minimize further deleterious changes in symptoms.

Corticosteroid Hormones

Introduction

The adrenal cortex produces two major classes of steroid hormones: the adrenal corticosteroids and the adrenal androgens. These two classes of steroid hormones are synthesized from cholesterol and secreted by cells within three distinct layers of the adrenal cortex. The outermost zona glomerulosa produces mineralocorticoids. Just beneath this outermost layer is the zona fasciculata, the source of glucocorticoid production. The innermost layer of the cortex is the zona reticularis, responsible for the production of adrenal androgens. This section will focus on cortisol, aldosterone, and their synthetic derivatives.

Cortisol (Chemical Structure 19.3) is the primary glucocorticoid synthesized and secreted by the adrenal cortex. Cortisol secretion is regulated by adrenocorticotropic hormone (ACTH) produced by the anterior pituitary. ACTH is, in turn, regulated by corticotropin-releasing hormone (CRH) produced by the hypothalamus. Cortisol exerts negative feedback control by inhibiting the secretion of CRH and ACTH. Cortisol and glucocorticoids prepare the body for stress by suppressing inflammation and increasing the availability of carbohydrates.

Aldosterone (Chemical Structure 19.4) is the primary mineralocorticoid synthesized and secreted by the adrenal cortex. Its secretion is regulated by the renin-angiotensin system (RAS). Briefly, baroreceptors in the kidney releases renin in response to decreased perfusion pressure due to intravascular volume depletion.

Renin converts angiotensinogen to angiotensin I, which is then converted by angiotensin-converting enzyme to angiotensin II. Angiotensin II restores blood pressure by vasoconstriction and by stimulation of aldosterone secretion. Aldosterone restores intravascular volume by increasing sodium and water reabsorption by the distal tubules and collecting ducts. Aldosterone and mineralocorticoids therefore play an important role in the maintenance of intravascular volume and sodium balance.

Drug Class and Mechanism of Action

All corticosteroids, natural or synthetic, enter cells and bind to an intracellular cytoplasmic receptor. This bound complex then enters the nucleus and stimulates DNA transcription resulting in protein production that mediates the effect of the steroid hormone. Transcription and translation into protein products takes time and the effects of corticosteroids are usually not immediate. Clinically, the beneficial effects of corticosteroids are generally seen several hours after drug delivery. However, there is evidence that corticosteroids may exert immediate effects by non-genomic mechanisms [9]. Examples of this include the ability of corticosteroids to augment the responsiveness to catecholamine-mediated vasoconstriction. The mechanisms of these actions are not well understood.

Several natural and synthetic derivatives of corticosteroids are commercially available. These drugs are classified by their relative mineralocorticoid versus glucocorticoid potency.

The actions of corticosteroid derivatives with strong glucocorticoid activity include:

- *Anti-inflammatory action*: This is perhaps the most sought after property of glucocorticoids. Although the exact mechanism is complex and not fully understood, glucocorticoids mediate anti-inflammation by inhibiting the production of interleukin-2 and suppressing the proliferation of T lymphocytes. Histamine and serotonin release from mast cells and platelets are suppressed. Inhibition of phospholipase A_2 blocks the formation of arachidonic acid and thereby decreases prostaglandin and leukotriene synthesis [10].
- *Increase resistance to stress*: Glucocorticoids increase gluconeogenesis, catabolism, and lipolysis. These actions in concert raise plasma glucose levels and provide the body with energy required to combat stress. Glucocorticoids also modestly raise the blood pressure by enhancing vasoconstrictor action of catecholamines on vascular endothelium.
- *Effects on other systems*: These are the adverse effects associated with glucocorticoids. Increase in gastric acid and pepsin production may cause peptic ulcers. Long-standing therapy may promote hypertension, diabetes, fluid retention, edema, weight gain, bone demineralization, emotional instability, and myopathy leading to muscle weakness.

Corticosteroid derivatives with strong mineralocorticoid activity tend to help control the body's water volume and concentration of electrolytes, especially sodium and potassium. The cellular mechanism of action is based on its activity on principles cells and alpha-intercalated cells of the nephron. Principle cells reside in the distal tubules and collecting ducts of the nephron. Activation of mineralocorticoids receptors located within the principal cells upregulates sodium/potassium pumps with resultant sodium and water reabsorption and potassium secretion. Mineralocorticoids acting on alpha-intercalated cells of the late distal tubule and collecting duct result in increased hydrogen ion secretion. The net effect is the restoration of intravascular volume and blood pressure.

Indications/Clinical Pearls

There are multiple clinical applications for corticosteroids. Common uses of corticosteroids are listed:

- *Primary adrenal insufficiency*: Caused by the primary impairment of the adrenal glands. The vast majority is due to autoimmune destruction. Other causes include adrenal hemorrhage, tumor destruction, infection, and amyloid infiltration. Patients with primary adrenal insufficiency require lifelong hormone replacement with both glucocorticoids and mineralocorticoids.
- *Secondary adrenal insufficiency*: Caused primarily by insufficiency ACTH secretion. The most common and clinically relevant cause of secondary adrenal insufficiency is chronic corticosteroid therapy. Chronic corticosteroid use suppresses the hypothalamus and anterior pituitary, resulting in decreased CRH and ACTH, respectively. Decreased activity of these trophic hormones causes atrophy of the zona fasciculata. During times of physiologic stress, these patients are unable to acutely increase glucocorticoid production, resulting in acute adrenal insufficiency. Mineralocorticoid deficiency is also seen but to a lesser degree. Patients with secondary adrenal insufficiency may require additional perioperative stress dose of corticosteroids [11].
- *Relief of inflammation*: This is the most common indication for corticosteroids and covers multiple disease processes where inflammation plays a significant role. In general, these include autoimmune diseases such as systemic lupus erythematosus, rheumatic disorders, vasculitic disorders, asthma, ocular inflammatory conditions, multiple sclerosis, cerebral edema secondary to tumors, dermatologic inflammatory conditions, and inflammatory gastrointestinal diseases such as ulcerative colitis.
- *Treatment of allergies*: These include anaphylaxis, drug hypersensitivity reactions, serum sickness, transfusion reactions, and atopic and contact dermatitis.
- *Treatment of severe sepsis and shock*: Accepted but controversial use of steroids [12].

- *Perioperative adjunct*: Antiemetic effect of glucocorticoids is well documented, although the mechanism is not well understood. Prophylactic glucocorticoid therapy has been shown to prevent post-extubation airway obstruction by limiting airway edema. The anti-inflammatory action of glucocorticoids also contributes to analgesia.
- *Diagnostic*: Dexamethasone suppression test.

Dosing Options

Due to the myriad of conditions treated by corticosteroids, specific dosing recommendations for each disease process are beyond the scope of this chapter. However, when considering the dosage of corticosteroids, factors such as glucocorticoid versus mineralocorticoid activity, duration of action, and type of preparation should be considered. These are summarized in Table 19.1. Furthermore, dosage requirements are often variable and must be individualized based on the disease process and response of the patient.

Common perioperative dosing of corticosteroids:

- *Airway edema* – Proven role in the management of croup. For patient with prolonged intubation in the ICU, dexamethasone 5 mg IV every 6 h for a total of four doses on the day preceding extubation has been shown to reduce post-extubation stridor. Available data regarding one-time dexamethasone dose in the OR has been equivocal.
- *Anaphylaxis* – While glucocorticoids are not helpful acutely, they may potentially help prevent recurrences and shorten the duration of the attack. Hydrocortisone 100 mg IV bolus can be given after airway, ventilation, and hemodynamic stability have been addressed.
- *Anti-emesis* – Dexamethasone 4 mg IV can be given at induction of anesthesia for postoperative nausea and vomiting prophylaxis.
- *Cerebral edema from primary or metastatic tumor* – During craniotomy for tumor resection, an intravenous loading dose of dexamethasone 10 mg followed by 4 mg every 6 h can be considered. For inoperable palliative maintenance therapy, oral doses of dexamethasone 4 mg twice or three times per day may be effective.

Controversy remains over whether supplemental perioperative steroids are required for patients on maintenance corticosteroids who undergo surgery. A 2009 Cochrane review concluded that there is inadequate evidence to support or refute the use of perioperative stress dose steroids [13]. In clinical practice, many clinicians routinely administer perioperative stress dose steroids to patients on maintenance corticosteroids. Obviously, careful consideration of patient comorbidities as well as the risk and benefits of steroid supplementation needs to be assessed on a case by case basis. A review of expert opinions in literature has the following recommendation [14]:

Table 19.1 Glucocorticoid equivalents of commonly prescribed corticosteroids

Corticosteroid	Relative glucocorticoid activity	Relative mineralo-corticoid activity	Equivalent glucocorticoid dose (mg)	Plasma half-life (min)
Hydrocortisone	1.0	1.0	20	90
Cortisone	0.8	0.8	25	30
Prednisone	4	0.8	5	60
Prednisolone	4	0.8	5	200
Triamcinolone	5	0	4	300
Methylprednisolone	5	0	4	180
Betamethasone	25	0	0.8	100–300
Dexamethasone	25	0	0.8	100–300
Fludrocortisone	10	125	2	200

Relative milligram comparisons with hydrocortisone (cortisol)

- *Minimal stress procedures* (<1 h under local anesthesia) – Continue the usual replacement corticosteroid.
- *For minor stress procedures* (colonoscopy, inguinal hernia repair) – Continue the usual replacement corticosteroids and administer hydrocortisone 25 mg IV at the start of the procedure.
- *For moderate stress procedures* (open cholecystectomy, joint replacement, lower-limb revascularization, abdominal hysterectomy) – Administer IV hydrocortisone 75 mg/day on the day of the procedure (25 mg IV every 8 h), and then taper over the next 1–2 days to usual replacement doses.
- *For severe stress procedures* (cardiothoracic, Whipple, liver resection) – Administer IV hydrocortisone 150 mg/day (50 mg IV every 8 h), then taper over the next 2–3 days to the usual replacement dose.

Drug Interactions

Etomidate – Inhibits cortisol secretion by inhibiting CYP11B1 activity. Current literature is unclear as to whether the use of etomidate is justified due to its propensity to suppress cortisol production [15].

Amphotericin B – Enhanced hypokalemia. Potassium levels should be check frequently and supplemented as needed.

Oral anticoagulants – Corticosteroids may potentiate or decrease the action of anticoagulants. INR levels should be closely monitored.

Insulin or oral hypoglycemics – Corticosteroids worsen glucose tolerance. Glucose levels should be closely monitored and dosage of insulin and oral hypoglycemic medication should be titrated up as necessary.

Digitalis – Potassium wasting effects of corticosteroids may enhance digitalis toxicity associated with hypokalemia.

Hepatic enzyme inducers (e.g., barbiturates, phenytoin, carbamazepine, rifampin) – P450 inducers will increase the metabolism of corticosteroids.

Diuretics (potassium-depleting) – Enhanced hypokalemia. Potassium levels should be checked frequently and supplemented as needed.

NSAIDs – Increases the ulcerogenic effect of corticosteroids.
Vaccines – Attenuated antibody response may occur in patients on corticosteroids.

Side Effect

Glucocorticoid adverse effects include hypertension, hyperglycemia, peptic ulcer-ation, impaired wound healing, impaired immune function, increased susceptibility to infection, weight gain, redistribution of body fat, acne, hirsutism, easy bruising, striae, cataracts, avascular necrosis of bone, loss of calcium and phosphorus result-ing in osteoporosis, and muscle wasting. Mineralocorticoid adverse effects include hypertension, sodium and water retention, peripheral edema, hypokalemic alkalo-sis, and congestive heart failure in patients with depressed myocardium.

Perhaps the most serious side effect is hypothalamic-pituitary-adrenal suppres-sion. Acute withdrawal of corticosteroids may cause acute adrenal insufficiency. Large treatment doses of steroids or chronic steroid therapy should be tapered to prevent secondary adrenal insufficiency.

Summary

Corticosteroids have a wide range of effects and play an integral part in the modulation of inflammation and maintenance of fluid balance. Corticosteroids have vital life-sus-taining roles in the management of adrenal insufficiency and proven roles in myriads of numerous inflammatory conditions. The clinically available natural and synthetic derivatives of corticosteroids are numerous. A thorough understanding of each agent's relative glucocorticoid versus mineralocorticoid activity and duration of action is para-mount in choosing the appropriate therapy to meet the patient's clinical needs.

Patients on chronic corticosteroid therapy may be susceptible to acute adrenal insufficiency in times of stress. Perioperative stress dose corticosteroids should be considered based on the anticipated level of perioperative stress.

Chemical Structures

Chemical Structure
19.1 L-thyroxine

Chemical Structure
19.2 L-3,5,3′-
triiodothyronine

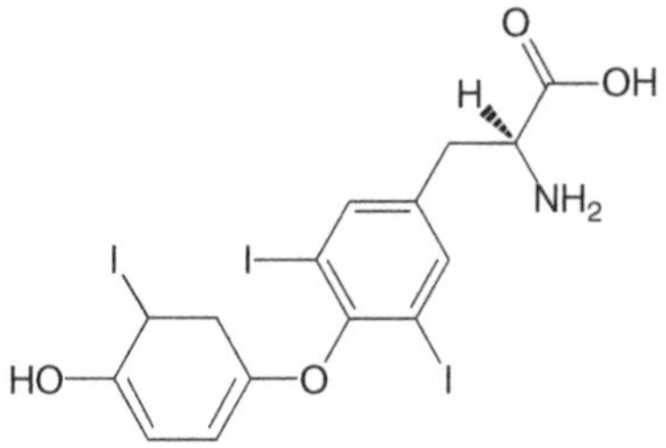

Chemical Structure
19.3 Cortisol

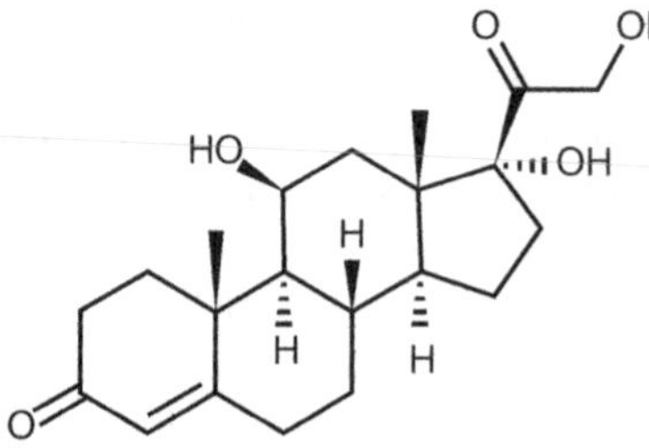

Chemical Structure
19.4 Aldosterone

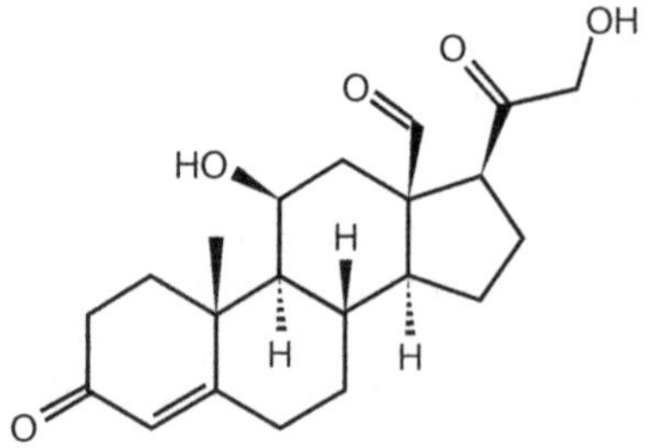

References

1. Bernal J. Thyroid hormone receptors in brain development and function. Nat Clin Pract Endocrinol Metab. 2007;3:249–59.
2. Kwaku MP, Burman KD. Myxedema coma. J Intensive Care Med. 2007;22:224–31.
3. Schussler GC. The thyroxine-binding proteins. Thyroid. 2000;10:141–9.
4. Visser WE, Friesema EC, Jansen J, Visser TJ. Thyroid hormone transport in and out of cells. Trends Endocrinol Metab. 2008;19:50–6.
5. Yen PM, Ando S, Feng X, Liu Y, Maruvada P, Xia X. Thyroid hormone action at the cellular, genomic and target gene levels. Mol Cell Endocrinol. 2006;246:121–7.
6. Kahaly GJ, Dillmann WH. Thyroid hormone action in the heart. Endocr Rev. 2005;26:704–28.
7. Grozinsky-Glasberg S, Fraser A, Nahshoni E, Weizman A, Leibovici L. Thyroxine-triiodothyronine combination therapy versus thyroxine monotherapy for clinical hypothyroidism: meta-analysis of randomized controlled trials. J Clin Endocrinol Metab. 2006;91:2592–9.
8. Hahner S, Loeffler M, Bleicken B, Dreschsler C, Milovanovic D, Fassnacht M, et al. Epidemiology of adrenal crisis in chronic adrenal insufficiency: the need for new prevention strategies. Eur J Endocrinol. 2010;162:597–602.

9. Stahn C, Buttgereit F. Genomic and nongenomic effects of glucocorticoids. Nat Clin Pract Rheumatol. 2008;4:525–33.
10. Chrousos GP. The hypothalamic-pituitary-adrenal axis and immune-mediated inflammation. N Engl J Med. 1995;332:1351–62.
11. Coursin DB, Wood KE. Corticosteroid supplementation for adrenal insufficiency. JAMA. 2002;287:L236–40.
12. Sprung CL, Annane D, Keh D, Moreno R, Singer M, Freivogel K, et al. Hydrocortisone therapy for patients with septic shock. N Engl J Med. 2008;358:111–24.
13. Yong SL, Marik P, Esposito M, Coulthard P. Supplemental perioperative steroids for surgical patients with adrenal insufficiency. Cochrane Database Syst Rev. 2009;7(4):CD005367.
14. Jung C, Inder WJ. Management of adrenal insufficiency during the stress of medical illness and surgery. Med J Aust. 2008;188:409–13.
15. Marik PE. Etomidate in critically ill patients. Is it safe? Crit Care Med. 2012;40:301–2.

Chapter 20
Hormones Part 2: Insulin and Other Glucose-Controlling Medications

Kumar Vivek, Shamantha Reddy, and Justo Gonzalez

Contents

Introduction to Hypoglycemics

Diabetes mellitus (DM) is an extremely common disease process worldwide. These patients often need surgical interventions for a wide variety of reasons. One of the differences between type 1 and type 2 DM is that patients with type 1 would die without insulin and is associated with an autoimmune attack on the patient's beta cells in the pancreas. Type II diabetes mellitus (T2DM) is characterized by insulin deficiency, insulin resistance, and increased hepatic glucose output [1–3]. The chronic state of elevated glucose levels affects the whole body at a macro- and microvascular level, ultimately leading to the deterioration of vital organs, such as the kidney, cardiac, and nervous system. Diabetes is the leading cause of renal insufficiency in the United States and is a strong risk factor for coronary artery disease. This chronic state affects many perioperative patients currently, and its prevalence is projected to increase substantially in the near future.

K. Vivek, MD (✉) • S. Reddy, MD • J. Gonzalez, MD
Department of Anesthesiology, Montefiore Medical Center, Albert Einstein College of
Medicine, Bronx, NY, USA
e-mail: kvivek@montefiore.org; jusgonza@montefiore.org

A.D. Kaye et al. (eds.), *Essentials of Pharmacology for Anesthesia,*
Pain Medicine, and Critical Care, DOI 10.1007/978-1-4614-8948-1_20,
© Springer Science+Business Media New York 2015

There is high-quality evidence to support the use of oral pharmacologic therapy in T2DM patients when hyperglycemia persists despite dietary changes, lifestyle modifications, and weight loss [4]. Hemoglobin A1c (HbA1C), or glycosylated hemoglobin, is a product of hemoglobin exposed to a high circulating blood glucose level. HbA1c serves as a marker for average plasma glucose levels over the previous 3 months. Achieving a HbA1c level less than 6.5 % is a primary objective of diabetes management. There are currently six different categories of oral hypoglycemic agents approved for use in the United States [5]. In addition, injectable non-insulin adjuvants, such as exenatide, allow for enhanced expression and sensitivity to endogenous insulin.

Yet with time, T2DM patients can become insulin deficient and have a need for direct insulin administration, as do type 1 diabetics who are unable to secrete insulin. In the acute setting, the stress response to illness in the diabetic patient usually causes acute hyperglycemia. This hyperglycemia is associated with impaired immune system, impaired wound healing, osmotic diuresis leading to infection, and overall poor outcome [6]. Various forms of insulin have been developed to control glucose levels, with the intent of maintaining euglycemia and avoiding the detrimental side effects of hypo- and hyperglycemia. Both the patient and physician must be familiar with insulin administration and the pitfalls involving the various insulin and non-insulin medications in order to ensure a safe perioperative environment. Dosing options are listed in Table 20.1.

Oral Medications

Drug Class

Sulfonylureas

Mechanism of Action

Sulfonylureas are insulin secretagogues which bind to pancreatic beta cell K^+-ATP complex, thereby resulting in membrane depolarization, calcium influx, and secretion of insulin.

Indications/Clinical Pearls

Sulfonylureas are inexpensive medications used to treat hyperglycemia in T2DM patients. They are utilized in combination with metformin for added control but can be used as monotherapy in patients who cannot tolerate metformin. They are expected to decrease HA1c by 1–2 %.

Drug Interactions

There is a moderate amount of drug interactions with sulfonylureas, and patients with difficult-to-treat glucose levels should have a review of medications to see whether certain agents may be enhancing or depressing the usual effects. The more

Table 20.1 Dosing options for non-insulin antidiabetic agents

Drug class	Drug	Brand names	Dosing option
Sulfonylureas	Glyburide	*Regular tablets* DiaBeta®	1.25–20 mg, 1–2 times/day
		Micronized tablets Glynase® PresTab®	1.5–12 mg, 1–2 times /day
	Glipizide	*Immediate release* Glucotrol®	5–20 mg, 1–2 times /day
		Extended release Glucotrol XL®	5–20 mg/day
	Glimepiride	Amaryl®	1–8 mg/day
Meglitinides	Repaglinide	Prandin®	0.5–4 mg/day
	Nateglinide	Starlix®	60–120 mg 3 times/day
Biguanide	Metformin	*Immediate release* Glucophage® Riomet® (liquid)	500–2,500 mg, 1–2 times/day
		Extended release Fortamet® Glumetza® Glucophage® XR	500–2,500 mg/day
Thiazolidinediones	Pioglitazone	Actos®	15–40 mg/day
	Rosiglitazone	Avandia	4–8 mg, 1–2 times/day
Alpha-glucosidase inhibitors	Miglitol	Glyset®	25–100 mg, 3 times/day
	Acarbose	Precose®	25–100 mg, 3 times/day
DPP-4 inhibitors	Sitagliptin	Januvia®	100 mg /day
	Saxagliptin	Onglyza™	2.5–5 mg /day
Bile acid sequestrants	Colesevelam	Welchol®	1,875–4,375 mg, 1–2 times/day
GLP-1 agonists	Exenatide	Bydureon™ Byetta®	Immediate release – 5–10 mcg twice daily
			Extended release – 2,000 mcg/week
	Liraglutide	Victoza®	0.6–1.8 mg/day
Amylin agonists	Pramlintide	Symlin®	60–120 mcg before meals

common drugs that can cause an increase in the occurrence of hypoglycemia when used in combination with sulfonylureas are salicylates, sulfonamides, fibric acid derivatives (such as gemfibrozil), and warfarin.

Side Effects/Black Box Warnings

Sulfonylureas are generally well tolerated. Hypoglycemia is the most common side effect, generally seen more frequently in longer-acting agents like glyburide. Sulfonylureas should be used with caution in elderly and renal patients. Weight gain and gastrointestinal disturbances may also occur. In addition, patients on sulfonylureas have been shown to have an increased odds ratio (OR = 2.77) for early mortality after acute MI and angioplasty [7]. It is known that ATP-dependent potassium channels exist on coronary vessels;

thus, sulfonylureas prevent vasodilation, causing further myocardial damage. Another possible mechanism is interference in ischemic preconditioning. Therefore, sulfonylureas should be avoided in acute cardiac conditions or patients admitted for cardiac procedures. However, newer generation sulfonylureas are selective for pancreatic sulfonylurea receptors and have been shown to have similar cardiac outcomes compared to other secretagogues [8].

Drug Class

Meglitinides

Mechanism of Action

Meglitinides block ATP-dependent K^+ channels, thereby depolarizing the pancreatic beta cell membrane and facilitating calcium entry through calcium channels. This increase in intracellular calcium stimulates insulin release from the pancreatic beta cells. Though similar to sulfonylureas in action, they work via different receptors. Meglitinide-induced insulin release is glucose dependent.

Indications/Clinical Pearls

Meglitinides increase insulin secretion with the expectation of lowering HA1c by 1–2 %. Monotherapy can be initiated, but in combination with metformin, it has superior glucose control. In comparison to sulfonylureas, the incidence of hypoglycemic episodes is lower.

Drug Interactions

Gemfibrozil combined with repaglinide has been show to enhance the hypoglycemic action.

Side Effects/Black Box Warnings

The most common adverse event is hypoglycemia (20 % with repaglinide, uncommon with nateglinide). Meglitinides should be used with caution in patients with renal and/or severe liver disease. Nateglinide is hepatically metabolized with active metabolites that are renally excreted; therefore, it is better avoided in the renal patient. Repaglinide is metabolized via the liver and less than 10 % is renally excreted; thus, it does not need dose adjustment in renal patients. Other side effects include headache, arthralgia, upper respiratory tract infection, chest pain (3 % with repaglinide), and cardiac ischemia (2 % with repaglinide).

Drug Class

Biguanide

Mechanism of Action

Biguanides decrease hepatic glucose output in the presence of insulin. They also increase insulin-mediated glucose utilization by peripheral tissues.

Indications/Clinical Pearls

Metformin is an inexpensive medication that decreases hepatic glucose production while not causing hypoglycemia or weight gain. The expectation is for a reduction in HA1c by 1–2 %. It is usually the first treatment to be started in patients who cannot control glucose levels with lifestyle changes. Often as the glucose levels become less manageable, other oral hypoglycemics are added or even insulin is combined. Metformin is also used off-label for the treatment of oligomenorrhea, hirsutism, infertility, obesity, and prevention of T2DM in polycystic ovarian syndrome patients.

Drug Interactions

Patients receiving radiographic contrast are placed at risk for lactic acidosis as are acute or chronic alcohol consumers. Azole antifungal agents, levofloxacin, and monoamine oxidase inhibitors may increase the risk for hypoglycemia. Furosemide and nifedipine may enhance metformin absorption. Cationic drugs (amiloride, cimetidine, cotrimoxazole, digoxin, morphine, procainamide, quinidine, quinine, ranitidine, triamterene, and vancomycin) increase the risk for lactic acidosis by interfering with the renal tubular transport of metformin but can be used with close monitoring.

Side Effects/Black Box Warnings

> Possible side effects include diarrhea and nausea, which are common (30 %). Vitamin B12 can be lowered and should be checked every 2–3 years. Lactic acidosis is a very rare complication. There is a lack of evidence for increased risk with the use of biguanides during the perioperative period [9]. Therefore, biguanide use should not be a cause for delay or cancelation of surgery. Despite this, use should probably be stopped in the surgical patient 24 h prior and avoided in patients with renal dysfunction and in those likely to receive IV contrast. Creatinine levels should be reassessed 2–3 days after contrast to rule out nephropathy prior to reinitiating. Metformin should also be held in patients with decreased tissue perfusion or hemodynamic instability due to infection, concurrent liver disease, alcohol abuse, or heart failure.

Drug Class

Thiazolidinediones

Mechanism of Action

Thiazolidinediones are peroxisome proliferator-activated receptor-gamma (PPARγ) agonists which lower blood glucose by improving target cell response to insulin without increasing pancreatic insulin secretion.

Indications/Clinical Pearls

Thiazolidinediones decrease insulin resistance and increase glucose utilization. They are expected to decrease HA1c by 0.5–1.4 %. Due to the associated increase in side effects and expense, they are used as second-line therapy in patients with high risk for hypoglycemia or intolerance of or contraindications to metformin or sulfonylureas.

Drug Interactions

Controversial data shows possible interactions with statin therapy via the cytochrome P450 system.

Side Effects/Black Box Warnings

Possible side effects include peripheral edema, congestive heart failure (CHF), weight gain, fractures, and macular edema. Rosiglitazone has been associated with increased risk for cardiovascular disease. Thiazolidinediones should be avoided in patients with CHF and liver disease (due to hepatotoxicity).

Drug Class

Alpha-glucosidase inhibitor

Mechanism of Action

The alpha-glucosidase inhibitors are competitive, reversible inhibitors of alpha-amylase, which is produced in the pancreas, and of alpha-glucosidase, which is located on the brush border of the small intestine. This inhibition results in reduced postprandial increases in blood glucose levels by delaying the digestion of dietary carbohydrates.

Indications/Clinical Pearls

It is helpful in reducing postprandial glycemia with the expectation of reducing HA1c by 0.5–0.8 %.

Drug Interactions

May reduce serum digoxin concentrations. Digestive enzymes and intestinal adsorbents, such as charcoal, should not be taken at the same time as the alpha-glucosidase inhibitors, as they will decrease the efficacy of the alpha-glucosidase inhibitors. Miglitol decreases the bioavailability of propranolol and ranitidine.

Side Effects/Black Box Warnings

Gastrointestinal effects are very common including abdominal pain, diarrhea, and flatulence. Patients may also experience changes in liver function tests. It should be avoided in patients with inflammatory bowel disease, intestinal obstruction or predisposition to obstruction, colon ulceration, or other disorders of digestion or absorption. Used alone, alpha-glucosidase inhibitors do not cause hypoglycemia. However, hypoglycemia can occur when combined with other diabetic medications. Hypoglycemia should be treated with oral dextrose and not sucrose, which will be unable to be absorbed.

Drug Class

Dipeptidyl peptidase-4 (DPP-4) inhibitor

Mechanism of Action

This medication prolongs action of endogenous glucagon-like peptide-1 (GLP-1) by deactivating DPP-4, an enzyme that deactivates various bioactive peptides.

Indications/Clinical Pearls

There is an expected reduction of HA1c by 0.5–1 % without causing hypoglycemia. Yet due to its expense and limited experience in practice, it has not played a large role in diabetic management.

Drug Interactions

Minimal drug reactions but may need to decrease sulfonylurea dose due to risk of hypoglycemia.

Side Effects/Black Box Warnings

One should consider reducing dose in renal patients. May increase risk for infection.

Drug Class

Bile Acid Sequestrants

Mechanism of Action

This medication works as a bile acid sequestrant that lowers LDL.

Indications/Clinical Pearls

In patients with hyperlipidemia, it is expected to decrease HA1c by 0.5 %.

Drug Interactions

This medication can interfere with absorption of other drugs such as glyburide, levothyroxine, and oral contraceptives containing ethinyl estradiol or norethindrone, by binding to them in the stomach and preventing their absorption into the body. It can also reduce phenytoin and warfarin activity. Drugs interacting with colesevelam should be given 4 h prior to its administration.

Side Effects/Black Box Warnings

Known side effects include constipation, dyspepsia, abdominal pain, nausea, and difficult triglyceride control. It should be avoided in patients with intestinal obstruction.

Non-insulin Injectables

Drug Class

Glucagon-like peptide (GLP)-1 agonists

Mechanism of Action

This medication increases insulin while decreasing glucagon and slowing gastric emptying.

Indications/Clinical Pearls

GLP-1 agonists result in satiety and weight loss with a projected decrease of HA1c by 0.5–1 %.

Drug Interactions

There is a risk of hypoglycemia with insulin secretagogues and other GI motility-slowing agents.

Side Effects/Black Box Warnings

Nausea is a known side effect. These drugs should be used with caution in patients with renal disease and pancreatitis.

Drug Class

Amylin agonists

Mechanism of Action

The mode of action includes slowing gastric emptying and decreasing glucagon secretion.

Indications/Clinical Pearls

This medication reduces postprandial glycemia and causes weight loss and with an expected HA1c decrease by 0.25–0.5 %.

Drug Interactions

There is a risk of hypoglycemia with coadministration of insulin. It should also be used with caution in drugs that slow gastrointestinal motility.

Side Effects/Black Box Warnings

Nausea is the most common side effect.

There are a number of black box warnings as summarized below (www.fda.gov):

- SYMLIN is used with insulin and particularly among patients who have type 1 diabetes appears to increase the risk of insulin-induced severe hypoglycemia.
- SYMLIN-associated severe hypoglycemia is seen within 3 h following injection.
- Severe hypoglycemia that occurs during high-risk activities (e.g., operating a motor vehicle or heavy machinery) can cause serious injuries.
- It is incumbent upon clinicians to select appropriate patients, provide clear and thorough instructions, and adjust insulin doses to reduce potential risk.

Injectable Insulin

Drug Class

Insulin, short and long acting (See Table 20.2).

Mechanism of Action

Insulin is produced by beta cells of the pancreas, and it lowers blood glucose by increasing peripheral glucose uptake (mostly into fat and skeletal muscle) and inhibiting hepatic gluconeogenesis.

Table 20.2 Pharmacology of insulin [9]

Drug class: generic (*trade name*)	Onset	Peak effect	Duration
Short acting and rapid acting			
Regular (*Novolin R, Humulin R*)	30–60 min	2–4 h	6–8 h
Lispro (*Humalog*)	5–15 min	30–90 min	4–6 h
Aspart (*Novolog*)	5–15 min	30–90 min	4–6 h
Glulisine (*Apidra*)	5–15 min	30–90 min	4–6 h
Intermediate acting			
NPH (*Novolin N, Humulin N-NF*)	2–4 h	4–10 h	10–16 h
Zinc insulin (*Lente*)	2–4 h	4–10 h	12–20 h
Extended zinc insulin (*Ultralente*)	6–10 h	10–16 h	18–24 h
Long acting (peakless)			
Glargine (*Lantus*)	2–4 h	None	20–24 h
Detemir (*Levemir*)	2–4 h	None	20–24 h
Mixed insulins (NPH + regular)			
70 % NPH/30 % regular (*Novolin 70/30, Humulin 70/30*)	30–90 min	Dual	10–16 h
50 % NPH/50 % regular (Humulin 50/50)	30–90 min	Dual	10–16 h
Mixed insulins (intermediate-acting + rapid-acting analogs)			
70 % Aspart protamine suspension/30 % Aspart (Novolog mix 70/30)	5–15 min	Dual	10–16 h
75 % Lispro protamine suspension/25 % Lispro (Humalog mix 75/25)	5–15 min	Dual	10–16 h
50 % Lispro protamine suspension/50 % Lispro (Humalog mix 50/50)	5–15 min	Dual	10–12 h

Indications/Clinical Pearls

As non-insulin agents become unable to control hyperglycemic symptoms, or as HA1c increases >8.5 %, adding an insulin regimen is recommended.

Drug Interactions

The following drugs may decrease the effectiveness of insulin, resulting in hyperglycemia: acetazolamide, albuterol, asparaginase, calcitonin, corticosteroids, cyclophosphamide, danazol, dextrothyroxine, diazoxide, diltiazem, diuretics, dobutamine, epinephrine, estrogens, ethacrynic acid, HIV antivirals, isoniazid, lithium, morphine, niacin, oral contraceptives, phenothiazines, phenytoin, somatropin, terbutaline, thiazide diuretics, and thyroid supplements.

The following drugs may increase the effectiveness of insulin, resulting in hypoglycemia: ACE inhibitors, alcohol, anabolic steroids, beta blockers, calcium, chloroquine, clofibrate, clonidine, disopyramide, fluoxetine, guanethidine, lithium, mebendazole, monoamine oxidase inhibitors, octreotide, pentamidine, phenylbutazone, propoxyphene, pyridoxine, salicylates, sulfinpyrazone, sulfonamides, and tetracyclines.

Side Effects/Black Box Warnings

> Hypoglycemia, hypokalemia, and lipodystrophy (which can be avoided by rotating the injection sites). Patients using protamine-derived insulin, which is made from fish sperm, may develop immunologic sensitization, which upon protamine reversal of heparin can cause anaphylaxis.

Perioperative Glucose Control

After taking a formal preoperative history and physical focusing on particular aspects pertinent to diabetics, one should review medications and recommend how to modify/discontinue these medications in preparation for the day of surgery. Glycosylation of the cervical joints can cause a stiff-neck syndrome, making intubation challenging. Concern about the degree of autonomic degeneration can be identified with a 3 min EKG tracing looking at loss of R-R variability. Usually oral hypoglycemic medications are stopped while NPO, e.g., day of surgery, and the patient should be scheduled as early as possible due to fluctuations in glucose levels while fasting. Ideally, insulin-dependent patients should have a dedicated IV through which an insulin-glucose infusion is started 2 h prior to surgery (also see Table 20.3). Once the patient resumes eating, they can be restarted on their regular medications, though medications may need adjustments due to a new postoperative physiologic state. When assessing the surgical patient in order to have an idea of the amount of insulin that may be required to control glucose levels, one needs to investigate how well controlled the patient is and how much insulin is usually taken. (See inpatient insulin therapy algorithm in Table 20.4.)

For elective surgery, one can use HbA1c to see how well controlled the patient has been over the past 3 months. As per the ADA guidelines, a goal of less than 7 % is deemed adequate control, though not infrequently many patients present to surgery not meeting that goal. For perspective, a HbA1c >10 % correlates with a daily glucose >250 mg/dL. At some institutions, this is the threshold above which elective surgery would not be performed, since improved glucose control is recommended prior to the stress of surgery. Serum glucose levels on the day of surgery are also important in determining a patient's readiness for surgery. In general, on the day of surgery, a patient with serum glucose greater than 270 mg/dL should have surgery delayed until his or her glucose levels are controlled with insulin. One should note that osmotic diuresis occurs when blood glucose exceeds approximately 180–250 mg/dL which is above the renal glucose threshold [10]. There are no fixed guidelines for the level of glucose control prior to surgery, but usually the goal is a glucose level approximately <180 mg/dL. Patients with serum glucose greater than 400 mg/dL should have elective surgery canceled [11]. Patients with baseline poorly controlled diabetes should be kept around their baseline due to the fact that their bodies may have an altered hypoglycemic response to euglycemia.

Table 20.3 Instructions to patient regarding preoperative insulin and non-insulin injectable administration [9]

Insulin regimen	Day before surgery	Day of surgery	Comments
Insulin pump	No change	No change	Use "sick day" or "sleep" basal rates
Long-acting, peakless insulins	No change	75–100 % of morning dose	Reduce nighttime dose if history of nocturnal or morning hypoglycemia On the day of surgery, the morning dose of basal insulin may be administered on arrival to the ambulatory surgery facility
Intermediate-acting insulins	No change in the daytime dose 75 % of dose if taken in the evening	50–75 % of morning dose or calculated as below	See the comments for long-acting insulins
Fixed combination insulins	No change	50–75 % of morning dose of intermediate-acting component or calculated as below	Lispro protamine only available in combination; therefore use NPH instead, on day of surgery See the comments for long-acting insulins
Short- and rapid-acting insulin	No change	Hold the dose	
Non-insulin injectables	No change	Hold the dose	

Adapted from Jacober and Vann

Note: Optional intermediate-acting insulin dose (ID) calculation

$$\frac{(\text{Dose interval (hrs)} - \text{Hours of fast during interval (hrs)})}{\text{Dose interval (hrs)}} = \text{Fraction of intermediate insulin to give}$$

For example, a patient on NPH insulin 12 units twice daily at 7 a.m. and 7 p.m. (24 units total) (dosing interval = 12 h) scheduled for 1 pm surgery (hours fasted from am dose = 6); thus, (12–6)/12 = ½ of dose to be taken, i.e., 12 units. If 24 units, NPH taken once per day in am (dosing interval = 24 h), (24–6)/24 = ¾ of 24 units [27, 28]

One area of controversy is how tightly glucose levels should be controlled. In 2001, Van den Berghe et al. published an initial landmark study involving a single-center randomized controlled trial comparing a treatment group with target glucose goals of 80–110 mg/dL versus a conventional treatment group using insulin infusion for blood glucose >215 mg/dL with target goals of 180–200 mg/dL. The trial followed 1,548 surgical patients in an ICU setting under mechanical ventilation [12]. The results showed a decrease in the primary outcome of ICU mortality from 8.0 to 4.6 % ($P < 0.04$) in the tightly controlled group. Other complications that were decreased included bloodstream infections, ARF requiring dialysis, red-cell transfusions, and polyneuropathy. Although impressive, these results have not been

Table 20.4 Inpatient insulin algorithm [26]

Goal BG: _____**mg/dL**

Standard Drip: Regular insulin 100 units/100 mL 0.9 % NaCl via infusion device

Initiating the infusion

Bolus dose: Regular insulin 0.1 unit/kg = _____units

Algorithm 1: Start here for most patients

Algorithm 2: Start here if w/p CABG, s/p solid organ transplant or islet cell transplant, receiving glucocorticoids, vasopressors, or diabetics receiving >80 units/day of insulin as an outpatient

Algorithm 1		Algorithm 2		Algorithm 3		Algorithm 4	
BG	**Units/h**	**BG**	**Units/h**	**BG**	**Units/h**	**BG**	**Units/h**
		<60	=	Hypoglycemia (see below for treatment)			
<70	Off	<70	Off	<70	Off	<70	Off
70–109	0.2	70–109	0.5	70–109	1	70–109	1.5
110–119	0.5	110–119	1	110–119	2	110–119	3
120–149	1	120–149	1.5	120–149	3	120–149	−5
150–179	1.5	150–179	2	150–179	4	150–179	7
180–209	2	180–209	3	180–209	5	180–209	9
210–239	2	210–239	4	210–239	6	210–239	12
240–269	3	240–269	5	240–269	8	240–269	16
270–299	3	270–299	6	270–299	10	270–299	20
300–329	4	300–329	7	300–329	12	300–329	24
330–359	4	330–359	8	330–359	14	>330	28
>360	6	>360	12	>360	16		

Moving from Algorithm to Algorithm

Moving up: An algorithm failure is defined as BG outside the goal range for 2 h (see above goal), and the level does not change by at least 60 mg/dL within 1 h

Moving down: When BG is <70 mg/dL for two checks or if BG decreases by >100 mg/dL in an hour

Tube feeds or TPN: Decrease infusion by 50 % if nutrition (tube feeds or TPN) is discontinued or significantly reduced. Reinstitute hourly BG checks every 4 h

Patient Monitoring: Check capillary BG every hour until it is within goal range for 4 h, then decrease to every 2 h for 4 h, and if it remains at goal, may decrease to every 4 h

Treatment of Hypoglycemia (BG <60 mg/dL)

Discontinue insulin drip and give D50W IV

Patient conscious: 25 mL (1/2 amp)

Patient unconscious: 50 mL (1 amp)

Recheck BG every 20 min and repeat 25 min of D50W IV if <60 mg/dL

Restart drip once BG is >70 mg/dL for two checks

Restart drip with lower algorithm (see moving down)

Intravenous Fluids Most patients will need 5–10 g of glucose per hour (D5W or D5 1/2 NS at 100–200 mL/h or equivalent [TPN, enteral feeds])

BG blood glucose, *CABG* coronary artery bypass graft, *TPN* total parenteral nutrition

reproduced, perhaps because of the following limitations: The study was unblinded and was performed at a single center with mainly cardiac surgery patients, which had a nurse-to-patient ratio of 1:1, allowing for close monitoring and treatment.

Subsequent studies have consistently showed the danger of hypoglycemia and have proven hypoglycemia as an independent predictor of mortality [13–17]. Furthermore, a meta-analysis of 29 randomized trials comparing intensive glycemic control versus conventional therapy failed to show an in-hospital mortality benefit, regardless of glucose goal or patient population [18]. Therefore, a reasonable glucose goal for perioperative control would be between 110 and 180 mg/dL, while aiming for minimal fluctuations.

Usually one unit of insulin is expected to decrease glucose by 25–30 mg/dL, but one should be able to estimate a person's sensitivity to insulin prior to administration. A useful rule of thumb is the "Rule of 1800 and 1500." After totaling the patient's insulin usual daily requirements, say the patient takes 50 units per day. For each unit of insulin, it would drop 36–50 mg/dL using the above rule (obtained by calculating 1,800/50 and 1,500/50, respectively).

The type of insulin chosen is usually ultrarapid, given subcutaneous, or regular, given IV. These have been shown to be equally effective. Actually ultrarapid insulin given hourly can match IV regular insulin infusion rates (it is discouraged to administer regular insulin via IV bolus because it peaks in 30–40 min). Ultrarapid insulin has the benefit of reaching peak sooner and not requiring the logistics of an infusion system.

In addition, while treating hyperglycemia, one should also be vigilant for signs of hypoglycemia, and it is usually recommended to check glucose levels every 1–2 h in cases greater than 2 h in length. It is also important to note when interpreting point-of-care monitoring in the ill that the results for the patient may be off by >20 % in 15 % of capillary blood samples and 7 % of whole blood samples. Hypotension was associated with discrepancy in values and also with hypoglycemia only corresponding 26 % for capillary blood and 56 % for arterial blood using glucometers, and 65 % for chemical analysis of blood gas [19]. Most errors tended to overestimate blood glucose levels. Preferentially blood glucose levels are drawn in order of most to least accurate: artery, vein, and capillary and be monitored by blood gas analyser or in laboratory [20]. Also most patients should have a glucose-containing infusion running while being given insulin while being NPO. If the patient becomes hypoglycemic (<60 mg/dL) or becomes symptomatic, then the patient should be treated with glucose either orally (e.g., 8 oz juice) or given D50 IV with 50 mL, usually raising the glucose by 100 mg/dL. If the patient is unconscious without IV access, then glucagon 1 mg subcutaneous may be administered.

Special Considerations

Diabetic ketoacidosis (DKA) and the hyperosmolar hyperglycemic state (HHS) are the two most serious acute metabolic complications of diabetes. Most patients with DKA have autoimmune type 1 diabetes; however, patients with type 2 diabetes are also at risk during the catabolic stress of acute illness such as trauma, surgery, or infections [21]. A complex understanding of these disorders is beyond the scope of this chapter. Successful treatment of DKA and HHS requires correction of dehydration, hyperglycemia, and electrolyte imbalances; identification of comorbid precipitating events; and above all, frequent patient monitoring. The mainstay in the treatment of these hyperglycemic disorders involves primarily correction of dehydration/hypovolemia by restoring intravascular volume with isotonic fluids and by the administration of regular insulin via continuous intravenous infusion or by frequent subcutaneous injections [22–24]. Note that the danger of correcting hyperglycemia prior to volume status correction can be catastrophic since glucose in this instance maintains osmotic pressure and intravascular volume and collapse can occur when glucose is driven back into the cells too quickly. Added to this are rapid changes in tonicity may cause cerebral edema, which is a serious and real complication [25]. After recovery of kidney function, electrolytes, such as potassium, should be supplemented. Although blood levels may be elevated, potassium is actually depleted systemically. Usually nonemergent surgery should be postponed until the metabolic derangement has been controlled, which could take several days.

In summary, patients taking agents to lower glucose need careful attention to detail. Frequent monitoring can reduce the likelihood of hyper- or hypoglycemia. Preoperative evaluation can facilitate a rational plan to ensure the best outcome for these patients.

Chemical Structures

**Chemical Structure
20.1** Metformin

Chemical Structure 20.2 Acarbose

References

1. Luna B, Feinglos MN. Oral agents in the management of type 2 diabetes mellitus. Am Fam Physician. 2001;63(9):1747–56.
2. DeFronzo RA. Pharmacologic therapy for type 2 diabetes mellitus. Ann Intern Med. 1999;131(4):281–303.
3. Feinglos MN, Bethel MA. Treatment of type 2 diabetes mellitus. Med Clin N Am. 1998;82(4):757–90.
4. Qaseem A, et al. Oral pharmacologic treatment of type 2 diabetes mellitus: a clinical practice guideline from the American College of Physicians. Ann Intern Med. 2012;156(3):218–31.
5. Alexander GC, et al. National trends in treatment of type 2 diabetes mellitus, 1994–2007. Arch Intern Med. 2008;168(19):2088–94.
6. Miller RD. Miller's anesthesia, 7th Edition, 2010, Churchill Livingstone/Elsevier, Philadelphia, PA;1716–21.
7. Garratt KN, et al. Sulfonylurea drugs increase early mortality in patients with diabetes mellitus after direct angioplasty for acute myocardial infarction. J Am Coll Cardiol. 1999;33(1):119–24.
8. Zeller M, et al. Impact of type of preadmission sulfonylureas on mortality and cardiovascular outcomes in diabetic patients with acute myocardial infarction. J Clin Endocrinol Metab. 2010;95(11):4993–5002.
9. Joshi GP, et al. Society for ambulatory anesthesia consensus statement on perioperative blood glucose management in diabetic patients undergoing ambulatory surgery. Anesth Analg. 2010;111(6):1378–87.
10. Longnecker D, et al. Anesthesiology, 1st Edition, 2008, McGraw-Hill Companies, Incorporated, New York, NY;187.
11. Hines RL, Marschall KE. Stoelting's anesthesia and co-existing disease, 5th Edition, 2008, Churchill Livingstone, Philadelphia, PA;375.
12. van den Berghe G, et al. Intensive insulin therapy in critically ill patients. N Engl J Med. 2001;345(19):1359–67.
13. Brunkhorst FM, et al. Intensive insulin therapy and pentastarch resuscitation in severe sepsis. N Engl J Med. 2008;358(2):125–39.
14. Finney SJ, et al. Glucose control and mortality in critically ill patients. JAMA. 2003; 290(15):2041–7.
15. Krinsley JS, Grover A. Severe hypoglycemia in critically ill patients: risk factors and outcomes. Crit Care Med. 2007;35(10):2262–7.
16. Preiser JC, et al. A prospective randomised multi-centre controlled trial on tight glucose control by intensive insulin therapy in adult intensive care units: the glucontrol study. Intensive Care Med. 2009;35(10):1738–48.
17. Lipshutz AK, Gropper MA. Perioperative glycemic control: an evidence-based review. Anesthesiology. 2009;110(2):408–21.
18. Wiener RS, Wiener DC, Larson RJ. Benefits and risks of tight glucose control in critically ill adults: a meta-analysis. JAMA. 2008;300(8):933–44.
19. Kanji S, et al. Reliability of point-of-care testing for glucose measurement in critically ill adults. Crit Care Med. 2005;33(12):2778–85.
20. Lena D, et al. Glycemic control in the intensive care unit and during the postoperative period. Anesthesiology. 2011;114(2):438–44.
21. Kitabchi AE, et al. Hyperglycemic crises in adult patients with diabetes. Diabetes Care. 2009;32(7):1335–43.
22. Alberti KG, Hockaday TD, Turner RC. Small doses of intramuscular insulin in the treatment of diabetic "coma". Lancet. 1973;2(7828):515–22.
23. Kitabchi AE, et al. Management of hyperglycemic crises in patients with diabetes. Diabetes Care. 2001;24(1):131–53.

24. Kitabchi AE, Ayyagari V, Guerra SM. The efficacy of low-dose versus conventional therapy of insulin for treatment of diabetic ketoacidosis. Ann Intern Med. 1976;84(6):633–8.
25. Barash PG, et al. Clinical anesthesia, 6th Edition, 2009, Lippincott Williams and Wilkins, a Wolters Kluwer Business, Philadelphia, PA;1300.
26. Hines RL, Marschall KE. Stoelting's anesthesia and co-existing disease, 5th Edition, 2008, Churchill Livingstone, Philadelphia, PA;377.
27. Jacober SJ, Sowers JR. An update on perioperative management of diabetes. Arch Intern Med. 1999;159(20):2405–11.
28. Vann MA. Perioperative management of ambulatory surgical patients with diabetes mellitus. Curr Opin Anaesthesiol. 2009;22(6):718–24.

Chapter 21
Antacids, Gastrointestinal Prokinetics, and Proton Pump Inhibitors

Sunitha Kanchi Kandadai and Mark V. Boswell

Contents

S.K. Kandadai, MD (✉) • M.V. Boswell, MD, PhD, MBA
Department of Anesthesiology and Perioperative Medicine,
University of Louisville School of Medicine,
530 S Jackson Street RM C2A01, Louisville, KY 40202, USA
e-mail: s0kanc03@louisville.edu, skanc03@exchange.louisville.edu;
mark.boswell@louisville.edu

A.D. Kaye et al. (eds.), *Essentials of Pharmacology for Anesthesia,*
Pain Medicine, and Critical Care, DOI 10.1007/978-1-4614-8948-1_21,
© Springer Science+Business Media New York 2015

Antacids

Physiology of Acid Secretion

Gastric acid is secreted by the proton pump (H+, K +-ATPase) located in the luminal membrane of parietal cells (also called oxyntic cells) in the stomach. H+, K +-ATPase stimulation is controlled by three regulatory mechanisms: neurocrine, paracrine, and endocrine. There are three phases of gastric secretion: cephalic, gastric, and intestinal phases [1]. In addition, there is a basal or interdigestive phase where there is constant basal acid secretion in the absence of food and other stimuli [2].

The cephalic phase accounts for 20–30 % of total acid secretion in the stomach, in response to signals arising from sight, smell, and/or thoughts of food that activate the vagal pathway via the cerebral cortex and hypothalamus. In turn, vagal nerves stimulate the enteric nervous system, inducing parietal cells to secrete gastric acid, through release of pituitary adenylate cyclase-activating polypeptide (PACAP) at gastric enteric neurons and consequent stimulation of the PACAP receptor (PAC1) on the surface of gastric ECL (enterochromaffin-like) cells [3].

The gastric phase is activated by antral distension, protein content of food, and pH >4 and accounts for most of the gastric acid secretion (50 %). The intestinal phase is responsible for about 5 % of total gastric acid secretion, activated by intestinal gastrin and absorbed amino acids. All phases lead to increased circulating gastrin.

Gastrin is released by antral G cells, endocrine cells located in the gastric epithelium, pancreas, and duodenum. Although gastrin directly stimulates gastrin receptors in the basal membrane of parietal cells, its major role is indirect gastric acid secretion via gastrin-induced ECL cell histamine release; histamine stimulates parietal cell H2 receptors (see Figs. 21.1 and 21.2) [4].

Drug Class and Mechanism of Action: Antacids

Antacids are inorganic, relatively insoluble weak bases that partially neutralize gastric hydrochloric acid, raising gastric pH [5]. Generally, large doses of antacids are needed to raise gastric pH significantly [6, 7]. Antacid potency is based on molar equivalency required to neutralize a known amount of acid. The acid neutralization capacity among different proprietary formulations of antacids varies with rate of dissolution, water solubility, and rate of gastric emptying [8, 9].

Indications for Antacids/Clinical Pearls

1. Only nonparticulate antacids (e.g., sodium citrate, magnesium trisilicate) should be used when antacids are indicated for selected patients for reducing the risk of pulmonary aspiration [10]. Bicitra® contains 100 g of sodium citrate/1,000 ml, i.e., 0.34 M [11]. Because antacids have a short duration of action, they must be administered every 1–2 h to achieve and maintain pH >3.5–4.0 [12, 13].

2. Antacids bind bile acids, stimulate epithelial regeneration, and increase the production of prostaglandins, which in turn have a protective effect on gastric

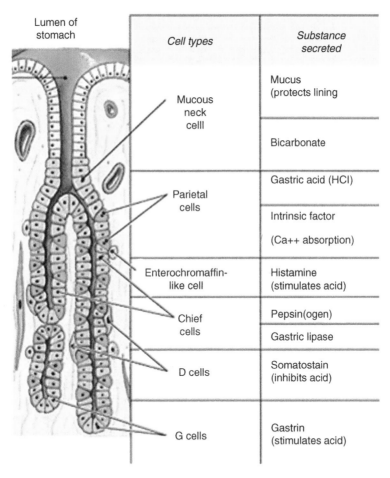

Fig. 21.1 Normally, acid secretion is mediated by a negative-feedback mechanism that is activated by lowered gastric pH; this negative-feedback system is mediated by somatostatin, secretin, prostaglandins, and a variety of other hormones. Somatostatin is secreted by the D cells which are also endocrine cells of the gastric epithelium. (**a**) Stomach cell types and substance secreted. (**b**) (From Yeo [103], Townsend [104], Copyright © 2012 Saunders, An Imprint of Elsevier)

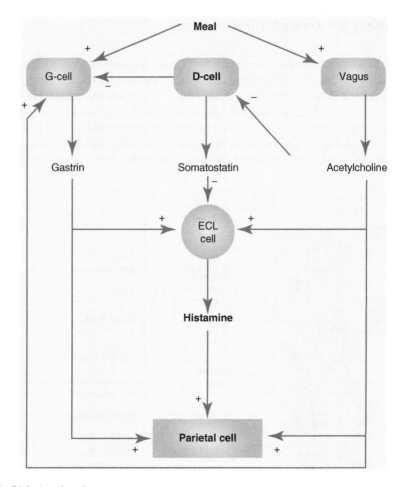

Fig. 21.1 (continued)

mucosa [12]. Antacids can be used for temporary relief of symptoms of duodenal ulcers, gastric ulcers, stress gastritis, and GERD.
3. Sodium hydroxide and aluminum hydroxide have been used to decrease steatorrhea in patients with pancreatic insufficiency [14]. Calcium and magnesium salts
   worsen steatorrhea [14, 15].
4. Aluminum (which binds bile acids more tightly than magnesium) and magnesium
   salts bind to bile acids and are effective in reducing cholerrheic diarrhea [16].
5. Among the antacids, calcium and aluminum salts are thought to cause constipation. However, studies have shown no evidence for this [17, 18]. Magnesium
   salts tend to cause diarrhea [19]. The absorbable antacid sodium bicarbonate
   does not affect stool frequency. The side effects of antacids may be used to
   advantage in particular patients. If the patient has a tendency to constipate, then

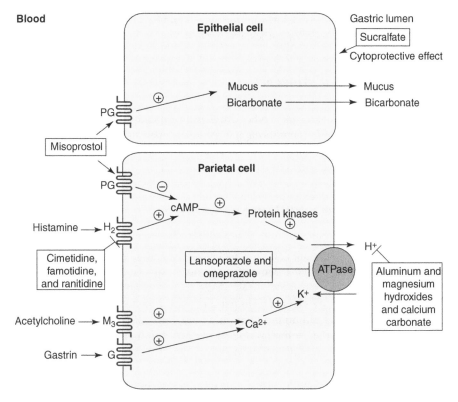

Fig. 21.2 H+, K+-ATPase is irreversibly blocked by the proton pump inhibitors (PPIs). The effect of histamine is blocked by H2 receptor antagonists (cimetidine, famotidine, and ranitidine). Prostaglandins (e.g., misoprostol) inhibit gastric acid secretion and stimulate secretion of mucus and bicarbonate by epithelial cells. Sucralfate binds to proteins of the ulcer crater and exerts a cytoprotective effect, whereas antacids (salts of aluminum, calcium, or magnesium) neutralize acid in the gastric lumen (From Brenner [105], Copyright © 2012 Saunders, An Imprint of Elsevier)

a magnesium antacid may be the best choice. In a patient with a tendency to loose stools, calcium or aluminum antacids may be preferable [20].

Dosing Options for Antacids

The dose for magnesium hydroxide and aluminum hydroxide is 600–1,200 mg three to four times daily. The dosage for calcium carbonate is 1–2 g daily, administered in 3–4 divided doses; the duration of action of antacids is very short and requires redosing. Sodium citrate 0.3 M has a pH of 8.4 and has a very unpleasant metallic taste. The nonparticulate antacid Bicitra® contains citric acid and sodium citrate with a pH of 5.2, lower than sodium citrate and so more palatable.

It is available in a 30 ml [3], 0.3 M solution and should be administered 15–30 min prior to induction of general anesthesia to prevent aspiration of gastric contents.

Drug Interactions of Antacids

Generally, it is advisable to space other drugs from antacids by 1–2 h. Drug interactions involving antacids occur through three mechanisms: (1) antacid binding of another drug in the gastrointestinal tract, (2) antacid-induced changes in gastrointestinal pH, and (3) changes in the urinary pH [21–27].

Side Effects of Antacids/Black Box Warnings

1. Side effects of aluminum antacids include constipation, belching, and flatulence; diarrhea is most common with magnesium-containing antacids [17–19].
2. Aluminum toxicity can occur in patients with impaired renal function with ingestion of aluminum-containing antacids [28]. Aluminum may accumulate in the brain producing acute aluminum neurotoxicity, manifested as rapidly progressive encephalopathy with confusion, seizures, myoclonus, and coma.

   Hypercalcemia can occur with prolonged ingestion of antacids, especially in patients with impaired renal function. Sodium-containing antacids used in excess may cause sodium overload in susceptible patients with congestive heart failure, ascites, and renal impairment. The milk–alkali syndrome, rarely observed currently, was originally reported as the triad of metabolic alkalosis, hypercalcemia, and renal insufficiency in patients with peptic ulcer disease who ingested large amounts of calcium and absorbable alkali [29].
3. Allergic reactions, including asthma and eosinophilic esophagitis, have been reported with the use of antacids [30].
4. Excessive use of gastric acid inhibitors including antacids increases the risk of intestinal infections [31].

Summary of Antacids

Antacids are inorganic salts available over the counter, which increase gastric pH and help improve some gastrointestinal disorders over the short term, but should not be used on a long-term basis as they are not completely benign medications. Their use or misuse is associated with serious side effects relating to mineral metabolism and allergic reactions, and patients and clinicians should use them judiciously.

Table 21.1 Prokinetic agents

Cholinergic agonists	Bethanechol, neostigmine, acotiamide
Dopamine antagonists	Metoclopramide, domperidone, itopride
Macrolides, motilin receptor agonists/motilides, ghrelin receptor agonists	Erythromycin, mitemcinal
Substituted benzamides	Cisapride, mosapride, renzapride, prucalopride
5-Hydroxytryptamine agonists/antagonists	Ondansetron, granisetron, tegaserod
Cholecystokinin receptor antagonists	Loxiglumide, dexloxiglumide
Gonadotropin-releasing hormone analogs	Leuprolide
Somatostatin analogs	Octreotide
Prostaglandins	Misoprostol, lubiprostone
Opioid receptor antagonists	Alvimopan, methylnaltrexone

Not all drugs in this table are currently available clinically

GI Prokinetics

Introduction

Gastrointestinal prokinetic drugs augment gastrointestinal motility by increasing peristaltic contractile force and frequency in the small bowel, thus accelerating transit in the gastrointestinal tract. Prokinetic drugs provide symptomatic relief of abdominal bloating due to delayed gastric emptying, as seen with gastroparesis. These agents are also of value in promoting gastric emptying in patients undergoing anesthesia and surgery.

Drug Class and Mechanism of Action

Gastrointestinal prokinetic drugs act on diverse receptors to stimulate motility in the gastrointestinal tract (Table 21.1).

Cholinergic Agonists: Bethanechol, Neostigmine, and Acotiamide

Bethanechol, an ester derivative of choline, stimulates muscarinic M2-type receptors on the gastrointestinal smooth muscle cell. Owing to their nonspecific action and inconsistent evidence for effectiveness in motility disorders, their use has nearly disappeared with the availability of newer agents.

Neostigmine, a reversible acetylcholine esterase inhibitor, facilitates parasympathetic and enteric stimulation of colonic motility. Neostigmine may be effective in producing rapid colonic decompression in those who failed conservative therapy in acute colonic pseudo-obstruction or Ogilvie's syndrome [32–34].

Evidence for improvement of postoperative ileus is less clear [35]. The dose of neostigmine in one randomized controlled trial was 0.5 mg administered subcutaneously twice daily [36]. Common adverse events include bradycardia, increased bronchotracheal secretions, and abdominal cramps; cardiac arrest has been reported [37]. Cardiovascular monitoring is indicated when using neostigmine, and atropine or glycopyrrolate must be available. Contraindications include recent myocardial infarction, acidosis, systolic blood pressure <90 mmHg, pulse <60 beats/min, bronchospasm requiring medical treatment, and creatinine >3 mg/dL.

Dopamine Antagonists: Metoclopramide, Domperidone, and Itopride

Metoclopramide

Metoclopramide, a para-aminobenzoic acid derivative, is an antiemetic and a gastrointestinal prokinetic agent that stimulates gastrointestinal smooth muscle by multiple mechanisms. It is an antagonist at central and peripheral dopamine DA2 receptors, has direct and indirect effects on cholinergic receptors, and is a mixed 5-HT3 antagonist and 5-HT4 agonist [38–40]. Indications for metoclopramide include gastroesophageal reflux, although the drug does not promote endoscopic healing of esophagitis [38]. Metoclopramide accelerates gastric emptying and is approved for short-term treatment (≤12 weeks) of gastroesophageal reflux and diabetic gastroparesis (≤8 weeks) [38, 40–42]. Metoclopramide may shorten the duration of ileus, but there is little evidence of its efficacy in pseudoobstruction [35].

Metoclopramide with or without H2 receptor blockers and antacids has been used to decrease the risk of pulmonary aspiration in patients with a full stomach, prior to the induction of general anesthesia. It has also shown to be useful as a prophylactic and a therapeutic antiemetic drug. The recommended dose of metoclopramide for most conditions is 10–15 mg orally before meals and at bedtime; the parenteral dose is 10 mg. Drug clearance is impaired in patients with cirrhosis and renal failure [43].

Metoclopramide may decrease the therapeutic effects of dopaminergic antiparkinsonian agents and increase the toxicity of antipsychotics, serotonergic agents, and tricyclic agents. Metoclopramide causes side effects in 10–20 % of patients, especially at higher doses and at the extremes of age. Mild side effects include mild anxiety, nervousness, and insomnia. More severe reactions include confusion, hallucinations, extrapyramidal symptoms and acute dystonic reactions [44], gynecomastia secondary to enhanced release of prolactin in adults [45], oculogyric crisis in children [46], neuroleptic malignant syndrome [47], and tardive dyskinesia [48]. Tardive dyskinesia (TD) is rarely reversible, and the FDA has required a black box warning associated with chronic use (>3 months) of metoclopramide. Advanced age, female gender, diabetes, renal failure, chronic alcohol intake, cirrhosis, tobacco use, schizophrenia, known organic CNS pathology, and concomitant use of dopaminergic neuroleptics are risk factors [48]. The annual incidence of metoclopramide-induced TD dramatically increased after the withdrawal of cisapride from the US market in 2000 [49]. Metoclopramide should be stopped immediately if TD is suspected, and alternative treatments of the gastrointestinal symptoms should be used. As a preventive measure, it is better to avoid continuous metoclopramide use for longer than 12 weeks. Dopamine antagonists may facilitate release of norepinephrine. Because monoamine oxidase (MAO) inhibitors impair metabolism of endogenous norepinephrine, dopamine antagonists should not be given in conjunction with MAOs [50].

Domperidone

Domperidone is an antiemetic and prokinetic agent that has peripheral dopamine DA2 receptor antagonist properties and unlike metoclopramide does not readily cross the blood–brain barrier. Thus, it is free from the troublesome central nervous system side effects associated with metoclopramide. Domperidone increases esophageal peristalsis and lower esophageal sphincter tone, increases gastric motility and peristalsis, facilitates gastric emptying, and decreases small bowel transit time. Domperidone is different from other prokinetic agents in that it has no cholinergic activity and its action is not inhibited by atropine [50, 51]. Currently, in the USA, domperidone requires an investigational new drug program request through the FDA.

Erythromycin

Erythromycin, a macrolide antibiotic, was the first nonpeptide compound for which agonism at the motilin receptors and gastroprokinetic properties were demonstrated [52–54]. Motilin, a hormone released from endocrine cells in the duodenal mucosal layer, stimulates gastric and duodenal motility via action on G-protein-coupled receptors called motilin receptors, which are localized in smooth muscle cells and nerve endings [55, 56].

Erythromycin is available in oral and intravenous forms. Oral erythromycin may improve gastric emptying and symptoms for several weeks, but its chronic use has been associated with tachyphylaxis due to downregulation of the motilin receptors [57]. The current off-label prokinetic indications for intravenous erythromycin are acute exacerbation of diabetic gastroparesis, optimizing small bowel feeding tube placement and optimizing endoscopy visualization for acute UGI bleeding [56]. It is recommended that the prescribed intravenous infusion be slow, over at least 60 min per dose. Erythromycin must be prescribed with caution in patients with renal and/ or hepatic impairment. Side effects/warnings for erythromycin include abdominal pain, nausea, vomiting at high doses by inducing spastic gut contractions, and the risk of sudden cardiac death by prolongation of the QT interval and torsade de pointes [58–61].

Substituted Benzamides

Cisapride is a serotonin 5-HT4 agonist and 5-HT3 antagonist that stimulates the release of acetylcholine from postsynaptic neurons in the enteric nervous system. It was initially introduced as a prokinetic in the 1990s and later withdrawn from the market in 2000 following reports of serious cardiac events (QTc prolongation, torsade de pointes, and cardiac arrest). Its current use is through a limited access protocol requiring special authorization from the FDA.

5-HT Agonists/Antagonists

Ondansetron, granisetron, and other similar 5-HT agonists/antagonists have both prokinetic and antiemetic effects; their primary use is as an antiemetic and is discussed in detail in the antiemetic section of this book. Prokinetic effects of these agents are moderate.

Somatostatin Analog: Octreotide

Octreotide is a synthetic analog of somatostatin with a longer duration of action. In low doses, it stimulates motility, primarily through the induction of migrating motor complexes (MMC) [62–64]. However, higher doses often are employed for its antisecretory effects, which may inhibit motility. Octreotide infusion increases LES pressure and esophageal body contraction [65, 66]. However, the net effect of octreotide on gastric emptying and intestinal transit remains controversial and may be dose related. Several studies have indicated that despite its MMC-stimulating effect, octreotide delays gastric emptying and intestinal transit. Octreotide has been shown to reduce the sensation of rectal distention through inhibition of visceral afferent pathways.

Indications for octreotide include severe dysmotility syndromes such as malignant intestinal pseudo-obstruction [63], bacterial overgrowth in scleroderma [65], and postoperative ileus [67].

The most common side effects include abdominal discomfort, diarrhea, biliary tract symptoms, impaired glucose tolerance, hypoglycemia (shortly after starting treatment), persistent hyperglycemia (during long-term treatment), gallstones (10–20 % of patients on long-term treatment), and pancreatitis (associated with gallstones).

Prostaglandins

The role of prostaglandins in gastrointestinal motility is complex and difficult to interpret, and the effect depends on the type of prostaglandin, dose, and the muscle layer studied [68]. Misoprostol, a PGE1 analog, hastens postprandial intestinal motility and accelerates orocecal transit time [69]. The NSAIDs diclofenac sodium and indomethacin do not appear to stimulate gastric motility in humans [70]. Lubiprostone, a bicyclic fatty acid derived from prostaglandin E1, activates the apical membrane of the chloride channel in the intestinal epithelium that stimulates intestinal fluid secretion, enhances and stimulates contraction in colonic as well as gastric muscles, and may act as a prokinetic agent [71, 72].

Lubiprostone is approved for the treatment of chronic idiopathic constipation and constipation predominant irritable bowel syndrome (IBS-C). Common side effects of lubiprostone include abdominal pain, nausea, vomiting, diarrhea, bloating, and, rarely, dyspnea [73].

Opioid Antagonists Used as Prokinetic Agents

Opiates regulate gastrointestinal motility through effects on the enteric nervous system by promoting an inhibitory effect on gastrointestinal motility [74]. Methylnaltrexone and alvimopan are two recently marketed peripherally acting mu-opioid receptor antagonists that do not readily cross the blood–brain barrier and used to treat opioid-induced bowel dysfunction and functional constipation [75]. Alvimopan is approved for short-term in-hospital treatment of postoperative ileus. The dose is 12 mg orally, taken up to 5 h preoperatively and twice daily postoperatively for up to 7 days (15 doses total). The efficacy and safety of these drugs for long-term use are not well understood [76]. These agents are contraindicated in patients with mechanical bowel obstruction. Methylnaltrexone is available as a subcutaneous formulation. The dose for an average adult patient is 12 mg (0.6 ml; 0.15 mg/kg) every other day. Side effects are similar to alvimopan.

Proton Pump Inhibitors: PPIs

Introduction of PPIs

Proton pump inhibitors (PPIs) are commonly prescribed medications for the treatment of several acid-related gastrointestinal disorders. As a class, PPIs are generally considered remarkably safe; however, there are increasing concerns about the consequences of long-term use, since numerous adverse effects have been associated with chronic therapy.

Drug Class and Mechanism of Action of PPIs

PPIs cause pronounced and long-lasting gastric acid suppression by irreversible inhibition of the proton pump (gastric H+/K + adenosine triphosphatase) via covalent binding to cysteine residues. The amount of H+/K + adenosine triphosphatase present in the parietal cell is maximum after a prolonged fast, and so PPIs are most effective when administered before the first meal of the day.

Indications of PPIs/Clinical Pearls

Indications for the use of PPIs are peptic ulcer disease (PUD), *Helicobacter pylori*, chronic nonsteroidal anti-inflammatory drug (NSAID) use, Barrett esophagitis, erosive esophagitis, and Zollinger–Ellison syndrome.

1. *Peptic ulcer disease (PUD)*: Clinical trials have consistently demonstrated that proton pump inhibitors are superior to standard doses of histamine2 receptor antagonists for GERD and PUD management [76]. Patients with bleeding peptic ulcers treated with PPIs have demonstrated decreases in the risk of rebleeding, the need for transfusions or surgery, and a reduction in length of hospital stay, although no evidence has been noted for an effect on mortality [77].
2. *H. pylori* is associated with gastric and duodenal ulcers. *H. pylori* must be eradicated to facilitate healing and to decrease the risk of ulcer recurrence; PPIs are used for this purpose as part of triple therapy (PPI + two antibiotics) or quadruple therapy (PPI + bismuth + two antibiotics).
3. *NSAID long-term use*: According to the American College of Gastroenterology 2009 guidelines, patients taking long-term daily NSAIDs should be considered for preventive therapy with daily PPIs [78].
4. *Barrett esophagitis*: PPIs are more effective than H2 antagonists in Barrett esophagitis in providing symptomatic relief, preventing stricture formation, and promoting effective and faster healing of esophagitis and esophageal ulcers. It is unknown whether high-dose PPI therapy helps reduce the risk of esophageal malignancy, and further studies are warranted to address this issue [79].
5. *Erosive esophagitis*: PPIs provide healing of erosive esophagitis and relief of symptoms in patients with GERD.
6. *Zollinger–Ellison syndrome*: PPI therapy is remarkably effective in controlling gastric acid hypersecretion, thereby reducing morbidity and potential mortality of this syndrome [80].

PPIs' Dosing Options, Pharmacodynamics, and Pharmacokinetics

PPIs differ in bioavailability, half-lives, metabolism, pKa, routes of excretion, peak plasma levels, and drug interactions (Table 21.2). Lansoprazole and pantoprazole have the greatest bioavailability and achieve the highest plasma levels. All PPIs have short half-lives, typically 1–2 h. All PPIs are metabolized via hepatic P450 enzymes, with CYP2C19 and CYP3A4 playing dominant and minor roles, respectively. Rabeprazole is the most potent PPI, metabolized mostly by CYP3A4,

Table 21.2 Comparison of proton pump inhibitors

Agent	Bioavailability %	T1/2; hours	Metabolism	pKa	Elimination	Dose; mg
Omeprazole	45	0.5–1	Hepatic	4	Renal	20–40
Lansoprazole	85	1.5	Hepatic	4	Renal/fecal	15–30
Rabeprazole	52	1–2	Hepatic	5	Renal	20
Pantoprazole	77	1	Hepatic	3.9	Renal	20–40
Esomeprazole	89	1–1.4	Hepatic	4.0	Renal	20–40

and has less drug interactions, whereas omeprazole is less potent, preferentially metabolized by CYP2C19, and has more drug interactions. Pantoprazole and esomeprazole are available as intravenous formulation in the USA. None of the PPIs require dose adjustment for hepatic or renal insufficiency. Several studies have shown that no PPI is superior to another. All patients should be maintained on the lowest possible dose that provides symptomatic relief.

Side Effects of PPIs/Black Box Warnings

PPIs are associated with primary adverse events, typically in the order of 1–5 %, and include nausea, diarrhea, headache, constipation, and rash. Secondary adverse effects associated with long-term use of PPIs include osteoporosis, increased risk of infections, formation of gastric polyps or carcinoid, interstitial nephritis, and altered metabolism of other medications. Other concerns associated with long-term PPI use are hypomagnesemia and reduced vitamin B12 and iron absorption.

1. *Osteoporosis*: Long-term PPI use causing profound acid suppression impairs calcium, folate, riboflavin, and vitamin B12 absorption, which in turn influences homocysteine levels, collagen cross-linking, with decreased bone mineral density and bone strength. Hypergastrinemia resulting from profound acid suppression also causes release of parathyroid hormone from hyperplastic parathyroid glands and contributes to increased bone resorption and decreased metabolic bone density [81]. PPIs may also act on the vacuolar proton pump located on osteoclasts [82], causing an acidic environment, protease activation, dissolution of bone matrix, decreased bone mineral density, osteoporosis, and increased risk of fractures. According to a recent review, the levels of risk reported have generally been low [83].
2. *Increased risk of infections*: Gastric acidity acts as a major defense mechanism of the body by sterilizing the contents entering the digestive tract, preventing bacterial colonization of the upper gastrointestinal tract, and influencing the normal intestinal flora composition. PPIs increase gastric pH, resulting in more bacterial overgrowth in the stomach and deconjugation of bile acids [84]. Chronic PPI use may also impair leukocyte function by increasing basal cytosolic calcium

concentrations in neutrophils and decreasing intracellular and extracellular reactive oxygen species impairing bactericidal activity [85]. PPIs may be associated with an increased risk of community-acquired pneumonia, an effect not demonstrated with long-term therapy [86, 87]. There is evidence that PPI therapy may increase the risk of enteric infection, especially with *Clostridium difficile*, *Salmonella*, and *Campylobacter* species [88].

3. *Formation of gastric polyps or carcinoid*: PPI use leads to diminished acid secretion, diminished somatostatin release, enterochromaffin-like cell hyperplasia, and increased G-cell release of gastrin. Gastric cells may become hyperplastic and form fundic gland polyps in 7–10 % of patients taking PPIs for more than 12 months. Such polyps are benign and typically regress with the discontinuation of PPI. Hypergastrinemia has raised the concern of long-term PPI use possibly predisposing some patients to the development of neuroendocrine tumors. Gastric carcinoids have been observed in rodents given PPIs, but the relationship of PPIs to carcinoid in humans is unclear.

4. *Intersitial nephritis*: PPI-related acute interstitial nephritis is a rare, idiosyncratic inflammatory reaction of the renal interstitium and tubules that may lead to renal failure. There is insufficient evidence to establish a causal relationship between the two, but there may be an association [89].

5. *Hypomagnesemia*: Several case series report severe hypomagnesemia, refractory to supplementation associated with long-term PPI use [90–96]. The cause of hypomagnesemia remains poorly understood but does not involve increased urinary excretion of magnesium [95, 97]. PPI use can inhibit active magnesium transport in the intestine. The FDA issued a warning in March 2011 that prescription PPIs may cause low serum magnesium levels if taken for prolonged periods of time and suggested that prescribers consider checking a baseline serum magnesium level in patients about to start PPI therapy, as well as periodic monitoring during therapy [100].

PPI Drug Interactions

PPIs and Clopidogrel

Concerns have been raised about a possible interaction between PPIs, especially omeprazole and clopidogrel that could decrease the antiplatelet efficacy of clopidogrel and increase the risk of cardiovascular (CV) events [99–101]. The FDA and the European Medicines Agency (EMA) have issued warnings regarding the concomitant use of these medications. PPIs can attenuate metabolism of clopidogrel to its active metabolite by inhibiting various hepatic CYP450 enzymes, especially CYP2C19. Concomitant use of a PPI with clopidogrel reduces clopidogrel active metabolite generation and subsequent platelet inhibition. Observational studies provide a mixed clinical picture of this drug interaction. The only randomized trial [102] studying the PPI–clopidogrel interaction did not demonstrate any difference in cardiovascular outcomes, but did show a reduction in gastrointestinal bleeding with the use of PPIs.

Several other drugs interact with PPIs and may increase or decrease the therapeutic effects of each other, and so the product information should be thoroughly read before PPI administration.

Summary of PPIs

The indications for PPI use include peptic ulcer disease, erosive and Barrett esophagitis, gastritis, and chronic NSAID use. Risks associated with PPI use include increased risk of fractures, infections, drug interactions, and low magnesium. PPIs should be used judiciously, and their long-term use reevaluated periodically.

Chemical Structures

**Chemical Structure
21.1** Omeprazole

Chemical Structure 21.2
Ondansetron

References

1. Wolfe MM, Soll AH. The physiology of gastric acid secretion. N Engl J Med. 1988;319:1707–15.
2. Feldman M. Gastric secretion: normal and abnormal. In: Feldman M, Scharschmidt BF, Sleisenger MH, editors. Gastrointestinal and liver disease. Philadelphia: Saunders; 1998. p. 587–603.
3. Zeng N, Athmann C, Kang T, et al. PACAP type I receptor activation regulates ECL cells and gastric acid secretion. J Clin Invest. 1999;104:1383–91.
4. Dubois A. Control of gastric acid secretion. In: Brandt LJ, editor. Clinical practice of gastroenterology. Philadelphia: Current Medicine; 1999. p. 180–8.

5. Fordtran JS, Collyns JAH. Antacid pharmacology in duodenal ulcer. Effect of antacids on postcibal gastric acidity and peptic activity. N Engl J Med. 1966;274:92–7.

6. AHFS drug information. In: Mc Evoy GK, editor. Bethesda: American Society of Health-System Pharmacists; 1998. p. 2374–9.

7. Littman A, Pine BH. Antacid and anticholinergic drugs. Ann Intern Med. 1975;82:544–15.

8. Mirrissey JF, Barreras RF. Antacid therapy. N Engl J Med. 1974;290:550–4.

9. Harvey SC. Gastric antacids and digestants. In: Goodman LS, Gillian A, Gillian AG, editors. The pharmacological basis of therapeutics. 6th ed. New York: Macmillan; 1980. p. 988–1001.

10. American Society of Anesthesiologists Committee. Practice guidelines for preoperative fasting and the use of pharmacologic agents to reduce the risk of pulmonary aspiration: application to healthy patients undergoing elective procedures: an updated report by the American Society of Anesthesiologists Committee on Standards and Practice Parameters. Anesthesiology. 2011;114(3):495–511.

11. James CF, Gibbs CP. Nonparticulate antacids. Anesth Analg. 1982;61(9):801.

12. Mutlu GM, Mutlu EA, Factor P. GI complications in patients receiving mechanical ventilation. Chest. 2001;119:1222–41.

13. Tryba M, Cook D. Current guidelines on stress ulcer prophylaxis. Drugs. 1997;54:581–96.

14. Graham DY, Patterson DJ. Double-blind comparison of liquid antacid and placebo in the treatment of symptomatic reflux esophagitic. Dig Dis Sci. 1983;28:559–63.

15. Regan PT, Malagelada JR, DiMagno EP, et al. Comparative effects of antacids, cimetidine and enteric coating on the therapeutic response to oral enzymes in severe pancreatic insufficiency. N Engl J Med. 1977;297:854–8.

16. Cousar GD, Gadacz TR. Comparison of antacids on the binding of bile salts. Arch Surg. 1984;119:1018–20.

17. Clemens JD, Feinstein AR. Calcium carbonate and constipation: a historical review of medical mythopoeia. Gastroenterology. 1977;72:957–61.

18. Saunders D, Sillery J, Chapman R. Effect of calcium carbonate and aluminum hydroxide on human intestinal function. Dig Dis Sci. 1988;33:409–13.

19. Strom M. Antacid side-effects on bowel habits. Scand J Gastroenterol. 1982;75(Suppl):54–5.

20. Maton PN, Burton ME. Antacids revisited, a review of their clinical pharmacology and recommended therapeutic use. Drugs. 1999;57(6):855–70.

21. Tatro DS. Drug interaction facts. Facts and comparisons. 3rd ed. St Louis; 1992.

22. Welling PG. Interactions affecting drug absorption. Clin Pharmacokinet. 1984;9:404–34.

23. Hurwitz A. Antacid therapy and drug kinetics. Clin Pharmacokinet. 1977;2:269–80.

24. Hansten PD, Horn JR, Koda-Kimble MA, et al., editors. Principles of antacid interaction. In: Drug interaction & updates quarterly. Vancouver: Applied Therapeutics, Inc.; 1993. p 69–72.

25. Hansten PD, Horn JR, Koda-Kimble MA, et al., editors. Antacid drug interactions. In: Drug interaction & updates quarterly. Vancouver: Applied Therapeutics, Inc.; 1993. p 137–51.

26. Gugler AH. Effects of antacids on the clinical pharmacokinetics of drugs: an update. Clin Pharmacokinet. 1990;18:210–9.

27. Lomaestro BM, Bailie GR. Absorption interactions with fluoroquinolones. Drug Saf. 1995;12:314–33.

28. Herzog P, Holtermüller KH. Antacid therapy—changes in mineral metabolism. Scand J Gastroenterol Suppl. 1982;75:56–62. [0085-5928] Herzog.

29. McMillan DE, Freeman RB. The milk alkali syndrome: a study of the acute disorder with comments on the development of the chronic condition. Medicine. 1965;44:485–501.

30. Merwat SN, Spechler SJ. Might the use of acid-suppressive medications predispose to the development of eosinophilic esophagitis? Am J Gastroenterol. 2009;104:1897–902.

31. Canani RB, Terrin G. Gastric acidity inhibitors and the risk of intestinal infections. Curr Opin Gastroenterol. 2010;26:31–5.

32. Ponec RJ, Saunders MD, Kimmey MB. Neostigmine for the treatment of acute colonic pseudo-obstruction. N Engl J Med. 1999;341:137.

33. Trevisani GT, Hyman NH, Church JM. Neostigmine: safe and effective treatment for acute colonic pseudo-obstruction. Dis Colon Rectum. 2000;43:599.

34. Loftus CG, Harewood GC, Baron TH. Assessment of predictors of response to neostigmine for acute colonic pseudo-obstruction. Am J Gastroenterol. 2002;97:3118–22.
35. Holte K, Kehlet H. Postoperative ileus: progress towards effective management. Drugs. 2002;62(18):2603–15.
36. Hallerbäck B, Ander S, Glise H. Effect of combined blockade of beta-adrenoceptors and acetylcholinesterase in the treatment of postoperative ileus after cholecystectomy. Scand J Gastroenterol. 1987;22(4):420–4.
37. Maher L, Young PJ. Cardiac arrest complicating neostigmine use for bowel opening in a critically ill patient. Crit Care Resusc. 2011;13(3):192–3.
38. Ramirez B, Richter JE. Review article: promotility drugs in the treatment of gastroesophageal reflux disease. Aliment Pharmacol Ther. 1993;7:5–20.
39. Albibi R, McCallum RW. Metoclopramide: pharmacology and clinical application. Ann Intern Med. 1983;98:86–95.
40. McCallum RW. Clinical pharmacology forum: motility agents and the gastrointestinal tract. Am J Med Sci. 1996;312:19–26.
41. Shaffer D, Butterfield M, Pamer C, Mackey AC. Tardive dyskinesia risks and metoclopramide use before and after U.S. market withdrawal of cisapride. J Am Pharm Assoc. 2004;44:661–5.
42. McCallum RW, Ricci DA, Rakatansky H, et al. A multicenter placebo-controlled clinical trial of oral metoclopramide in diabetic gastroparesis. Diabetes Care. 1983;6:463–7.
43. Bateman DN. Clinical pharmacokinetics of metoclopramide. Clin Pharmacokinet. 1983;8(6):523–9.
44. Walker M, Samii A. Chronic severe dystonia after single exposure to antiemetics. Am J Emerg Med. 2006;24:125–7.
45. McCallum RW, Sowers JR, Hershman JM, Sturdevant RAL. Metoclopramide stimulates prolactin secretion in man. J Clin Endocrinol Metab. 1976;42:1148–52.
46. Edwards M, Koo MW, Tse RK. Oculogyric crisis after metoclopramide therapy. Optom Vis Sci. 1989;66:179–80.
47. Nonino F, Campomori A. Neuroleptic malignant syndrome associated with metoclopramide. Ann Pharmacother. 1999;33(5):644–5.
48. Rao AS, Camilleri M. Review article: metoclopramide and tardive dyskinesia. Aliment Pharmacol Ther. 2010;31:11–9.
49. Kenney C, Hunter C, Davidson A, Jankovic J. Metoclopramide, an increasingly recognized cause of tardive dyskinesia. J Clin Pharmacol. 2008;48:379–84.
50. Reddymasu SC M.D., Soykan I M.D., McCallum RW M.D. Domperidone: review of pharmacology and clinical applications in gastroenterology. Am J Gastroenterol. 2007;102:2036–45.
51. Reynolds JC. Prokinetic agents: a key in the future of gastroenterology. Gastroenterol Clin N Am. 1989;18:437–57.
52. Weber Jr FH, Richards RD, McCallum RW. Erythromycin: a motilin agonist and gastro intestinal prokinetic agent. Am J Gastroenterol. 1993;88(4):485–90.
53. Moayyedi P, Soo S, Deeks J, Delaney B, Innes M, Forman D. Pharmacological interventions for non-ulcer dyspepsia. Cochrane Database Syst Rev. 2006;18:CD001960.
54. Karamanolis G, Tack J. Promotility medications—now and in the future. Dig Dis. 2006;24:297–307.
55. Itoh Z. Motilin and clinical application. Peptides. 1997;18:593–608.
56. Galligan JJ, Vanner S. Basic and clinical pharmacology of new motility promoting agents. Neurogastroenterol Motil. 2005;17:643–53.
57. Camilleri M, et al. Clinical guideline: management of gastroparesis. Am J Gastroenterol. 2013;108:18–37.
58. De Ponti F, Poluzzi E, Montanaro N. QT-interval prolongation by non-cardiac drugs: lessons to be learned from recent experience. Eur J Clin Pharmacol. 2000;56:1–18.
59. Drici MD, Knollmann BC, Wang WX, Woosley RL. Cardiac actions of erythromycin: influence of female sex. JAMA. 1998;280:1774–6.
60. Shaffer D, Singer S, Korvick J, Honig P. Concomitant risk factors in reports of torsades de pointes associated with macrolide use: review of the United States Food and Drug Administration Adverse Event Reporting System. Clin Infect Dis. 2002;35:197–200.

61. Berthet S, Charpiat B, Mabrut JY. Erythromycin as a prokinetic agent: risk factors. J Visceral Surg. 2010;147:e13–8.
62. Thompson JS M.D., Quigley EMM M.D. Prokinetic agents in the surgical patient. Am J Surg (Omaha, NE). 1999;177:508–14.
63. Mercadante S, Porzio G. Octreotide for malignant bowel obstruction: twenty years after. Crit Rev Oncol Hematol. 2012;83(3):388–92.
64. Owyang C. Octreotide in gastrointestinal motility disorders. Gut. 1994;35 Suppl 3:S11–4.
65. Soudah HC, Hasler WL, Owyang C. Effect of octreotide on intestinal motility and bacterial overgrowth in scleroderma. NEJM. 1991;325:1461–7.
66. Gunshefski LA, Rifley WJ, Slattery DW, et al. Somatostatin stimulation of the normal esophagus. Am J Surg. 1992;163:59–62.
67. Cullen JJ, Eagon C, Dozois EJ, Kelly KA. Treatment of acute postoperative ileus with octreotide. Am J Surg. 1993;165:113–20.
68. Waller SL. Prostaglandins and the gastrointestinal tract. Gut. 1973;14(5):402–17.
69. Soffer EE, Launspack J. Effect of misoprostol on postprandial intestinal motility and orocecal transit time in humans. Dig Dis Sci. 1993;18:851–5.
70. Bassotti G, Bucaneve G, Furno P, et al. Double blind, placebo controlled study on the effects of diclofenac sodium and indomethacin on postprandial gastric motility in man. Dig Dis Sci. 1998;42:1172–6.
71. Kapoor S. Lubiprostone: clinical applications beyond constipation. World J Gastroenterol. 2009;15(9):1147–7.
72. Bassil AK, Borman RA, Jarvie EM, McArthur-Wilson RJ, Thangiah R, Sung EZ, Lee K, Sanger GJ. Activation of prostaglandin EP receptors by lubiprostone in rat and human stomach and colon. Br J Pharmacol. 2008;154:126–35.
73. Chamberlain SM, Rao SS. Safety evaluation of lubiprostone in the treatment of constipation and irritable bowel syndrome. Expert Opin Drug Saf. 2012;11(5):841–50.
74. Wood JD, Galligan JJ. Function of opioids in the enteric nervous system. Neurogastroenterol Motil. 2004;16 Suppl 2:17–28.
75. Neyens R, Jackson KC. Novel opioid antagonists for opioid-induced bowel dysfunction and postoperative ileus. J Pain Palliat Care Pharmacother. 2007;21:27–33.
76. Lambert R. Review article: current practice and future perspectives in the management of gastro-oesophageal reflux disease. Aliment Pharmacol Ther. 1997;11:651–62.
77. Leontiadis GI, Sharma VK, Howden CW. Proton pump inhibitor therapy for peptic ulcer bleeding: cochrane collaboration meta-analysis of randomized controlled trials. Mayo Clin Proc. 2007;82:286–96.
78. Lanza FL, Chan FK, Quigley EM, Practice parameters committee of the American College of Gastroenterology. Guidelines for prevention of NSAID-related ulcer complications. Am J Gastroenterol. 2009;104:728–38.
79. Chubineh S M.D., Birk J M.D. Proton pump inhibitors: the good, the bad, and the unwanted. South Med J. 2012;105(11):613–8.
80. Wilcox CM, Hirschowitz BI. Treatment strategies for Zollinger–Ellison syndrome. Expert Opin Pharmacother. 2009;10(7):1145–57.
81. Neena S. Abraham, proton pump inhibitors: potential adverse effects. Curr Opin Gastroenterol. 2012;28:615–20.
82. Jefferies KC, Cipriano DJ, Forgac M. Function, structure and regulation of the vacuolar (H+)-ATPases. Arch Biochem Biophys. 2008;476:33–42.
83. Chen J, Yuan YC, Leontiadis GI, Howden CW. Recent safety concerns with proton pump inhibitors. J Clin Gastroenterol. 2012;46:93–114.
84. Theisen J, Nehra D, Citron D, et al. Suppression of gastric acid secretion in patients with gastro esophageal reflux disease results in gastric bacterial overgrowth and deconjugation of bile acids. J Gastrointest Surg. 2000;4:50–4.
85. Zedtwitz-Liebenstein K, Wenisch C, Patruta S, et al. Omeprazole treatment diminishes intra- and extracellular neutrophil reactive oxygen production and bactericidal activity. Crit Care Med. 2002;30:1118–22.

86. Sarkar M, Hennessy S, Yang YX. Proton-pump inhibitor use and the risk for community-acquired pneumonia. Ann Intern Med. 2008;149(6):391–8.
87. Giuliano C, Wilhelm SM, Kale-Pradhan PB. Are proton pump inhibitors associated with the development of community-acquired pneumonia? A meta-analysis. Expert Rev Clin Pharmacol. 2012;5(3):337–44.
88. Moayyedi P, Leontiadis GI. The risks of PPI therapy. Nat Rev Gastroenterol Hepatol. 2012;9:132–9.
89. Sierra F, Suarez M, Rey M, Vela MF. Systematic review: proton pump inhibitor associated acute interstitial nephritis. Aliment Pharmacol Ther. 2007;26:545–53.
90. Epstein M, McGrath S, Law F. Proton-pump inhibitors and hypomagnesemic hypoparathyroidism. N Eng J Med. 2006;355:1834–6.
91. Broeren MA, Geerdink EA, Vader HL, van den Wall Bake AW. Hypomagnesemia induced by several proton-pump inhibitors. Ann Intern Med. 2009;151:755–6.
92. Dornebal J, Bijlsma R, Brouer RML. An unrecognized potential side effect of proton pump inhibitors: hypomagnesaemia. Ned Tidjschr Geenesk. 2009;153:A711.
93. Kuipers MT, Thang HD, Arntzenius AB. Hypomagnesaemia due to use of proton pump inhibitors – a review. Neth J Med. 2009;67:169–72.
94. Hoorn EJ, van der Hoek J, de Man RA, et al. A case series of proton pump inhibitor-induced hypomagnesemia. Am J Kidney Dis. 2010;56:112–6.
95. Regolisti G, Cabassi A, Parenti E, et al. Severe hypomagnesemia during long-term treatment with a proton pump inhibitor. Am J Kidney Dis. 2010;56:168–74.
96. Mackay JD, Bladon PT. Hypomagnesaemia due to proton-pump inhibitor therapy: a clinical case series. QJM. 2010;103:387–95.
97. Shabajee N, Lamb EJ, Sturgess I, et al. Omeprazole and refractory hypomagnesaemia. BMJ. 2008;337:a42.
98. Administration US FDA. FDA Drug Safety Communication: low magnesium levels can be associated with long-term use of Proton Pump Inhibitor drugs (PPIs). 2011. http://www.fda.gov/Drugs/DrugSafety/ucm245011.htm.
99. Gilard M, Arnaud B, Cornily JC, et al. Influence of omeprazole on the antiplatelet action of clopidogrel associated with aspirin: the randomized, double-blind OCLA (Omeprazole CLopidogrel Aspirin) study. J Am Coll Cardiol. 2008;51:256–60.
100. Pezalla E, Day D, Pulliadath I. Initial assessment of clinical impact of a drug interaction between clopidogrel and proton pump inhibitors. J Am Coll Cardiol. 2008;52:1038–9.
101. Juurlink DN, Gomes T, Ko DT, et al. A population-based study of the drug interaction between proton pump inhibitors and clopidogrel. CMAJ. 2009;180:713–8.
102. Bhatt DL, Cryer BL, Contant CF, Cohen M, Lanas A, Schnitzer TJ, Shook TL, Lapuerta P, Goldsmith MA, Laine L, Scirica BM, Murphy SA, Cannon CP, COGENT Investigators. Clopidogrel with or without omeprazole in coronary artery disease. N Engl J Med. 2010;363(20):1909–17.
103. Yeo C. Shackelford's surgery of the alimentary tract. 6th ed. Philadelphia: WB Saunders; 2007.
104. Townsend CM. Sabiston textbook of surgery. 19th ed. Philadelphia: Saunders Elsevier; 2012.
105. Brenner GM. Pharmacology. 4th ed. Philadelphia: Saunders Elsevier; 2012.

Chapter 22
Histamine Modulators

Michael Yarborough and Judy G. Johnson

Contents

Introduction

Discovery of certain chemicals to counteract the effects of histamine occurred in the early twentieth century. The development of a drug that would alleviate allergic reactions such as itchy, watery eyes, and a runny nose from a cold or hay fever had an astronomical effect on the medical community. By the 1950s, antihistamines were being mass-produced in the USA and prescribed extensively as the drug of choice for those suffering from allergies. The public perceived antihistamines as the "wonder drug" and with the misconception that it was a "cure all" to the common cold. Eventually, scientist began to discover additional indications for the use of antihistamines. These compounds continue to be one of the most universal drugs lining the shelves of local pharmacies. However, the plethora of roles that antihistamines play in the treatment of the human condition is much more extensive, including suppression of allergy symptoms, sedative agents, and antiemetic actions to name a few.

M. Yarborough, MD
Department of Anesthesiology, Tulane Medical Center, New Orleans, LA, USA
e-mail: myarboro@tulane.edu

J.G. Johnson, MD (✉)
Department of Anesthesiology, Louisiana State University, New Orleans, LA, USA

A.D. Kaye et al. (eds.), *Essentials of Pharmacology for Anesthesia,*
Pain Medicine, and Critical Care, DOI 10.1007/978-1-4614-8948-1_22,
© Springer Science+Business Media New York 2015

Drug Class and Mechanism of Action

Histamine is involved in local immune responses as well as regulation of physiologic functions in the gut. It can also act as a neurotransmitter. Histamine is made and released by different cells, i.e., basophils, mast cells, platelets, histaminergic neurons, lymphocytes, and enterochromaffin cells. It is stored in vesicles or granules awaiting release upon stimulation [1]. As part of an immune response to foreign pathogens, histamine increases the permeability of capillaries to white blood cells and other proteins in order to allow them to engage foreign invaders in the infected tissues. Clinical effects of histamine result in increased vascular permeability and leakage of plasma proteins, causing fluid to escape from capillaries into the tissues [2]. This leads to the classic symptoms of an allergic reaction such as a localized rash, itching, puffy and watery eyes, nasal congestion, and rhinorrhea.

There are four known human histamine receptors that have been identified (Table 22.1). These receptors belong to the G-protein-coupled receptors family. They are signified as H_1, H_2, H_3, and H_4. Stimulation of the H_1 receptor can activate intracellular signaling pathways leading to the development of classic allergic symptoms [1].

Historically, antihistamines were noted to cause a parallel displacement in the histamine concentration/response. This behavior was consistent with a competitive inhibition for histamine receptors, lending to the classification as the H_1 receptor antagonists. With further research, it was found that the antihistamines are in the class that are now called inverse agonists

Table 22.1 Histamine receptors classification

Receptor type	Tissue location	Intracellular function
H_1	Airway and vascular smooth muscles, endothelial, central nervous system (nerve cells), neutrophils, eosinophils, monocytes	Cause bronchial smooth muscle contraction, separation of endothelial cells causing hives, pain, and itching. Allergic reaction symptoms, motion sickness, and regulation of sleep
H_2	Nerve cells, vascular smooth muscles and parietal cells, hepatocytes, endothelial cells, epithelial cells, neutrophils, eosinophils, monocytes	Vasodilation and stimulation of gastric acid secretion
H_3	Histaminergic neurons, eosinophils. Found primarily in the central nervous system, low expression in peripheral tissues	Inhibits histamine release and synthesis. Decreases release of serotonin, acetylcholine, and norepinephrine
H_4	High expression in bone marrow and peripheral hematopoietic cells. Low expression in nerve cells, hepatocytes, spleen, thymus, small intestine, colon, heart	Stimulates chemotaxis of eosinophils and mast cells

Table 22.2 Chemical classifications of antihistamines

Alkylamines	Brompheniramine, chlorpheniramine, dexchlorpheniramine, pheniramine, triprolidine
Ethanolamines	Carbinoxamine, clemastine, dimenhydrinate, diphenhydramine, doxylamine, orphenadrine
Ethylenediamines	Pyrilamine, tripelennamine
Phenothiazines	Methdilazine, promethazine, trimeprazine
Piperidines	Cyproheptadine, fexofenadine, desloratadine, loratadine
	Terfenadine and astemizole recalled by FDA
Piperazines	Cetirizine, cyclizine, hydroxyzine, levocetirizine, meclizine

Modified from Nicolas [5]

As an inverse agonist, the compound preferably binds to the inactive state of the histamine receptor, stabilizing the receptor in the inactive conformation, and moves the equilibrium shift in the direction of the inactive state. Since H_1 antihistamines have been discovered as inverse agonist, the adoption of the term "H_1 antihistamines" has been contemplated [1, 3]. The chemical structure of antihistamines can be varied (Table 22.2).

Indications and Clinical Pearls

H_1 antihistamines are used to relieve or prevent allergy symptoms. Suppression of allergic inflammation in the mucous membranes and reduction of the size of wheal (swelling) and flare (vasodilation) response will help alleviate symptoms such as itching, rhinorrhea, sneezing, urticaria, and congestion [4]. The effect on airway smooth muscle is that of bronchodilation. H_1 antihistamines can be grouped into two classifications: First-generation (sedative) antihistamines and second-generation (nonsedating) antihistamines. First-generation H_1 antihistamines include chlorpheniramine (Chlor-Trimeton), clemastine (Tavist), dexchlorpheniramine (Polaramine), dimenhydrinate (Dramamine), dimetindene (Fenistil), doxylamine (Unisom – used as the sedative in NyQuil), diphenhydramine (Benadryl), hydroxyzine (Vistaril), meclizine (Antivert), orphenadrine (Norflex), pheniramine (Avil), and promethazine (Phenergan).

First-generation H_1 antihistamines cross the blood-brain barrier due to their lipophilic molecular structure leading to the possible unwarranted effect of sedation. Adverse reactions may be due to their inhibition on muscarinic, serotonergic, and adrenergic receptors (Table 22.3). Reports of toxicity with overdose, whether intentional or accidental, have been reported.

Antiemetic effects may be elicited due to blockade of the histaminergic signal from the vestibular nucleus to the vomiting center in the medulla [6]. Clinical uses can extend beyond the treatment of allergic symptoms to the treatment of vestibular disorders, sedatives, sleeping aids, and antiemetics. These agents are usually administered in three to four daily doses (Table 22.4).

Table 22.3 H$_1$ antihistamine adverse effects on various receptors

Adverse effect of first-generation H$_1$ antihistamines		
H$_1$ receptor	$\geq$	CNS neurotransmission reduction, sedation, cognitive and neuropsychomotor performance reduction, appetite↑
Muscarinic receptor	$\geq$	Tachycardia, urinary retention
α-adrenergic receptor	$\geq$	Hypotension, dizziness, reflex tachycardia
Serotonin receptor	$\geq$	Appetite increase
Cardiac channels	$\geq$	Prolongation of the QT interval, ventricular arrhythmia

Modified from [1, 5]

Second-generation antihistamines include acrivastine (Semprex), cetirizine (Zyrtec), desloratadine (Clarinex), ebastine (Kestine), fexofenadine (Allegra), levo-cetirizine (Xyzal), and loratadine (Claritin). The Food and Drug Administration (FDA) removed terfenadine (Seldane) and astemizole (Hismanal) from the US market.

With development over the last two decades of the newer second-generation H$_1$ antihistamines, advantages over the earlier drugs have been seen. Less sedation and fewer anticholinergic side effects have lead to their significant advance in the pharmacologic treatment of allergic symptoms. Second-generation H$_1$ antihistamines differ from the first generation because of their high specificity and affinity for peripheral H$_1$ receptors [5]. These newer advanced drugs have much less effect on the central nervous system and do not have sedating effects (Table 22.5). They are rapidly absorbed and peak plasma concentrations are reached after 1–3 h. Once- to possibly twice-daily dosing administration schedules are recommended. Of note, most show significant renal clearance lending to the need to adjust dosing in patients with renal impairment.

Suppression of stomach acid secretion occurs due to prevention of histamine action on the H$_2$ receptor found in the gastric mucosa parietal cells. Like the H$_1$ antihistamines, the H$_2$ antihistamines are inverse agonist rather that true receptor antagonists. Their uses are for treatment of acid-related gastrointestinal conditions, i.e., dyspepsia, gastroesophageal reflux, and peptic ulcer disease. Prevention of stress ulcers has also been described along with a decrease in vascular permeability. H$_2$ receptors are also found in smooth muscle, cardiac cells, and the central nervous system [6].

All four H$_2$ blockers, including cimetidine, ranitidine, famotidine, and nizatidine, are available over the counter in the USA. Most are well tolerated due to the selectivity. They do not block H$_1$ receptors or have antimuscarinic activity (Table 22.6).

Table 22.4 First-generation H₁ antihistamines

Drug	Treatment usage	Dosage	Special precautions	Special diet	Side effects	Availability
Diphenhydramine Benadryl©	Allergy symptoms Motion sickness Insomnia Dystonia in early Parkinson's disease	25–50 mg PO q4–6 h; 10–50 mg IV/IM (total of 400 mg/day) (Tabs, capsules, liquid, rapidly dissolving tab or strip, IV)		Normal	Dry mouth Drowsiness Dizziness Nausea/vomiting Constipation Increase in chest congestion Headaches photosensitivity Urinary retention	Over the counter
Hydroxyzine Vistaril©	Allergy symptoms Nausea/vomiting Motion sickness Anxiety Alcohol withdrawal	25 mg po TID–QID 25–100 mg IM q 4–6 h (Capsules, oral suspension, IM)		Normal	Dry mouth drowsiness Dizziness Chest congestion Headache Muscle weakness Increased anxiety	Prescribed
Orphenadrine Norflex©	Pain (muscle spasms), headache Migraines Parkinson's disease	60–100 mg PO q 8 h, 60 mg PO, IM, IV for Parkinson's disease (Tabs, oral solution, IM/IV)		Normal	Dry mouth Drowsiness Dizziness Restlessness Constipation Increase in chest congestion Urinary retention Euphoria	Prescribed

(continued)

Table 22.4 (continued)

Drug	Treatment usage	Dosage	Special precautions	Special diet	Side effects	Availability
Promethazine© *Phenergan*	Allergy symptoms	6.25–12.5 mg PO qd, 12.5–25 mg IV q 4–6 h (tabs, rectal supp, IV)	Precaution in the elderly and children	Normal	Dry mouth	Prescribed
	Motion sickness Insomnia		Not to be given to children under 2 years of age		Drowsiness Nausea/vomiting Blurred vision Nightmares Nervousness Restless, hyperactivity Respiratory depression Confusion	

Modified from Lin [6]

Table 22.5 Second-generation H$_1$ antihistamines

Drug	Treatment usage	Dosage	Special precautions	Special diet	Side effects	Availability
Cetirizine © Zyrtec ©	Seasonal allergic rhinitis Chronic idiopathic urticaria	5–10 mg PO q day (tablets, chewable tabs, syrup)	Dosing adjustment for renal, hepatic impairment and the elderly	Normal	Somnolence Fatigue Dry mouth Pharyngitis Stomach pain Diarrhea Vomiting	Over the counter
Desloratadine © Clarinex ©	Seasonal allergic rhinitis Chronic idiopathic urticaria	5 mg PO q day (Tablets, orally disintegrating tabs, syrup)	Dosing adjustment for renal or hepatic impairment	Normal	Pharyngitis Dry mouth Myalgia Fatigue Somnolence Headache	Prescribed
Fexofenadine © Allegra ©	Seasonal allergic rhinitis Chronic idiopathic urticaria Motion sickness Insomnia	60 mg PO BID or 180 mg PO q day (Tablet, orally disintegrating tabs, suspension)	Dosing adjustment for renal impairment	Decreased absorption from fruit juices: grapefruit, orange, and apple	Dry mouth Nausea Dizziness Weakness Headache Aggression	Over the counter
Levocetirizine © Xyzal ©	Seasonal allergic rhinitis Chronic idiopathic urticaria	5 mg PO q day (Tablet, oral solution)	Dosing adjustment for renal impairment	Normal	Dry mouth Pharyngitis Somnolence Fatigue Nasopharyngitis	Prescribed

(continued)

Table 22.5 (continued)

Drug	Treatment usage	Dosage	Special precautions	Special diet	Side effects	Availability
Loratadine Claritin©	Seasonal allergic rhinitis Chronic idiopathic urticaria	10 mg PO q day (Tablet, orally disintegrating tabs, syrup)	Dosing adjustment for hepatic and renal impairment	Increased plasma levels noted with CYP inhibitors	Headache Dry mouth Somnolence Blurred vision Fatigue	Over the counter

Modified from Lin [6]

Table 22.6 H₂ antihistamines

Drug	Treatment usage	Dosage	Special precautions	Special diet	Side effects	Availability
Cimetidine © *Tagamet* ©	Dyspepsia Peptic ulcer disease (PUD) Gastroesophageal reflux (GERD) Prevention of stress ulcers	300 mg PO q day – twice daily for OTC, 300 mg q 6–8 h PO or maximum 2.4 g/day (Tablet, liquid, IV/IM)	Inhibits hepatic oxidative metabolism by most cytochrome P450 enzymes leading to drug interactions	30 min prior to meals and bedtime	Confusion Headache Diarrhea Dizziness Drowsiness Depression	Over the counter, some prescribed formulations
Famotidine © *Pepcid* ©	Dyspepsia PUD GERD Prevention of stress ulcers	20 mg PO q day, twice daily for OTC, 20 mg up to four times/day (tablet, chewable tabs, capsule, liquid, IV)	Does not interfere with hepatic oxidation	15–60 min prior to meals and bedtime	Headache Dizziness Constipation Diarrhea	Over the counter, some prescribed formulations
Ranitidine © *Zantac* ©	Dyspepsia PUD GERD Prevention of stress ulcers	150 mg PO twice daily, 50 mg IV/IM q 6–8 h (tablet, effervescent tabs, granules, syrup, capsule, IV)	Does not interfere with hepatic oxidation	30–60 min prior to meals and bedtime	Headache Diarrhea Constipation Nausea/vomiting Stomach pain	Over the counter, some prescribed formulations
Nizatidine © *Axid* ©	Dyspepsia PUD GERD Prevention of stress ulcers (Experimental use with weight gain)	150 mg PO q day, twice daily (tablets, capsule)	Does not interfere with hepatic oxidation, increase in liver enzymes noted in some patients.	30–60 min prior to meals and bedtime	Headache Dizziness Constipation Diarrhea Sweating Stomach pain	Over the counter, some prescribed formulations, last H2 antihistamine before "proton pump inhibitors"

Modified from Lin [6]

Drug Interactions/Side Effects/Black Box Warnings

Cardiac Effects

Concerns over the development of ventricular arrhythmias have been reported, and the metabolic profile and susceptibility with other drug interactions among some of these second-generation compounds exist. Potassium channels in the heart may be blocked by various substrates lending to a prolongation of the QT interval of the electrocardiogram resulting in lethal arrhythmias [7].

Metabolism is emerging as an important part of second-generation antihistamines. In order to understand the risk of cardiac arrhythmias, an understanding of CYP3A4 antihistamine metabolism and other drug interactions, i.e., inhibitors, substrates, and inducers, must be understood. Compounds such as the second-generation antihistamines have very low plasma levels secondary to high tissue uptake and first-pass liver metabolism. These compounds are metabolized to pharmacologically active agents. The metabolic pathway is mediated primarily by CYP3A4, an isoenzyme belonging to the cytochrome P450 (CYP) superfamily. CYP3A4 is responsible for 30 % of total CYP metabolism in the liver and 70 % in the intestine. Besides antihistamines, CYP3A4 can accommodate a large variety of structurally diverse exogenous and endogenous compounds. It should be noted the CYP3A4 can be inhibited or induced by a number of drugs; hence it is implicated in many drug interactions [1, 5].

An example of potential risk is found in the concomitant usage of erythromycin and ketoconazole with terfenadine. These compounds hinder the metabolic clearance of terfenadine, thereby inducing its accumulation triggering a cardiac response. These effects are thought to be due to the potency of terfenadine to block cardiac potassium channels leading to QT interval prolongation and possible fatal arrhythmias. Subsequent investigations have shown other substrates and/or inhibitors have lead to cardiac events with terfenadine. The FDA removed this drug from the US market in 1997. Astemizole also has been shown to have arrhythmogenic potential [5] resulting in its withdrawal from the US market in 1999.

In contrast, cetirizine, epinastine, and fexofenadine are on the other side of the metabolic hurdle, and most of the dose is eliminated as unchanged drug. No active metabolites have been reported for these agents [1].

Grapefruit juice and tonic water containing quinine may interfere with antihistamine metabolism by inhibition of CYP3A4-dependent first-pass metabolism at the intestinal level. FDA warnings about interactions with astemizole and quinine have been established. As for grapefruit juice, the magnitude of the interaction may be unpredictable and dependent on factors of individual susceptibility, type and amount of juice consumed, and timing of administration [1, 5, 6].

In addition, variability among humans with the lowest CYP activities may be at risk for development of high concentrations of antihistamines even with recommended dosing and no interfering drugs. Metabolic pathways and concomitant drug usage may affect the safety of these drugs. Terfenadine and astemizole are examples of potential concern. It has been suggested that three questions should guide the physician when prescribing H_1 antihistamines [7]:

- Is there a history of organic heart disease, cardiac arrhythmias, electrolyte disturbances, or hepatic disease?
- Is there a possibility of concomitant use of macrolides, anti-arrhythmics, antipsychotics, opiates, imidazole compounds, or migraine medications?
- Are there any special diets requiring grapefruit juice or tonic water?

CNS Effects

Studies have shown that CNS impairment such as somnolence or cognitive and psychomotor impairment can occur when cerebral H_1 receptors are at least 50 % occupied. Cyproheptadine unlike most antihistamines antagonizes serotonin receptors. With only weak anticholinergic properties, its ability to compete with serotonin at receptor sites produces both antiemetic effects and stimulates appetite. Orphenadrine binds to both H_1 and NMDA receptors. The medication is marketed for use in acute, painful, musculoskeletal conditions due to its reported relaxing effect on skeletal muscle spasms [8, 9]. Chlorpheniramine plasma levels showed cerebral H_1 receptor occupation exceeding 50 % resulting in perceived central adverse manifestations. For an H_1 antihistamine to be considered as not having sedative effects, they must not exceed 20 % cerebral H_1 receptor occupation when using maximum dosages [1]. Second-generation H_1 antihistamines do not appear to have significant receptor occupation leading to adverse CNS effects. Tolerance of adverse CNS effects among these first-generation H1 antihistamines has been found to occur after consecutive use over 5 days.

In the CNS, histamine (H_1 and H_2) modulates activities such as arousal, thermoregulation, neuroendocrine, and cognitive functions. Blockade of central H_2 receptors can cause delirium, confusion, agitation, and rarely seizures. H_2 antihistamines rarely cause CNS toxicity even in large dosing regimens.

Cimetidine is the exception and has been implicated in adverse drug reactions including hypotension, headaches, dizziness, confusion, loss of libido, and impotence in males. A study of African Americans found that long-term use of H_2 blockers appeared to increase the risk of cognitive impairment [10]. A relationship between H_2 blocker utilization in patients over 65 and depression has been reported.

Age

Second-generation H_1 antihistamines are effective with safety profiles superior in the treatment of allergic symptoms [11]. Risk of psychomotor impairment may have negative impacts on children. Concern over the sedative effects related to many of the first-generation antihistamine agents should prompt caution in the elderly and children. Hydroxyzine and chlorpheniramine have been accepted for children over the age of two. Desloratadine, fexofenadine, and levocetirizine can be used in children between the ages of 1–2 [1].

Gestation and Lactation

The FDA has listed some H_1 first- and second-generation antihistamines as Category B, which may be used in the first trimester of pregnancy. Third trimester antihistamines usage has been associated with a risk of neonatal seizures, and, therefore, Category C compounds such as diphenhydramine, hydroxyzine, clemastine, fexofenadine, and ebastine should be avoided. Advisements from drug manufacturers have been published warning lactating mothers to avoid H_1 antihistamine use due to infant irritability, sedation, and a reduction in the production of breast milk. Some second-generation antihistamines have been noted to have minimal amounts present in the mother's milk supply and can be used without concern [11].

The H_2 antagonists cimetidine, ranitidine, and famotidine have been assigned Category B by the FDA in association with pregnancy, while nizatidine was assigned Category C. In a recent meta-analysis, it was felt that the use of H_2 antagonists was considered safe for the treatment of acid reflux and managing heartburn in pregnancy [12].

Metabolism

With regard to pharmacokinetics, cimetidine also inhibits hepatic oxidative metabolism through the liver cytochrome P450 pathway. By altering the metabolism of other drugs through enzyme pathways, cimetidine can increase the serum levels leading to possible toxicity. A variety of drugs including warfarin, propranolol, labetalol, metoprolol, phenytoin, lidocaine, benzodiazepines, quinidine, theophylline, certain tricyclic antidepressants, and serotonin reuptake inhibitors can be affected [13]. The more recently developed H_2 receptor antagonists are less likely to alter CYP metabolism. Ranitidine is not as potent a CYP inhibitor but still may interact with warfarin, theophylline, phenytoin, metoprolol, and midazolam [14]. Famotidine has little effect on the CYP system and appears to have no significant interactions. Rare cases of bradycardia, tachycardia, and A-V heart block have been reported with H_2 receptor antagonists.

Black Box Warnings

In 2009, the US Food and Drug Administration began telling manufacturers of the drug promethazine to include a boxed warning regarding the injectable form of the drug. The warning, under FDA's authority to require safety-labeling changes, highlights the risk of serious tissue injury when this drug is administered incorrectly. Promethazine should neither be administered into an artery nor administered under the skin because of the risk of severe tissue injury, including gangrene, the boxed warning says. There is also a risk that the drug can leach out from the vein during intravenous administration and cause serious damage to the surrounding tissue. As a result of these risks, the preferred route of administration is injecting the drug deep into the muscle [15]. An additional FDA safety alert from April of 2006 reminded physicians of the antihistamines ability to produce fatal respiratory depression and that the medication is not intended to be used in children under 2 years of age.

Summary

Histamine receptor modulators are some of the most utilized, prescribed and over the counter, medications in the world. Their varied uses and relatively limited side effect profiles make them readily available either by prescription or via over-the-counter preparations. This prevalence makes it paramount for practitioners to understand the mechanism of actions of these medications and the potentially undesirable and dangerous side effects including cardiac manifestations, nervous system interactions, alterations in the metabolism of other medications, and age-related side effects to name a few. Remarkably, with all of the varied medications and chemical structures, there is only one histamine modulator that has received a box warning from the FDA, promethazine. In addition, that warning is related to the delivery of the injectable medication.

Chemical Structures

Chemical Structure
22.1 Chlorphenamine

Chemical Structure
22.2 Hydroxyzine

Chemical Structure
22.3 Promethazine

Chemical Structure
22.4 Cimetidine

Chemical Structure
22.5 Ranitidine

References

1. Criado PR, Criado RFJ, Maruta CW, et al. Histamine, histamine receptors and antihistamines: new concepts. Braz Annals Dermatol. 2010;85(2):195–210.
2. Jutel M, Blaser K, Akdis CA. Histamine in chronic allergic responses. J Invest Allergy Clin Immunol. 2005;15:1–8.
3. Leurs R, Church MK, Taglialatela M. H1-antihistamines: inverse agonism, anti-inflammatory actions and cardiac effects. Clin Exp Allergy. 2002;32:489–98.

4. Monroe E, Daly A, Shalhoub R M.D. Appraisal of the validity of histamine-induced wheal and flare is used to predict the clinical efficacy of antihistamines. J Allergy Clin Immunol. 1997;99(2):S789–806.

5. Nicolas JM. The metabolic profile of second-generation antihistamines. Allergy. 2000;55 Suppl 60:46–52.

6. Lin S. Antihistamines. In: Sinatra R, Jahr J, Watkins-Pitchford J, editors. The essence of analgesia and analgesics. New York: Cambridge University Press; 2011. p. 391–6.

7. Davila I, Sastre J, Bartra J, del Cuvillo A, Jauregui I, Montoro J, et al. Effect of H1 antihistamines upon the cardiovascular system. J Investig Allergol Clin Immunol. 2006;16 Suppl 1:13–23.

8. Rumore MM, Schlichting DA. Analgesic effects of antihistaminics. Life Sci. 1985;36(5):403–16.

9. Kornhuber J, Parson CG, Hartnamm S, et al. Orphenadrine is an uncompetitive N-methyl-D-aspartate (NMDA) receptor antagonist: binding and patch clamp studies. J Neural Transm Gen Sect. 1995;102(3):237–46.

10. Boustani M, Hall KS, Lane KA, et al. The association between cognition and histamine-2 receptor antagonists in African Americans. J Am Geriatr Soc. 2007;55(8):1248–53.

11. Powell RJ, Du Toit GI, Siddique N, Leech SC, Dixon TA, Clark AT, British Society for Allergy and Clinical Immunology (BSACI), et al. BSACI guidelines for the management of chronic urticaria and angio-oedema. Clin Exp Allergy. 2007;37:631–50.

12. Gill SK, O'Brien L, Koren G. The safety of histamine 2 (H2) blockers in pregnancy: a meta-analysis. Dig Dis Sci. 2009;54:1835–8.

13. Humphries TJ, Merritt GJ. Review article: drug interactions with agents used to treat acid-related diseases. Aliment Pharmacol Ther. 1999;13 Suppl 3:18–26.

14. Kirch W, Hoensch H, Janisch HD. Interactions and non-interactions with ranitidine. Clin Pharmacokinet. 1984;9(6):493–510.

15. U.S. Food and Drug Administration[Internet]. Postmarket drug safety information for patients and providers. Information for healthcare professionals – intravenous promethazine and severe tissue injury, including gangrene. (updated 09/16/2009). Available from http://www.fda.gov/Drugs/DrugSafety/PostmarketDrugSafetyInformationforPatientsandProviders/DrugSafetyInformationforHeathcareProfessionals/ucm182169.htm.

Chapter 23
Central Nervous System Stimulants

Eric S. Hsu

Contents

Introduction

It has been estimated that 1.5 % of the general population complains of excessive daytime sleepiness or excessive sleep amounts consistent with a hypersomnia disorder. Narcolepsy is a neurological disorder affecting the regulation of sleep and

E.S. Hsu, MD
Anesthesiology Pain Medicine Center, UCLA–School of Medicine, University of California, Los Angeles, CA, USA
e-mail: ehsu@mednet.ucla.edu

A.D. Kaye et al. (eds.), *Essentials of Pharmacology for Anesthesia, Pain Medicine, and Critical Care*, DOI 10.1007/978-1-4614-8948-1_23,
© Springer Science+Business Media New York 2015

wakefulness. It is characterized by excessive daytime sleepiness, cataplexy (sudden temporary inability to move), and other rapid eye movement (REM) sleep-associated manifestations (e.g., hypnagogic hallucinations and sleep paralysis).

The diagnoses of primary hypersomnolence are made after eliminating sleep deprivation, sleep apnea, disturbed nocturnal sleep, and psychiatric comorbidities as the main cause of daytime sleepiness.

Clinical syndromes with primary hypersomnolence can be divided into three groups according to the *Diagnostic and Statistical Manual of Mental Disorders*, 5th edition (DSM-V): (1) narcolepsy caused by hypocretin (orexin) deficiency, a disorder associated with human leukocyte antigen (HLA) marker DQB1*06:02 and believed to be autoimmune (almost all cases with cataplexy); (2) Kleine-Levin syndrome (KLS), a periodic hypersomnia associated with cognitive and behavioral abnormalities (KLS are considered a separate entity with separate therapeutic protocols); and (3) non-hypocretin-related hypersomnia syndromes (generally without cataplexy) which are diagnoses of exclusion. This is the most challenging and the most frequent diagnosis [1].

Narcolepsy caused by hypocretin deficiency is called "type 1 narcolepsy" in the *International Sleep Disorder Classification*, 3rd edition (ICSD3), while other hypersomnias (not likely due to hypocretin abnormalities) are subdivided into "type 2 narcolepsy" in the presence of a positive multiple sleep latency test (MSLT) with multiple sleep-onset REM periods (SOREMPs) versus idiopathic hypersomnias otherwise [2].

Shift work disorder (SWD) is characterized by symptoms of excessive sleepiness during work hours or insomnia during allotted daytime sleep hours, as well as by a disruption of the circadian rhythm. Many shift workers with SWD experience significant social, behavioral, and health problems as a result of this disorder. SWD is often associated with a higher risk of occupational and motor vehicle accidents. SWD in health-care providers may present additional risk for public health [3].

A diagnosis of attention deficit hyperactivity disorder (ADHD; DSM-IV) implies the presence of hyperactive-impulsive symptoms that caused impairment and were present before age 7 years. The symptoms must cause clinically significant impairment, e.g., in social, academic, or occupational functioning, and be present in two or more settings, e.g., school (or work) and at home.

Drug Class and Mechanism of Action

Amphetamine (Adderall) is a CNS stimulant. The chemical name for amphetamine is 1-phenylpropan-2-amine. The molecular formula is $C_9H_{13}N$. See Chemical Structure 23.1 at the end of the chapter.

Amphetamine (Adderall) increases monoamine release (such as dopamine, norepinephrine, and serotonin). Primary effects of amphetamine may be due to reverse efflux of dopamine through the dopamine transporter (DAT). Higher doses of amphetamine interfere with monoamine storage through the vesicular monoamine transporter (VMAT) and other effects. The D-isomer is more specific for dopamine transmission and is a better stimulant compound. Some effects on cataplexy (especially for the L-isomer), secondary to adrenergic effects, occur at higher doses. Amphetamine is available as racemic mixture or as pure D-isomer and various time-release formulations. Addiction potential is high for immediate-release formulation. High doses cause increased blood pressure and possible cardiac complications.

Modafinil (Provigil) is a wakefulness-promoting agent for oral administration. Modafinil is a racemic compound. The chemical name for modafinil is 2-[(diphenylmethyl) sulfinyl] acetamide. The molecular formula is $C15H15NO2S$ and the molecular weight is 273.35. See Chemical Structure 23.2 at the end of the chapter.

The precise mechanism(s) through which modafinil promotes wakefulness is unknown. Modafinil has wake-promoting actions similar to sympathomimetic agents like amphetamine and methylphenidate. However, the pharmacologic profile of modafinil is not identical to sympathomimetic amines. Modafinil has weak to negligible interactions with receptors for norepinephrine, serotonin, dopamine, gamma-aminobutyric acid (GABA), adenosine, histamine-3, melatonin, and benzodiazepines. Modafinil does not inhibit the activities of monoamine oxidase (MAO)-B or phosphodiesterases II–V. Modafinil-induced wakefulness can be attenuated by the alpha (α) 1-adrenergic receptor antagonist prazosin; however, modafinil is inactive in other in vitro assay systems known to be responsive to a-adrenergic agonists, such as the rat vas deferens preparation.

Modafinil is not a direct- or indirect-acting dopamine receptor agonist. However, modafinil binds to the dopamine transporter and inhibits dopamine reuptake in vitro. This activity has been associated in vivo with increased extracellular dopamine levels in some brain regions of animals. In genetically engineered mice lacking the dopamine transporter (DAT), modafinil lacked wake-promoting activity, suggesting that this activity was DAT-dependent.

However, the wake-promoting effects of modafinil, unlike those of amphetamine, were not antagonized by the dopamine receptor antagonist haloperidol in rats.

In the cat, equal wakefulness-promoting doses of methylphenidate and amphetamine increased neuronal activation throughout the brain. Modafinil at an equivalent wakefulness-promoting dose selectively and prominently increased neuronal activation in more discrete regions of the brain. The relationship of this finding in cats to the effects of modafinil in humans is unknown.

Modafinil produces psychoactive and euphoric effects such as alterations in mood, perception, thinking, and feelings typical of other CNS stimulants in humans. Modafinil has two major metabolites, modafinil acid and modafinil sulfone, that do not appear to contribute to the CNS-activating properties.

Armodafinil (Nuvigil) is a wakefulness-promoting agent for oral administration. Armodafinil is the R-enantiomer of modafinil which is a mixture of the R- and S-enantiomers. The chemical name for armodafinil is 2-[(R)-(diphenylmethyl) sulfinyl] acetamide. The molecular formula is $C15H15NO2S$ and the molecular weight is 273.35. See Chemical Structure 23.3 at the end of the chapter.

The precise mechanism(s) through which armodafinil (R-enantiomer) or modafinil (mixture of R- and S-enantiomers) promotes wakefulness is unknown.

However, armodafinil and modafinil have shown similar pharmacological properties in nonclinical animal and in vitro studies. At pharmacologically relevant concentrations, armodafinil does not bind to or inhibit several receptors and enzymes potentially relevant for sleep/wake regulation.

The chemical name for Caffeine is 1, 3, 7-trimethylxanthine. Its molecular formula is $C_8H_{10}N_4O_2$. See Chemical Structure 23.4 at the end of the chapter.

Caffeine is a widely consumed stimulant and treatment of hypersomnia. The wake-promoting potency of caffeine is often not strong enough yet high doses may induce side effects. Caffeine is an adenosine A1 and A2 receptor antagonist. Caffeine is metabolized to paraxanthine, theobromine, and theophylline. Paraxanthine is a central nervous stimulant and exhibits higher potency at A1 and A2 receptors. Paraxanthine had lower toxicity and lesser anxiogenic effects than caffeine *as studied in Orexin/Ataxin-3 transgenic narcoleptic mice model* [4].

Methylphenidate (Ritalin) hydrochloride is a mild central nervous system (CNS) stimulant. It is available as tablets of 5, 10, and 20 mg for oral administration. Ritalin-SR is available as sustained-release tablets of 20 mg for oral administration. The chemical formula for methylphenidate is methyl α-phenyl-2-piperidineacetate hydrochloride. The molecular formula is C14 H19 NO2. See Chemical Structure 23.5 at the end of the chapter.

The mode of action in man is not completely understood. Methylphenidate likely activates the brain stem arousal system and cortex to produce its stimulant effect. There is no specific evidence to establish the effect or mechanism in CNS how methylphenidate produces its mental and behavioral effects in children. It has short half-life. It is available as racemic mixture or as pure D-isomer and in various time-release formulations. Addiction potential is notable for immediate-release methylphenidate.

Methylphenidate (Ritalin) blocks monoamine (such as dopamine, norepinephrine, serotonin) uptake in nonclinical animal and in vitro studies. There is no effect on reverse efflux or on vesicular monoamine transporter (VMAT).

Atomoxetine (Strattera) HCl is a selective norepinephrine reuptake inhibitor. Atomoxetine HCl is the $R(-)$ isomer as determined by X-ray diffraction. The chemical name for atomoxetine is (-)-*N*-Methyl-3-phenyl-3-(*o*-tolyloxy)-propylamine hydrochloride. The molecular formula is C17H21NO•HCl, which corresponds to a molecular weight of 291.82. See Chemical Structure 23.6 at the end of the chapter.

The precise mechanism by which atomoxetine produces its therapeutic effects in ADHD is unknown. It is thought to be related to selective inhibition of the presynaptic norepinephrine transporter, as determined in ex vivo uptake and neurotransmitter depletion studies.

Sodium oxybate, a CNS depressant, is the active ingredient in Xyrem. The chemical name for sodium oxybate is sodium 4-hydroxybutyrate. The molecular formula is C4H7NaO3, and the molecular weight is 126.09. See Chemical Structure 23.7 at the end of the chapter.

Sodium oxybate (Xyrem) is a CNS depressant. Sodium oxybate has therapeutic effect on excessive daytime sleepiness. Its mechanism of action is unknown. Sodium oxybate is the sodium salt of gamma hydroxybutyrate, an endogenous compound and metabolite of the neurotransmitter gamma-aminobutyric acid (GABA).

It is hypothesized that the therapeutic effects of sodium oxybate are mediated through GABA-B actions at noradrenergic and dopaminergic neurons, as well as at thalamocortical neurons. Sodium oxybate reduces dopamine release in nonclinical animal and in vitro studies.

Indications/Clinical Pearls

Amphetamine (ADDERALL XR) is indicated for the treatment of ADHD:

- Children (ages 6–12): Efficacy was established in one 3-week outpatient, controlled trial and one analog classroom, controlled trial in children with ADHD.
- Adolescents (ages 13–17): Efficacy was established in one 4-week controlled trial in adolescents with ADHD.
- Adults: Efficacy was established in one 4-week controlled trial in adults with ADHD.

Modafinil (Provigil) is indicated to improve wakefulness in adult patients with excessive sleepiness associated with narcolepsy, obstructive sleep apnea (OSA), and shift work disorder (SWD). Modafinil is indicated as an adjunct to standard treatment(s) for the underlying obstruction in OSA. Careful attention to the diagnosis and treatment of underlying sleep disorder(s) is of utmost importance in all cases of excessive sleepiness. A maximal effort to treat with continuous positive airway pressure (CPAP) for an adequate period of time should be made prior to initiating modafinil. The encouragement and periodic assessment of CPAP compliance is necessary, while modafinil is used as adjunctive treatment.

The effectiveness of modafinil in long-term use (greater than 9 weeks in narcolepsy clinical trials and 12 weeks in OSA and SWD clinical trials) has not been systematically evaluated in placebo-controlled trials. Periodical reevaluation is recommended for long-term use of modafinil in patients with narcolepsy, OSA, or SWD.

Armodafinil (Nuvigil) is indicated to improve wakefulness in patients with excessive sleepiness associated with OSA, narcolepsy, and SWD. In OSA, armodafinil is indicated as an adjunct to standard treatment(s) for the underlying obstruction. The effectiveness of armodafinil in long-term use (greater than 12 weeks) has not been systematically evaluated in placebo-controlled trials. Periodical reevaluation of efficacy is highly recommended for long-term use of armodafinil in narcolepsy, OSA, or SWD.

Caffeine has a potential role in promoting alertness during times of desired wakefulness in persons with SWD or jet lag sleep disorder [5].

Methylphenidate (Ritalin) is indicated for attention deficit hyperactivity disorder (ADHD; DSM-IV) and narcolepsy. Methylphenidate is indicated as an integral part of a total treatment program on ADHD. It typically includes other remedial measures (psychological, educational, and social) for a stabilizing effect in children with a behavioral syndrome characterized by the following group of developmentally inappropriate symptoms: moderate-to-severe distractibility, short attention span, hyperactivity, emotional lability, and impulsivity. The diagnosis of ADHD should not be made with definiteness when these symptoms are only of comparatively recent origin.

Atomoxetine (Strattera) is indicated for the treatment of ADHD. The efficacy of atomoxetine capsules was established in seven clinical trials in outpatients with ADHD: four 6–9-week trials in pediatric patients (ages 6–18), two 10-week trial in adults, and one trial for maintenance in pediatrics (ages 6–15).

Sodium oxybate (Xyrem) oral solution is indicated for the treatment of cataplexy in narcolepsy and excessive daytime sleepiness (EDS) in narcolepsy. Sodium oxybate may only be dispensed to patients enrolled in the Xyrem Success Program.

Sodium oxybate needs at minimum bi-nightly dosing with immediate effects on disturbed nocturnal sleep. Therapeutic effects of sodium oxybate on cataplexy and daytime sleepiness can be delayed weeks to months. Nausea, weight loss, and psychiatric complications are possible side effects. As for any sedative, use with caution in the presence of hypoventilation or sleep apnea.

Dosing Options

Amphetamine (Adderall XR)

- Pediatric patients (ages 6–17): 10 mg once daily in the morning. The maximum dose for children 6–12 is 30 mg once daily.
- Adults: 20 mg once daily in the morning.

Modafinil (Provigil)

Modafinil is available as 100 and 200 mg as racemic mixture. It is administered once or twice a day (morning and noon), with a maximum of 400 mg/day. It is also available as R-modafinil (50, 150, and 250 mg) which is approximately twice more potent than racemic modafinil per mg. Headache is a common side effect but is usually avoidable by increasing the dose slowly. It is advisable to monitor allergic side effects due to modafinil notably in children. Modafinil has not been approved by Food and Drug Administration (FDA) for pediatrics.

Armodafinil (Nuvigil)

The recommended dose of armodafinil for patients with obstructive sleep apnea (OSA) or narcolepsy is 150 or 250 mg given as a single dose in the morning. There is no consistent evidence that 250 mg/day of armodafinil confers additional benefit beyond 150 mg/day in patients with OSA.

The recommended dose of armodafinil for patients with shift work disorder (SWD) is 150 mg given daily approximately 1 h prior to the start of their work shift. Dosage adjustment should be considered for concomitant medications that are substrates for CYP3A4/5, such as steroidal contraceptives, triazolam, and cyclosporine. Drugs that are largely eliminated via CYP2C19 metabolism, such as diazepam, propranolol, and phenytoin, may have prolonged elimination upon coadministration with armodafinil and may require dosage reduction and monitoring for toxicity.

Armodafinil should be administered at a reduced dose in patients with severe hepatic impairment. There is inadequate information to determine safety and efficacy of armodafinil dosing in patients with severe renal impairment.

In elderly patients, elimination of armodafinil and its metabolites may be reduced as a consequence of aging. Therefore, consideration should be given to the use of lower doses in elderly.

Caffeine

Caffeine increases nighttime alertness but has little effect on daytime sleep. It has been recommended for patients with SWD. According to practice parameters from the American Academy of Sleep Medicine (AASM), caffeine is recommended to enhance alertness during the night shift in patients with SWD. In a study of healthy adults, caffeine equivalent to 2–4 cups of coffee was shown to be effective in reducing sleepiness and improving alertness. The alerting effect of caffeine was described as equivalent to a 3.5 h nap, and it persisted for 5.5–7.5 h [6].

In a study of healthy volunteers undergoing a simulated night-shift schedule for five nights, caffeine decreased sleep tendency during the night shift compared with placebo, and fewer subjects receiving caffeine were sleepy across the first three nights of the study. A laboratory study of healthy subjects under conditions of simulated night shifts demonstrated that caffeine, alone or in combination with napping, improved alertness and performance as measured by the Maintenance of Wakefulness Test and Psychomotor Vigilance Task. In a related field study with shift workers working night shifts or rotating shifts, caffeine plus napping improved performance and decreased reports of sleepiness in the night-shift workers [7].

Methylphenidate (Ritalin)

Methylphenidate (Ritalin) may be more effective and potent than modafinil and low cost. Methylphenidate can substitute for modafinil when using long-acting formulations of the racemic mixture of any single isomer typically 20–40 mg/day. Various preparations and formulations can have substantially different interindividual effects. As base preparation, immediate release (5–10 mg) can be helpful, either to alleviate sleep drunkenness in hypersomnia, to bridge gaps in alertness during the daytime (postprandial dose), or to use when necessary in case of emergency (e.g., need to drive to the hospital)

Sodium Oxybate (Xyrem)

Administration of sodium oxybate at night is effective in consolidating sleep in patients with disturbed sleep due to insomnia, excessive activity during rapid eye movement sleep, hypnagogic hallucinations, and sleep paralysis. Effect of sodium oxybate on cataplexy and daytime sleepiness is evident soon after treatment begins and builds further along several weeks.

The recommended starting dose is 4.5 g (g) per night administered orally in two equal, divided doses: 2.25 g at bedtime and 2.25 g taken 2.5–4 h later.

Increase the dose by 1.5 g per night at weekly intervals (additional 0.75 g at bedtime and 0.75 g taken 2.5–4 h later) to the effective dose range of 6–9 g per night orally. Doses higher than 9 g per night have not been studied and should not ordinarily be administered.

Take the first dose of sodium oxybate (Xyrem) at least 2 h after eating because food significantly reduces the bioavailability of sodium oxybate.

Prepare both doses of sodium oxybate prior to bedtime. Prior to ingestion, each dose of sodium oxybate should be diluted with approximately ¼ cup (approximately 60 mL) of water in the empty pharmacy vials provided. Patients should take sodium oxybate while in bed and lie down immediately after dosing as sodium oxybate may cause them to fall asleep abruptly without first feeling drowsy. Patients will often fall asleep within 5–15 min of taking sodium oxybate, though the time it takes any individual patient to fall asleep may vary from night to night. Therefore, patients should remain in bed following ingestion of the first dose and should not take the second dose until 2.5–4 h later. Patients may need to set an alarm to awaken for the second dose.

Drug Interactions

Monoamine oxidase inhibitors (MAOI) antidepressants may slow amphetamine metabolism. A variety of toxic neurological effects and malignant hyperpyrexia can occur with fatal results. Do not administer amphetamine during or within 14 days following the administration of MAOI.

Coadministration of amphetamine with gastrointestinal alkalinizing agents (such as antacids) or urinary alkalinizing agents (acetazolamide, some thiazides) increases blood levels and potentiates the actions of amphetamines. Gastrointestinal acidifying agents (e.g., guanethidine, reserpine, glutamic acid HCl, ascorbic acid) and urinary acidifying agents (e.g., ammonium chloride, sodium acid phosphate, methenamine salts) may lower blood levels and efficacy of amphetamines.

Amphetamines may enhance the activity of tricyclic antidepressants or sympathomimetic agents; d-amphetamine with desipramine or protriptyline and possibly other tricyclics cause striking and sustained increases in the concentration of d-amphetamine in the brain; cardiovascular effects can be potentiated.

Amphetamines potentiate the analgesic effect of meperidine. Amphetamines may enhance the adrenergic effect of norepinephrine. Haloperidol blocks dopamine receptors, thus inhibiting the central stimulant effects of amphetamines. The anorectic and stimulatory effects of amphetamines may be inhibited by lithium carbonate. Coadministration of ADDERALL XR and proton pump inhibitors (PPI) should be monitored for changes in clinical effect.

Modafinil (Provigil)

In a single-dose study in healthy volunteers, coadministration of modafinil (200 mg) with methylphenidate (40 mg) did not cause any significant alterations in the pharmacokinetics of either drug. However, the absorption of modafinil may be delayed by approximately one hour when coadministered with methylphenidate. In a multiple-dose, steady-state study in healthy volunteers, modafinil was administered once daily at 200 mg/day for 7 days followed by 400 mg/day for 21 days. Coadministration of methylphenidate (20 mg/day) during days 22–28 of modafinil treatment 8 h after the daily dose of modafinil did not cause any significant alterations in the pharmacokinetics of modafinil.

Chronic modafinil treatment did not show a significant effect on the single-dose pharmacokinetics of warfarin (substrate of CYP2C9) in clinical study on healthy volunteers. Coadministration with modafinil in drugs that are largely eliminated via CYP2C19 metabolism (such as diazepam, propranolol, and phenytoin) may result in prolonged elimination. Modafinil may raise the levels of tricyclic antidepressants (TCA) in patients that are deficient in CYP2D6 yet dependent more on CYP2C19 metabolism. Therefore, a reduction in the dose of TCA might be needed in these patients.

In addition, due to the partial involvement of CYP3A4 in the metabolic elimination of modafinil, coadministration of potent inducers of CYP3A4 (e.g., carbamazepine, phenobarbital, rifampin) or inhibitors of CYP3A4 (e.g., ketoconazole, itraconazole) could alter the plasma levels of modafinil. The effect of armodafinil on CYP1A2 activity was not observed clinically in an interaction study performed with caffeine.

Armodafinil (Nuvigil)

Chronic administration of armodafinil resulted in moderate induction of CYP3A activity. Hence, the effectiveness of drugs that are substrates for CYP3A enzymes (e.g., cyclosporine, ethinyl estradiol, midazolam, and triazolam) may be reduced after coadministration with armodafinil. Dose adjustment may be required.

Administration of armodafinil resulted in moderate inhibition of CYP2C19 activity. Hence, dosage reduction may be required for some drugs that are substrates for CYP2C19 (e.g., phenytoin, diazepam, propranolol, omeprazole, and clomipramine) when used concurrently with armodafinil.

Data specific to armodafinil drug-drug interaction potential with CNS active drugs are not available. However, the following available drug-drug interaction information on modafinil should be applicable to armodafinil. Concomitant administration of modafinil with methylphenidate or dextroamphetamine produced no significant alterations on the pharmacokinetic profile of modafinil or either stimulant, even though the absorption of modafinil was delayed for approximately 1 h.

Methylphenidate (Ritalin) should not be used in patients being treated (currently or within the preceding 2 weeks) with monoamine oxidase inhibitors (MAOI) inhibitors. Methylphenidate should be used cautiously with pressor agents because of possible effects on blood pressure. Methylphenidate may decrease the effectiveness of drugs used to treat hypertension.

Methylphenidate is metabolized primarily to ritalinic acid by de-esterification and not through oxidative pathways. Human pharmacologic studies have shown that racemic methylphenidate may inhibit the metabolism of Coumadin anticoagulants, anticonvulsants (e.g., phenobarbital, phenytoin, primidone), and tricyclic drugs (e.g., imipramine, clomipramine, desipramine). Downward dose adjustments of these drugs may be required when given concomitantly with methylphenidate. It may be necessary to adjust the dosage and monitor plasma drug concentration when initiating or discontinuing methylphenidate.

Sodium oxybate (Xyrem) is a CNS depressant. Sodium oxybate should not be used in combination with alcohol or sedative hypnotics. Obtundation and clinically significant respiratory depression occurred in clinical trials at recommended doses. Almost all of the patients who received sodium oxybate during clinical trials in narcolepsy were receiving CNS stimulants.

Side Effects/Black Box Warnings

Black Box Warning
Amphetamine (Adderall) has a high potential for abuse. Prolonged administration of amphetamine may lead to drug dependence and must be avoided. Misuse of amphetamine may cause serious cardiovascular adverse reactions and sudden death. Amphetamines should be prescribed and dispensed sparingly.

Modafinil (Provigil) and armodafinil (Nuvigil) may cause serious rash, including Stevens-Johnson syndrome (SJS). Serious rash requiring hospitalization and discontinuation of treatment has been reported in adults and children in association with the use of modafinil. Modafinil and armodafinil are not approved for use in pediatric patients for any indication.

The median time to rash that resulted in discontinuation was 13 days in pediatric clinical trials. No serious skin rashes have been reported in adult clinical trials (0 per 4,264) of modafinil. Rare cases of serious or life-threatening rash, including SJS, toxic epidermal necrolysis (TEN), and drug rash with eosinophilia and systemic symptoms (DRESS) have been reported in adults and children in worldwide post-marketing experience. Estimates of the background incidence rate for these serious skin reactions in the general population range between 1 and 2 cases per million person-years.

There are no factors that are known to predict the risk of occurrence or the severity of rash associated with modafinil. Nearly all cases of serious rash associated with modafinil occurred within 1–5 weeks after treatment initiation. However, isolated cases have been reported after prolonged treatment (e.g., 3 months).

Accordingly, duration of therapy cannot be relied upon as a means to predict the potential risk heralded by the first appearance of a rash.

Although benign rashes also occur with modafinil, it is not possible to reliably predict which rashes will prove to be serious. Accordingly, modafinil should ordinarily be discontinued at the first sign of rash, unless the rash is clearly not drug related.

Other possible adverse events of modafinil and armodafinil may include angioedema and anaphylactoid reactions, multiorgan hypersensitivity reactions, persistent sleepiness, and psychiatric symptoms.

Methylphenidate (Ritalin) should be given cautiously to patients with a history of drug dependence or alcoholism. Chronic abuse can lead to marked tolerance and psychological dependence with varying degrees of abnormal behavior. Frank psychotic episodes can occur, especially with parenteral abuse. Careful supervision is required during withdrawal from abuse since severe depression may occur. Withdrawal following chronic therapeutic use may unmask symptoms of the underlying disorder that may require follow-up.

Sodium oxybate is a Schedule III controlled substance because of the risks of CNS depression, abuse, and misuse. Sodium oxybate is the sodium salt of gamma hydroxybutyrate (GHB). Abuse of GHB is associated with CNS adverse reactions including seizure, respiratory depression, decreases in the level of consciousness, coma, and death. Sodium oxybate is available only through a restricted distribution program called the Xyrem Success Program using a centralized pharmacy. Prescribers and patients must enroll in the Xyrem Success Program.

Most common side effects of sodium oxybate are nausea and loss of appetite, usually beneficial, but occasionally leading to reduced weight that becomes problematic. Psychiatric side effects are possible, notably in patients with an anxious premorbid personality; specific serotonin uptake blocker can occasionally be added to mitigate these.

Anesthesia Considerations

Methylphenidate actively induced emergence from isoflurane general anesthesia by increasing arousal and respiratory drive in clinical research, possibly through activation of dopaminergic and adrenergic arousal circuits. Methylphenidate may emerge as a valuable agent to reverse general anesthetic-induced unconsciousness and respiratory depression toward the end of surgery [8].

Methylphenidate decreased time to emergence after a single dose of propofol and induced emergence during continuous propofol anesthesia in rats. Further study may be warranted to test the hypothesis that methylphenidate induces emergence from propofol general anesthesia in humans [9].

Modafinil (200 mg) significantly reduced fatigue and improved the feelings of alertness and energy in clinical study on postoperative care. Patients recovering from general anesthesia may significantly benefit from the administration of modafinil [10].

There were 60 patients in a clinical study who received similar sedation and analgesia for extracorporeal shock wave lithotripsy. Modafinil did reduce patient-reported tiredness after sedation and analgesia versus placebo. However, modafinil did not improve recovery in terms of objective measures of patients' psychomotor skills [11].

There were 34 children in a clinical study who took stimulants for ADHD and continued medications to the day of surgery. There was no alteration in bispectral index (BIS) or depth of anesthesia at 1 MAC of sevoflurane. These results did not support the common consensus for a change in anesthetic practice for children who continued stimulants up to the day of surgery, in terms of either increasing the amount of anesthetics given or monitoring of anesthesia depth [12].

There was a case study on anesthetic management of a narcoleptic patient performed using sevoflurane-remifentanil with BIS monitoring. The use of BIS monitoring for titrating sevoflurane concentration was useful for preventing not only over sedation but also intraoperative awareness caused by the preoperative medication [13].

A 1-year retrospective chart review of 11 patients was done for opioid-induced sedation receiving modafinil. A significant decrease Epworth Sleepiness Scale (ESS) measurement was observed between pretreatment and posttreatment with modafinil. The results suggested that modafinil may be beneficial for opioid-induced sedation in chronic nonmalignant pain syndromes [14].

Summary

There is a robust need for safe and effective treatment for hypersomnia disorders.

Whereas a large number of safe hypnotics are available, clinicians have very few options for wake-promotion beside dopamine-acting compounds, such as modafinil and amphetamine-like stimulants. Detailed knowledge of the pharmacological profile of each compound is needed to optimize the practice of CNS stimulants.

The treatment of narcolepsy/hypocretin deficiency involves pharmacotherapies using sodium oxybate, stimulants, antidepressants, and behavioral modifications.

Hypersomnia patients without hypocretin deficiency should receive conservative therapy (such as modafinil, atomoxetine, behavioral modifications). The more aggressive (high-dose stimulants and sodium oxybate) can be considered on a case-by-case, empirical trial basis.

It is important to challenge diagnosis and therapy over time as cause and evolution are unknown in hypersomnia. The possibility of tolerance and stimulant addiction must be kept in mind while treating hypersomnia [1].

Shift work disorder (SWD) describes dyssynchrony between the internal clock and the external light-dark cycle. The American Academy of Sleep Medicine and the British Society of Psychopharmacology have developed guidelines for the diagnosis and treatment of SWD. Chronobiotics such as melatonin may cause phase adjustment of the body clock. Non-pharmacologic interventions include optimizing the sleep environment, by strategic avoidance of and exposure to light, napping, and behavioral modifications. Pharmacologic agents such as modafinil, armodafinil, and caffeine may promote nighttime alertness in SWD. Prudent identification and management of SWD will likely reduce its *negative sequelae, including occupational or motor vehicle accidents* and improve the quality of life [15].

With regard to Black Box warnings (www.fda.gov):

- Amphetamines have a high potential for abuse. Therefore, it is noted that the administration of amphetamines for prolonged periods of time may lead to drug dependence, and, therefore, this must be avoided.
- Given the high abuse potential, patients obtaining amphetamines need to be monitored for and carefully screened that they are using them for non-therapeutic use or distribution to others, and as a general rule, the drugs should be prescribed or dispensed sparingly.
- Misuse may cause a number of untoward effects, including serious cardiovascular-related events and sudden death.
- Particular attention should be paid to the possibility of subjects obtaining amphetamines for nontherapeutic use or distribution to others.
- Amphetamines should be prescribed or dispensed sparingly.

Drug Dependence

Give methylphenidate cautiously to emotionally unstable patients such as those with a history of drug dependence or alcoholism, because such patients may increase dosage at their own initiative.

Long-term abusive use can lead to marked tolerance and psychological dependence with varying degrees of abnormal behavior. Frank psychotic episodes can occur, especially with parenteral abuse. Careful supervision is required during withdrawal, because severe depression as well as the effects of chronic overactivity can be unmasked. Withdrawal following long-term therapeutic use may unmask symptoms of the underlying disorder that may require follow-up. Long-term follow-up may be required because of the patient's basic personality disturbances.

Chemical Structures

Chemical Structure
23.1 Amphetamine
(Adderall)

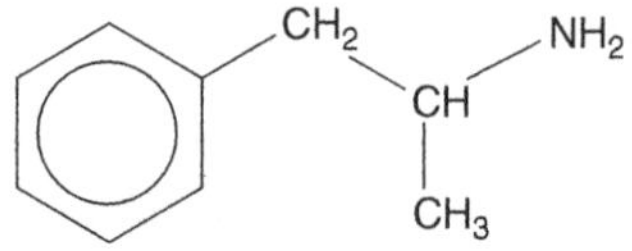

Chemical Structure
23.2 Modafinil (Provigil)

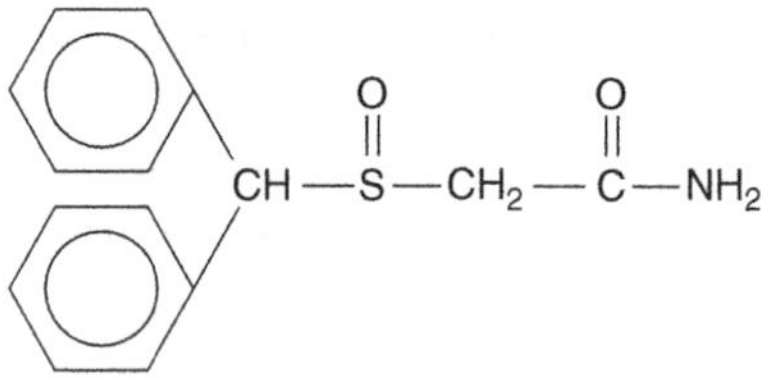

Chemical Structure
23.3 Armodafinil (Nuvigil)

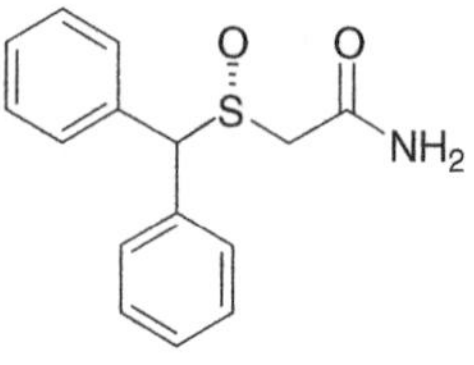

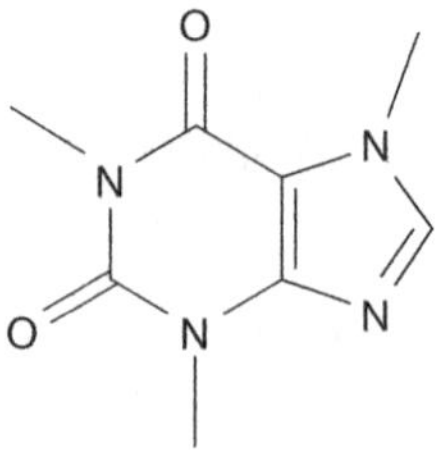

Chemical Structure
23.4 Caffeine

Chemical Structure
23.5 Methylphenidate
(Ritalin)

Chemical Structure
23.6 Atomoxetine (Strattera)
HCl

Chemical Structure
23.7 Sodium oxybate

Chemical Structure
23.8 Methylphenidate

References

1. Mignot EJ. A practical guide to the therapy of narcolepsy and hypersomnia syndromes. Neurotherapeutics. 2012;9(4):739–52.
2. Sonka K, Susta M. Diagnosis and management of central hypersomnias. Ther Adv Neurol Disord. 2012;5(5):297–305.
3. Thorpy M. Understanding and diagnosing shift work disorder. Postgrad Med. 2011;123(5):96–105.
4. Okuro M, Fujiki N, Kotorii N, Ishimaru Y, Sokoloff P, Nishino S. Effects of paraxanthine and caffeine on sleep, locomotor activity, and body temperature in orexin/ataxin-3 transgenic narcoleptic mice. Sleep. 2010;33(7):930–42.
5. Kolla BP, Auger RR. Jet lag and shift work sleep disorders: how to help reset the internal clock. Cleve Clin J Med. 2011;78(10):675–84.
6. Muehlbach MJ, Walsh JK. The effects of caffeine on simulated night-shift work and subsequent daytime sleep. Sleep. 1995;18(1):22–9.
7. Ker K, Edwards PJ, Felix LM, Blackhall K, Roberts I. Caffeine for the prevention of injuries and errors in shift workers. Cochrane Database Syst Rev. 2010;(5):CD008508.
8. Solt K, Cotten JF, Cimenser A, Wong KF, Chemali JJ, Brown EN. Methylphenidate actively induces emergence from general anesthesia. Anesthesiology. 2011;115(4):791–803.
9. Chemali JJ, Van Dort CJ, Brown EN, Solt K. Active emergence from propofol general anesthesia is induced by methylphenidate. Anesthesiology. 2012;116(5):998–1005.

10. Larijani GE, Goldberg ME, Hojat M, Khaleghi B, Dunn JB, Marr AT. Modafinil improves recovery after general anesthesia. Anesth Analg. 2004;98(4):976–81.
11. Galvin E, Boesjes H, Hol J, Ubben JF, Klein J, Verbrugge SJ. Modafinil reduces patient-reported tiredness after sedation/analgesia but does not improve patient psychomotor skills. Acta Anaesthesiol Scand. 2010;54(2):154–61.
12. Chambers NA, Pascoe E, Kaplanian S, Forsyth I. Ingestion of stimulant medications does not alter bispectral index or clinical depth of anesthesia at 1 MAC sevoflurane in children. Paediatr Anaesth. 2012;22(4):341–4.
13. Morimoto Y, Nogami Y, Harada K, Shiramoto H, Moguchi T. Anesthetic management of a patient with narcolepsy. J Anesth. 2011;25(3):435–7.
14. Webster L, Andrews M, Stoddard G. Modafinil treatment of opioid-induced sedation. Pain Med. 2003;4(2):135–40.
15. Roth T. Appropriate therapeutic selection for patients with shift work disorder. Sleep Med. 2012;13(4):335–41.

Chapter 24
Anticoagulant Drugs

Subarna Biswas, Jun Sasaki, and Michelle Braunfeld

Contents

Anticoagulation has been established as effective therapy for preventing stroke in atrial fibrillation, preventing and limiting venous thrombosis and embolism, and preventing extension of arterial thrombosis in both acute coronary syndrome and peripheral vascular disease. As well, it is mandatory for surgeries which require interruption of arterial flow and is necessary when blood is exposed to a foreign surface such as a cardiopulmonary bypass machine. Anticoagulants are thus used in both acute and chronic settings, and their mode of delivery (oral, intermittent injection, or intravenous) generally dictates their utility.

S. Biswas, MD (✉)
UCLA Department of Surgery, UCLA Medical Center, Los Angeles, CA, USA
e-mail: sbiswas@mednet.ucla.edu

J. Sasaki, MD • M. Braunfeld, MD
UCLA Department of Anesthesiology, David Geffen School of Medicine at UCLA, Los Angeles, CA, USA
e-mail: jsasaki@gmail.com; mbraunfeld@mednet.ucla.edu

A.D. Kaye et al. (eds.), *Essentials of Pharmacology for Anesthesia,*
Pain Medicine, and Critical Care, DOI 10.1007/978-1-4614-8948-1_24,
© Springer Science+Business Media New York 2015

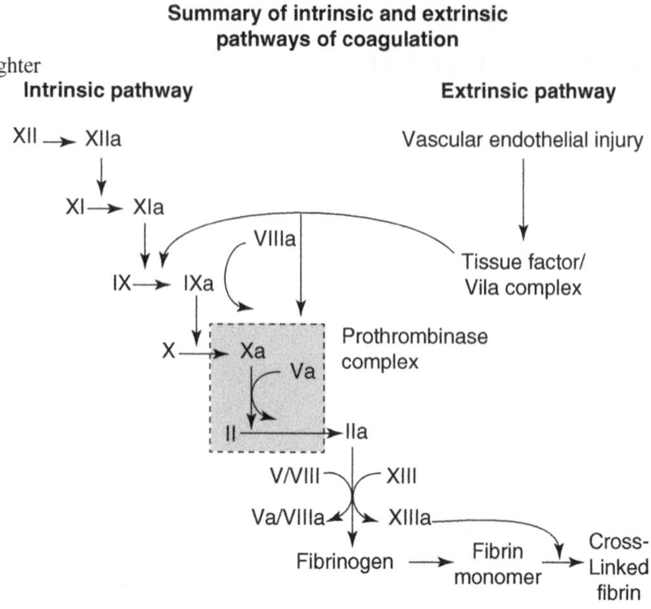

Fig. 24.1 Factor-based (historic) model of coagulation. From Slaughter [1]

Summary of intrinsic and extrinsic pathways of coagulation

The process of coagulation has been described and revised throughout the past century. Beginning in 1905 with the idea that a few coagulation factors could be serially enzymatically converted to end in the formation of a fibrin plug, the discovery of an ever-increasing number of additional factors in the process led to the concept of a veritable cascade of reactions culminating in the cross-linking of fibrin strands to form a functional clot. This series of reactions was separated into two pathways, described as the extrinsic (initiated by tissue factor, which resides external to blood flow) and intrinsic (thought to be entirely composed of factors within circulating blood). The extrinsic and intrinsic pathways converged into a final, common pathway at the point of activation of factor X which then continued to the production of fibrin. The function of the platelet in this "coagulation cascade" scenario was in a parallel role, both as a "first responder" to injury and subsequently as a structural component of the clot, enmeshed in cross-linked fibrin.

More recently it has been recognized that the separation of the coagulation process into extrinsic and intrinsic systems is an artificial construct that furthermore does not describe the very central role of platelets in clot formation. Nonetheless, the classic cascade scheme of the coagulation process is helpful in conceptualizing the process and understanding at which points different anticoagulants exert their effects (Fig. 24.1).

The coagulation process is divided into three phases: initiation, amplification, and propagation (Fig. 24.2).

Although coagulation is initiated by the extrinsic pathway, subsequent reactions reflect overlapping contributions from both the extrinsic and intrinsic

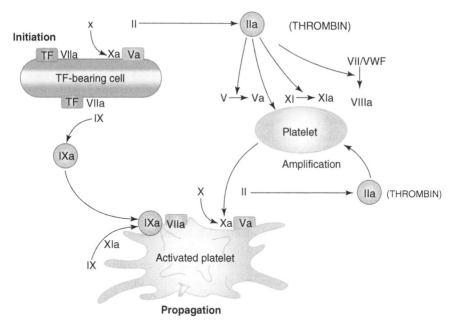

Fig. 24.2 Cell-based (contemporary) model of coagulation. From Woodruff et al. [2]

pathways. In initiation, an exposed tissue-factor-bearing cell (normally external to the circulation) binds to factor VII, activating it and leading to the production of a small amount of thrombin. This small amount of thrombin is the catalyst for several events in the amplification phase: activation of platelets to stick to the damaged vessel, activation of platelet-derived factors V and VIII (which complex to factors Xa and IXa, respectively), and activation of factor XI to initiate the intrinsic pathway and increase the supply of factor IX. The propagation phase is marked by explosive generation of thrombin, driven by the activated coagulation factors assembled on the platelet surface. Thrombin cleaves fibrinogen to form soluble fibrin strands, which then polymerize into cross-linked, insoluble fibrin. Clot is subsequently revised and limited by plasmin, which is generated from the cleavage of plasminogen by plasminogen activators. Plasmin cleaves fibrin into fibrin degradation products of varying molecular weights, the most clinically relevant being D-dimer.

Clinically available drugs that affect the clot formation and revision process can be divided into the following groups by mechanism: vitamin K antagonists (coumarin derivatives), direct and indirect thrombin inhibitors, direct factor Xa inhibitors, fibrinolytics, and antiplatelet agents. The ideal agent would be one with clinical efficacy over a wide range of indications at a once a day dose that does not require monitoring, but does have an easily assessed means of quantitating clinical effect that is not toxic, has a low incidence of bleeding complications, and can easily be reversed. All currently available agents have some of these qualities, but unfortunately, none has all.

Vitamin K Antagonists

Vitamin K antagonists (VKAs) inhibit vitamin K reductase and vitamin K epoxide reductase, preventing the vitamin K-mediated gamma-carboxylation of coagulation factors II, VII, IX, and X and anticoagulants protein S and protein C. Without carboxylation, these factors are nonfunctional. Since this is a posttranslational step, VKAs affect only factors synthesized after their administration. Those synthesized before are still fully functional. Because the half-lives of the already formulated vitamin K-dependent factors may range from 6 (factor VII) to 72 (factor II) hours, the anticoagulant effect is not immediate and makes dose titration cumbersome. It should be kept in mind that the relatively short half-life of protein C creates an initial imbalance favoring thrombosis on initiation of warfarin therapy. Thus the patient should be treated with another anticoagulant (typically unfractionated or low-molecular-weight heparin) until therapeutic INR is reached.

Vitamin K antagonists are approved for use in primary and secondary prevention of venous thromboembolism, for prevention of systemic embolism in patients with prosthetic heart valves or atrial fibrillation, for prevention of stroke, for prevention of acute myocardial infarction (AMI) in patients with peripheral arterial disease, and for prevention of recurrent MI or death in patients with AMI [3]. The classic vitamin K antagonist is warfarin. Warfarin is an oral agent that is readily absorbed and highly protein bound (99 %) [4]. It is essentially entirely eliminated by hepatic metabolism via the microsomal enzyme cytochrome P450-C29. Genetic mutations in this enzyme or alterations in hepatic function may increase sensitivity to warfarin. Conversely, genetic mutation of vitamin K epoxide reductase may account for observed resistance to warfarin [5]. The list of foods, drugs, and clinical conditions that may affect the metabolism of vitamin K or warfarin (and thus the state of anticoagulation) is lengthy and includes antibiotics, antimycotics, antidepressants, antiepilepsy drugs, antiarrythmics, statins, and food plants which contain the plant-based vitamin K, phylloquinone.

The vitamin K-dependent coagulation factors are all part of the extrinsic/common pathway and accordingly are monitored for clinical effect by measurement of the prothrombin time (PT). PT varies by the thromboplastin used in the assay and thus for the purposes of standardization is adjusted for the particular thromboplastin used and reported as the INR. Target INR recommended by the American Academy of Chest Physicians is 2.0–3.0. Options for reversal of VKAs include withholding the drug and/or administration of vitamin K, fresh-frozen plasma (FFP), or prothrombin complex concentrates (PCCs) [6]. While it is recommended that patients may routinely receive vitamin K for an INR >10.0 without evidence of bleeding, the use of FFP or PCC should be reserved for clinically significant bleeding. In the case of severe, life-threatening bleeding, a PCC may be preferable to FFP administration [7], and if available a four-factor complex is preferable to a three-factor complex [8]. In countries where four-factor complexes are not available (e.g., the United States), there is evidence that a three-factor complex plus RVIIa [9], three-factor complex plus FFP and vitamin K [10], or possibly RVIIa alone may control bleeding [6].

Indirect Thrombin Inhibitors

Currently available indirect thrombin inhibitors include unfractionated heparin (UFH), low-molecular-weight heparin (LMWH), and fondaparinux. UFH, LMWH, and fondaparinux may all be administered subcutaneously, but only UFH may be administered as a continuous infusion.

Heparin is a mucopolysaccharide that binds to, and potentiates the activity of the naturally occurring serine protease inhibitor, antithrombin III (ATIII). Many of the coagulation factors are serine proteases, and thus the heparin/ATIII complex inactivates several coagulation factors, most importantly thrombin (factor IIa) and factor Xa. Heparin/ATIII binding occurs via a unique pentasaccharide sequence present on only some heparin molecules, accounting for some of the variability in dose-response among patients.

The clinical effect of heparin is monitored with the activated prothrombin time (aPTT) or activated clotting time (ACT). Although there are no randomized prospective trials examining the appropriate aPTT target for prevention of recurrent VTE, a range of 1.5–2.5 times control is generally accepted [11]. This acceptance is complicated by the fact that the measured aPTT varies by the reagents and instruments used to obtain it. Heparin resistance is the state characterized by the requirement of unusually high doses of heparin to achieve a therapeutic aPTT. This may be caused by ATIII deficiency (in which the patient paradoxically requires FFP to achieve anticoagulation because of the ATIII it provides) or increased heparin clearance or heparin binding. UFH may be reversed by protamine sulfate in a ratio of 1 mg per 100 units of UFH.

Unfractionated heparin consists of molecules ranging in molecular weight from 3,000 to 30,000 kDa. Only about one-third of these molecules contain the requisite ATIII-binding pentasaccharide sequence. Within this fraction, smaller heparin molecules containing fewer than 18 saccharide units (roughly 6,000 kDa) are not sufficiently long to mediate ATIII binding to thrombin, but can still catalyze ATIII/factor Xa inactivation. Since factor Xa inactivation is not reflected in the aPTT, this may be another reason for variability in observed patient response. UFH is cleared by both a rapid, saturable reticuloendothelial system and slower, largely renal mechanism. Although a large proportion of clearance is nonrenal, patients with severe renal disease may require dosage adjustment. Because of this two-system clearance, UFH has a context-sensitive half-life ranging from 30 min after an IV bolus of 25 U/kg to 150 min with a bolus of 400 U/kg [11].

Among the feared complications of heparin administration is heparin-induced thrombocytopenia. This is an immune-mediated, prothrombotic phenomenon caused by the production of IgG antibodies against a heparin-platelet factor 4 (PF4) complex. These antibodies are capable of platelet activation, followed by thrombin generation, further platelet consumption, and culminating in the clinical picture of thrombocytopenia and thrombosis. Because the formation of a heparin/PF4 complex depends on the size of the heparin molecule, the incidence of HIT with UFH is three times higher than with LMWH [12].

Low-molecular-weight heparin molecules range in molecular weight from 2,000 to 9,000 kDa. Compared to UFH fewer of these molecules are sufficiently long to bridge ATIII to thrombin, thus LMWH exerts more of its effect by inactivating factor Xa. With 90 % bioavailability, lack of significant protein binding, and a 3–6 h half-life, LMWH is appropriate for subcutaneous injection and is approved for VTE prophylaxis and treatment in addition to treatment of non-ST elevation acute coronary syndromes [11]. It is typically administered in a fixed or weight-adjusted dose depending on indication. The predictability of LMWH makes monitoring generally considered unnecessary, but if needed the anti-Xa level is the test of choice.

Elimination of LMWH is largely renal, and there is uncertainty when and how to adjust dosing in the setting of renal insufficiency. It is recommended that consideration be given either to an alternate agent or to dose adjustment and monitoring with anti-Xa levels for patients with a creatinine clearance of <30 cc/min [11]. Protamine sulfate has only partial efficacy in reversing the effects of LMWH, neutralizing its antithrombin activity but only a portion of its anti-Xa activity. Nonetheless, it is recommended that in the event reversal is required within 8 h of a dose of LMWH, protamine be administered in a ratio of 1 mg per 100 anti-Xa units of LMWH [11].

Fondaparinux is a synthetic pentasaccharide developed to mimic the action of the necessary ATIII-binding pentasaccharide present in UFH and LMWH. The molecular weight of fondaparinux is 1,728 kDa. Thus it is not sufficiently long to bridge ATIII and thrombin to inactivate thrombin, but is capable of anti-Xa activity. The half-life of fondaparinux is 17 h, and it is almost entirely eliminated by renal excretion. Like LMWH fondaparinux has high bioavailability after subcutaneous injection and negligible binding to plasma proteins other than ATIII, not only making monitoring unnecessary but also making it appropriate for once a day administration. However, almost exclusive renal elimination mandates dose adjustment in moderate renal impairment and avoidance in severe renal insufficiency (creatinine clearance <30 mL/min). Reversal is problematic as well because fondaparinux does not bind protamine. Fondaparinux is indicated for VTE prophylaxis in joint replacement or abdominal surgery. Evidence for the association of fondaparinux with HIT is on the order of isolated case reports. Nonetheless it is not recommended for use in HIT [13].

Direct Thrombin Inhibitors

Direct thrombin inhibitors exert their action without the involvement of ATII and by directly binding thrombin. There are four drugs of this class commercially available: hirudin, bivalirudin, argatroban, and dabigatran. Of these, only dabigatran is administered orally. The rest are parenteral agents. The parenteral direct thrombin inhibitors are primarily used to treat patients with HIT or who require anticoagulation and are considered at risk to develop HIT. Dabigatran is poised to rival warfarin as the agent of choice for chronic anticoagulation.

Of the two hirudin derivatives, lepirudin and desirudin, only desirudin is currently still available. The hirudins may be administered either intravenously or subcutaneously, with half-lives of 60 and 120 min, respectively [11, 14]. They bind to both free and fibrin-bound thrombin in an essentially irreversible complex which makes reversal problematic in the acute setting. Desirudin is approved for postoperative thromboprophylaxis in hip replacement surgery and in that role does not require monitoring [15]. The hirudins are almost exclusively cleared by the kidneys and thus must be dose-adjusted when creatinine clearance is below 60 mL/min. Additionally, they are highly immunogenic and have been associated with anaphylactoid reactions [16].

Bivalirudin is a hirudin analog with two advantages over the hirudins: it is less dependent on renal excretion, which accounts for 20 % of its elimination, and it has a half-life of 25 min [15]. It is approved as an alternative to heparin for patients who either have or are at risk for HIT and are undergoing percutaneous cardiac intervention. The currently recommended dose regimen is a bolus of 0.75 mg/kg followed by an infusion of 1.75 mg/kg/h. Bivalirudin may be monitored by aPTT measurement, with a target of 1.5–2.5 times control [17].

Argatroban is a small molecule derived from L-arginine that reversibly binds to thrombin at its active catalytic site. It is approved for treatment and prevention of HIT and as an alternative to heparin in patients undergoing percutaneous cardiac intervention who have HIT or who are considered at risk to develop HIT. It has a plasma half-life of 45 min and is metabolized in the liver by the P450 3A4/5 system. Thus it is particularly attractive for patients with renal impairment. Argatroban is administered as an intravenous infusion of 1–2 mcg/kg/min and titrated to an aPTT of 1.5–2.5 times control.

Dabigatran is an oral direct thrombin inhibitor that binds reversibly to the active site of thrombin. Although it is under evaluation for VTE prophylaxis after joint replacement, for secondary prevention of VTE, and for use in acute coronary syndromes, in the United States and Canada it is currently approved only for the prevention of stroke or systemic embolism in non-valvular atrial fibrillation. The pivotal trial supporting this was the Randomized Evaluation of Long-Term Anticoagulation (RE-LY) trial, which concluded that when used for stroke prevention in non-valvular atrial fibrillation, dabigatran at a dose of 150 mg twice a day was more effective than warfarin and associated with a similar rate of major hemorrhage. At a dose of 110 mg twice a day, dabigatran was as effective as warfarin and associated with lower rates of major hemorrhage [18].

Dabigatran is not well absorbed after oral administration and so is given as the prodrug dabigatran etexilate. Dabigatran is predominantly excreted by the kidneys and has a plasma half-life of 12–14 h [19]. Gender and body weight do not affect pharmacokinetics, but renal insufficiency and age do. Although age >75 years was not a condition of exclusion in RE-LY, a creatinine clearance of <30 mL/min was. Thus dabigatran is contraindicated in severe renal insufficiency, but dose adjustment may be appropriate in the elderly.

Unlike warfarin, dabigatran has no interactions with foods, is not metabolized by any enzymes of the cytochrome P450 complex, and has few drug interactions. For these reasons, monitoring is felt to be unnecessary. However, in the setting of emergency surgery or major hemorrhage, standard coagulation tests are likely to be inadequate to define drug effect. Although dabigatran prolongs aPTT and ACT, there is poor correlation between dabigatran plasma levels and measured aPTT or ACT. Thrombin time (TT) is overly sensitive to dabigatran, but may be used to determine presence of the drug. Both ecarin clotting time (ECT) and the proprietary HEMOCLOT thrombin inhibitor assay show a linear correlation between assay measurements and plasma concentrations of dabigatran at clinically relevant levels [20, 21]. However, neither is currently readily available.

Also problematic is the lack of a reversal agent for dabigatran. In the setting of major hemorrhage or emergency surgery, unlike the intravenous direct thrombin inhibitors, the half-life of dabigatran is sufficiently long that withdrawing the drug and waiting for the effect to dissipate may not be an option. Treatment is anecdotal and empirical but on the basis of animal studies, it appears that while 3- or 4-factor PCC, RVIIa, or an activated prothrombin complex concentrate (aPCC, e.g., FEIBA) may all be considered for reversal of catastrophic bleeding related to dabigatran, aPCC may be preferred if available [22–25]. Other measures to consider are activated charcoal in the setting of recent ingestion and dialysis since dabigatran is not highly protein bound. An open label study of a single dose dabigatran in patients with end-stage renal failure on dialysis found a mean difference in drug levels of 62 % between inlet and outlet lines after 2 h of dialysis [26].

Factor Xa Inhibitors

The limitations of warfarin prompted the development of new oral anticoagulants that target factor Xa. Factor Xa binds platelet-bound Va to form prothrombinase, the complex that converts prothrombin to thrombin. Each molecule of factor Xa generates about 1,000 molecules of thrombin through the prothrombinase complex in a key amplification step that results in a flare of thrombin generation at sites of injury [27]. These drugs are unaffected by dietary vitamin K intake, have a wide therapeutic index, and can be administered in fixed doses without routine coagulation monitoring [3, 8].

Oral factor Xa inhibitors are active compounds that interact with the catalytic pocket of factor Xa. They have mixed renal and fecal excretion and a rapid onset of action with good oral bioavailability [28]. Factor Xa inhibitors do not require monitoring and theoretically do not prevent the generation of sufficient amounts of thrombin for hemostasis.

In the orthopedic setting, rivaroxaban at 10 mg daily has been compared with enoxaparin for thromboprophylaxis in the four trials (Regulation of Coagulation in Orthopedic Surgery to Prevent Deep Vein Thrombosis and Pulmonary Embolism, RECORD 1, 2, 3, and 4). The rate of venous thromboembolism was significantly lower with rivaroxaban than with enoxaparin in patients undergoing elective hip or knee arthroplasty [29–32] with no significant increase in life-threatening hemorrhage. However, in a trial of medically ill patients (Venous Thromboembolic Event Prophylaxis in Medically Ill Patients, MAGELLAN), the rate of VTE was reduced with extended rivaroxaban prophylaxis, but this group also experienced more bleeding complications [33]. In patients with atrial fibrillation (Rivaroxaban Once Daily Oral Direct Factor Xa Inhibitor Compared with Vitamin K Antagonism for Prevention of Stroke and Embolism Trial in Atrial Fibrillation, ROCKET-AF), Rivaroxaban at 10 mg daily has been found to work as well as warfarin in the prevention of stroke or system embolism and significantly lowers rates of hemorrhagic stroke and fatal bleeding [34]. Rivaroxaban is licensed in the United States as an alternative to warfarin for stroke prevention in AF and for VTE prophylaxis after elective hip or knee arthroplasty.

Apixaban has also been evaluated for stroke prevention in AF (Apixaban for the Prevention of Stroke in Subjects with Atrial Fibrillation, ARISTOTLE). Compared with warfarin, apixaban at 5 mg daily was superior in preventing stroke or systemic embolism and produced significantly less major bleeding [35]. Compared to aspirin in the AVERROES trial, apixaban was also better at preventing stroke or systemic embolism in patients with AF and had similar rates of bleeding [36]. For thromboprophylaxis in the orthopedic setting (ADVANCE 1, 2, 3), apixaban was better than enoxaparin in patients undergoing knee or hip replacement surgery at preventing clots. Rates of bleeding were not significantly different [37–39]. Apixaban is FDA approved for use in stroke prevention in AF and in Canada and Europe for VTE prophylaxis after hip or knee arthroplasty.

Both agents are partially excreted by the kidneys, and the drugs are contraindicated in patients with a creatinine clearance (CrCl) less than 30 mL/min for VTE prophylaxis and less than 15 mL/min in AF. Rivaroxaban is excreted partially by the liver in a CYP-dependent manner. It has strong interactions with azole drugs such as ketoconazole and fluconazole. Amiodarone, diltiazem, and azithromycin are expected inhibitors of rivaroxaban metabolism, while rifampin, Dilantin, and St. John's wort are potential inducers. Apixaban does not affect CYP enzymes and is expected to have few drug-drug interactions, though this has not been directly studied [40]. Factor Xa inhibitors should be stopped 24 h prior to procedures in patients with normal renal function and 2 days earlier for those with CrCl less than 50.

There is currently no reversal protocol for bleeding patients on these new agents. Use should be avoided in patients with hepatic disease associated with coagulopathy. They are highly protein bound and hemodialysis is ineffective. Activated charcoal can be used as an antidote to the drugs if recently ingested. A small study of healthy volunteers given rivaroxaban was able to show immediate reversal of drug and normalization of PT, PTT, and endogenous thrombin potential with nonactivated prothrombin complex concentrate (PCC) [41], though this has yet to be replicated in a larger clinical setting.

Fibrinolytic Drugs

Thrombolytic agents lyse fibrin by initiating the conversion of plasminogen to plasmin, which then degrades fibrin and fibrinogen. Several enzymes found in urine, blood, and tissues serve as physiologic activators of thrombolysis and served as a basis to develop the first generation of fibrinolytic drugs.

Of these, streptokinase is indicated for use in lysis of pulmonary emboli, extensive deep vein thromboses, and arterial emboli. In the setting of acute myocardial infarction, it has shown associated improvement in ventricular function and a mortality benefit when used to lyse intracoronary clots. Streptokinase may also be used to clear occluded arteriovenous cannulae. The streptokinase protein is derived from hemolytic streptococci and initiates fibrinolysis by forming an active complex with plasminogen. It is highly antigenic due to its bacterial origin, which limits its use. Another major limitation is the potential to cause life-threatening bleeding due to its systemic fibrinolytic activity [42]. Streptokinase has largely been supplanted by newer agents.

Anistreplase, a complex of human plasminogen and acetylated streptokinase, has a longer half-life than streptokinase and requires only a single bolus injection. Once spontaneous hydrolysis of the acyl group occurs, the complex is activated and thrombolysis begins. A randomized, double-blind clinical trial (GREAT study) has shown a mortality benefit and a cost advantage to prehospital thrombolysis with anistreplase in acute MI. Like streptokinase, anistreplase does have immunogenic properties, though the presence of neutralizing antibodies has been theorized to dampen its systemic effects [43].

Though at present there is no agent available that completely avoids systemic fibrinolysis, alteplase has greater fibrin specificity than streptokinase and anistreplase. Alteplase is an unmodified human tissue-type plasminogen activator that has been manufactured by recombinant DNA technology. In comparison with streptokinase and heparin, patients with evolving MI who received t-PA and heparin had a 14 % reduction in mortality and a lower combined endpoint of death or disabling stroke. Vessel patency at 90 min was also highest with t-PA and heparin together [44]. For acute, ischemic stroke, one trial of alteplase versus placebo showed an improvement in disability at 3 months with t-PA treatment initiated within 3 h of symptom onset; however mortality rates at 3 months were not different, and rates of intracerebral bleeding were higher [45].

Reteplase is a modified recombinant version of t-PA with a nonglycosylated deletion. It has a longer half-life and greater specificity for fibrin than alteplase. Angiographic patency of coronary vessels treated with reteplase appears better than alteplase. In a large randomized clinical trial, reteplase was non-inferior to alteplase when used for reperfusion in acute MI, with a similar low rate of bleeding complications [46]. Reteplase has the advantage of bolus dosing. It is approved by the FDA for use in myocardial revascularization.

Tenecteplase is also a recombinant t-PA engineered in mammalian cells with modifications at three sites, allowing for a longer half-life and bolus dosing, with high resistance to physiologic inhibitors. Results have been shown to be similar to alteplase infusion in acute MI, with equivalent 30 day mortality benefits and an equally low incidence of bleeding and hemorrhagic stroke [47]. In acute stroke, a recent trial has shown that tenecteplase at high doses (0.25 mg/kg) is superior to alteplase in terms of radiographic improvement in lesions and in clinical improvement at 24 h, with a similar rate of adverse events [48]. Tenecteplase is currently FDA approved only for use in acute MI.

Antiplatelet Agents

Platelets that adhere to injured endothelium release adenosine diphosphate and thromboxane Ax, both of which trigger platelet aggregation. Thromboxane A2 is also a potent vasoconstrictor. In addition to aspirin, more recently developed antiplatelet agents are available.

Ticlopidine is an adenosine diphosphate receptor inhibitor in the thienopyridine family. It is approved for use in stroke prophylaxis and in prevention of coronary stent thrombosis, but it has been associated with a low rate of thrombotic thrombocytopenic purpura and severe neutropenia and requires initial monitoring of white cell counts. The use of ticlopidine has largely been supplanted by newer agents.

Clopidogrel is a thienopyridine derivative that selectively inhibits adenylate cyclase, leading to inhibition of platelet aggregation. The efficacy of clopidogrel has been compared to aspirin in reducing the combined risk of ischemic stroke, MI, or vascular death. There was an additional 8.7 % risk reduction with clopidogrel, with no significant differences in side effects including neutropenia [49]. Clopidogrel is approved by the FDA for prevention of stroke, MI, and vascular disease in patients with documented atherosclerotic disease.

Prasugrel, a newer thienopyridine with a more rapid onset, has been compared with clopidogrel in a large randomized clinical trial of patients with acute coronary syndromes undergoing scheduled percutaneous coronary intervention. Though there were significantly lower rates of ischemic events and stent thrombosis with prasugrel therapy, there was also an increased risk of major bleeding, with similar overall mortality rates [50]. In patients who were medically managed, there were no significant benefits to the use of prasugrel. Prasugrel is indicated for reduction of thrombotic cardiovascular events in patients managed with percutaneous coronary intervention.

Abciximab is a monoclonal antibody that targets the integrin glycoprotein IIb/IIIa receptor complex, which induces platelet aggregation by cross-linking receptors on nearby platelets when activated. A randomized double-blind clinical trial evaluated abciximab as an adjunct to heparin and aspirin to prevent acute vessel closure in patients undergoing percutaneous transluminal coronary angioplasty or atherectomy. When abciximab was given as a bolus and infusion at the time of intervention, outcomes were improved for up to 3 years [51] Abciximab is approved for high-risk angioplasty and atherectomy procedures by the FDA. It is antigenic, especially with repeated administrations.

Eptifibatide is a cyclic heptapeptide and a reversible antagonist of the GPIIb/IIIa receptor. Unlike abciximab it reverses within a few hours of cessation. In a trial assessing eptifibatide's efficacy in preventing restenosis in patients undergoing coronary intervention, there was no evidence of antigenicity with this drug and no increased risk of bleeding [52]. Eptifibatide was approved by the FDA 4 years after abciximab, for use in patients undergoing percutaneous coronary interventions and for treatment of acute coronary syndrome.

Another reversible antagonist of the GPIIb/IIIa is tirofiban, nonpeptide molecule. Two studies have shown a mortality benefit in using tirofiban with aspirin or heparin in patients with acute coronary syndrome. There appears to be little risk of bleeding complications or antigenicity in these studies [53]. Tirofiban is approved for treatment of patients with unstable angina or non-Q-wave MI.

Phosphodiesterase Inhibitors

Dipyridamole is a cyclic adenosine monophosphate (cAMP)-phosphodiesterase inhibitor which increases cAMP and leads to vascular smooth muscle relaxation and vasodilation. It also inhibits platelet aggregation by inhibiting cyclooxygenase and phospholipase. Extended-release dipyridamole is used in combination with aspirin (under the trade name Aggrenox) to prevent stroke in patients with cerebrovascular disease, which in some meta-analyses is better than aspirin alone [54]. Dipyridamole alone may be used to prevent thrombosis after cardiac valve replacement, in conjunction with warfarin. Absorption is pH dependent and inhibited by gastric acid suppression. Bleeding events, though otherwise rare, have been increased with concomitant use of aspirin and clopidogrel. Aminophylline can reverse the hemodynamic effects of dipyridamole, but there is no antidote to the antiplatelet actions.

Pentoxifylline and Pletal are nonselective phosphodiesterase inhibitors which similarly cause vasodilation and inhibit platelet aggregation. In patients with chronic lower extremity peripheral arterial occlusive disease, cilostazol has been shown to improve ankle-brachial indices and clinically increase maximum walking distance [55]. Both drugs are approved for treatment of symptoms of intermittent claudication and are increasingly also used in vascular dementia and Peyronie's disease.

Summary

Coagulation is a dynamic, intricate system that limits blood loss and repairs injury while maintaining blood flow. It can be modified through several mechanisms, and novel agents continue to provide active areas of study and development. The pharmacokinetic properties [56] of drugs described in this chapter follow (Table 24.1).

Table 24.1 Summary of drugs

	Dose	Oral bioavailability	Time to peak activity	Half-life	Renal clearance
Warfarin	1–10 mg po daily	100 %	4–5 days	40 h	None
Heparin	varies	None	5–10 min	1–2 h	<10 %
LMWH	30 mg SQ BID	None	3–5 h	3–6 h	>80 %
Fondaparinux	2.5 mg SQ BID	None	2–4 h	17 h	Near 100 %
Desirudin	15 mg/kg SQ	None	1–2 h	2 h	100 %
Bivalirudin	0.75 mg/kg bolus then 1.75 mg/kg/h	None	Minutes	25 min	20 %
Argatroban	1–10 ucg/kg/h	None	Minutes	45 min	NS
Dabigatran	150 mg po BID	6–7 % (prodrug)	1–3 h	14–17 h	100 %
Rivaroxaban	10 mg po daily	50 %	1–2 h	12 h	25 %
Apixaban	5 mg po daily	80 %	2–3 h	7–11 h	33 %
Streptokinase	MI: 1.5 mil U iv PE: 250,000 U iv then 100,000 U/h	None	30 min	20 min	None
Alteplase	0.9 mg/kg iv	None	30–60 min	5 min	None
Tenecteplase	0.5 mg/kg iv bolus	None	Minutes	90 min	None
Reteplase	10 U iv q30 min × 2	None	2 h	13–16 min	60 %
Ticlopidine	250 mg po	80 %	2 h	12 h	None
Clopidogrel	75 mg po daily (300 mg loading dose)	50 %	4–6 h with loading dose, 3–5 days without	6 h	50 %
Prasugrel	60 mg po loading, then 10 mg daily	80 %	4 h	3–4 h	None
Ticagrelor	180 mg po loading, then 90 mg twice daily	36 %	1.5 h	7 h	None
Abciximab	250 mcg iv, then 0.125 mcg/kg/min	None	2 h	30 min	None
Eptifibatide	180 mcg/kg bolus, then 2 mcg/kg/min infusion	None	2 min	2.5 h	50 %
Tirofiban	0.4 mcg/kg/min for 30 min, then 0.1 mcg/kg/min	None	30 min	2 h	65 %
Dipyridamole	200 mg po given with 25 mg Aspirin BID	37 %	2 h	13–15 h	5 %
Pentoxifylline	400 mg po daily	100 %	1–4 h	1–2 h	60 %
Cilostazol	100 mg po BID	90 %	2–4 h	11–13 h	30 %

Chemical Structures

**Chemical Structure
24.1** Warfarin

**Chemical Structure
24.2** Dipyridamole

**Chemical Structure
24.3** Dabigatran etexilate

References

1. Slaughter T. Atlas of cardiothoracic anesthesia, Current Medicine Group, Philadelphia PA. vol 1, chapter 11. 2009.
2. Woodruff B, Sullenger B, Becker RC. Antithrombotic therapy in acute coronary syndrome: how far up the coagulation cascade will we go? Curr Cardiol Rep. 2010;12(4):315–20.
3. Hirsch J, Warkentin TE, Shaughnessy SG, Anand SS, Halperin JL, Raschke R, et al. Heparin and low-molecular-weight heparin. Chest. 2001;119:64S–94.
4. Jacobs LG. Warfarin pharmacology, clinical management, and evaluation of hemorrhagic risk for the elderly. Cardiol Clin. 2008;26:157–67.
5. Dzik W. Reversal of drug-induced anticoagulation: old solutions and new problems. Transfusion. 2012;52:45S–55.
6. Ageno W, Gallus AS, Wittkowsky A, Crowther M, Hylek EM, Palareti G. Oral anticoagulant therapy. Chest. 2012;141(2):e44S–88.
7. Guyatt GH, Akl EA, Crowther M, Gutterman DD, Schunemann HJ. Executive summary antithrombotic therapy and prevention of thrombosis, 9th ed: American college of chest physicians evidence-based clinical practice guidelines. Chest. 2012;141(2):7s–47.
8. Voils SA, Baird B. Systematic review: 3-factor versus 4-factor prothrombin complex concentrate for warfarin reversal: does it matter? Thromb Res. 2012;130:833–40.
9. Sarode R, Matevosyan K, Bhagat R, Rutherford C, Madden C, Beshay JE. Rapid warfarin reversal: a 3-factor prothrombin complex concentrate and recombinant factor VIIa cocktail for intracerebral hemorrhage. J Neurosurg. 2012;116:491–7.
10. Cabral KP, Fraser GL, Duprey J, Gibbons BA, Hayes T, Florman JE, et al. Prothrombin complex concentrates to reverse warfarin-induced coagulopathy in patients with intracranial bleeding. Clin Neurol Neurosurg. 2013;115(6):770–4.
11. Garcia DA, Baglin TP, Weitz JI, Samama MM. Parenteral anticoagulants. Chest. 2012;141(2): e24S–43.
12. Warkentin TE, Levine MN, Hirsh J, Horsewood P, Roberts RS, Gent M, et al. Heparin- induced thrombocytopenia in patients treated with low-molecular-weight heparin or unfractionated heparin. N Engl J Med. 1995;332:1330–5.
13. Linkins L, Dans AL, Moores LK, Bona R, Davidson BL, Schulman S, et al. Treatment and prevention of heparin-induced thrombocytopenia. Chest. 2012;141(2):e495S–530.
14. Harder S, Klinkhardt U, Alvarez JM. Avoidance of bleeding during surgery in patients receiving anticoagulant and/or antiplatelet therapy. Clin Pharmacokinet. 2004;43(14):963–81.
15. Warkentin TE. Bivalent direct thrombin inhibitors: hirudin and bivalirudin. Best Prac Res Clin Haematol. 2004;17:105–25.
16. Greinacher P, Lubenow N, Eichler P. Anaphylactic and anaphylactoid reactions associated with lepirudin in patients with heparin-induced thrombocytopenia. Circulation. 2003;108:2062–5.
17. Kelton JG, Arnold DM, Bates SM. Nonheparin anticoagulants for heparin-induced thrombocytopenia. N Engl J Med. 2013;368:737–44.
18. Connolly SJ, Ezekowitz MD, Yusuf S, Eikelboom J, Oldgren J, Parekh A. Dabigatran versus warfarin in patients with atrial fibrillation. N Engl J Med. 2009;361:1139–51.
19. Stangier J, Clemens A. Pharmacology, pharmacokinetics, and pharmacodynamics of dabigatran etexilate an oral direct thrombin inhibitor. Clin Appl Thromb Hemost. 2009;15(1S):9S–16.
20. Van Ryn J, Stangier J, Haertter S, Liesenfeld K, Wienen W, Feuring M, et al. Dabigatran etexilate – a novel, reversible, oral direct thrombin inhibitor: interpretation of coagulation assays and reversal of anticoagulant activity. Thromb Haemost. 2010;103:1116–27.
21. Tripodi A, Di Iorio G, Lippi G, Testa S, Manotti C. Position paper on laboratory testing for patients taking new oral anticoagulants. Clin Chem Lab Med. 2012;50:2137–40.
22. Siegal DM, Cuker A. Reversal of novel oral anticoagulants in patients with major bleeding. J Thromb Thrombolysis. 2013;35(3):391–8.
23. Miyares MA, Davis K. Newer oral anticoagulants: a review of laboratory monitoring options and reversal agents in the hemorrhagic patient. Am J Health Syst Pharm. 2012;69:1473–84.

24. Khoo TL, Weatherburn C, Kershaw G, Reddel CJ, Curnow J, Dunkley S. The use of FEIBA in the correction of coagulation abnormalities induced by dabigatran. Int J Lab Hematol. 2013. doi:10.1111/ijlh.12005. Epub 2012 Sep 28.

25. Harinstein LM, Morgan JW, Russo N. Treatment of dabigatran-associated bleeding: case report and review of the literature. J Pharm Prac. 2013;26(3):264–9.

26. Stangier J, Rathgen K, Stahle H, Mazur D. Influence of renal impairment on the pharmacokinetics and pharmacodynamics of oral dabigatran etexilate. Clin Pharmacokinet. 2010;49:259–68.

27. Mann KG, Butenas S, Brummel K. The dynamics of thrombin formation. Arterioscler Thromb Vasc Biol. 2003;23:17–25.

28. Yeh CH, Frendenburgh JC, Weitz JI. Oral direct factor Xa inhibitors. Circ Res. 2012;111: 1069–78.

29. Eriksson BI, Borris LC, Friedman RJ, Haas S, Huisman MV, Kakkar AK, Bandel TJ, Beckmann H, Muehlhofer E, Misselwitz F, Geerts W. Rivaroxaban versus enoxaparin for thromboprophylaxis after hip arthroplasty. N Engl J Med. 2008;358:2765–75.

30. Kakkar AK, Brenner B, Dahl OE, Eriksson BI, Mouret P, Muntz J, Soglian AG, Pap AF, Misselwitz F, Haas RECORD2 Investigators. Extended duration of rivaroxaban versus short term enoxaparin for prevention of venous thromboembolism after total hip arthroplasty: a double-blind, randomised controlled trial. Lancet. 2008;372:31–9.

31. Lassen MR, Ageno W, Borris LC, Lieberman JR, Rosencher N, Bandel TJ, Misselwitz F, Turpie AG, RECORD3 Investigators. Rivaroxaban versus enoxaparin for thromboprophylaxis after total knee arthroplasty. N Engl J Med. 2008;358:2776–86.

32. Turpie AG, Lassen MR, Davidson BL, Bauer KA, Gent M, Kwong LM, Cushner FD, Lotke PA, Berkowitz S, Bandel TJ, Benson A, Misselwitz F, Fisher W, RECORD4 Investigators. Rivaroxaban versus enoxaparin for thromboprophylaxis after total knee arthroplasty: a randomised trial. Lancet. 2009;373:1673–80.

33. Cohen AT, Spiro TE, Büller HR, Haskell L, Hu D, Hull R, Mebazaa A, Merli G, Schellong S, Spyropoulos AC, Tapson V. Rivaroxaban for thromboprophylaxis in acutely ill medical patients. N Engl J Med. 2013;368:513–23.

34. Patel MR, Mahaffey KW, Garg J, et al. and for the ROCKET AF Investigators and the ROCKET AF Steering Committee. Rivaroxaban versus warfarin in nonvalvular atrial fibrillation. N Engl J Med. 2011;385(10):883–91.

35. Granger CB, Alexander JH, McMurray JJ, Lopes RD, Hylek EM, Hanna M, Al-Khalidi HR, Ansell J, Atar D, Avezum A, Bahit MC, Diaz R, Easton JD, Ezekowitz JA, Flaker G, Garcia D, Geraldes M, Gersh BJ, Golitsyn S, Goto S, Hermosillo AG, Hohnloser SH, Horowitz J. Apixaban versus warfarin in patients with atrial fibrillation. N Engl J Med. 2011;11:981–92.

36. Connolly SJ, Eikelboom J, Joyner C, Diener HC, Hart R, Golitsyn S, Flaker G, Avezum A, Hohnloser SH, Diaz R, Talajic M, Zhu J, Pais P, Budaj A, Parkhomenko A, Jansky P, Commerford P, Tan RS, Sim KH, Lewis BS, Van Mieghem W, Lip GY, Kim JH, Lanas-Zanetti F. Apixaban in patients with atrial fibrillation. N Essngl J Med. 2011;364(9):806–17.

37. Lassen MR, Raskob GE, Gallus A, Pineo G, Chen D, Portman RJ. Apixaban or enoxaparin for thromboprophylaxis after knee replacement. N Engl J Med. 2009;361:594–604.

38. Lassen MR, Gallus A, Raskob GE, Pineo G, Chen D, Ramirez LM. Apixaban versus enoxaparin for thromboprophylaxis after hip replacement. N Engl J Med. 2010;363:2487–98.

39. Lassen MR, Raskob GE, Gallus A, Pineo G, Chen D, Hornick P. Apixaban versus enoxaparin for thromboprophylaxis after knee replacement (ADVANCE-2): a randomised double-blind trial. Lancet. 2010;375:807–15.

40. Garcia D, Libby E, Crowther MA. The new oral anticoagulants. Blood. 2010;15(1):15–20.

41. Eerenberg E. Reversal of rivaroxaban and dabigatran by PCC. Circulation. 2011;124:1573–9.

42. Frangos SG, Chen AH, Sumpio B. Vascular drugs in the new millennium. J Am Coll Surg. 2000;191(1):76–92.

43. Rawles J. Magnitude of benefit from earlier thrombolytic treatment in acute myocardial infarction: new evidence from Grampian region early anistreplase trial (GREAT). BMJ. 1996; 312(7025):212–5.

44. Investigators, The GUSTO. An international randomized trial comparing four thrombolytic strategies for acute myocardial infarction. N Engl J Med. 1993;329:673–82.
45. The National Institute of Neurological Disorders and Stroke rt-PA Stroke Study Group. Tissue plasminogen activator for acute stroke. N Engl J Med. 1995;333(24):1581–7.
46. Investigators, GUSTO III. A comparison of reteplase with alteplase for acute myocardial infarction. N Engl J Med. 1997;337:1118–23.
47. Investigators, ASSENT-2. Single-bolus tenecteplase compared with front-loaded alteplase in acute myocardial infarction: the ASSENT-2 double-blind randomised trial. Lancet. 1999;354(9180):716–22.
48. Parsons M, Spratt N, Bivard A, Campbell B, Chung K, Miteff F, O'Brien B, Bladin C, McElduff P, Allen C, Bateman G, Donnan GM. A randomized trial of tenecteplase versus alteplase for acute ischemic stroke. N Engl J Med. 2012;366:1099–107.
49. Committee, CAPRIE Steering. A randomised, blinded, trial of clopidogrel versus aspirin in patients at risk of ischaemic events (CAPRIE). CAPRIE Steering Committee. Lancet. 1996;348(9038):1329–39.
50. Wiviott SD, Braunwald E, McCabe CH, Montalescot G, Ruzyllo W, Gottlieb S, et al. Prasugrel versus clopidogrel in patients with acute coronary syndromes. N Engl J Med. 2007;357:2001–15.
51. Investigators, EPIC. Use of a monoclonal antibody directed against the platelet glycoprotein IIb/IIIa receptor in high-risk coronary angioplasty. The EPIC Investigation. N Engl J Med. 1994;330(14):956–61.
52. Group, IMPACT Study. Randomised placebo-controlled trial of effect of eptifibatide on complications of percutaneous coronary intervention: IMPACT-II. Integrilin to minimise platelet aggregation and coronary thrombosis-II. Lancet. 1997;349(9063):1422–8.
53. Investigators, PRISM-PLUS Study. Inhibition of the platelet glycoprotein IIb/IIIa receptor with tirofiban in unstable angina and Non–Q-wave myocardial infarction. N Engl J Med. 1998;338:1488–97.
54. Group, ESPRIT Study. Aspirin plus dipyridamole versus aspirin alone after cerebral ischaemia of arterial origin (ESPRIT): randomised controlled trial. Lancet. 2006;367(9523):1665–73.
55. Dawson DL, Cutler BS, Meissner MH, et al. Cilostazol has beneficial effects in treatment of intermittent claudication: results from a multicenter, randomized, prospective, double-blind trial. Circulation. 1998;98:679–86.
56. Federal Drug Bibliography Administration, Drugs@DFA. 2012. http://www.accessdata.fda.gov/scripts/cder/drugsatfda/index.cfm. Accessed 27 Mar 2013.

Chapter 25
Hemostatic Agents

John S. McNeil and M. Dustin Boone

Contents

Introduction

Excessive bleeding during the perioperative period increases morbidity and mortality. Thus, significant effort has been focused on a variety of methods for controlling blood loss. In addition to traditional methods, drugs have been developed to interact at specific sites along the coagulation cascade to enhance clotting and reduce bleeding. These drugs are known as hemostatic agents. In certain populations at high risk for bleeding, such as patients undergoing major cardiac and orthopedic procedures, as well as trauma patients and those who refuse blood transfusion, the administration of hemostatic drugs may be indicated.

J.S. McNeil, MD (✉) • M.D. Boone, MD
Department of Anesthesia, Harvard Medical School, Boston, MA, USA

Department of Anesthesia, Critical Care and Pain Medicine,
Beth Israel Deaconess Medical Center, Boston, MA 02215, USA
e-mail: jsmcneil@bidmc.harvard.edu; mboone@bidmc.harvard.edu

A.D. Kaye et al. (eds.), *Essentials of Pharmacology for Anesthesia,*
Pain Medicine, and Critical Care, DOI 10.1007/978-1-4614-8948-1_25,
© Springer Science+Business Media New York 2015

Drug Class and Mechanism of Action

Antifibrinolytics are analogs or derivatives of the amino acid lysine. They induce a structural change in plasminogen, which inhibits its conversion to plasmin. A potent enzyme, plasmin degrades many proteins in the blood especially fibrin clots, a process known as fibrinolysis. Aminocaproic acid and tranexamic acid (TXA) are the two most commonly used medications in this class. TXA is six to ten times as potent as aminocaproic acid, which is commonly known by the trade name Amicar.

Aprotinin has a different mechanism of action. It inhibits several other proteases in addition to plasmin including chymotrypsin, kallikrein, tissue plasminogen activator, and trypsin,

In cases of severe bleeding and/or coagulopathy, these medications often will be given after transfusion of products such as fresh frozen plasma or cryoprecipitate; these modalities are covered in detail in Chap. 24.

Indications/Clinical Pearls

Antifibrinolytics are used to treat excess intraoperative and postoperative bleeding related to fibrinolysis. They are particularly useful as prophylaxis in major cardiac and orthopedic surgeries when large blood loss is anticipated. They may be used in other situations when bleeding occurs: in thrombophilic patients (especially mucosal bleeding), in women with excess menstrual bleeding, and in liver transplantation. Antifibrinolytics may be indicated as an antidote to excessive fibrinolysis (i.e., tissue plasminogen activator overdose).

It is well established that tranexamic acid reduces bleeding and transfusion rates in a wide variety of surgeries. A meta-analysis looking at 129 different trials found that transfusion rates were one-third less with TXA [1]. This reduction helps avoid the many side effects associated with blood product transfusion.

The use of these agents has been widely studied in cardiac surgery, and their beneficial effects on blood loss reduction and decreased transfusion rates have been well documented [2]. Although many centers now employ antifibrinolytics universally with cardiopulmonary bypass, it is most beneficial in situations when excess bleeding may occur. Examples include repeat operations, surgeries without blood transfusion (i.e., Jehovah's Witnesses), and patients with pre-existing coagulopathy or recent use of gpIIb/IIIa inhibitors [3].

In orthopedic surgery, antifibrinolytics decrease blood loss and transfusions [4], but additional studies are needed to evaluate overall outcomes. Topical use of antifibrinolytics is one promising application that early studies show may help reduce bleeding with the potential for less systemic side effects [5].

These agents can also be used in trauma. The large CRASH-2 study found that TXA reduced mortality in bleeding trauma patients without increasing the risk of adverse events [6]. TXA should be given as early as possible and within 3 h of injury. Treatment later than 3 h may actually increase the risk of death from bleeding.

Dosing Options

Aminocaproic acid must be diluted, usually in 250 mL of diluent. It is typically administered as an intravenous bolus of 4–5 g followed by a 1 g per hour infusion. Alternatively, the loading dose can be between 50 and 75 mg/kg with an infusion of 25 mg/kg/h.

Tranexamic acid is most commonly bolused at 10 mg/kg followed by a 1–5 mg/kg/h infusion. In some cases, particularly in orthopedics, a bolus alone may suffice. Lower doses should be given in patients with renal failure to limit accumulation.

In cardiac cases, antifibrinolytics are usually stopped before chest closure. In noncardiac cases, it is recommended that the infusion be continued for 8 h or until bleeding stops.

Aminocaproic acid can also be administered orally for mucosal bleeding.

Drug Interactions

In theory, antifibrinolytics may interfere with heparin during cardiac bypass, posing a risk of thrombosis. However, this concern has not been observed clinically. Administration of antifibrinolytics does not need to be delayed until after heparinization [7].

Side Effects/Black Box Warnings (If Any)

Both aminocaproic acid and TXA are relatively safe. The theoretical risk of excess thrombosis has not been born out in studies. One meta-analysis found no higher incidence of deep vein thrombosis or pulmonary embolus in patients undergoing total knee replacements on TXA as compared to placebo [1, 8]. In patients with a history of thromboembolic disease or active coronary artery disease, a careful risk/benefit analysis must be performed.

Amicar and TXA both lack black box warnings. Anaphylaxis is rare. They are both generally well tolerated with nausea, vomiting, headache, and dizziness as the most common side effects. TXA has been linked to colorblindness in case reports and should be used with caution in patients with pre-existing colorblindness.

Although it has become generally accepted in cardiac surgery that aprotinin poses a higher risk of mortality and renal failure compared to other antifibrinolytics [9], recent studies are conflicting. A Cochrane review in 2011 found a higher rate of mortality with aprotinin, although it was associated with less blood loss [10]. A 2013 large meta-analysis [11] found no difference between aprotinin and other antifibrinolytics. Because of this uncertainty, it is no longer widely used in the USA. It also has a black box warning against re-exposure within a year of initial dose due to a possible increased risk of hypersensitivity reactions.

Other Hemostatic Drugs

Other drugs that interact along the coagulation cascade, such as Factor VIIa, have been demonstrated to reduce bleeding in certain situations. Factor VIIa induces clot formation by binding to tissue factor, which is exposed during injury. It is approved for use in patients with hemophilia A or B with inhibitors to Factors VIII or IX and in those with congenital Factor VII deficiency. However, several off-label indications have been investigated: acute reversal of warfarin-induced coagulopathy in patients with intracerebral hemorrhage and in the trauma population. In trauma victims who become coagulopathic, Factor VIIa may be useful if bleeding persists despite conventional measures. Of note, Factor VIIa is contraindicated in patients with intracerebral hemorrhage as a result of isolated head trauma. The administration of Factor VIIa is not without risk; studies have demonstrated a higher risk of arterial thromboembolic events and should be avoided in patients who are at risk for clot formation. Table 25.1 outlines the indications and dosage for Factor VII in our center. Recently,

Table 25.1 BIDMC indications and dosing recommendations for rVIIa

	Comments	Dose (IV)	Frequency
FDA approved use			
Hemophilia A or B with inhibitors	rVIIa is first-line therapy	90 mcg/kg	Every 2–3 h initially, with subsequent dosing per hematology service
Congenital FVII deficiency	rVIIa is first-line therapy	15–30 mcg/kg	Every 2–3 h initially, with subsequent dosing per hematology service
BIDMC approved use			
Acquired inhibitors to FVIII, IX (V, VII, X, XI)	Use in the setting of life- or limb-threatening bleeding	90 mcg/kg	Subsequent dosing to be determined in consultation with the hematology and transfusion medicine services
Glanzmann's thrombasthenia	In the presence of platelet transfusion refractoriness with documented antibodies to GPIIb-IIIa	90 mcg/kg	Subsequent dosing to be determined in consultation with the hematology and transfusion medicine services
Life-threatening hemorrhage	Continued hemorrhage despite adequate blood product replacement, reversal agents, surgical hemostasis, and other procoagulant therapies	40 mcg/kg	Subsequent dosing to be determined in consultation with the hematology and transfusion medicine services

WARNING: patients with known thromboembolic or vaso-occlusive disease, disseminated intravascular coagulation (DIC), crush injury, advanced atherosclerotic disease, septicemia, or concomitant treatment with prothrombin complex concentrates may have an increased risk of developing thrombotic events
NOTE: all requests for rVIIa must be approved by the Transfusion Medicine Service (pager: 30003)
Approved by: Pharmacy & Therapeutics Committee: 06/13/07

the FDA approved a four-factor prothrombin complex concentrate, KCentra (CSL Behring), for acute warfarin reversal in patients with major bleeding. KCentra contains non-activated Factors II, VII, IX, and X and proteins C and S.

Desmopressin (DDAVP) is a synthetic analog of vasopressin and is used to reduce bleeding in patients with hemophilia and von Willebrand's disease (although it must be used with caution in subtype 2B as it can induce thrombocytopenia). It is also used to reduce bleeding time in patients who are taking antiplatelet medications such as aspirin and clopidogrel. DDAVP stimulates the release of von Willebrand factor as well as Factor VIII from the endothelium. In the kidney, DDAVP binds to V2 receptors and increases free water absorption, which is the basis for its use in patients with central diabetes insipidus. Of note, DDAVP has no activity at V1 receptors and thus does not promote vasoconstriction. It can be administered orally, intranasally, or intravenously. The intravenous dose of DDAVP to reverse platelet dysfunction from aspirin or clopidogrel is 0.3 mcg/kg over 30 min.

Summary

Antifibrinolytic agents interact along the coagulation cascade to improve clot formation and reduce bleeding. In patient populations where significant blood loss is anticipated, prophylaxis with these drugs may reduce the need for blood product transfusion. This is significant due to the expense and possible risks associated with transfusion.

Chemical Structures

Chemical Structure
25.1 Aminocaproic acid

References

1. Ker K, Edwards P, Perel P, Shakur H, Roberts I. Effect of tranexamic acid on surgical bleeding: systematic review and cumulative meta-analysis. BMJ. 2012;344:e3054.
2. Brown JR, Birkmeyer NJ, O'Connor GT. Meta-analysis comparing the effectiveness and adverse outcomes of antifibrinolytic agents in cardiac surgery. Circulation. 2007;115(22):2801–13.
3. Butterwork JF, Mackey DC, Wasnick JD. Morgan & Mikhail's clinical anesthesiology. 5th ed. New York: McGraw Hill; 2013.
4. Zufferey P, Merquiol F, Laporte S, Decousus H, Mismetti P, Auboyer C, et al. Do antifibrinolytics reduce allogeneic blood transfusion in orthopedic surgery? Anesthesiology. 2006;105(5):1034–46.
5. Ipema HJ, Tanzi MG. Use of topical tranexamic or aminocaproic acid to prevent bleeding after major surgical procedures. Ann Pharmacother. 2012;46(1):97–107.

6. Roberts I, Shakur H, Ker K, Coats T, CRASH-2 Trial Collaborators. Antifibrinolytic drugs for acute traumatic injury. Cochrane Database Syst Rev. 2012;12:CD004896.

7. Kluger R, Olive DJ, Steward AB, Blyth CM. Epsilon-aminocaproic acid in coronary artery bypass graft surgery: preincision or postheparin? Anesthesiology. 2003;99(6):1263–9.

8. Yang ZG, Chen WP, Wu LD. Effectiveness and safety of tranexamic acid in reducing blood loss in total knee arthroplasty: a meta-analysis. J Bone Joint Surg Am. 2012;94(13):1153–9.

9. Hutton B, Joseph L, Fergusson D, Mazer CD, Shapiro S, Tinmouth A. Risks of harms using antifibrinolytics in cardiac surgery: systematic review and network meta-analysis of randomised and observational studies. BMJ. 2012;345:e5798.

10. Henry DA, Carless PA, Moxey AJ, O'Connell D, Stokes BJ, Fergusson DA, Ker K. Antifibrinolytic use for minimising perioperative allogeneic blood transfusion. Cochrane Database Syst Rev. 2011;3, CD001886.

11. Howell N, Senanayake E, Freemantle N, Pagano D. Putting the record straight on aprotinin as safe and effective: results from a mixed treatment meta-analysis of trials of aprotinin. J Thorac Cardiovasc Surg. 2013;145(1):234–40.

Chapter 26
Blood, Blood Products, and Substitutes

Molly Chung, Laura Mayer, Hamid Nourmand,
Michelle You, and Jonathan S. Jahr

Contents

Introduction

Blood and blood products have long been available from blood banks for restoration of oxygen carrying potential and replacement of coagulation factors and platelets. This chapter will review the current use of these products, with specific focus on risk/benefits, and then introduce blood substitutes that may eventually replace or augment the use of the donated products with safer, more efficient uses and improved

M. Chung, MD • L. Mayer, MD • H. Nourmand, MD • M. You • J.S. Jahr, MD (✉)
Department of Anesthesiology, David Geffen School of Medicine at UCLA,
Ronald Reagan UCLA Medical Center, 757 Westwood Plaza, Suite 3325,
Los Angeles, CA 90095, USA
e-mail: mchung@mednet.ucla.edu; hnourmand@mednet.ucla.edu;
you.michelle@hotmail.com; jsjahr@mednet.ucla.edu

A.D. Kaye et al. (eds.), *Essentials of Pharmacology for Anesthesia,*
Pain Medicine, and Critical Care, DOI 10.1007/978-1-4614-8948-1_26,
© Springer Science+Business Media New York 2015

outcomes. The chapter will be divided into two major sections of blood and blood products, and substitutes, and further divided into subsections that mirror other chapters in this textbook. However, there are differences from pharmaceuticals and biologicals, and as such, exact replication of the format for pharmaceuticals is not possible for a chapter as this.

Blood and Blood Products

Approximately 15 million units of red blood cells is transfused annually in the USA, and about 85 million units is transfused annually worldwide [1]. Physicians commonly use hemoglobin values as well as symptoms of anemia to decide when to transfuse. Optimal use of red blood cells involves transfusing enough product to maximize the clinical impact of transfusion (increasing oxygen carrying capacity) while avoiding unnecessary transfusions that increase cost and patient exposure to risks such as infection and immune reactions.

Intraoperative and postoperative management of blood loss includes monitoring the amount of blood loss, interpreting the hemoglobin or hematocrit level in the clinical context, and assessing for signs of inadequate perfusion and oxygenation of vital organs [2]. These factors help direct the transfusion of allogeneic blood components or autologous blood. The literature is insufficient to evaluate the efficacy of any particular monitoring technique for evaluating inadequate perfusion and oxygenation of vital organs or as an indicator for transfusion of red blood cells [2]. However, practice guidelines and recommendations have been published by organizations such as the American Society of Anesthesiologists (ASA) and the American Association of Blood Banks (AABB).

In addition to management of blood loss, intraoperative and postoperative management of coagulopathy is important. Assessment of coagulopathy includes visual assessment of the surgical field for presence of microvascular bleeding, laboratory testing (e.g., platelet count, PT, aPTT, fibrinogen), and administration of platelets, fresh frozen plasma (FFP), cryoprecipitate, and adjuvant pharmacologic agents such as desmopressin, topical hemostatics, and recombinant factor VII [2]. The adjuvant pharmacologic agents are discussed separately in another chapter in this text.

Drug Class and Mechanism of Action

(i) *Whole blood* – Whole blood contains red blood cells, white blood cells, and platelets suspended in plasma [3]. As patients seldom need all components of whole blood, separating red blood cells, platelets, and plasma allows more specific intervention for the individual patient and allows more than one patient to benefit from one donated unit of whole blood [3].

(ii) *PRBC* – Red blood cells contain hemoglobin, an iron-containing protein, and serves to carry oxygen throughout the body [3].

(iii) *Plasma* – Plasma, the liquid portion of blood, accounts for 55 % of the total blood volume and consists of albumin, fibrinogen, globulins, and other clotting proteins [3]. Plasma may be separated into albumin, specific clotting factor concentrates, intravenous immune globulin (IVIG), or frozen within hours of donation to preserve clotting factors as fresh frozen plasma (FFP) [3].

(iv) *Platelets* – Platelets are a cellular component of blood that promotes coagulation by adhering to the lining of blood vessels [3].

(v) *Cryoprecipitate* – Cryoprecipitate is a portion of plasma that is rich in factor VII, fibrinogen, von Willebrand factor, and factor XIII [3]. Each unit of cryoprecipitate contains 150–250 mg fibrinogen. In comparison, each unit of FFP contains 2–4 mg of fibrinogen/ml, equivalent to 2 units of cryoprecipitate [2].

Indications/Clinical Pearls

(i) *PRBC* – The ASA task force recommends transfusion of red blood cells when hemoglobin level is less than 6 g/dl and states that red blood cell transfusion is usually unnecessary when hemoglobin level is above 10 g/dl [2]. Determining whether to transfuse in the intermediate zone of hemoglobin levels between 6 and 10 g/dl proves a challenge and is influenced by potential or actual ongoing bleeding, indications of organ ischemia, intravascular fluid status, and patient comorbidities that signify higher risk of complications from inadequate oxygenation. Patients who have low cardiopulmonary reserve or who have higher oxygen consumption, such as pregnant patients, fall into this latter category [2]. The AABB recommends consideration of transfusion for hemodynamically stable adult and pediatric ICU patients at hemoglobin 7 g/dl or less, based on the TRICC and TRIPICU trials, and for postsurgical patients at hemoglobin 8 g/dl or less or for symptoms of chest pain, hypotension or tachycardia unresponsive to fluid resuscitation, or congestive heart failure, based on the FOCUS trial [1]. Other indications include exchange transfusion (e.g., hemolytic disease of newborn) or red cell exchange (acute chest syndrome in sickle cell disease) [4].

(ii) *FFP* – The ASA recommends FFP transfusion in a bleeding patient when PT is greater than 1.5 times normal, INR greater than 2, or aPTT is greater than 2 times normal for correction of microvascular bleeding [2]. Additionally, other indications for FFP transfusion include urgent reversal of warfarin, coagulation factor deficiency after massive transfusion of red blood cells (more than one blood volume), and heparin resistance (antithrombin III deficiency) in a patient requiring heparin [2]. One unit of FFP provides an equivalent amount of coagulation factors as four to five platelet concentrates, 1 unit single-donor apheresis platelets, or 1 unit of fresh whole blood [2]. Albumin is discussed separately in another chapter within this textbook.

(iii) *Platelets* – The ASA recommends transfusion of platelets when the platelet count is less than 50,000 cells/mm^3 [2]. As such, a platelet count should be obtained if possible before transfusion. Additionally, a test of platelet function may be considered in patients with suspected platelet dysfunction (e.g., on aspirin or clopidogrel therapy). It is rarely indicated to transfuse when platelet count is above 100,000 cells/mm^3 [2]. Transfusion between 50,000 and 100,000 cells/mm^3 is based on potential for platelet dysfunction (e.g., after cardiopulmonary bypass), ongoing bleeding, and risk of bleeding into a confined space (e.g., intracranial) [2]. If thrombocytopenia is due to ongoing platelet destruction, transfusion of platelets is not effective.

(iv) *Cryoprecipitate* – The ASA recommends administration of cryoprecipitate when fibrinogen concentrations are less than 80–100 mg/dl in the presence of excessive microvascular bleeding [2]. Additional indications include microvascular bleeding in the presence of massive transfusion and congenital fibrinogen deficiency. If specific concentrates are not available to treat bleeding patients with von Willebrand's disease or hemophilia, cryoprecipitate may be indicated [2].

Dosing Options (See Table 26.1)

Table 26.1 Blood and blood products: indication, dosing, and relative contraindications

Blood product	Indication	Dosing	Relative contraindication
Whole blood	Autologous donated units for elective surgery, large volume hemorrhage, neonatal exchange transfusion		Volume overload
PRBC	Increase oxygen carrying capacity to tissues, exchange transfusion, red cell exchange	10–20 ml/kg	Iron overload, volume overload, chronic asymptomatic anemia
FFP	Active bleeding due to deficiency of multiple coagulation factors, risk of bleeding due to deficiency of coagulation factors, urgent reversal of warfarin, massive transfusion	10–20 ml/kg	Normalizing abnormal coagulation screen tests in absence of bleeding

Table 26.1 (continued)

Blood product	Indication	Dosing	Relative contraindication
Platelets	Bleeding due to insufficient circulating platelet count or abnormally functioning platelets; prophylactic to prevent bleeding in patients undergoing invasive procedures	10–15 ml/kg	40 u filter, hypothermia, risk of thrombosis, bypass circuit, autoimmune thrombocytopenia, thrombotic thrombocytopenic purpura
Cryoprecipitate	Bleeding associated with fibrinogen deficiency or factor XIII deficiency, hemophilia A, or von Willebrand's disease if specific concentrates unavailable	1 unit/10 kg	

PRBC – 1 unit of PRBC will increase hemoglobin in the average adult who is not bleeding or hemolyzing by about 1 g/dl or hematocrit by about 3 % [4]. For pediatric patients, the dose is generally 10–20 ml/kg [5].

FFP – A dose of 10–20 ml/kg is usually sufficient to achieve a plasma factor concentration of 30 % of normal [4, 5].

Platelet – One plateletpheresis unit ($\geq 3 \times 10^{11}$ platelets) or 4–10 pooled platelet units ($\geq 5.5 \times 10^{10}$ platelets) for adults or 10–15 ml/kg for pediatric patients should raise platelet count by 50,000–100,000/mm^3 [4, 5].

Cryoprecipitate – 1 unit per 10 kg will raise fibrinogen by about 50 mg/dl in the absence of continued consumption or massive bleeding [4].

Drug Interactions

There are no known drug interactions with blood products; however, citrate toxicity may result from rapid infusion, especially in the setting of liver disease [4]. Citrate, an anticoagulant used in blood products, is normally metabolized quickly by the liver and binds calcium and magnesium. As such, calcium-containing carrier fluids (e.g., lactated Ringer's solution) should not be used due to a theoretical risk of clot formation.

Side Effects/Black Box Warnings

(i) *Immune reactions* – These reactions may be hemolytic or nonhemolytic. Signs of hemolytic immune reaction include urticaria, hypotension, tachycardia, increased airway pressure, hyperthermia, decreased urine output, hemoglobinuria, and microvascular bleeding [4]. Risk of death from severe hemolytic reaction is about one in one million [1].

(ii) *Infection risk from handling* – Bacterial contamination of blood products is most frequently associated with platelets and is the leading cause of death related to transfusions [2]. This risk is related to storage temperatures of platelets above 20–24 °C. Contaminated platelets may be suspected if a patient develops a fever within 6 h after receiving platelets.

(iii) *TRALI* – Transfusion-related acute lung injury is a non-cardiogenic pulmonary edema resulting from leukocyte antibodies from transfused blood products. The risk is about 1 in 10,000 [1]. It usually manifests 1–2 h after transfusion with peak effect within 6 h. Recovery is usual in 96 h; however, TRALI is one of the three most common causes of transfusion-related deaths [2], and case fatality rate has been reported between 5 and 10 % [6].

(iv) *Infectious disease transmission from donors* – Hepatitis C and HIV transmission rates from blood transfusion are now rare (one in one million) [1], because these diseases can be detected by nucleic acid technology. Risk of hepatitis B transmission is about 1 in 300,000 [1]. Currently, malaria, Chagas disease, and variant Creutzfeldt-Jakob disease cannot be detected [1].

Blood Substitutes

Introduction/Description/History

Transfusion of blood products is vital for when lifesaving resuscitation measures are needed. However, packed red blood cells have limitations and additional risks as discussed above. The development of blood substitutes have been studied for over 50 years in hopes to create an infusible product that serves as an alternative to pRBC [7]. Patients who would most benefit are those with an immediate need for resuscitation products, who are immunoreactive to all blood types, and who reside in areas where pRBCs are difficult to obtain and store or which lack blood banks and in areas where there is increased prevalence of donor blood-borne disease transmittance [8].

Hemoglobin-based oxygen carriers (HBOCs) are blood substitutes that are constructed from human or bovine blood cells. HBOCs use the natural O2 delivery system of hemoglobin, which is removed from the red cell, purified, and re-polymerized [7]. Hemoglobin consists of two alpha and two beta subunit chains, each of which contains an iron atom that binds oxygen. Some preparations of HBOCs are presented

Table 26.2 Clinical studies on HBOCs

Name	Company	Chemical/genetic modification	Proposed application	Status
HemAssist	Baxter	α-α intra-tetramer cross-linked human Hba	Trauma, stroke	Suspended – USA 2008
Hemopure	Biopure (now OPK Biotech)	α-α intra- and inter-tetramer cross-linked bovine Hba	Surgery, sickle cell crisis, trauma	Phase III – US FDA denied further clinical trials, 2008
PolyHeme	Northfield Laboratories (closed activities)	Inter-tetramer cross-linked human Hba	Trauma	Phase III – completed with FDA approval denied, 2008
Hemospan	Sangart	PEGylated human Hba	Elective orthopedic surgery as blood expander	Phase III, completed in Europe. Results under evaluation
Hemolink	Hemosol	Inter-tetramer cross-linked human Hba	Elective surgery	Phase II – suspended, 2004
PEG-Hb	Enzon	PEGylated bovine Hba	Tumor therapy	Phase Ib – suspended in USA, 1997
PHP/ Hemoximer	Apex Bioscience/ Curacyte	PEGylated Hba	Septic shock (NO scavenging)	Phase III – undergoing in Europe

Modified from Bettati et al. [8]

as bags of red colored liquid, and others come in powder form and are to be mixed with an IV fluid for use as an intravenous infusion. Early generations of HBOCs that had high amounts of hemoglobin dimmers and tetramers (no longer in testing) were filtered through renal glomerulus and excreted through the kidneys, while newer versions are too large to be filtered and are metabolized the same way free hemoglobin is, via breakdown in the liver to usable iron, proteins, and bilirubin. Currently, there are three HBOC versions in active testing: polymerized, conjugated, and cross-linked [9]. Preliminary studies suggest that patients treated with certain HBOCs have safely avoided the need for blood transfusion [8, 10]. However, there have been considerable setbacks in the development of these products including renal failure, increased mortality, systemic and pulmonary hypertension, myocardial infarction, hemolysis, and chemical pancreatitis [11]. Although there are no currently approved blood substitutes in the USA for human use, further investigations and clinical trials are underway in hopes of providing efficacious HBOCs with minimal complications (see Table 26.2). One product is approved for veterinary use in the USA and European Union since 1997 and 1998, respectively (Oxyglobin®, hemoglobin glutamer 301 (bovine), OPK Biotech, Cambridge, MA), and one product is approved for human use in South Africa and Russia since 2001 and 2010, respectively (Hemopure®, hemoglobin glutamer 201 (bovine), OPK Biotech, Cambridge, MA).

HBOCs May Offer Advantages Over pRBCs

- Maintaining and processing the units is easier and more cost effective.
- HBOCs may be stored at room temperature, ideal for locations where refrigeration is not available such as battlefields, third world countries, or for trauma in ambulances and helicopters.
- HBOCs may be easily produced and readily available, especially in the event of blood shortages as seen in natural disasters or low donor recruitment (bovine blood is more easily and safely procured).
- HBOCs have a long shelf life of up to 3 years [13] compared to pRBCs which expire after 42 days [14].
- HBOCs may be more amenable to persons with religious objections [15].
- Since the antigens and other immune markers are removed with the red cell membrane, the patient does not need to be cross matched and will have less of a propensity to cause an immunogenic reaction (hemoglobin itself tends to be less antigenic as multiple species eat other species and are not immunized against foreign hemoglobin). Also, there will be fewer complications due to human error in transfusing the wrong blood.
- The risk of donor-related disease transmission (including hepatitis B and C and HIV) and bacterial contamination is decreased. This is especially relevant in areas in which HIV/AIDS is prevalent such as Southern Africa (processes for removing bacteria, viruses, prions, parasites, and other infectious materials are well validated and documented).
- There is a decrease in proinflammatory markers as HBOCs are not exposed to white blood cells in their preparation.
- The oxygen affinity is increased due to a depletion of 2,3-diphosphoglycerate (2,3,DPG) during the separation of Hg from the red blood cell and a decrease in the partial pressure of HBOC (approx. 5–14 mmHg) compared to that of pRBCs (approx. 27 mmHg in adults) (this is true for the newest generation of HBOCs; earlier versions have an increased P50).
- There is also a reduction in transfusion reactions including TRALI, electrolyte imbalances, hemolytic reactions, and TACO.

HBOCs May Have Some Disadvantages Compared to pRBCs

- The RBC contains methemoglobin reductase which protects the hemoglobin from oxidation. The HBOCs do not have this enzyme and have a higher incidence of oxidation which causes increased levels of methemoglobin and free radicals [15].

- The endothelium is exposed to the free Hb of the HBOC and binds nitric oxide which produces vasoconstriction and hypertension. This may in turn stimulate catecholamine release, limit tissue perfusion, cause pulmonary hypertension, and decrease cardiac output. This is particularly concerning in the setting of hypovolemia or hypotension [9].
- Earlier engineered HBOC substrates have led to nephrotoxicity, myocardial infarction, hemolysis, and pancreatitis [12, 13].
- May cause problems with platelet aggregation and adhesion [15].
- HBOCs demonstrated immunosuppression in some animal trials [9].

Table 26.3 compares and contrasts blood and blood products with HBOCs. Figure 26.1 demonstrates the relative sizes and configurations of the different types of blood substitutes.

Table 26.3 Risk benefit comparison of PRBCs and HBOCs

Issues	HBOCs	pRBCs
Complications	Nephrotoxic/myocardial effects	Acute
	Possible vasoconstrictor effects	Acute hemolytic reaction
	Decreased tissue perfusion (P50 decreased, left shift of Hb-O2 curve)	Allergic reaction
	Pulmonary HTN	Anaphylactic reaction
	Increased risk of methemoglobinemia	Coagulation problems in massive transfusion
		Electrolyte abnormalities
		Febrile nonhemolytic reaction
		Metabolic derangements
		Mistransfusion (transfusion of the incorrect product to the incorrect recipient)
		Septic or bacterial contamination
		Transfusion-associated circulatory overload
		Transfusion-related acute lung injury
		Urticarial reaction
		Disease transmission including HIV, West Nile, hepatitis B and C
		Delayed
		Delayed hemolytic reaction
		Iron overload
		Microchimerism
		Overtransfusion or undertransfusion
		Posttransfusion purpura
		Transfusion-associated graft-versus-host disease
		Transfusion-related immunomodulation

(continued)

Table 26.3 (continued)

Issues	HBOCs	pRBCs
Contraindications	Unknown	Religious objections
Duration of activity	Maximum 3 days	70 % or less pRBC stays within circulation for 24 h
Onset of action	Immediate	Requires 2,3-DPG for oxygen release
Oxygen affinity	Increased	Decreased
Preparation	None	Cross matching, donor screening
P50	12–14 mmHg	27 mmHg
Reproducibility	Can be rapidly made	Requires donor donation, screening, and processing of blood
Shelf life	1–3 years	42 days
Storage	Can be stored at room temperature	Requires refrigeration
Viscosity	Low	High

Modified from Sharma et al. [17]
Data from Refs. [10, 13, 14, 16, 18, 19]

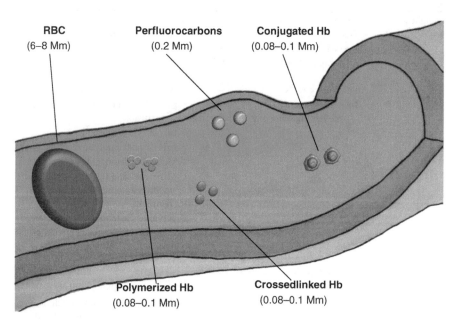

RBC
(6–8 Mm)

Perfluorocarbons
(0.2 Mm)

Conjugated Hb
(0.08–0.1 Mm)

Polymerized Hb
(0.08–0.1 Mm)

Crossedlinked Hb
(0.08–0.1 Mm)

Fig. 26.1 The relative sizes and configurations of the different types of blood substitutes

Conclusion and Summary

Blood and blood products have long been administered to patients with apparent benefit, but no double blind, randomized trials in large groups of patients or volunteers in diverse patient populations have been performed. In fact, if blood or blood products were presented to regulatory bodies today, it would be challenging for them to be approved. Nonetheless, these products are used in high amounts worldwide with apparent benefit. As such, it makes intuitive sense that a blood substitute should be developed that may take the place of red cells and clotting factors and platelets. However, except in veterinary medicine and in South Africa and Russia for humans, no alternatives are available to date. After 50 years of extensive work, no one product or development strategy has emerged to fill this unmet need. Hopefully, continued research and funding from governmental agencies, and collaboration between industry, investigators, and regulatory agencies, will enable products to be developed, tested, and eventually made available for use [20, 21].

References

1. Carson JL, Grossman BJ, Kleinman S, Tinmouth AT, Marques MB, Fung MK, Holcomb JH, Illoh O, Kaplan LJ, Katz LM, Rao SV, Roback JD, Shander A, Tobian AAR, Weinstein R, McLaughlin LGS, Djulbegovic B. Red blood cell transfusion: a clinical practice guideline from the AABB. Ann Intern Med. 2012;1:E-429.
2. American Society of Anesthesiologists Task Force on Perioperative Blood Transfusion and Adjuvant Therapies. Practice guidelines for perioperative blood transfusion and adjuvant therapies. Anesthesiology. 2006;105:198–208.
3. Whole blood and blood components. http://www.aabb.org/resources/bct/bloodfacts/pages/fabloodwhole.aspx. Accessed on 4 Mar 2013.
4. Practice guidelines for blood transfusion. 2nd ed. American Red Cross; 2007. http://www.sld.cu/galerias/pdf/sitios/anestesiologia/practical_guidelines_blood_transfusion.pdf. Accessed on 4 Mar 2013.
5. Hillyer C, Strauss R, Luban N. Handbook of pediatric transfusion. San Diego: Elsevier Academic Press; 2004.
6. Vamvakas E, Blajchman M. Transfusion-related mortality: the ongoing risks of allogeneic blood transfusion and the available strategies for their prevention. Blood. 2009;113(15):3406–17.
7. Jahr JS, Zimmerman D. Blood substitutes. In: Singh-Radcliff N, Gupta A, editors. The 5-minute anesthesia consult. Philadelphia: WoltersKlumer – LWW; 2012. p. 132–3.
8. Bettati S, Bruno S, Faggiano S, Mozzarelli A, Ronda L. Haemoglobin-based oxygen carriers: research and reality towards an alternative to blood transfusions. Blood Transfus. 2010;8:59–68. http://www.ncbi.nlm.nih.gov/pmc/articles/PMC2897202/. Accessed 27 Mar 2013.
9. Dong Q, Stowell C. Blood substitutes. What they are and how they might be used. Am J Clin Pathol. 2002;118:S71–80.
10. Jahr JS, Mackenzie C, Pearce B, Pitman A, Greenburg AG. HBOC-201 as an alternative to blood transfusion: efficacy and safety evaluation in a multicenter phase III trial in elective orthopedic surgery. J Trauma Inj Infect Crit Care. 2008;64(6):1484–97.
11. Levy J. Blood substitutes. Hemoglobin-based oxygen carriers. The American Council of Science and Health. 2009. http://www.acsh.org/wp-content/uploads/2012/04/20090721_blood_substitutes.pdf. Accessed 24 Mar 2013.
12. Kleinman S, Silvergleid A, Tirnauer J. Use of red blood cells for transfusion. UpToDate, Inc. Updated 4 Mar 2013. http://www.uptodate.com/contents/use-of-red-blood-cells-for-transfusion?source=search_result&search=the+use+for+red+blood+cell+transfusion&selectedTitle=3%7E150. Accessed 22 Mar 2013.
13. Jahr JS, SadighiAkha A, Doherty L, Li A, Kim HW. Chapter 22: Hemoglobin-based oxygen carriers: history, limits, brief summary of the state of the art, including clinical trials. In: Andrea M, Stefano B, editors. Chemistry and biochemistry of oxygen therapeutics: from transfusion to artificial blood. 1st ed. London: Wiley; 2011. p. 301–16.

14. Fridey J, Silvergleid A, Tirnauer J. Oxygen carriers as alternatives to red cell transfusion. UpToDate, Inc. Updated 8 May 2012. http://www.uptodate.com/contents/oxygen-carriers-as-alternatives-to-red-cell-transfusion?source=search_result&search=Oxygen+carriers+as+alternatives+to+red+cell+transfusion&selectedTitle=1%7E150. Accessed 22 Mar 2013.

15. Dorman S, Kenny C, Miller L, Hirsch R, Harrington J. Role of redox potential of hemoglobin-based oxygen carriers on methemoglobin reduction by plasma components. Artif Cells Blood Substit Immobil Biotechnol. 2002;30(1):39–51.

16. Jahr JS, Liu H, Albert O, Gull A, Moallempour M, Lim J, Gosselin R. Does HBOC-201 (Hemopure®) affect platelet function in orthopedic surgery: a single site analysis from a multicenter study. Am J Ther. 2010;17:140–7.

17. Sharma S, Poonam S, Tyler L. Transfusion of blood and blood products: indications and complications. Am Fam Physician. 2011;83(6):719–24.

18. Werlin E, McQuinn G, Lepine G, Ophardt R. Hemoglobin-based oxygen carriers. Brown University. 2005. http://biomed.brown.edu/Courses/BI108/BI108_2005_Groups/10/webpages/HBOClink.htm. Accessed 1 Mar 2013.

19. Chantigian R, Hall B. Anesthesia. A comprehensive review. 4th ed. Maryland Heights: Mosby Elsevier; 2010. p. 133.

20. Jahr JS, Koch CG, Smith CE. Strategies for treatment of coagulopathy associated with hemorrhage. Am Soc Anesthesiol Newsl. 2012;76:12–4.

21. Kim HW, Mozzarelli A, Sakai H, Jahr JS. Chapter 29: Academia – industry collaboration in blood substitute development – issues, case histories and a proposal. In: Mozzarelli A, Bettati S, editors. Chemistry and biochemistry of oxygen therapeutics: from transfusion to artificial blood. 1st ed. London: Wiley; 2011. p. 413–28.

Chapter 27
Antipyretics: Acetaminophen, Arachidonic Acid Agents, and COX1 and COX2 Inhibitors

My Tu, Karina Gritsenko, Boleslav Kosharskyy, and Naum Shaparin

Contents

M. Tu, MD (✉) • B. Kosharskyy, MD
Department of Anesthesiology, Albert Einstein School of Medicine – Yeshiva University,
Montefiore Medical Center, Bronx, NY, USA
e-mail: mtu@montefiore.org; bkoshars@montefiore.org

K. Gritsenko, MD • N. Shaparin, MD
Department of Anesthesiology, Albert Einstein School of Medicine – Yeshiva University,
Montefiore Medical Center, Bronx, NY, USA

Department of Family and Social Medicine,
Albert Einstein School of Medicine – Yeshiva University,
Montefiore Medical Center, Bronx, NY, USA
e-mail: karinagritsenko@googlemail.com; nshapari@montefiore.org

A.D. Kaye et al. (eds.), *Essentials of Pharmacology for Anesthesia,*
Pain Medicine, and Critical Care, DOI 10.1007/978-1-4614-8948-1_27,
© Springer Science+Business Media New York 2015

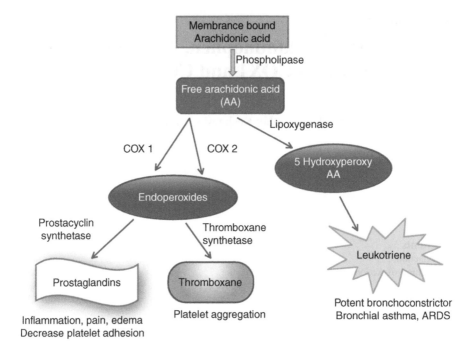

Fig. 27.1 Arachidonic acid (on cell membrane) activated by phospholipase enzyme to become free arachidonic acid (*AA*) which goes to one of two pathways. (*1*) 5-hydroxyperoxy-arachidonic acid by lipoxygenase producing leukotriene. (*2*) Endoperoxides by COX, prostacyclin synthetase to prostaglandin, thromboxane synthetase to become thromboxane

Introduction

This chapter is intended to provide an overview of fundamentals of nonsteroidal anti-inflammatory drugs (NSAIDs). They are one of the most commonly prescribed medications, with an estimated 70 million number of prescriptions written annually written and $6.8 billion spent worldwide [1, 2].

NSAIDs are grouped into categories depending on their interactions with prostaglandin synthase enzymes along the inflammation pathway (Fig. 27.1). There are two prostaglandin synthase enzymes which are commonly known as cyclooxygenase-1 and cyclooxygenase-2 (COX-1 and COX-2). Inhibition of cyclooxygenase-2 (COX-2) is responsible for the antipyretic, analgesic, and anti-inflammatory effects, while adverse gastropathies are thought to be mediated through inhibition of cyclooxygenase-1 (COX-1) [3].

The common over-the-counter NSAIDS are known as traditional NSAIDS (tNSAIDS) [4]. Traditional NSAIDS reversibly compete with free arachidonic acid (AA) at the active site of COX-1 and COX-2 enzymes. Propionic acid derivatives (ibuprofen, naproxen), acetic acid derivatives (indomethacin), and enolic acids (piroxicam) are a few examples of tNSAIDS [4]. Aspirin (ASA) acetylates both

COX enzymes causing an irreversible inhibition of their activity. Acetaminophen provides fever reduction with analgesic properties. It has less gastrointestinal (GI) side effects, but has only minimal anti-inflammatory activity [4].

Mechanism of Action

Inhibition of Cyclooxygenases

The therapeutic effects of NSAIDs are due to their ability to inhibit prostaglandin (PG) production. The key enzyme in the PG pathway is collectively known as prostaglandin synthase, commonly known as cyclooxygenases (COX), cyclooxygenase-1 and cyclooxygenase-2 [4]. These two enzymes convert free arachidonic acid (AA) to endoperoxides which will produce either thromboxanes or prostaglandins (Fig. 27.1).

Two forms of COX exist, COX-1 and COX-2. Both contribute to prostaglandin formation, inflammation, and pain. COX-2 is induced by cytokines, shear stress, and tumor promoters. COX-1 is expressed constitutively in most cells primarily for housekeeping functions, such as gastric epithelial cells and hemostasis. It is the cytoprotective PG [3]. Thus, inhibition of COX-1 is the underlying mechanism for the adverse gastrointestinal effects that frequently accompany tNSAID therapy.

Selective COX-2 inhibitors are Y-shaped in structure and were created to avoid the adverse gastrointestinal side effects seen with tNSAID therapy. The selective COX-2 inhibitors have a bulky side group which fits into a large "side pocket" along the COX-2 enzyme. This large side group prevents its access into the smaller binding channel of COX-1 [4]. Celecoxib (Celebrex) is currently the only COX-2 inhibitor licensed for use in the USA. Other coxibs have been withdrawn from the market due to significant adverse events. For example, rofecoxib (Vioxx) is associated with an increased incidence of myocardial infarction and cerebral vascular accidents [5].

Acetaminophen, a very weak anti-inflammatory agent, is associated with a reduced incidence of gastrointestinal adverse effects compared to tNSAIDs. At 1,000 mg, acetaminophen inhibits both COXs by approximately 50 % [4].

The lipoxygenase (LOX) pathway is not affected by any NSAIDS; therefore, leukotriene formation is not suppressed (Fig. 27.1).

Aspirin's Irreversible Inhibition

Aspirin acetylates and, hence, irreversibly inhibits the activity of both cyclooxygenase enzymes. The significance of the difference in mechanism of action is that the recovery of enzymes is dependent on the turnover rate of the prostaglandin enzymes [4]. The duration of effect for the reversible, competitive drugs is dependent on the time course of drug disposition. Arachidonic acid metabolite formation is therefore also dependent on the turnover of COX enzymes [4].

Importantly, platelet activity is affected. Platelets, being anucleated, have a limited capacity for protein synthesis [4]. Whereas other arachidonic acid metabolites such as prostacyclin, made primarily in the reticuloendothelial cells of the gut, are nucleated and will maintain levels, resulting in a change in the ratio between platelet aggregation and disaggregation. Inhibition of platelet COX-1 lasts for the lifetime of the platelet (COX-2 is expressed in megakaryocytes). Therefore, COX-1 inhibition disrupts the formation of thromboxane A_2, decreasing vasoconstriction and secondary platelet aggregation. Inhibition of platelet COX-1-dependent thromboxane formation is cumulative with repeated doses of aspirin (as low as 30 mg/day). It takes approximately 8–12 days for platelets to turnover and to fully recover once aspirin is discontinued. A few days after the last aspirin dose, there may be some normal functioning platelets, sufficient enough hemostasis allowing for some elective surgery to proceed [4].

The antiplatelet effect of aspirin is exploited in its use as a cardioprotective agent. Aspirin use has consistently demonstrated a pattern of reduced mortality in all primary prevention trials [6]. Even a small dose of aspirin (81 mg daily) provides adequate cardioprotection in patients who are at high risk (i.e., history of myocardial infarction) for thrombotic vascular events. Caution is advised as use of low-dose aspirin minimizes, not eliminates, the potential associated adverse GI events. Placebo-controlled trials demonstrate that aspirin, at any dose, increases the incidence of serious GI bleeds and intracranial bleeds [4]. The benefits of aspirin's antiplatelet effect are also appreciated in treatment of Kawasaki disease in children (see Sect. 6).

Pharmacology

Absorption

Traditional NSAIDs are generally weak acids with pK_a 3–5 and are well absorbed in the stomach and intestinal mucosa [4, 5]. Peak plasma concentration is reached at 2–3 h [4]. Concomitant food intake can delay absorption and may decreases systemic availability. Antacids that commonly are taken with NSAIDs may contribute to variable delays of absorption, but will not usually reduce absorption. Some compounds (e.g., diclofenac, nabumetone) undergo first-pass or pre-systemic elimination. Acetaminophen is metabolized to a small extent during absorption. Aspirin begins to acetylate platelets within minutes of reaching the pre-systemic circulation [4].

Distribution

The majority of NSAIDs are highly protein bound (95–99 %), usually to albumin [4]. Caution is advised in patients with disease states that decrease protein concentrations (cirrhosis) as they are at increased risk of toxicity due to an increased free fraction of the drug. Plasma protein binding often is concentration dependent (i.e., naproxen, ibuprofen), saturated at high concentrations, and can displace other drugs. Most NSAIDs are distributed widely throughout the body and can be readily found in synovial fluid after repeated dosing [7]. Counterintuitively, drugs with short half-lives stay in the synovial fluid longer than predicted from their half-lives, while drugs with longer half-lives are cleared from the synovial space at a rate proportional to their half-lives [7]. Most NSAIDs are lipophilic; therefore, they can achieve sufficient concentrations in the CNS which is responsible for its central analgesic effect. Celecoxib is particularly lipophilic and accumulates in fat and is readily transported into the CNS [4]. The lipophilic property also enables them to access the hydrophobic arachidonate binding channel [4]. Aspirin and acetaminophen are an exception [4].

Elimination

Plasma $t_{1/2}$ is highly inconsistent among the NSAIDS. The primary route of elimination is via hepatic biotransformation and renal excretion. Some have active metabolites. For example, acetaminophen, at therapeutic doses, is oxidized to form traces of the highly reactive metabolite, *N*-acetyl-*p*-benzoquinone imine (NAPQI) [4]. When overdosed (usually >10 g of acetaminophen), the metabolic pathways are saturated, and hepatotoxic NAPQI concentrations can be formed [4]. If renal excretion is compromised or competition for renal excretion of other drugs exists, some NSAIDs can be hydrolyzed back to the parent compound. This is true for the propionic acid derivatives naproxen and ketoprofen [4]. Elimination can thus be significantly prolonged. Because NSAIDs are extensively protein bound, they cannot be removed with dialysis; salicylic acids are the exception. NSAIDs should, therefore, be avoided in patients with severe hepatic or renal impairment.

Therapeutic Uses

All NSAIDs, including selective COX-2 inhibitors, are antipyretic, analgesic, and anti-inflammatory, with the exception of acetaminophen, which is an antipyretic and analgesic, but possesses minimal anti-inflammatory activity [4].

Due to their ability to penetrate into the synovial space, the anti-inflammatory effect of NSAIDs is useful in treatment of musculoskeletal disorders, such as rheumatoid arthritis and osteoarthritis. They provide symptomatic relief from pain and inflammation associated with such diseases [8].

The antipyretic effect is indicated in patients in whom fever in itself may be deleterious and for those who experience considerable relief when fever is lowered [4]. Fever prevention may obscure the clinical picture and must be considered in diagnostic evaluation. Although NSAIDs reduce fever in pathological states, this category of medications does not alter the circadian variation in temperature or the rise in response to exercise or to increased ambient temperature [4].

According to the WHO step ladder for cancer pain management, NSAIDs are the first line of therapy [9]. Unfortunately, their analgesic property is limited and only effective for pain of low to moderate degree. Concomitant use of NSAIDs with opioids is indicated in the second and third step of the WHO step ladder [9]. The advantage of this combination is the potential reduction in the amount of opioids required – potentially avoiding adverse opioid effects including respiratory depression, pruritus, nausea, and vomiting.

NSAIDs do not change the perception of sensory modalities other than pain [3, 4]. They are only effective when inflammation has caused peripheral and/or central sensitization of pain perception [3, 4]. Thus, postoperative discomfort or pain arising from inflammation, such as arthritic pain, is controlled well by NSAIDs, whereas visceral pain is not relieved. Menstrual pain is an exception. Prostaglandins released by the endometrium during menstruation result in menstrual cramps and other symptoms of primary dysmenorrhea [4]. This etiology of visceral pain and discomfort can therefore be effectively treated with NSAIDs. NSAIDs are also used as first-line therapy to treat migraines and can be combined with second-line drugs, such as the triptans. NSAIDs have no effect against neuropathic pain.

NSAIDs are also commonly indicated for closure of a persistent patent ductus arteriosus in the neonatal period. Prostaglandins keep the ductus arteriosus open; inhibiting its formation will enable closure of the patent ductus. Indomethacin and ibuprofen and other tNSAIDs have been used for such purpose.

Adverse Effects of NSAID Therapy

Common effects and adverse events are summarized in Table 27.1. As a general rule, age is associated with an increased likelihood of developing serious adverse reactions. Caution should be taken in the initial starting dose for elderly patients.

Numerous cases of epidural hematoma during central neuraxial blocks in combination with aspirin and other COX-1 inhibitor NSAID have been published. However, the 2010 American Society of Regional Anesthesia (ASRA) guidelines, third edition, state, "nonsteroidal anti-inflammatory drugs seem to represent no added significant risk for the development of spinal hematoma in patients having epidural or spinal anesthesia. Nonsteroidal anti-inflammatory drugs (including aspirin) do not create a level of risk that will interfere with the performance of neuraxial blocks [10]." ASRA does, however, recommend against performing neuraxial techniques in patients who are concurrently on NSAIDs and any anticoagulants [10].

The risk of epidural hematoma is estimated to be 1 in 150,000, and is increased 15-fold in patients on anticoagulant therapy [11]. Many herbals, over-the-counter agents, and drugs in general (e.g., fish oil, SSRIs) possess additive anticoagulant risks. A prudent clinician would minimize the use of any of these agents when

Table 27.1 Drug effects and adverse events [4, 7]

System	Effect	PE	Test
CV	Hypertension Congestive heart failure Thrombotic events Closure of ductus arteriosus	BP, edema, rales, chest pain	CXR, EKG
Resp	Asthma Bronchospasm	Wheezing	Chest auscultation, PFT
Hepatic	Elevated LFTs	Jaundice	LFTs
GI	Gastropathies (nausea, vomiting) Abdominal pain GI bleeding Esophageal disease Pancreatitis		Stool heme, Hgb, upper endoscopy, colonoscopy
Heme	Inhibited platelet activation Neutropenia Propensity for bruising Increased risk of hemorrhage	Pallor	Bleeding time, Hgb
Derm	Pruritus Urticaria Erythema multiforme Rash	Visible skin pathology	
GU	Renal insufficiency Sodium/fluid retention Papillary necrosis Interstitial nephritis	BP, edema, weight changes	$\uparrow$ K$^+$/BUN/Cr, $\downarrow$ UO, biopsy
CNS	Headache Vertigo Dizziness Confusion Hyperventilation (salicylates) Aseptic meningitis Hearing disturbances (tinnitus)	Somnolence, confusion	CSF

surgery or interventional pain procedures are planned electively, thereby reducing any risk of bleeding and potential complications.

Pediatric and Geriatric

In children, few studies have been performed. Pediatric patients have relatively larger surface area and prolonged emptying time of the gastrointestinal tract, higher percentage of total body water, lower percentage of body fat, decreased amount of plasma protein, and immature Phase I and II metabolism. These physiological differences could be explained by the ongoing maturation of the body and organ function in pediatric patients. Therefore, the pediatric drug absorption and disposition process might be correlated with age and/or body size such as height, weight, or body surface area, the effects of which are ultimately reflected in the pediatric dosing regimens [12]. Any pharmacokinetic studies that were performed involved patients >2 years of age and therefore cannot be applied directly to neonates and infants. The systemic bioavailability of rectal acetaminophen in neonates and preterm babies is higher than in older patients. Acetaminophen clearance is reduced in preterm neonates probably due to their immature hepatic function. Because of the reduced clearance time, acetaminophen dosing intervals should be extended (8–12 h) or daily doses reduced to avoid accumulation and liver toxicity [4].

Importantly, aspirin should be avoided in children as it may cause Reye's syndrome. Reye's syndrome is a severe and often fatal disease characterized by the acute onset of encephalopathy, liver dysfunction, and fatty infiltration of the liver and other viscera [4]. The one exception to aspirin's contraindication in children is in those afflicted with Kawasaki disease. "Kawasaki disease is characterized by a febrile, exanthematous, multisystem vasculitis that exists worldwide. If untreated, approximately 20 % of children may develop coronary artery abnormalities, including aneurysms. Approximately 80 % of cases of Kawasaki disease occur in children younger than 5 years of age" [13].

Aspirin is used for anti-inflammatory and antithrombotic actions, although aspirin alone does not decrease risk of coronary artery abnormalities [13]. The optimal dose or duration of aspirin treatment is unknown. Aspirin is administered in doses of 80–100 mg/kg per day in four divided doses once the diagnosis is made followed by low dose in the subacute phase [13]. Aspirin is discontinued if no coronary artery abnormalities have been detected by 6–8 weeks after onset of illness. Low-dose aspirin therapy should be continued indefinitely for people in whom coronary artery abnormalities are present. In general, ibuprofen should be avoided in children with coronary aneurysms taking aspirin for its antiplatelet effects, because ibuprofen antagonizes the platelet inhibition that is induced by aspirin [13].

In the elderly population, the clearance of NSAIDs may be reduced due to slower hepatic metabolism. NSAIDs with long $t_{1/2}$ can have elevated plasma concentrations. Albumin's binding capacity may also be diminished in older patients and may result in higher free fractions of NSAIDs which may result in toxicity. For example, free naproxen concentrations are markedly increased in older patients, although total plasma concentrations essentially are unchanged [4]. The elevated free fraction and plasma concentration also puts this population at an increased risk of GI complications [4]. As a general rule, for most medications prescribed to the elderly population one should "start low and go slow."

Summary

Therapeutic effects of traditional NSAIDS, selective COX-2 inhibitors, aspirin, and acetaminophen are in their ability to prevent prostaglandin synthesis. They each inhibit the prostaglandin synthesis via different mechanisms with variable side effect profiles. Traditional NSAIDS inhibit both cyclooxygenase enzymes, causing a significant amount of gastropathies. Selective COX-2 inhibitors provide analgesic and anti-inflammatory effects while sparing adverse gastrointestinal effects. Aspirin causes an irreversible inhibition of cyclooxygenases and hence renders platelet activity dependent on the turnover rate of COX enzymes. Acetaminophen is a very weak anti-inflammatory agent with very minimally COX enzyme inhibition and hence associated with a reduced incidence of gastrointestinal adverse effects.

Generally, NSAIDs are well absorbed via the gastrointestinal tract. Caution should be exercised in patients who have disease states that decrease protein concentrations as toxic doses can occur from an increase in free fraction. The drugs are primarily eliminated via hepatic transformation and renal excretion. Due to altered hepatic and renal function in the elderly and children, accumulation of metabolites and drugs may occur. Again, dosing recommendations for the neonates and infants are extrapolated from adult data; clinical judgment is advised.

Although NSAIDs are popularly used for its antipyretic, analgesic, and anti-pyretic effects, they are effective for other uses. Aspirin's antiplatelet side effect profile has proven it to be useful in cardiac protection against ischemia. Indomethacin and ibuprofen are used to close a patent ductus arteriosus in the neonatal period. NSAID use plays a key role in a multimodal approach to chronic pain management as it aids to reduce the amount of opioid consumption.

Clinical Pearls

1. Discontinue any NSAID, aspirin, or concomitant herbal, fish oil, or drug that can increase bleeding risk for elective surgery or an interventional pain procedure.
2. Current recommendations for acetaminophen have recently been reduced to approximately 2,600–2,800 mg/day to minimize liver toxicity.
3. A significant number of people suffer NSAID-mediated GI bleeds. Between 60 and 80 % of individuals that bleed do so without any symptoms, resulting in the potential for morbidity and mortality.
4. Intravenous acetaminophen is available in many hospitals and can be utilized in a number of pathological processes, including pain.
5. COX-2 inhibitors and acetaminophen have been studied and demonstrated positive results as agents in multimodal therapies and preemptive analgesia.

Chemical Structures

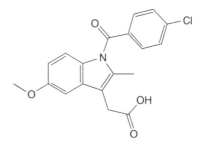

Chemical Structure
27.1 Indomethacin

Chemical Structure
27.2 Piroxicam

Chemical Structure
27.3 Aspirin

References

1. Warner TD, Giuliano F, Vojnovic I, Bukasa A, Mitchell JA, Vane JR. Nonsteroid drug selectivities for cyclo-oxygenase-1 rather than cyclo-oxygenase-2 are associated with human gastrointestinal toxicity: a full in vitro analysis. Proc Natl Acad Sci U S A. 1999;96:7563–8.
2. Bleumink GS, Feenstra J, Sturkenboom MC, Stricker BH. Nonsteroidal anti-inflammatory drugs and heart failure. Drugs. 2003;63:525–34.
3. Rathmell JP, Fields HL. Chapter 11. Pain: pathophysiology and management. In: Longo DL, Fauci AS, Kasper DL, Hauser SL, Jameson JL, Loscalzo J, editors. Harrison's principles of internal medicine. 18th ed. New York: McGraw-Hill; 2012. http://www.accessmedicine.com/content.aspx?aID=9094544. Accessed 12 Mar 2013.
4. Grosser T, Smyth E, FitzGerald GA. Goodman & Gilman's the pharmacological basis of therapeutics, 12e. Section IV. Inflammation, immunomodulation, and hematopoiesis. Chapter 34. Anti-inflammatory, antipyretic, and analgesic agents; pharmacotherapy of gout. New York: McGraw-Hill Education, LLC; 2011.
5. Thorsteinsson SB, Sigvaldason H, Einarsdottir R, et al. Rofecoxib, but not celecoxib, increases the risk of thromboembolic cardiovascular events in young adults-a nationwide registry-based study. Eur J Clin Pharmacol. 2010;66(6):619–25. doi:10.1007/s00228-010-0789-2. Epub 2010 Feb 16. Gudbjornsson Source Centre for Rheumatology Research, Landspitali University Hospital, Reykjavik, Iceland. bjorngu@landspitali.is.
6. Raju N, Sobieraj-Tieague M, Hirsh J, et al. Effect of aspirin on mortality in the primary prevention of cardiovascular disease. MsCc haematology unit, Queensland Pathology and Department of Internal Medicine, Prince Charles Hospital, Brisbane, Australia SA Pathology, Flinders Medical Centre, Adelaide, Australia Thrombosis Medicine, McMaster University, Hamilton.
7. Furst DE, Ulrich RW, Prakash S. Chapter 36. Nonsteroidal anti-inflammatory drugs, disease-modifying antirheumatic drugs, nonopioid analgesics, & drugs used in gout. In: Katzung BG, Masters SB, Trevor AJ, editors. Basic & clinical pharmacology. 12th ed. New York: McGraw-Hill; 2012. http://www.accessmedicine.com/content.aspx?aID=55827134. Accessed 12 Mar 2013.
8. Wyatt JE, Pettit J, Harirforoosh S. Pharmacogenetics of nonsteroidal anti-inflammatory drugs. Pharmacogenomics J. 2012;12:462–7.

9. World Health Organization (WHO). National Cancer Control Programmes: policies and managerial guidelines. 3rd ed. Geneva; 2002. Available from: http://whqlibdoc.who.int/hq/2002/9241545577.pdf. Last access on 14 Feb 2013.
10. Horlocker TT, Wedel DJ, Rowlingson JC, et al. Regional anesthesia in the patient receiving antithrombotic or thrombolytic therapy: American Society of regional anesthesia and pain medicine evidence-based guidelines (3rd ed). Reg Anesth Pain Med. 2010;35(1):64–101.
11. Rosenecher N, Bottet M, Sessler D. Selected new antithrombotic agents and neuraxial anesthesia for major orthopaedic surgery: management strategies. Anaesthesia. 2007;62:1154–60.
12. Novak E, Allen PJ. Prescribing medications in pediatrics: concerns regarding FDA approval and pharmacokinetics. Pediatr Nurs. 2007;33:64–70.
13. Committee on Infectious Diseases, American Academy of Pediatrics. Pickering LK, editor. 2012. Red Book®: 2012 Report of the Committee on infectious diseases – 29th ed. 2012. Printed in the United States of America. American Academy of Pediatrics. ISBN-10: 1-58110-703-X, ISBN-13: 978-1-58110-703-6. ISSN: 1080-0131. STAT!Ref Online Electronic Medical Library. http://online.statref.com/document.aspx?fxid=76&docid=58. 2/13/2013 4:12:28PM CST (UTC -06:00).

Chapter 28
Antiemetic Agents

Aaron M. Fields

Contents

Introduction

Fifty-two percent of all surgical patients will experience postoperative nausea and vomiting (PONV) when no antiemetics are used. Risk factors include female sex, nonsmoker, having a history of motion sickness, or PONV. Anesthetic risk factors include not receiving a total intravenous anesthetic (TIVA), receiving opioids,

A.M. Fields, MD
Department of Anesthesiology, Tripler Army Medical Center, Honolulu, HI, USA
e-mail: afieldsmd@yahoo.com

A.D. Kaye et al. (eds.), *Essentials of Pharmacology for Anesthesia,*
Pain Medicine, and Critical Care, DOI 10.1007/978-1-4614-8948-1_28,
© Springer Science+Business Media New York 2015

exposure to nitrous oxide, and the length of the anesthetic. Class/type of antiemetic or not using a triggering anesthetic technique was associated with the same decrease in PONV, and to each was attributed a 26 % decrease in PONV [1]. Additionally, patients are willing to pay between $56 and $100 out of pocket to receive an antiemetic that is completely effective [2]. Neostigmine has been found to be a triggering agent at a dose above 2.5 mg in some studies, but other studies have failed to show any correlation between neostigmine and PONV [3]. A recent meta-analysis showed that inhaled isopropyl alcohol was more effective than placebo, but less effective than standard antiemetics [4].

The chemoreceptor trigger zone is located outside the blood-brain barrier in the medulla and is responsible for beginning the emesis process. Lesions of the area do not prevent emesis due to vagal stimulation or motion [5]. The CTZ is rich in chemical receptors, and antagonists to these receptors have become the mainstay of PONV prevention. While not well studied, PONV in diabetic patients with gastroparesis can be treated with metoclopramide.

Drug Class and Mechanism of Action

Serotonin Receptor Antagonists (see Fig. 28.1)

Serotonin released from enterochromaffin cells of the small intestinal mucosa binds to the 5-hydroxytryptamine type 3 (5-HT_3) in the CTZ. Most of the 5-HT3 blockers (ondansetron, granisetron) competitively antagonize these receptors and receptors in the gut [6]. The newest 5-HT3 antagonist (palonosetron) allosterically binds and causes downregulation of this type of serotonin receptor, possibly contributing to its long half-life [7]. It may also inhibit the emetic response caused by substance P, a characteristic shared by the NK1 receptor antagonists [8]. In a recent study, it was shown to be as effective as other 5-HT3 blockers plus dexamethasone and more effective than the others alone [9].

Corticosteroids

Dexamethasone and other corticosteroids stabilize liposomal membranes and interfere with the synthesis of prostaglandins [10].

Anticholinergics

Scopolamine

While there are many anticholinergic agents, only scopolamine is used in the prevention of PONV by inhibiting the binding of acetylcholine in the vestibular

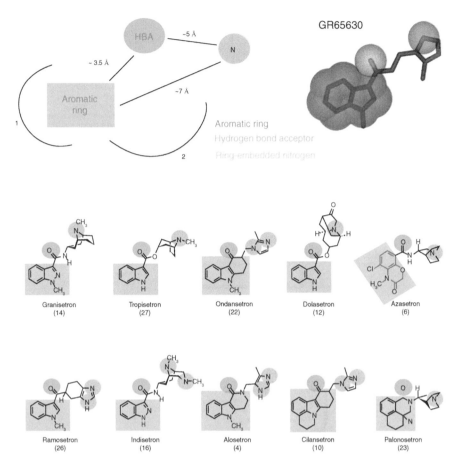

Fig. 28.1 5-hydroxytryptamine3 (5-HT3) receptor antagonists Thompson [22]

system [11] and the cortex and pons [12]. It is available in IV or transdermal formulations. It has been shown to be effective across a wide range of surgery times as a preventative agent as opposed to a rescue medication. Additionally, patients receiving this antiemetic reported much higher satisfaction scores than those in other treatment groups despite a high incidence of side effects [13].

Substance P Receptor (NK1) Antagonists

Aprepitant has been found to be more effective than ondansetron at preventing PONV in the perioperative period [14]. It has been found to exert its effects via a final, more common pathway of the emetic centers after crossing the blood-brain barrier [15]. In fact, there were no improved outcomes when scopolamine and aprepitant were combined [16]. However, it has not led to complete abolishment of nausea, so other mechanisms may be involved.

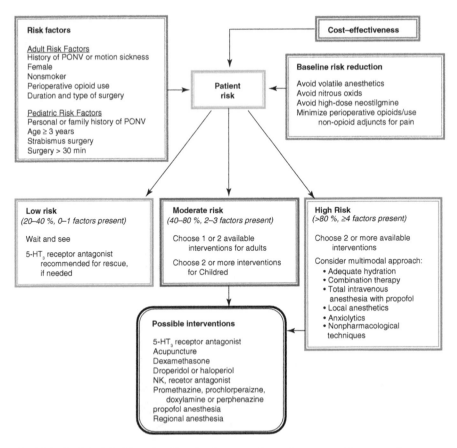

Fig. 28.2 A clinical decision algorithm for the prevention and treatment of postoperative nausea and vomiting (PONV) Le and Gan [18]

Dopamine Antagonists

Droperidol and promethazine block the effects of dopamine on the CTZ, and promethazine has additional histamine-blocking properties [17].

Indications/Clinical Pearls

- Le and Gan have developed an algorithm for the prevention of PONV based on risk factors. Risk factors include female sex, nonsmoker, having a history of motion sickness or PONV, and the use of opioids. For 0–1 risk factors, no antiemetics are recommended. For 2–3 risk factors, give one or two antiemetics, and if four or more risk factors are present, consider two or more antiemetics. TIVA can be used in place of one antiemetic [18] (See Fig. 28.2).

- As mentioned, alcohol has been shown to be effective in the clinical setting. Owing to its parasympathetic mediation, nausea can be rapidly treated successfully with two alcohol pads in each nostril with four deep breaths through the nose. The mechanism is believed to be the noxious smell creating a sympathetic overdrive response, and it should be seen within 30 s to a minute.

Dosing Options [17]

Ondansetron should be given in 4 mg doses. Dexamethasone should be administered at a dose of 8 mg [17] and it should be given at least 2 h prior to the end of surgery [19]. Scopolamine transdermal patch (1.5 mg) should be applied the night before surgery and removed 24 h after surgery. Aprepitant should be given in a dose of 40 mg [14]. Droperidol should be administered in a dose of 0.625 mg.

Drug Interactions (Package Inserts)

Ondansetron should not be given with apomorphine or any agent that prolongs QTc. Dexamethasone has no interaction with commonly used operating room drugs. Scopolamine levels may be increased by ipratropium, magnesium sulfate, and droperidol. Aprepitant may increase the levels of corticosteroids. Droperidol should not be given with MAO inhibitors or other agents that prolong the QTc.

Side Effects/Black Box Warnings

Headaches and constipation are the most common side effects associated with ondansetron, and it has a black box warning for QTc prolongation, most commonly associated with high doses. Dexamethasone has many side effects, but rarely are any of them a concern with a single injection with the exception of perineal burning after rapid IV injection [20]. Aprepitant is associated with fatigue, constipation, weakness, and hiccups. Droperidol was issued a block box warning for prolonged QT syndrome. However, this is rarely seen in the low doses used to prevent PONV [21].

Summary

PONV is a frequent problem that rarely leads to hospital admission. Most of the antiemetics today are inexpensive and have a very favorable side effect profile. All classes of antiemetics have been shown to be somewhat efficacious, but much of the data is contradictory given the complex nature of PONV. Nausea and emesis are multifactorial, and, therefore, no one agent is likely to prevent PONV in all patients. A large number of patients need to be studied to best sort out individual variables. Identifying patients who are at high risk and giving appropriate preventative anti-emetics can decrease PACU stays and increase patient comfort.

Disclosure The opinions expressed in this manuscript are the opinions of the author and do not necessarily reflect the opinions of the US Air Force, Army, or government.

Chemical Structures

**Chemical Structure
28.1** Dexamethasone

**Chemical Structure
28.2** Scopolamine

References

1. Apfel CC, Korttila K, Abdalla M, et al. A factorial trial of six interventions for the prevention of postoperative nausea and vomiting. N Engl J Med. 2004;350(24):2441–51.
2. Gan T, Sloan F, Dear Gde L, et al. How much are patients willing to pay to avoid postoperative nausea and vomiting? Anesth Analg. 2001;92(2):393–400.
3. Cheng CR, Sessler DI, Apfel CC. Does neostigmine administration produce a clinically important increase in postoperative nausea and vomiting? Anesth Analg. 2005;101:1349–55.
4. Hines S, Steels E, Chang A, et al. Aromatherapy for treatment of postoperative nausea and vomiting. Cochrane Database Syst Rev. 2012;4:CD007598.
5. Miller AD, Leslie RA. The area postrema and vomiting. Front Neuroendocrinol. 1994;15(4): 301–20.
6. Andrews P, Rapeport W, Sanger G. Neuropharmacology of emesis induced by anti-cancer therapy. Trends Pharmacol Sci. 1988;9:334–41.
7. Rojas C, Stathis M, Thomas AG, et al. Palonosetron exhibits unique molecular interactions with the 5-HT3 receptor. Anesth Analg. 2008;107:469–78.
8. Rojas C, Li Y, Zhang J, et al. The antiemetic 5-HT3 receptor antagonist palonosetron inhibits substance P-mediated responses in vitro and in vivo. J Pharmacol Exp Ther. 2010;335:362–8.

9. Moon YE, Joo J, Kim JE, Lee Y. Anti-emetic effect of ondansetron and palonosetron in thyroidectomy: a prospective, randomized, double-blind study. Br J Anaesth. 2012;108:417–22.

10. Rich W, Abdulhayoglu G, Di Saia PJ. Methylprednisolone as antiemetic during cancer chemotherapy: a pilot study. Gynecol Oncol. 1980;9:193–8.

11. Pergolizzi JV, Philip BK, Leslie JB, Taylor R, Raffa RB. Perspectives on transdermal scopolamine for the treatment of postoperative nausea and vomiting. J Clin Anesth. 2012;24(4):334–45.

12. McCarthy BG, Peroutka SJ. Differentiation of muscarinic cholinergic receptor subtypes in human cortex and pons: implications for anti-motion sickness therapy. Aviat Space Environ Med. 1988;59(1):63–6.

13. Kranke P, Morin A, Roewer N, et al. The efficacy and safety of transdermal scopolamine for the prevention of postoperative nausea and vomiting: a quantitative systematic review. Anesth Analg. 2002;95:133–43.

14. Diemunsch P, Apfel C, Gan TJ, et al. Preventing postoperative nausea and vomiting: post hoc analysis of pooled data from two randomized active-controlled trials of aprepitant. Curr Med Res Opin. 2007;23(10):2559–65.

15. Minami M, Endo T, Kikuchi K, et al. Antiemetic effects of sendide, a peptide tachykinin NK1 receptor antagonist, in the ferret. Eur J Pharmacol. 1998;363:49–55.

16. Green MS, Green P, Malayaman SN, et al. Randomized, double-blind comparison of oral aprepitant alone compared with aprepitant and transdermal scopolamine for prevention of postoperative nausea and vomiting. Br J Anaesth. 2012;109(5):716–22.

17. Scuderi PE. Pharmacology of antiemetics. Int Anesthesiol Clin. 2003;41(4):41–66.

18. Le TP, Gan TJ. Update on the management of postoperative nausea and vomiting and postdischarge nausea and vomiting in ambulatory surgery. Anesthesiol Clin. 2010;28(2):225–49.

19. Elhakim M, Nafie M, Mahmoud K, et al. Dexamethasone 8 mg in combination with ondansetron 4 mg appears to be the optimal dose for the prevention of nausea and vomiting after laparoscopic cholecystectomy. Can J Anaesth. 2002;49:922–6.

20. Wang JJ, Ho ST, Tzeng JI, et al. The effect of timing of dexamethasone administration on its efficacy as a prophylactic antiemetic for postoperative nausea and vomiting. Anesth Analg. 2000;91(1):136–9.

21. White PF. Droperidol: a cost-effective antiemetic for over thirty years. Anesth Analg. 2002;95(4):789–90.

22. Thompson AJ. Recent developments in 5-HT3 receptor pharmacology. Trends Pharmacol Sci. 2013;34(2):100–9. doi:10.1016/j.tips.2012.12.002. ISSN 0165-6147.

Chapter 29
Antiepileptic Agents

Angelika Kosse and Heesung Kang

Contents

A. Kosse, MD (✉) • H. Kang, MD
Department of Anesthesiology, Montefiore Medical Center,
University Hospital of Albert Einstein College of Medicine
of Yeshiva University, Bronx, NY, USA
e-mail: akosse@montefiore.org; hkang@montefiore.org

A.D. Kaye et al. (eds.), *Essentials of Pharmacology for Anesthesia,*
Pain Medicine, and Critical Care, DOI 10.1007/978-1-4614-8948-1_29,
© Springer Science+Business Media New York 2015

This chapter provides an overview of the currently available antiepileptic drugs. At this time, there are 24 antiepileptic drugs approved by the FDA, several only recently [1]. Some drugs have more than one mechanism of action [2]. Some of these agents have only one particular indication, while others have a broad spectrum of action [3]. A few are approved only for adjunct therapy. A common classification is by generation [2, 4–6]:

First generation: hydantoins, barbiturates, carbamazepine, succinimides, valproic acid, and benzodiazepines [7]
Second generation: lamotrigine, oxcarbazepine, topiramate, gabapentin, levetiracetam, felbamate, pregabalin, tiagabine, and zonisamide [7]

Epilepsy

Epilepsy is a brain disorder causing recurrent seizures. Among possible etiologies for their occurrence are a genetic predisposition, head trauma, stroke, brain tumor, metabolic abnormalities, drug and alcohol withdrawal, and CNS infection [8–10]. Seizures are due to electrical disturbances of cortical neurons leading to a sudden imbalance between excitatory and inhibitory activity resulting in a net excitation [1, 4, 9]. The symptoms depend on the location and function of the epileptic focus. There are several types of seizures [6, 10]:

Partial (focal) seizures (about 60 % of all seizures), which are divided into *simple*, if consciousness does not get affected, or *complex* if it does (temporal or psychomotor seizures)
Generalized seizures (about 40 % of all seizures) with bilateral symmetric electrical activity resulting in abnormal motor activity and/or loss of consciousness. Inhibitory or nonconvulsive seizures include atonic (petit mal) seizures, with transient lapse in consciousness, and absence seizures that are characterized by a loss of consciousness and staring spells. Excitatory and convulsive seizures include myoclonic (brief involuntary muscle twitches), clonic (series of muscle contractions), and tonic-clonic (grand mal) seizures with tonic-clonic motor activity and loss of consciousness. Partial seizures can progress to secondarily generalized tonic-clonic seizures.
Unclassified Seizures

Seizures also are categorized as epileptic syndrome, including seizure type, etiology, age of onset, etc. There are more than 50 such syndromes.

Mechanism of Action

Antiepileptics change the excitation or inhibition of neurotransmission via an effect on ion channels, receptors, or neurotransmitter metabolism [1–4, 6, 9, 11].

1. Blockade of voltage-gated Na channel

   The sodium channels are responsible for the depolarization phase of the neuronal action potential by allowing sodium influx. This active phase is followed by an inactive refractory period. Some antiepileptics stabilize the inactive state and block the depolarization of the nerve terminal and subsequent release of neurotransmitter and prevent the high-frequency neuronal firing leading to seizures [3, 4, 6, 7].

2. Potentiation of inhibition by GABA

   Gamma-aminobutyric acid is the main inhibitory transmitter in the brain [3]. It binds to GABA-A and GABA-B receptors. GABA-A receptors are coupled to chloride channels [4], where chloride influx decreases the excitability of the postsynaptic membrane [4]. GABA-B receptors are coupled to presynaptic potassium channels which indirectly may inhibit the release of neurotransmitter.

   The inhibition of GABA transaminase increases the amount of released GABA [1, 4, 7].

   Also the reuptake of GABA can be blocked and its effect thereby increased.

3. Blockade of calcium channels

   T-type calcium channels in the thalamic neurons play a role in "spike and wave" discharges typical for absence seizures [2, 3]. Their blockade is effective against absence seizures. Effects on other voltage-gated calcium channels are less studied. Many antiepileptics act on different calcium channels; effect on N-type and P/Q-type seems to contribute to antiepileptic effect and effect on neuropathic pain of drugs, including gabapentin and pregabalin [3, 4, 7].

4. Action on alpha-amino-3-hydroxy-5-methyl-4-isoxazolepropionic acid (AMPA)/ kainite/N-methyl-D-aspartate (NMDA)

   They are glutamate receptor sites, which bind glutamate, an excitatory CNS neurotransmitter, activating influx of sodium and calcium ions and outflow of potassium ions leading to excitation. Glutamate antagonists modify these receptors [2, 4, 12–14].

5. Modulation of serotonergic transmission

   Serotonin (5-hydroxytryptamine) is a neurotransmitter modulating mood and behavior. Increased extracellular serotonin levels (i.e., by blockade of reuptake) inhibit seizures. Activation of some serotonin receptor subtypes also inhibits seizures. 5-HT2C depolarizes GABAergic neurons; 5-HT1A hyperpolarizes glutamatergic neurons [3, 4, 7, 15].

6. Effect on potassium current

   The outward potassium current is at least partially responsible for the refractory period after an action potential. Modifying this outward potassium current to flow faster and longer will enhance the refractory period that can slow the repetitive firing of neurons [1, 3, 4, 16].

7. Modulation of SV2A

   SV2A is a synaptic vesicle protein involved in vesicle exocytosis and ejection of stored neurotransmitters. Modulation of the SV2A can lead to decreased action potential-dependent neurotransmission [1, 2, 4, 17].

Drugs

Since 2008, the FDA mandated that all antiepileptic package inserts have to state that they increase the risk of suicidal thoughts/action [1, 5, 7, 18, 19]. Some of these warnings are modest: for example, the risk of suicidal thoughts for gabapentin is 4/10,000 versus 3/10,000 for placebo. Since then studies have cited odds ratios (>1 = increased suicidal risk) for topiramate (OR = 2.53), lamotrigine (OR = 2.08), valproate (OR = 1.4), carbamazepine (OR = 0.65–1.4), gabapentin (OR = 0.9), levetiracetam (OR = 0.7), pregabalin (OR = 0.2), and clonazepam (OR = 2.1) but also questioned if the warning is warranted [20–22]. After initiation of therapy, roughly 50 % of patients experience full control of their seizure activity, and 25 % experience improvement. To decrease toxicity, therapy with one drug is preferred [6]. For some AED drugs, it is recommended to slowly titrate the dose up to avoid or to decrease side effects. First-generation AEDs have been shown to increase the risk of fetal malformations two- to threefold if taken in the first trimester [3, 8]; many induce liver enzymes and increase metabolism of other drugs.

Phenytoin

This agent is a first-line therapy for partial and tonic-clonic seizures, status epilepticus, and prevention of seizures after neurosurgery. It blocks the ion influx and slows the recovery rate of voltage-gated sodium channels. It is 90 % protein bound (more free drug in neonate, hypoalbuminemia, uremia), 95 % of the drug is metabolized in the hepatic endoplasmic reticulum by CYP2C9/10/19, its metabolite is inactive, and its elimination is not linear but varies with its plasma concentration. By inducing liver enzymes (CYPs), phenytoin enhances the metabolism of other drugs (contraceptives, neuromuscular blockers) [2, 5, 6].

Dose

Adult dose is initially 100 mg three times a day, with max 600 mg/day. Loading dose for rapid therapeutic level is 1,000 mg (400, 300,300 mg 2 h apart) or 10–15 mg/kg IV at maximum 50 mg/min or 1–3 mg/kg/min, then 100 mg IV or PO every 6–8 h.

Compatible with normal saline and may precipitate with IV solutions/other drugs.

Therapeutic Level

10–20 mcg/ml; in neonates, 7.5–15 mcg/ml

Onset

1–2 h (IV), 2–24 h (PO)

Half-Life

10–15 h (IV), 22 h (PO)

Fosphenytoin

It is a water-soluble prodrug of phenytoin, and 75 mg of fosphenytoin is equivalent to 50 mg of phenytoin. The level can be checked 2 h after an IV dose.

Dose

15–20 mg/kg IV at max 150 mg/min, then maintenance dose 4–6 mg/kg/day given once daily or divided two times a day; if switching from phenytoin, same daily dose.

Therapeutic Level

10–20 mcg/ml phenytoin

Half-Life

15 min

Side Effects

For fosphenytoin, arrhythmias are less frequent with its IV use; acute overdose shows mostly cerebellar and vestibular signs; very high doses can lead to cerebellar atrophy, GI symptoms, gingival hyperplasia (about 20 %), osteomalacia, megalo-blastic anemia, hirsutism, transient increase in liver enzymes (although this by itself is no reason to change therapy), skin reactions like rashes and Steven-Johnson's syndrome, SLE, fatal hepatic necrosis, leukopenia, mild thrombocytopenia, lymph-adenopathy and malignant lymphoma due to decreased IGA production, and hem-orrhage in newborns of mothers on phenytoin (can be prophylactically dosed with vitamin K); many side effects can be lowered with dose adjustments. Abrupt with-drawal can elicit seizures.

Black Box Warning

Cardiovascular symptoms such as severe hypotension and arrhythmias are possible with rapid infusion. If given IV, patients should be on cardiac monitor [23].

Other Uses

Trigeminal and other neuralgias and cardiac (ventricular) arrhythmias

Barbiturates

Phenobarbital (Luminal) inhibits seizures by binding to specific GABA-A receptor site and prolonging chloride channel opening. It is 40–60 % protein bound, with hepatic metabolism by CYP2C9/19, and 25 % renal excretion. It induces liver enzymes (UGT, CYP2C, 3A). It is used for therapy of secondarily generalized tonic-clonic and partial seizures and status epilepticus [4, 6].

Dose

Adults, 1–4 mg/kg/day up to 200–240 mg/day or divided twice a day [5, 8]

Neonates, 3–5 mg/kg/day IV/PO; infants, 5–6 mg/kg/day; 1–5 years, 6–8 mg/kg/day; 6–12 years, 4–6 mg/kg/day; >12 years, 1–3 mg/kg/day; for status epilepticus in infants and children, 15–20 mg/kg IV once, not faster than 30 mg/min; and in adults, 10–20 mg/kg once at 25–100 mg/min

Therapeutic Level

10–40 mcg/ml

Onset

After IV administration, 5–12 min, with peak levels at 30 min. If given orally, drug reaches steady state after 2–3 weeks.

Half-Life

50–120 h, in infants up to 400 h. Half-life is increased in pregnancy.

Side Effects

Sedation (but tolerance develops with time), rash, hypothrombinemia with hemorrhage in newborns, megaloblastic anemia, osteomalacia, irritability and hyperactivity in children, agitation and confusion in elderly, ataxia and nystagmus at excessive doses (>60 mcg/ml), respiratory depression with large doses, withdrawal seizures if stopped abruptly; injectable solution is highly alkaline – tissue necrosis can occur with extravasation [5, 6, 8].

Contraindication

Porphyria, severe liver disease, and lactation

Iminostilbenes

Carbamazepine (Tegretol, Carbatrol) slows recovery of inactivated sodium channels. It is 75 % protein bound, is metabolized in the liver to active 10,11-epoxide which metabolizes to an inactive compound, and is excreted in urine. Carbamazepine induces liver enzymes. It is used for all partial and generalized tonic-clonic seizures [4, 6, 8].

Dose

Initially 200 mg twice daily, suspension 100 mg four times daily, with maximum of 1,200 mg/day, rarely 1,600 mg/day. For ages 12–15 years, 1,000 mg divided into three or four daily doses; for ages under 6 years, 10–20 mg/kg/day in two or three doses [5, 8].

Therapeutic Level

4–12 mcg/ml, autoinduction starts 3–4 weeks after start, decreasing level

Onset

Plasma peak time: regular tab 4.5 h; oral suspension, 1.5 h; 3–12 h extended release tab

Half-Life

25–65 h at first, then decreasing to 12–17 h

Side Effects

Antidiuretic effect (increased antidiuretic hormone), CNS side effects start at 9 mcg/ml, drowsiness, ataxia, diplopia, aplastic anemia (1:200,000), agranulocytosis, eosinophilia, lymphadenopathy, splenomegaly, transient increase of liver enzymes (5–10 %) that resolves in 4 months, mild leukopenia, and thrombocytopenia. Renal and hepatic function need to be monitored.

The black box warning (www.fda.gov) include [24]:

- Concern over occasionally serious dermatologic reactions, which can include mucous membrane ulcers (including Stevens-Johnson syndrome and toxic epidermal necrolysis), painful rash, and elevated temperature (1–6 per 10,000 new users in countries with mainly white populations, but the risk with an almost exclusive Asian allele HLA-B*1502 is much higher, and epidemiological data in some Asian countries estimates risk to be approximately ten times higher).
- Aplastic anemia and agranulocytosis are very rare, but therapy may be halted if there is bone marrow suppression (the risk is 5–8 times greater than in the general population, and the overall risk of these reactions in the untreated general population is minimal, approximately six patients per one million population per year for agranulocytosis and two patients per one million population per year for aplastic anemia).

Contraindication

Sensitivity to tricyclic antidepressives, history of bone marrow depression, and no coadministration with MAO inhibitors (stop MAOI for 14 days) and nefazodone

Other Uses

Trigeminal and glossopharyngeal neuralgia, bipolar disorder, and lightning-type pain with bodily wasting [2, 5, 8, 25–28]

Oxcarbazepine is a prodrug and is a keto-analogue of carbamazepine that becomes converted to active 10-monohydroxy derivative (MHD). It is inactivated by glucuronide conjugation with renal excretion; it is 38 % protein bound and a less potent liver enzyme inducer. It is utilized for mono- or adjunct therapy of partial seizures in adults, monotherapy of partial seizures in children 4–16 years, adjunct therapy in children 2–4 years old, and used also for neuropathies and bipolar disorder.

Dose

Starting dose 300 mg twice daily, recommended 1,200 mg/day, can slowly be increased to up to 2,400 mg/day, but often not tolerated (CNS effects); for children aged 2–4 years, 8–10 mg/kg/day in divided doses up to 600 mg, then slowly increase up to 60 mg/kg/day; if <20 kg, start with 16–20 mg/kg/day; for 4–16 years, 8–10 mg/kg/day in two doses, then titrate over 2 weeks up depending on weight: 20–29 kg, 450 mg twice daily; 29–39 kg, 600 mg twice daily; >39 kg, 900 mg twice daily. Decrease initial dose with renal impairment.

Therapeutic Level

15–35 mcg/ml of active MHD

Onset

Peak drug level after 1–3 h; of active MHD, 4–12 h

Half-Life

1–3 h for oxcarbazepine and 8–10 h for MHD

Side Effects

Antidiuretic action leading to water retention and hyponatremia, especially in elderly patients (7.4 %) and in the first 3 months of therapy, somnolence, dizziness, GI disturbances, alopecia, anaphylaxis, angioedema, epidermal necrolysis, can worsen absence and myoclonic seizures and juvenile idiopathic generalized epilepsy, and diplopia. 25–30 % of those patients that are allergic to carbamazepine will also be allergic to oxcarbazepine.

Contraindications

Hypersensitivity to oxcarbazepine

Succinimides

Ethosuximide (*Zarontin*) is the primary and most selective agent for absence seizures (petit mal). It works by decreasing low-threshold T-type calcium currents in thalamic neurons. It has no significant protein binding; 25 % gets excreted unchanged in urine, and the rest is metabolized by hepatic microsomal enzymes into a major metabolite, hydroxyethyl derivative. Forty percent of drug excreted as glucuronides in urine [4, 5].

Dose

For ages 3–6 years, initial dose 250 mg/day. For 6 years and older, initial 500 mg once, and then optimal dose 20 mg/kg/day in divided doses

Therapeutic Level

40–100 mcg/ml, plasma concentration averages ~2 mcg/ml per 1 mg/kg

Onset

Peak plasma time 4 h

Half-Life

40–60 h, in children 30 h

Side Effects

Most common side effects include nausea and vomiting, anorexia, drowsiness, lethargy, euphoria, headaches, hiccough, occasional Parkinson-like symptoms, photophobia, restlessness, agitation inability to concentrate, lupus, blood dyscrasias, and abnormal renal and hepatic function.

Contraindication

Hypersensitivity

Valproic Acid (Depakote)

Valproic acid is different because it acts against absence as well as complex partial and generalized tonic-clonic seizures and is also used for migraine and bipolar disorder. It acts by increasing the amount of GABA by inhibiting its metabolism, and the drug also acts on sodium channels and on T-type calcium channels. It is metabolized in the liver and exhibits high protein binding and molarity, displacing other drugs from albumin. It inhibits enzyme CYP2C9 and UGT and decreases the metabolism of other drugs [2–5, 8, 13].

Dose

Initially 10–15 mg/kg, increased weekly by 5–10 mg/kg up to max 60 mg/kg, divided doses over 250 mg/day in adults and children. IV dilution is 100 mg/ml, and the IV dose and frequency is the same as PO doses. However, IV doses should be infused over 60 min at <20 mg/min.

Therapeutic Level

30–100 mcg/ml, but poor correlation of concentration and effect

Onset

Peak plasma time, 1–4 h; extended release, 7–14 h

Half-Life

6–16 h; in neonates, 10–67 h

Side Effects

GI symptoms, anorexia in 16 %, sedation, ataxia, occasional tremor, rash, alopecia, increased appetite, 40 % get increase of liver enzymes, asymptomatic, thrombocytopenia, increased bleeding time, weight loss, hyperammonemia, and multiorgan hypersensitivity reaction; use with clonazepam can trigger absence seizures and, rarely, absence status epilepticus.

> **Black Box Warning**
> Hepatotoxicity, hepatic failure especially in children under 2 years and if on multiple drugs or with metabolic disorders, risk decreases for 2–10 year olds and even more for older kids and adults (1:50,000). Serious or fatal hepatotoxicity may be preceded by nonspecific symptoms such as anorexia, facial edema, lethargy, malaise, vomiting, and weakness. Liver damage usually occurs in the first 6 months, and therefore, liver function tests prior to therapy and at frequent intervals are recommended, especially during the first 6 months. A second black box warning is pancreatitis, which can be hemorrhagic and rapidly progressing and may be fatal in both children and in adults. It should be noted that reported cases involve incidence shortly after initial use as well as after several years of use. A third black box warning is teratogenicity. The drug can cause neural tube defects (e.g., spina bifida) with poor cognitive outcome. This risk is greater than with other AEDs [29].

Contraindication

Liver disease, pancreatitis, pregnancy (especially in the first trimester), and urea cycle disorder

Benzodiazepines

Benzodiazepines approved for long-term therapy are *clonazepam* (Klonopin) and *clorazepate* (Tranxene), and those used for status epilepticus are *diazepam* (Valium) and *lorazepam* (Ativan). Benzodiazepines bind to a specific GABA-A receptor subunit and modulate chloride currents by increasing the frequency (but not the duration) of channel openings, increasing the GABA-mediated inhibition of the action potential. At higher doses, they may also act on sodium channels [2–6].

Diazepam is metabolized by hepatic enzymes, and a major metabolite is the partial agonist N-desmethyldiazepam. Both diazepam and its metabolite get hydroxylated into another active metabolite, oxazepam. It is highly lipid soluble and 99 % protein bound. It is used in status epilepticus but can also be used as an anxiolytic, a hypnotic, a muscle relaxant, and a treatment for alcohol withdrawal. Its main disadvantage is its relatively short duration of action [30].

Dose

2–10 mg PO every 6–12 h. For status epilepticus, 5–10 mg IV every 10–15 min up to 30 mg

Therapeutic Level

0.2–0.2 mcg/ml for other uses; for seizures, by effect

Onset

Prompt with rapid redistribution due to high lipid solubility

Half-Life

20–70 h

Side Effects

Sedation, confusion, anterograde amnesia, respiratory depression, ataxia, nausea, vomiting urinary retention, hypotension, increased CNS effects in elderly, dependence and withdrawal symptoms with abrupt cessation, and phlebitis with IV administration

Contraindication

Hypersensitivity, severe hepatic impairment, myasthenia gravis (with exceptions), and acute alcohol intoxication [2, 6]

Clonazepam has a higher affinity for the GABA-A receptor site than diazepam. It is metabolized in the liver to an inactive metabolite, and less than 1 % is excreted unchanged in urine. It is the drug of choice for myoclonic seizures and, to a lesser degree, subcortical myoclonus. It is also effective in status epilepticus. It can also be used for anxiety and panic disorders. Tolerance develops usually after 1–6 months, and once tolerance is developed, the drug has no effect at any dose. It is available in IV and PO form.

Dose

In adults, initially <1.5 mg/day, increase every 3 days by 0.5–1.0 mg/day to max 20 mg/day. In children, 0.01–0.03 mg/kg/day, increase every 3 days by 0.25–0.5 mg/day to max 0.2 mg/kg/day. Side effects are less if given in divided doses.

Therapeutic Level

Tolerance makes plasma concentration of limited value.

Onset

20–60 min, prompt after IV dose

Half-Life

18–60 h; 22–33 h in children

Side Effects

Sedation; anterograde amnesia; drowsiness; lethargy; muscular incoordination; ataxia; hypotonia; dysarthria; behavioral disturbances like aggression, hyperactivity, irritability, and difficulty to concentrate; anorexia or hyperphagia; increased salivation and bronchial secretions; seizure exacerbation; and status epilepticus if stopped abruptly (even after only a few weeks on the drug)

Contraindication

Same as for diazepam, narrow-angle glaucoma

Clorazepate has the same mechanism of action as the previous two benzodiazepines. It is metabolized in liver to desmethyldiazepam and oxazepam, which are excreted in urine. It is used for adjunct therapy of partial seizures, but is not approved for use in children under 9 years of age. It is also used for anxiety and alcohol withdrawal.

Dose

For seizures in children aged 9–12 years, 7.5 mg twice daily, then increase by <7.5 mg every week up to 60 mg/day. For ages 12 years and older, 7.5 mg three times daily, then increase weekly by <7.5 mg up to 90 mg/day. For anxiety and withdrawal, the starting doses are higher – about 30 mg.

Therapeutic Level

Not established

Onset

1–2 h

Half-Life

50–70 h

Side Effects

CNS depression, dry mouth, anterograde amnesia, blurred vision, withdrawal symptoms with abrupt cessation, and respiratory depression

Contraindication

Hypersensitivity and narrow-angle glaucoma

Lorazepam is also metabolized in the liver to inactive metabolites that are excreted in urine. It is 85 % protein bound in plasma. It is used as therapy for status epilepticus, anxiety, sedation, and chemotherapy-induced nausea and vomiting.

Dose

IV for status epilepticus – 4 mg IV, with range of 2–8 mg, repeat every 5–15 min, with maximum dose of 20 mg/h. In children, the dose is 0.05–0.1 mg/kg IV over 2–5 min, up to 4 mg. Repeat every 10–15 min if needed. For anxiety/sedation, 2–3 mg PO every 8–12 h, then 2–6 mg/day in divided doses or 0.02–0.06 mg/kg IV or 0.01–0.1 mg/kg/h; for children, 0.05 mg/kg PO every 4–8 h. With chemotherapy 1–2.5 mg PO or IV half an hour before treatment, then every 4 h if needed; in children, 0.05 mg/kg IV, and repeat every 6 h as needed.

Therapeutic Level

Peak plasma level after 2 mg is 20 ng/ml.

Onset

IV, 1–5 min; IM, 15–30 min

Half-Life

12–18 h

Side Effects

CNS depression, respiratory depression, extrapyramidal symptoms, changes in vision and appetite, increase of liver enzymes, and withdrawal symptoms with abrupt cessation

Contraindication

Hypersensitivity and narrow-angle glaucoma

Clobazam is approved for adjunctive therapy of LGS in patients 2 years and older. It binds also to GABA-A receptor, potentiating GABAergic neurotransmission.

Dose

Adults: Start 10 mg/day and increase up to 40 mg/day over at least 2 weeks. Pediatric: If under 30 kg, start 5 mg/day and then increase up to 20 mg/day. If over 30 kg, dose according to adult dosage [1, 2, 31].

Therapeutic Level

237–285 ng/ml

Onset

30 min to 4 h

Half-Life

36–42 h, but its metabolite, N-desmethylclobazam, has about 70–80 h.

Side Effects

Sedation: avoid other depressants, alcohol, and abrupt discontinuation (withdrawal).

Contraindications

Hypersensitivity: caution with myasthenia gravis.

Gabapentin (Neurontin) and Pregabalin (Lyrica)

Gabapentin is believed to have an effect on calcium channels as it binds to the a2δ subunit of calcium channels. It is highly lipid soluble, but is not metabolized and excreted unchanged in urine. It is not protein bound and does not induce hepatic enzymes. It is used for adjunct therapy of partial seizures with or without secondary generalized seizures. Other uses include migraine, chronic pain, postherpetic neuralgia, bipolar disorder, and other neuropathic pain states [2–6, 8].

Dose

Initially 300 mg PO every 8 h, up to 600 mg every 8 h, with maximum up to 3,600 mg/day. Adjust dose with renal impairment. For partial seizures age 3–12 years, 10–15 mg/kg/day in three doses. Titrate up to maintenance dose for ages 3–4 years old 40 mg/kg/day in three doses, and for 5–12 years, 25–35 mg/kg/day; for ages 12 and older, dosing is the same as adults'. For neuralgia in adults, titrate up to 600 mg three times daily.

Therapeutic Level

Not very helpful, effect at 2–20 mcg/ml, occasionally up to 80 mcg/ml as necessary

Onset

Peak serum level at 2–4 h

Half-Life

5–7 h

Side Effects

Somnolence, ataxia, dizziness, nystagmus, tremor, and diplopia: usually resolves after 2 weeks. Eighty-six percent of patients do not meet target doses because of side effects; a new gastroretentive formulation (Gralise) has similar efficacy with significantly improved side effect profile.

Contraindication

Hypersensitivity

Pregabalin is used for adjunctive therapy of partial seizures and also for neuropathies and fibromyalgia. It works similar to gabapentin, is excreted unchanged in urine, and is not protein bound.

Dose

For adults, start 150 mg/day up to 600 mg/day. Safety in pediatric population is not established.

Therapeutic Level

0.5–16 mcg/ml

Onset

Peak serum level at 1.5 h

Half-Life

6.3 h

Side Effects

Dizziness, peripheral edema, somnolence, ataxia, nystagmus, and tremor

Contraindication

Hypersensitivity

Lamotrigine (Lamictal)

Lamotrigine acts on sodium channels and is metabolized by glucuronidation in the liver. It is used for partial or secondary generalized tonic-clonic seizures, Lennox-Gastaut syndrome, tonic-clonic seizures, and absence seizures in children [2–5, 32].

Dose

If the patient is taking a hepatic enzyme-inducing medication, initial dose is 50 mg/day for 2 weeks, then increase up to 300–500 mg/day over several weeks, divided in two doses. If the patient is taking valproate alone, start with 25 mg/day and increase up to 200 mg/day over several weeks. If on none of those medications, start at 25 mg/day and increase the dose up to 375 mg/day over several weeks.

Therapeutic Level

Has not been established for Lamictal. Dose based on effects.

Onset

Peak serum level at 1.4–4.8 h

Half-Life

24–34 h for monotherapy; 13.5 h if adjunct therapy with enzyme-inducing drugs

Side Effects

Adverse effects include dizziness, ataxia, blurred or double vision, and nausea vomiting.

Black Box Warning
Severe life-threatening skin rashes, including Stevens-Johnson syndrome, and serious toxic epidermal necrolysis can occur, usually after 2–8 weeks. Rashes are more common in children (0.8 %) than in adults (0.3 %). Coadministration with valproic acid requires a reduction in the dose by 50 % to minimize the risk of Stevens-Johnson syndrome and toxic epidermal necrolysis. The incidence has been reported to be approximately 0.8 % (8/1,000) in pediatric patients (2–16 years of age) receiving lamotrigine for epilepsy and 0.3 % (3/1,000) in adults receiving therapy for epilepsy. Benign rashes can occur, and therefore, with any signs of rash, the most reasonable course of action is discontinuation of the agent [33].

Contraindication

Hypersensitivity

Levetiracetam (Keppra)

Levetiracetam is approved for adjunct therapy of myoclonic seizures and partial seizures with or without secondary generalized tonic-clonic seizures and for monotherapy of primary generalized tonic-clonic seizures in adults and children from 4 years and older. It acts on the synaptic vesicle protein SV2 to stop the release of excitatory neurotransmitters. It is not protein bound; about 66 % of the drug is excreted unchanged in the urine. There is no induction of hepatic enzymes.

Dose

For monotherapy in adults, 1,000–3,000 mg/day in both PO and IV forms. (PO and IV doses are interchangeable.) In children under 16, the initial dose is 20 mg/kg/day divided into two doses, up to 60 mg/kg/day. In renal patients, from 500 mg/day up to 1,500 mg/day [2–5, 8, 32, 34].

Therapeutic Level

Not established

Onset

1 h PO, 15 min IV

Half-Life

6–8 h; in renal failure patients, 11 h; in children, 5–6 h

Side Effects

Somnolence, asthenia, dizziness, and nasopharyngitis. Rarely, rashes and even seizures may occur; withdrawal symptoms with abrupt cessation [32].

Contraindications

Hypersensitivity

Tiagabine (Gabitril)

Tiagabine is approved for adjunct therapy of partial seizures in adults. It likely inhibits GABA transporter GAT-1, promoting more GABA binding to neurons. It is metabolized by hepatic CYP3A [4, 5].

Dose

In adults, initially 4 mg/day, and titrate up to 56 mg/day over 8 weeks. Safety not established for children under 12 years of age.

Therapeutic Level

20–100 mcg/l

Onset

45 min

Half-Life

About 8 h, but 2–3 h if taken with enzyme-inducing drugs

Side Effects

Dizziness, somnolence, mild tremor, nervousness, and inability to concentrate. Tiagabine is contraindicated in absence seizures. Most serious adverse effect may be nonconvulsive status epilepticus and withdrawal symptoms with abrupt cessation.

Contraindications

Hypersensitivity and absence seizures (exacerbates spike and wave discharges)

Topiramate (Topamax)

Topiramate is used for monotherapy of partial, primary generalized tonic-clonic seizures and Lennox-Gastaut syndrome. Other uses are for bipolar disorder, eating disorder, addiction disorders, migraine headaches, and chronic pain. It works on sodium and potassium channels and GABA and AMPA/kainate receptors. The drug undergoes little protein binding (10–20 %) and is mainly excreted unchanged in urine [2–5, 35–37].

Dose

For adults, initially 50 mg/day up to 400 mg/day divided into two doses; for children, 10–25 mg/kg/day divided into two doses

Therapeutic Level

10 mcg/ml

Onset

6–8 h

Half-Life

19–23 h

Side Effects

Somnolence, fatigue, weight loss, nervousness, change of taste of carbonated beverages, renal calculi, cognitive impairment, aphasia, metabolic acidosis, and hypohidrosis.

Contraindications

Hypersensitivity, history of kidney stones, and patients on high doses of vitamin C

Felbamate (Felbatol)

Felbamate is approved for adjunct therapy of partial seizures and drop attacks in Lennox-Gastaut syndrome. It works by potentiation of GABA-A receptor currents and blocking of NMDA receptor currents; it inhibits the liver enzyme CYP2C19 [2–5, 14, 38, 39].

Dose

Its recommended dose is 1,200–3,600 mg/day and should be titrated up weekly to achieve the desired dosage. In children, 15 mg/kg/day.

Therapeutic Level

30–60 mcg/ml

Onset

1–4 h

Half-Life

20–23 h

Side Effects

Nausea and vomiting, dizziness, headaches, insomnia, and gastric irritation

> **Black Box Warning**
> A black box warning for this agent is aplastic anemia (drug increases the risk 100-fold with a fatality rate of 20–30 %) and hepatic failure (see below). The drug should only be used for severe epilepsy. Risk of death varies with severity and etiology, and due to this drugs reported association with acute hepatic failure, it should not be used with any history of hepatic impairment. Monitor LFTs at baseline, then periodically, and discontinue therapy if LFTs increase or double or clinical signs or symptoms of hepatic failure occur [40].

Contraindication

Hypersensitivity, blood dyscrasias, and hepatic impairment

Zonisamide (Zonegran)

It is approved for adjunct therapy of partial seizures and secondary tonic-clonic seizures in adults. It inhibits T-type calcium currents and also sodium channel currents. 85 % of the drug is excreted unchanged in urine. The rest is metabolized by CYP3A4 and excreted as a glucuronide [2, 4, 5, 8, 9].

Dose

100–400 mg/day and titrated over several weeks. Not used for children under the age of 16. Adjust for renal failure.

Therapeutic Level

10–40 mcg/ml

Onset

2–4 h

Half-Life

63–69 h

Side Effects

Somnolence, ataxia, anorexia, and nervousness. More serious side effects include renal calculi, metabolic acidosis, aphasia, and cognitive impairment.

Contraindication

Hypersensitivity

Lacosamide (Vimpat)

It is approved for adjunct therapy of partial-onset seizures in patients older than 17 years. It acts by enhancing a slow inactivation of voltage-gated sodium channels (as opposed to fast inactivation by other antiepileptics); more than 40 % of the drug is excreted unchanged in urine, the rest as inactive metabolite. It does not induce liver enzymes [1, 2, 5, 9, 41–45].

Dose

200–400 mg/day orally. IV dose is the same as the oral dose.

Therapeutic Level

0.5–50 ng/ml

Onset

1–2 h PO; if IV, at the end of infusion (over 30 min)

Half-Life

13 h

Side Effects

Dizziness, ataxia, diplopia, and possible PR-interval prolongation (EKG prior to therapy)

Contraindications

Hypersensitivity

Rufinamide (Banzel)

It is approved for adjunct therapy of Lennox-Gastaut syndrome, tonic-clonic seizures, and atonic seizures. The exact mechanism of action is unknown, but it is presumed to inhibit high-frequency sodium channel currents. Rufinamide undergoes hepatic metabolism and inhibits CYP2E1. Otherwise, it is a weak inducer of liver enzymes [1, 5, 9, 46].

Dose

Initially 400 mg/day, max up to 3,200 mg/day divided into two doses. In children, 10 mg/kg/day; titrate up to 45 mg/kg/day.

Therapeutic Level

1–50 mcg/ml

Onset

3.4 h

Half-Life

6–10 h

Side Effects

Headaches, dizziness, fatigue, QT-interval shortening, and withdrawal seizures with abrupt cessation

Contraindication

Hypersensitivity and familial short QT syndrome

Vigabatrin (Sabril)

Vigabatrin is approved for adjunct therapy of refractory partial complex seizures in adults and of infantile spasms. It acts by irreversible inhibition of GABA transaminase, increasing the concentration of GABA. It induces some hepatic enzymes, is not protein bound and not metabolized in the liver, and is excreted in urine [1, 3, 47].

Dose

For adults, 1,000 mg/day in two doses; titrate up by 500 mg/d daily up to 3,000 mg/day in two doses. For infantile spasms, 50 mg/kg/day in two doses; titrate up by 25–50 mg/kg/day up to 150 mg/kg/day in two doses.

Therapeutic Level

Not known

Onset

1–2 h

Half-Life

5.3–7.4 h

Side Effects

Fatigue, somnolence, peripheral neuropathy, edema, weight gain, and MRI abnormalities, often transient

> **Black Box Warning**
> Progressive and permanent bilateral concentric visual field loss in 30 % of patients. Therefore, the use of vigabatrin is limited for refractory seizures and can only be prescribed through the SHARE program [48].

Contraindication

Hypersensitivity

Ezogabine

Ezogabine is used for adjunct therapy of partial-onset seizures refractory to other therapy. It works by potentiating the potassium channels' M-current. It primarily undergoes hepatic glucuronidation with an active metabolite, does not induce liver enzymes, and is excreted in urine (85 %) and feces (15 %) [1, 2, 16].

Dose

100 mg three times daily up to 1,200 mg/day divided in three doses; it is not approved for use in children.

Therapeutic Level

0.1–2 mcg/ml

Onset

0.5–2 h

Half-Life

8 h

Side Effects

Fatigue, dizziness, urinary retention, neuropsychiatric effects including psychotic symptoms that resolve after cessation of ezogabine, and increased QT interval.

Contraindication

Hypersensitivity

Anesthetic Considerations and Clinical Pearls

- It is important to realize some of the interactions of antiepileptic drugs and anesthetics. When patients are asked to fast prior to surgery, the provider should ask them to continue their antiepileptics to maintain a therapeutic plasma drug level during the perioperative period. If patients are not able to take their medication for a period exceeding the half-life of the antiepileptic medication, the patients' medications should be continued in an intravenous form, if the form is available for the drug [49].
- Some antiepileptic drugs are potent cytochrome P450 isoenzyme inducers, especially phenytoin, carbamazepine, phenobarbital, and primidone, which is metabolized into phenobarbital and the active phenylethylmalonamide. Weaker inducers are oxcarbazepine and topiramate in a dose-dependent fashion. This leads to exaggerated metabolism and lower plasma levels of drugs like oral contraceptives, beta-blockers, calcium channel antagonists, corticosteroids, warfarin, digoxin, other antiepileptic drugs, opioids, propofol, and non-depolarizing muscle relaxants. Valproic acid inhibits the hepatic microsomal enzyme system and leads to a slower clearance of drugs like phenytoin and phenobarbital (up to 50 %). Appropriate dose adjustments may be needed when taking these drugs. Gabapentin, lamotrigine, levetiracetam, tiagabine, and vigabatrin do not affect the enzyme system [2, 6].
- Metabolic changes as well as changes in serum pH and albumin levels during anesthesia can affect the serum drug level and possibly precipitate seizures up to 72 h postoperatively. Hypoxia, hyperventilation and hypocapnia, hypotension, and hyponatremia lower the seizure threshold and should be avoided as well as anesthetics that may provoke seizures [26].

- Among the inhalational anesthetics, halothane, isoflurane, and desflurane are potent anticonvulsants and can safely be used in epileptic patients. Sevoflurane has been reported to provoke seizures, especially in high doses and combined with hypocapnia. Enflurane as well can provoke seizure activity. Both sevoflurane and enflurane should not be used in epileptic patients. Nitrous oxide has not shown to have any effect [50].
- Opioids can increase seizure activity depending on the dose given. Meperidine can have neuroexcitatory effects via its metabolite normeperidine. Whenever it accumulates (i.e., renal disease, prolonged use), seizures may occur. Morphine can safely be used in epileptic patients but has provoked seizures in epileptic patients when given in the epidural space. The phenylpiperidine derivatives fentanyl, alfentanil, remifentanil, and sufentanil have been reported to have epileptogenic properties [50]. They can be useful in localizing epileptic foci. If alfentanil is added to propofol for electroconvulsive therapy, the seizure duration increases. High doses may be avoided in epileptic patients.
- Benzodiazepines are all anticonvulsant. Its antagonist flumazenil, if used to reverse sedation after a short procedure under sedation with a benzodiazepine, can produce seizures and should only be used with extreme caution in epileptic patients [51].
- Methohexital, ketamine, and etomidate can produce excitatory activity and myoclonus and activate an epileptogenic focus and may best not be used in epileptic patients [51].
- Dexmedetomidine has no anti- or proconvulsant effects and can safely be used in epileptic patients [51].
- Local anesthetics cross the blood-brain barrier and decrease cerebral metabolism and electrical activity, which causes sedating and analgesic effects and, at high plasma levels, a convulsant effect. This can happen due to accidental intravascular injection or with use in highly vascular areas (especially pelvic and oral regions) and rapid absorption. Systemic toxicity after regional anesthesia appears in 5/10,000 patients. Seizure threshold seems to be lower in patients who had a recent seizure [51].
- The neuromuscular drugs do not have an epileptogenic effect, but the metabolite of atracurium, laudanosine, causes seizures in animals that are not seen in humans. However, the possibility of seizures from laudanosine may have to be considered in patients with hepatic failure [51].
- Atropine and scopolamine can cause central cholinergic block, which can lead to agitation, seizures, stupor, and coma, which can be treated with physostigmine. Glycopyrrolate does not have that effect, since it does not cross the blood-brain barrier [51].
- In convulsive status epilepticus, the drug of first choice is lorazepam, but if, after 30–60 min, the drug therapy fails, general anesthesia may be required with midazolam, propofol, and thiopental, without the use of opioids. Desflurane and isoflurane may also be used [51].
- In general, Niesen et al. [52]. have found that the more antiseizure medication a person is on, and the longer the person is on the medications, the more likely the patient will have a seizure during the perioperative period. This is due to missed doses and/or decreased doses that lower the threshold for seizures. This fact is

independent on the type of surgery or anesthesia the patient receives. It is imperative that the anesthesiologist be aware of these risks in a patient with seizure disorder and be prepared to treat them during the perioperative period [52].

- When patients are anxious before the day of surgery and do not sleep well, the lack of sleep in itself may be a contributing factor to the lowered seizure thresholds [52].
- Seizures caused by anesthetic drugs are most commonly seen during induction and emergence from anesthesia. Careful monitoring of the vital signs may provide the first clues to an imminent seizure for the anesthesiologist.
- Preoperative oral dose (1,200 mg) of gabapentin has shown to decrease the need for narcotics and to decrease the MAC for inhalational anesthetics during surgery [53].
- Among the antiemetic drugs given perioperatively by anesthesiologists, dopamine antagonists may cause extrapyramidal side effects that may be confused for seizures. These drugs, such as prochlorperazine, droperidol, and metoclopramide, should be avoided.

Summary

As many antiepileptic drugs have unpleasant and also serious side effects, the search will go on for more specific and better tolerable therapies. Roughly 2 % of the population have some form of epilepsy, and it will hopefully be possible to treat all effectively someday. For those who have epilepsy refractory to medical therapy, implantation of a vagal nerve stimulator or surgery are options that may provide improvement.

Chemical Structures

Chemical Structure 29.1 Gabapentin

Chemical Structure 29.2 Phenytoin

Chemical Structure 29.3 Carbamazepine

Chemical Structure 29.4 Lamotrigine

Chemical Structure 29.5 Levetiracetam

Chemical Structure 29.6 Topiramate

Chemical Structure 29.7 Ethosuximide

References

1. Sirven JI, Noe K, Hoerth M, Drazkowski J. Antieplileptic drugs 2012: recent advances and trends. Mayo Clin Proc. 2012;87(9):879–89.
2. Ochoa JG, Benbadi SR, Riche W, Passaro EA, Talavera F. Antiepileptic drugs. Medscape Reference © 2011 WebMD, LLC [updated 25 Oct 2012]
3. Perucca E. An introduction to antiepileptic drugs. Epilepsia. 2005;46(Suppl 4):31-37
4. White HS, Smith MD, Wilcox KS. Mechanisms of action of antiepileptic drugs. Int Rev Neurobiol. 2007;81:85–110.
5. Woelfel JA, Cupp M. Comparison of antiepileptic drugs. Pharmacist's Letter/Prescriber's Letter, Detail-Document #250707. 2009;25#250707:1–24
6. Brunton LL, Chabner B, Knollman BC. 12e. Section 2. Neuropharmacology. Chapter 21. Pharmacotherapy of the epilepsies. In: Goodman and Gilman's pharmacological basis of therapeutics. New York: McGraw-Hill; 2011.
7. Perucca P, Mula M. Antiepileptic drug effects on mood and behavior: molecular targets. Epilepsy Behav. 2012. Available from: http://dx.doi.org/10.1016/j.yebeh.2012.09.018.
8. Hung C, Chen JW. Treatment of post-traumatic epilepsy. Curr Treat Options Neurol. 2012;14:293–306.
9. Bialer M, White HS. Key factors in the discovery and development of new antiepileptic drugs. Nat Rev Drug Discov. 2010;9:68–82.
10. Cavazos JE, Benbadis SR, Diaz-Arrastia R, Spitz M, Talavera F. Epilepsy and seizures. Medscape Reference ©2011WebMD, LLC [updated 25 Oct 2012]
11. Wang SP, Mintzer S, Skidmore CT, Zhan T, Stuckert E, Nei M, et al. Seizure recurrence and remission after switching antiepileptic drugs. Epilepsia. 2013;54:187–93.
12. Löscher W, Schmidt D. Perampanel – new promise for refractory epilepsy? Nat Rev Neurol. 2012;13:1–2.
13. Wasterlain CG, Chen JW. Mechanistic and pharmacologic aspects of status epilepticus and its treatment with new antiepileptic drugs. Epilepsia. 2008;49 Suppl 9:63–73.
14. Kleckner NW, Glazewski JC, Chen CC, Moscrip TD. Subtype-selective antagonism of N-Methyl-D-Aspartate receptors by felbamate: insights into the mechanism of action. J Pharmacol Exp Ther. 1999;289(2):886–94.
15. Ohno Y, Sofue N, Imaoku T, Morishita E, Kumafuji K, Sasa M, et al. Serotonergic modulation of absence-like seizures in groggy rats: a novel rat model of absence epilepsy. J Pharmacol Sci. 2012;114:99–105.
16. Ezogabine FE. A new angle on potassium gates. Epilepsy Curr. 2011;11(3):75–8.
17. Son YJ, Scranton TW, Sunderland WJ, Baek SJ, Miner JH, Sanes JR, et al. The synaptic vesicle protein SV2 is complexed with an α5-containing laminin on the nerve terminal surface. J Biol Chem. 2000;275(1):451–60.
18. Mula M, Kanner AM, Schmitz B, Schachter S. Antiepileptic drugs and suicidality: an expert consensus statement from the task force on therapeutic strategies of the ILAE commission on neuropsychobiology. Epilepsia. 2013;54:199–203.
19. Andersohn F, Schade R, Willich SN, Garbe E. Use of antiepileptic drugs in epilepsy and the risk of self-harm or suicidal behavior. Neurology. 2010;75:335–9.
20. Arana A, Wentworth CE, Ayuso-Mateos JL, et al. Suicide-related events in patients treated with antiepileptic drugs. N Engl J Med. 2010;363(6):542–51.
21. Olesen JB, Hansen PR, Erdal J, Abildstrom SZ, Weeke P, Fosbol EL, et al. Antiepileptic drugs and risk of suicide: a nationwide study. Pharmacoepidemiol Drug Saf. 2010;19(5):518–24.
22. Hesdorffer DC, Kanner AM. The FDA alert on suicidality and antiepileptic drugs: fire or false alarm? Epilepsia. 2009;50(5):978–86.
23. Internet Browser, Nov 2011, available from http://www.fda.gov/Safety/MedWatch/SafetyInformation/ucm243476.htm
24. Internet Browser, NDA 20-712/S-029 http://www.fda.gov/downloads/Drugs/DrugSafety/DrugSafetyNewsletter/UCM148014.pdf

25. Gil-Nagel A, Elger C, Ben-Menachem E, Halász P, Lopes-Lima J, Gabbai A, et al. Efficacy and safety of eslicarbazepine acetate as add-on treatment in patients with focal-onset seizures: integrated analysis of pooled data from double-blind phase III clinical studies. Epilepsia. 2013;54:98–107.
26. Dong X, Leppik IE, White J, Rarick J. Hyponatremia from oxcarbazepine and carbamazepine. Neurology. 2005;65:1976–8.
27. Mazza M, Marca GD, Nicola MD, Martinotti G, Pozzi G, Janiri L, et al. Oxcarbazepine improves mood in patients with epilepsy. Epilepsy Behav. 2007;10:397–401.
28. Ghaemi SN, Berv DA, Klugman J, Rosenquist KJ, Hsu DJ. Oxcarbazepine treatment of bipolar disorder. J Clin Psychiatry. 2003;64(8):943–5.
29. Internet Browser http://www.fda.gov/downloads/safety/medwatch/safetyinformation/safety-alertsforhumanmedicalproducts/ucm174647.pdf
30. Tassinari CA, Michelucci R, Riguzzi P, Volpi L, Dravet C, Cano JP, et al. The use of diazepam and clonazepam in epilepsy. Epilepsia. 1998;39 Suppl 1:S7–14.
31. Ng YT, Conry JA, Drummond R, Stolle J, Weinberg MA. Randomized, phase III study results of clobazam in Lennox-Gastaut syndrome. Neurology. 2011;77:1473–81.
32. Abou-Khalil B, Schmidt D. Antiepileptic drugs: advantages and disadvantages. Handb Clin Neurol. 2012;108:723–39.
33. Internet Browser http://www.ncbi.nlm.nih.gov/books/NBK55551/
34. Ulloa CM, Towfigh A, Safdieh J. Review of levetiracetam, with a focus on the extended release formulation, as adjuvant therapy in controlling partial-onset seizures. Neuropsychiatr Dis Treat. 2009;5:467–76.
35. Synowiec AS, Yandora KA, Yenugadhati V, Valeriano JP, Schramke CJ, Kelly KM. The efficacy of topiramate in adult refractory status epilepticus: experience of a tertiary care center. Epilepsy Res. 2012;98:232–7.
36. Shank RP, Gardocki JF, Streeter AJ, Maryanoff BE. An overview of the preclinical aspects of topiramate: pharmacology, pharmacokinetics, and mechanism of action. Epilepsia. 2000;41 Suppl 1:S3–9.
37. Patsalos PN. Properties of antiepileptic drugs in the treatment of idiopathic generalized epilepsies. Epilepsia. 2005;46 Suppl 9:140–8.
38. Devinsky O, Faught RE, Wilder BJ, Kanner AM, Kamin M, Kramer LD, et al. Efficacy of felbamate monotherapy in patients undergoing presurgical evaluation of partial seizures. Epilepsy Res. 1995;20:241–6.
39. Subramaniam S, Rho JM, Penix L, Donevan SD, Fielding RP, Rogawski MA. Felbamate block of the N-methyl-D-aspartate receptor. J Pharmacol Exp Ther. 1995;273(2):878–86.
40. Internet Browser https://online.epocrates.com/u/10a740/felbamate
41. Chung S, Sperling MR, Biton V, Krauss G, Hebert D, Rudd GD, et al. Lacosamide as adjunctive therapy for partial-onset seizures: a randomized controlled trial. Epilepsia. 2010;51(6):958–67.
42. Mnatsakanyan L, Chung JM, Tsimerinov EI, Eliashiv DS. Intravenous lacosamide in refractory nonconvulsive status epilepticus. Seizure. 2012;21:198–201.
43. Miró J, Toledo M, Santamarina E, Ricciardi AC, Villanueva V, Pato A, et al. Efficacy of intravenous lacosamide as an add-on treatment in refractory status epilepticus: a multicentric prospective study. Seizure [Internet]. 2012. Available from: http://dx.doi.org/10.1016/j.seizure.2012.10.004.
44. Ben-Menachem E, Biton V, Jatuzis D, Abou-Khalil B, Doty P, Rudd GD. Efficacy and safety of oral lacosamide as adjunctive therapy in adults with partial-onset seizures. Epilepsia. 2007;48(7):1308–17.
45. Errington AC, Coyne L, Stöhr T, Selve N, Lees G. Seeking a mechanism of action for the novel anticonvulsant lacosamide. Neuropharmacology. 2006;50:1016–29.
46. Brodie MJ, Rosenfeld WE, Vazquez B, Sachdeo R, Perdomo C, Mann A, et al. Rufinamide for the adjunctive treatment of partial seizures in adults and adolescents: a randomized placebo-controlled trial. Epilepsia. 2009;50(8):1899–909.

47. Dean C, Mosier M, Penry K. Dose-response study of vigabatrin as add-on therapy in patients with uncontrolled complex partial seizures. Epilepsia. 1999;40(1):74–82.
48. Internet Browser http://sabril.net/hcp/vision_loss_data/other_side_effects/
49. Perks Cheema S, Mohanraj R. Anaesthesia and epilepsy. Br J Anaesth. 2012;108(4):562–71.
50. Perks A, Cheema S, Mohanraj R. Anaesthesia and epilepsy. Br J Anesth. 2012;108:562–71.
51. Maranhao MVM, Gomes EA, de Carvalho PE. Epilepsy and anesthesia. Rev Bras Anestesiol. 2011;61(2):232–54.
52. Niesen AD, Jacob AK, Aho LE, Botten EJ, Nase KE, Nelson JM, et al. Perioperative seizures in patients with a history of a seizure disorder. Anesth Analg. 2010;111(3):729–35.
53. Doha NM, Rady A, El Azab SR. Preoperative use of gabapentin decreases the anesthetic and analgesic requirements in patients undergoing radical mastectomy. Egypt J Anesth. 2010;26(4):287–91.

Chapter 30
Neuropharmacologic Agents for Neurologic Conditions

Maria Bustillo and Tricia Vecchione

Contents

M. Bustillo, MD (✉) • T. Vecchione, MD
Department of Anesthesiology, Montefiore Medical Center,
Albert Einstein College of Medicine, Bronx, NY, USA
e-mail: mariabusri@aol.com; tvecchio@montefiore.org

A.D. Kaye et al. (eds.), *Essentials of Pharmacology for Anesthesia,*
Pain Medicine, and Critical Care, DOI 10.1007/978-1-4614-8948-1_30,
© Springer Science+Business Media New York 2015

Introduction

A variety of neurologic conditions may influence the selection and conduction of anesthesia. The pharmacodynamics of many anesthetics are often directly altered by neurologic disorders. Most anesthetic agents are reversibly neurotoxic, and thus monitoring the recovery of neurologic function after anesthesia becomes complicated. In addition, many neurologic disorders are rare resulting in limited anesthetic reports in the literature. The combination of these factors requires maximum caution in planning the administration of anesthesia.

Parkinson's Disease

Parkinson's disease is a progressive neurodegenerative disease caused by a loss of dopaminergic fibers in the basal ganglia resulting in unopposed cholinergic activation. It is characterized by impairment of voluntary movement (hypokinesia), resting tremor, rigidity, and postural instability. Parkinson's disease is an important cause of perioperative morbidity, and anesthetic considerations should include the interactions between antiparkinsonian drugs and anesthetic drugs [1].

Dopamine Precursors

Dopamine precursors act to restore dopamine levels in the basal ganglia. Levodopa crosses the blood-brain barrier where it is converted to dopamine by dopa decarboxylase. Carbidopa is a decarboxylase inhibitor, administered with levodopa, which does not cross the blood-brain barrier. It prevents the peripheral conversion of levodopa to dopamine, thereby increasing the amount of levodopa available in the central nervous system. A combination of carbidopa/levodopa is available in 1:10 and 1:4 ratios [3].

Indications

Motor symptoms generally respond better than extramotor symptoms. However, effectiveness diminishes after 2–5 years of treatment.

Dosing

Carbidopa/levodopa 60–600 mg/day.

Drug Interactions

Monoamine oxidase inhibitors are contraindicated with levodopa therapy, and sympathomimetics should be used with caution as these can result in acute rises in blood pressure. Drugs that may precipitate extrapyramidal symptoms, including phenothiazines (promethazine), butyrophenones (droperidol), and metoclopramide, are contraindicated. Halothane should be avoided because it can precipitate arrhythmias. Anticholinergic drugs act synergistically with levodopa.

Side Effects

Side effects of levodopa administration include nausea/vomiting, orthostatic hypotension, cardiac dysrhythmias, abnormal involuntary movements, psychiatric disturbances (elderly most vulnerable), and increased prolactin secretion and increased plasma levels of aldosterone. The side effects of levodopa administration are related to increased system levels of dopamine and are therefore decreased by the coadministration of carbidopa [8].

Catechol-O-methyltransferase (COMT) Inhibitors

COMT plays a role in the peripheral breakdown of levodopa. Tolcapone and entacapone block COMT enzyme activity, which slows the elimination of carbidopa/levodopa.

Indication

COMT inhibitors result in prolongation and potentiation of levodopa effects.

Dosing

Entacapone 200 mg with levodopa. Tolcapone 100–200 mg three times per day.

Drug Interactions

MAO inhibitors (rarely used at present).

Side Effects

Side effects include nausea/vomiting, dyskinesias, hepatotoxicity (liver disease may be a relative contraindication), rhabdomyolysis, orange urine, and piloerection [9].

Dopamine Agonists

Dopamine agonists, including bromocriptine, cabergoline, pramipexole, ropinirole, apomorphine, and rotigotine, act directly on postsynaptic dopamine receptors.

Indications

These drugs are used as levodopa-sparing monotherapy for younger patients with fewer "on-off" fluctuations and less dyskinesia than with levodopa.

Dosing

Initial dose: bromocriptine, 2.5 mg 3x/day; rotigotine, transdermal one 2 mg patch per day; pramipexole, 0.125 mg 3x/day; ropinirole, 0.25 mg 2x/day.

Side Effects

Side effects include visual and auditory hallucinations, hypotension, dyskinesia, pulmonary fibrosis, vertigo, increase in serum transaminases and alkaline phosphatase, nausea, and compulsive behavior such as gambling and hypersexuality [8].

Anticholinergics

Anticholinergic drugs blunt the effects of acetylcholine, thereby correcting the balance between dopamine and acetylcholine.

Indications

These drugs are most useful in patients under the age of 70 with minimal akinesia or gait disturbances. They may be used as adjuncts for persistent tremor.

Dosing

Initial dose: benzatropine, 0.5 mg 2x/day; trihexyphenidyl, 1–2 mg/day.

Drug Interactions

Alcohol, thorazine, antihistamines, and haloperidol.

Side Effects

Side effects include memory disturbances (relatively contraindicated in the elderly), sedation, mydriasis, and peripheral antimuscarinic effects [8].

Monoamine Oxidase B (MAO-B) Inhibitors

Selegiline and rasagiline irreversibly inhibit MAO-B, which inhibits the breakdown of dopamine.

Indications

MAO-B inhibitors have weak antiparkinsonian effects when used alone but may have modest effects when used in conjunction with carbidopa/levodopa.

Dosing

Selegiline, 5 mg 2×/day; rasagiline, 0.5 mg once a day.

Drug Interactions

These drugs should be used with caution with concomitant SSRIs and TCAs. They do not precipitate hypertension with tyramine ingestion.

Side Effects

Side effects include nausea, headache, diarrhea, confusion in the elderly, and insomnia (selegiline's amphetamine metabolite) [8].

Antivirals

Amantadine produces mild antiparkinsonian activity by unknown mechanisms.

Indications

Amantadine may be used as monotherapy for mild disease or to reduce levodopa-induced dyskinesia and motor fluctuations.

Dosing

Amantadine initial dose: 100 mg 2–3×/day.

Side Effects

Side effects are rare in monotherapy but may include hallucinations, livedo reticularis, confusion, and nightmares. CNS side effects are more common when used as an adjunct [8].

Anesthetic Drugs

Thiopental has been associated with dyskinesia. Propofol has been linked to dyskinesias but has also been noted to diminish tremor in the postoperative period. Ketamine has been widely used without incident. Inhaled anesthetics may increase postoperative rigidity. Patients with Parkinson's disease appear to have normal sensitivity to nondepolarizing neuromuscular blockers. There is conflicting data on the use of succinylcholine in Parkinson's disease. Opioids should be used with caution as they may exacerbate muscle rigidity [5, 6].

Huntington's Disease

Huntington's disease (HD) is an autosomal dominant disease characterized by choreoathetoid movements, cognitive decline, and psychiatric disturbances. Depression in these patients is typically treated with tricyclic antidepressants (TCAs) or selective serotonin reuptake inhibitors (SSRIs). Data regarding anesthetic management of patients with HD is limited, but few case reports suggest that abnormal responses to anesthetics may be of concern [1, 3].

Tricyclic Antidepressants (TCAs)

The antidepressant effects of TCAs result from blocking the reuptake of serotonin and norepinephrine at presynaptic terminals. TCAs are highly lipid soluble, and peak plasma levels usually occur within 2–8 h after oral administration. They undergo liver metabolism.

Indications

Nortriptyline and amitriptyline have been used in patients with HD. TCAs are highly effective at treating depression but are no longer as first-line therapy due to their unfavorable side effects, narrow therapeutic index, and lethal overdose.

Drug Interactions

TCAs produce an exaggerated response to indirect acting sympathomimetics, such as ephedrine; therefore, smaller doses should be titrated in slowly. TCA use with certain anesthetics may increase the risk of cardiac dysrhythmias. Concurrent use with anticholinergics may produce central anticholinergic syndrome. Opioid use may result in increased respiratory depression in patients taking TCAs.

Side Effects

Side effects include anticholinergic effects, orthostatic hypotension, increases in heart rate, widening of the QRS complex on ECG, and sedation [8].

Selective Serotonin Reuptake Inhibitors (SSRIs)

SSRIs selectively inhibit the reuptake of serotonin. They have a greater safety profile when taken in overdose compared to TCAs.

Indications

Fluoxetine, sertraline, and paroxetine have been used to treat mild to moderate depression in patients with HD.

Dosing

Initial dose: fluoxetine, 10–20 mg/day; sertraline, 25–50 mg/day; paroxetine, 20 mg/day.

Drug Interactions

Certain SSRIs (i.e., fluoxetine) inhibit cytochrome P450 enzymes and may increase plasma concentrations of drugs that depend on hepatic metabolism for clearance. When used with MAO inhibitors, SSRIs may result in serotonin syndrome.

Side Effects

Compared with TCAs, SSRIs do not have anticholinergic properties and do not produce orthostatic hypotension or cardiac dysrhythmias. However, side effects include nausea, anorexia, insomnia, agitation, and sexual dysfunction [8].

Anesthetic Drugs

No clear contraindications exist to the use of common anesthetic drugs. However, delayed emergence with thiopental was reported in one case report. Studies on the incidence of atypical pseudocholinesterase in patients with HD have been contradictory. There is only a single case report of delayed recovery after the administration of succinylcholine. Drugs that act on central dopamine receptors, such as metoclopramide, should be avoided because these drugs can worsen chorea symptoms [2, 3].

Dystonias

Dystonias are a group of muscle disorders characterized by involuntary muscle contractions, which lead to repetitive movements or abnormal postures. There are no medications to treat or slow the progression of dystonia; however, anticholinergic agents, GABAergic agents, and dopaminergic agents have been used "off-label" to ease some of the symptoms [1, 3].

Anticholinergic Drugs

Anticholinergic drugs competitively antagonize the effects of acetylcholine cholinergic postganglionic site. They blunt the effects of acetylcholine, thereby correcting the balance between dopamine and acetylcholine.

Indications

Trihexyphenidyl and benzatropine are anticholinergic drugs used frequently to reduce the side effects of antipsychotic treatment, such as pseudoparkinsonism and dystonia. Tetrabenazine is also available in the USA as an orphan drug.

Dosing

See section "Parkinson's Disease."

Drug Interactions

See "Parkinson's Disease."

Side Effects

Side effects of synthetic anticholinergics are less pronounced than atropine but may include memory disturbances (relatively contraindicated in the elderly), sedation, mydriasis, and peripheral antimuscarinic effects. Physostigmine is the specific treatment for side effects and overdose [8].

Anesthetic Drugs

No anesthetic agents are contraindicated. Neuromuscular blocking drugs and inhaled nitrous oxide concentrations greater than 50 % may relieve spasms [3, 5].

Multiple Sclerosis

Multiple sclerosis (MS) is an inflammatory autoimmune disorder characterized by demyelination of axonal sheaths in the CNS and subsequent development of sclerotic lesions in the brain leading to neurodegeneration. Current therapies including gluco-corticoid therapy, adrenocorticotropic hormone (ACTH), and immunosuppressive agents aim to ameliorate symptoms and reduce the number of exacerbations [1, 3].

Corticosteroids

Glucocorticoids bind to cytoplasmic receptors to stimulate changes in transcription of DNA and, consequently, the synthesis of proteins.

Indications

Used for anti-inflammatory and immunosuppressive effects.

Dosing

There is no clear consensus on the best route of administration or dosing schedule.

Drug Interactions

Patients on chronic corticosteroid therapy should receive an increased dose when undergoing a surgical procedure because of the risk of circulatory collapse.

Side Effects

Side effects include suppression of the HPA axis, electrolyte and metabolic changes, osteoporosis, skeletal muscle myopathy, central nervous system dysfunction, and weight gain [8].

Adrenocorticotropic Hormone (ACTH)

ACTH stimulated corticosteroid secretion, primarily cortisol, from the adrenal cortex.

Indications

Used to treat patients with optic neuritis [8].

Immunosuppressive Agents

Cyclophosphamide is a nitrogen mustard DNA alkylating agent. It forms DNA cross-links leading to cell death. Cytarabine is a pyrimidine analogue that interferes with DNA synthesis.

Indication

Used to prevent the number and severity of relapses in patients with MS.

Dosing

There are multiple reports describing different pulse therapy protocols of cyclophosphamide for the treatment of multiple sclerosis. Methylprednisolone is administered prior to cyclophosphamide, and the dose is adjusted by WBC count drawn just prior to schedule treatment.

Drug Interactions

Cyclophosphamide is a substrate or inhibitor of CYP450 2B6; its administration may increase plasma concentration of drugs metabolized by CYP450 2B6 like bupropion.

Side Effects

Side effects of cyclophosphamide include nausea/vomiting, anorexia, alopecia, hypersensitivity reactions, fibrosing pneumonitis, pericarditis, bone marrow suppression, and hemorrhagic cystitis. Side effects of cytarabine include nausea/vomiting, anorexia, myelosuppression, hepatic impairment, and thrombophlebitis at the site of infusion [10].

Anesthetic Drugs

There is no evidence that the types of anesthetic or particular anesthetic agents are associated with exacerbation of the disease. Volatile agents are the most commonly used anesthetic agent. Local anesthetics should be avoided intrathecally, but no problems have been reported given epidurally. The use of depolarizing muscle relaxants carries a theoretical risk of hyperkalemia in MS patients and should therefore be used with caution. Both increased and decreased sensitivities to nondepolarizing muscle relaxants have been reported [3, 5].

Guillain-Barre Syndrome

Guillain-Barre syndrome is an autoimmune disorder resulting in an immunologic response against peripheral nerves. It is characterized by paresthesias, numbness, progressive symmetric muscular weakness, and autonomic dysfunction. Current treatment is primarily supportive, and current evidence does not support the use of corticosteroids or interferon-beta. However, multiple studies do support the use of plasmapheresis and IVIG [1, 4].

Anesthetic Drugs

Succinylcholine should be avoided because of the significant risk of hyperkalemia. This risk may persist after clinical resolution of the disease. These patients may vary from overly sensitive to nondepolarizing neuromuscular blocking drugs (NMBDs) to resistance depending on the phase of the disease [5, 7].

Amyotrophic Lateral Sclerosis

Amyotrophic lateral sclerosis (ALS) is a progressive neurodegenerative disorder involving both upper and lower motor neurons. It is characterized by hyperreflexia, spasticity, rapidly progressive muscle weakness, muscle atrophy, and fasciculations. The most common presenting symptom is asymmetric limb weakness, while the minority of patients present with bulbar symptoms. Quinine used to be the therapy of choice for ALS, but due to its safety profile, its use has been eliminated. Antiepileptic drugs, including carbamazepine and phenytoin, have been suggested in its place. Riluzole remains the only agent with proven mortality benefit in ALS [1, 5].

Antiepileptic Drugs

Carbamazepine and phenytoin are a sodium ion channel blocker.

Indications

Carbamazepine and phenytoin, while used occasionally for symptomatic therapy of *amyotrophic lateral sclerosis (ALS)*, are still among the most frequently used agents in the treatment of epilepsy.

Dosing

The dose of carbamazepine is 10–40 mg/kg/day given in three to four divided doses. The dose of phenytoin is 3–5 mg/kg/day in two to three divided doses.

Drug Interactions

Carbamazepine and phenytoin are enzyme-inducing (P450 activity) drugs. Patients taking these drugs may require increased doses of propofol, thiopental, midazolam, opioids, and nondepolarizing (NMBDs).

Side Effects

Side effects of carbamazepine include vertigo, drowsiness, agranulocytosis, allergic dermatitis, Stevens-Johnson syndrome, hepatotoxic effects, pancreatitis, and teratogenicity. Side effects of phenytoin include nystagmus, ataxia, gingival hyperplasia, megaloblastic anemia, agranulocytosis, allergic dermatitis, Stevens-Johnson syndrome, hepatotoxic effects, hirsutism teratogenicity, and Dupuytren's contractures [8].

The black box warnings (www.fda.gov) include:

- *Serious dermatologic reactions and HLA-B*1502 allele*
  Concern over rare but potentially serious dermatologic reactions. These can include mucous membrane ulcers (including Stevens-Johnson syndrome and toxic epidermal necrolysis), painful rash, and elevated temperature (1–6 per 10,000 new users in countries with mainly white populations, but the risk with an almost exclusive Asian allele, HLA-B*1502, is much higher, and epidemiological data in some Asian countries estimates risk to be approximately 10 times higher).
- *Aplastic anemia and agranulocytosis*
  Additionally, aplastic anemia and agranulocytosis are rare, but therapy may be halted if there is bone marrow suppression (the risk is five to eight times greater than in the general population, and the overall risk of these reactions in the untreated general population is minimal, approximately six patients per one million population per year for agranulocytosis and two patients per one million population per year for aplastic anemia).

Riluzole

Riluzole is a sodium channel blocker with anti-NDMA activity and is thought to attenuate glutamate-induced excitotoxicity.

Indications

Shown to improve mortality in patients with ALS. Riluzole slows the progress of ALS and delays the need for a tracheostomy.

Dosing

50 mg orally twice a day.

Drug Interactions

Riluzole is metabolized by cytochrome P450 enzyme and may be affected by drugs that inhibit or induce this enzyme.

Side Effects

Side effects include weakness, dizziness, GI upset, and increases in transaminases [8].

Anesthetic Drugs

There are no absolute contraindications to any anesthetic technique in patients with ALS. However, succinylcholine should be avoided due to an increased risk of hyperkalemia. Patients with ALS may have increased sensitivity to nondepolarizing NMBDs and should be used with caution.

Myasthenia Gravis

Myasthenia gravis (MG) is an autoimmune neuromuscular disorder caused by antibodies to postsynaptic nicotinic acetylcholine receptors. It is characterized by fluctuating muscle weakness and fatigability. Myasthenia may be treated with anticholinesterase inhibitors, steroids, or immunosuppressive drugs depending on the severity of the disease. Various medications may trigger life-threatening exacerbations of MG, including antibiotics aminoglycosides, erythromycin, and ampicillin. Other medications including chloroquine, procaine, lithium, phenytoin, beta-blockers, procainamide, and statins also should be avoided or at least used cautiously. Recent evaluation of postmarketing reports from the US FDA produced warnings that included the contraindication of fluoroquinolones in MG patients. Clinicians treating MG patients should avoid this class entirely: levofloxacin, moxifloxacin, ciprofloxacin, and ofloxacin. These agents should be avoided in myasthenia gravis due to reports that they have profound neuromuscular blocking activity that has led to several deaths and severe exacerbations [1, 3].

Corticosteroids

See "Corticosteroids" under "Multiple Sclerosis."

Dosing

Prednisone 1 mg/kg on alternate days.

Anticholinesterase Inhibitors

Neostigmine and pyridostigmine reversibly inhibit the enzyme acetylcholinesterase resulting in increased availability of acetylcholine at the neuromuscular junction.

Indications

Used for symptomatic treatment in MG.

Dosing

Pyridostigmine: oral 60 mg, IV 2 mg, IM 2–4 mg. Neostigmine: oral 15 mg, IV 0.5 mg, IM 0.7–1 mg.

Drug Interactions

Corticosteroids may decrease the effect of anticholinesterases.

Side Effects

Side effects include bradycardia, nausea, bronchoconstriction, and miosis [8].

Nonsteroidal Drugs Producing Immunosuppression

Cyclosporin selectively inhibits helper T-lymphocyte-mediated immune response by blocking the transcription of cytokine genes. It has a narrow therapeutic index, and thus blood concentrations must be monitored closely.

Indication

Used to treat and decrease relapsing.

Dosing

5 mg/kg/day in divided doses.

Drug Interactions

Cyclosporine is extensively metabolized by cytochrome P450 3A.

Drugs that increase cyclosporin concentrations are diltiazem, nicardipine, verapamil, fluconazole, itraconazole, ketoconazole, azithromycin, clarithromycin, erythromycin, methylprednisolone, allopurinol, amiodarone, bromocriptine, colchicine, metoclopramide, and oral contraceptives. Drugs that will decrease cyclosporine concentrations are nafcillin, rifampin, carbamazepine, phenobarbital, phenytoin, octreotide, and ticlopidine.

Side Effects

Side effects include nephrotoxicity, systemic hypertension, seizures, cholestasis, allergic reactions, gingival hyperplasia, and hyperglycemia [11].

Immunosuppressants

Azathioprine antagonizes purine synthesis, thereby inhibiting DNA synthesis and consequently suppressing the proliferation of T and B lymphocytes. Mycophenolate mofetil is a reversible inhibitor of inosine monophosphate dehydrogenase, which is necessary for the growth of B- and T-lymphocyte proliferation.

Indications

Used to treat symptoms of a variety of autoimmune diseases.

Dosing

The median dose is 100 mg daily (range 75–200 mg; 1.5–3 mg/kg).

Drug Interactions

Azathioprine decreases the effects of warfarin and nondepolarizing NMBDs but increases the effects of depolarizing muscle relaxants.

Side Effects

Side effects of azathioprine include bone marrow suppression, infection, fever, GI hypersensitivity reactions, nausea/vomiting, anorexia, hepatotoxicity, and malignancy. Side effects of mycophenolate mofetil include nausea/vomiting, fever, dyspnea/cough, myelosuppression, immunosuppression, infection, malignancy/lymphoma, interstitial lung disease, GI bleeding, and progressive multifocal leuko-encephalopathy [12].

Anesthetic Drugs

Patients with MG are less susceptible to succinylcholine and more susceptible to nondepolarizing NMBDs. Therefore, quantitative twitch monitoring and careful titration of nondepolarizing NMBDs are important [4, 7].

Lambert-Eaton Myasthenic Syndrome

Lambert-Eaton syndrome is an autoimmune syndrome characterized by proximal muscle weakness that improves with repetitive effort. It is typically seen with small cell carcinoma of the lung but may be seen with other malignancies. It is associated with antibodies to voltage-gated calcium channels in presynaptic nerve terminals resulting in decreased release of acetylcholine at the neuromuscular junction. Guanidine therapy enhances acetylcholine release thereby improving muscle strength but is no longer recommended. If the syndrome is associated with a cancer, treatment of the cancer often relieves symptoms.

Anesthetic Drugs

Patients with Lambert-Eaton syndrome have increased sensitivity to both depolarizing and nondepolarizing NMBDs. Volatile agents alone usually provide sufficient muscle relaxation [3, 7].

Stroke

Stroke is characterized by a sudden loss of neurologic function due to ischemia (80 %) or hemorrhage (20 %). Ischemic strokes may be classified as thrombotic and embolic or as a result of systemic hypoperfusion, while hemorrhagic strokes may be classified as intracerebral (15 %) or subarachnoid (85 %). It is the third leading cause of death in the USA and the leading cause of long-term disability. Approximately 795,000 people suffer a stroke each year. Women have lower stroke rates than men up to the age of 85.

The initial therapy of acute ischemic stroke usually begins with aspirin. Intravenous recombinant tissue plasminogen activator may be used in eligible patients. Direct infusion of thrombolytic drugs into the occluded blood vessel is also an option. Medical management also includes controlling the patient's airway, oxygenation, ventilation, systemic blood pressure, blood glucose, and body temperature. Surgical decompression may have a role in a small percentage of stroke patients.

Assessment of neurologic function and vital signs is essential to the preoperative anesthesia evaluation. The anesthesiologists should also pay particular attention to comorbid conditions and current medications including cardiovascular medications, anticoagulants, and antiplatelet medications.

Collaboration between the patient, anesthesiologist, and surgeon may be necessary to determine whether general or regional anesthesia is best for the procedure. There is no general anesthetic regimen that is best for preserving cerebral perfusion and hemostasis for carotid endarterectomy or stenting. Volatile anesthetics decrease cerebral metabolic rate of oxygen consumption and increase cerebral blood flow. Etomidate has been shown to worsen ischemic injury in animal studies and should not be used as a cerebral protectant. Esmolol, labetalol, hydralazine, phenylephrine, ephedrine, and nitroglycerine may be used to modulate blood pressure and heart rate [13].

Chemical Structures

Chemical Structure
30.1 Levodopa

Chemical Structure
30.2 Benzatropine

Chemical Structure
30.3 Cyclophosphamide

Chemical Structure
30.4 Riluzole

Chemical Structure
30.5 Azathioprine

References

1. Dierdorf SF, Walton JS. Rare and coexisting diseases. In: Barash PG, Cullen BF, Stoelting RK, Cahalan MK, Stock MC, editors. Clinical anesthesia. 6th ed. Philadelphia: Lippincott Williams & Wilkins; 2009. p. 622–43.
2. Kivela JE, Sprung J, Southorn PA, Watson JC, Weingarten TN. Anesthetic management of patients with Huntington disease. Anesth Analg. 2010;110(2):515.
3. Pasternak JJ, Lanier WL. Diseases affecting the brain. In: Hines RL, Marschall KE, editors. Stoelting's anesthesia and co-existing disease. 5th ed. Philadelphia: Churchill Livingstone; 2008. p. 199–237.
4. Pasternak JJ, Lanier WL. Spinal cord disorders. In: Hines RL, Marschall KE, editors. Stoelting's anesthesia and co-existing disease. 5th ed. Philadelphia: Churchill Livingstone; 2008. p. 239–47.
5. Roizen MF, Fleisher LA. Anesthetic implications of concurrent disease. In: Miller RD, editor. Miller's anesthesia. 7th ed. Philadelphia: Churchill Livingstone; 2010. p. 1067–149.
6. Shaikh S, Verma H. Parkinson's disease and anesthesia. Indian J Anaesth. 2011;55(3):228–34.
7. Scott BK, Baranov D. Neurologic diseases. In: Fleisher LA, editor. Anesthesia and uncommon diseases. 6th ed. Philadelphia: Elsevier Saunders; 2012. p. 251–94.
8. Stoelting RK, Hillier SC. Pharmacology and physiology in anesthetic practice. 4th ed. Philadelphia: Lippincott Williams & Wilkins; 2006.
9. Ruottinen HM, Rinne UK. COMT inhibition in the treatment of Parkinson's disease. J Neurol. 1998;245(11 Suppl 3):25–34.
10. Thrower BW. Relapse management in multiple sclerosis. Neurologist. 2009;15(1):1–5.
11. Campana C, Regazzi MB, Buggia I, Molinaro M. Clinically significant drug interactions with cyclosporine. Clin Pharmacokinet. 1996;30(2):141–79.
12. Fonseca V, Harvard CW. Long term treatment of myasthenia gravis with azathioprine. Postgrad Med J. 1990;66(772):102–5.
13. Kaye AD, Lasala MF, Baluch A. Preanesthetic assessment of the patient with a Stroke. Anesthesia News. 2012;39(2):19–23.

Chapter 31
Chemotherapeutic Agents

Adrienne B. Warrick, Karina Gritsenko, and Melinda Aquino

Contents

A.B. Warrick, MD (✉) • M. Aquino, MD
Department of Anesthesiology, Montefiore Medical Center,
Albert Einstein College of Medicine – Yeshiva University, Bronx, NY, USA
e-mail: adrienne.m.buckman@gmail.com; maquino@montefiore.org

K. Gritsenko, MD
Department of Family and Social Medicine, Montefiore Medical Center,
Albert Einstein College of Medicine – Yeshiva University, Bronx, NY, USA
e-mail: karinagritsenko@googlemail.com

A.D. Kaye et al. (eds.), *Essentials of Pharmacology for Anesthesia,*
Pain Medicine, and Critical Care, DOI 10.1007/978-1-4614-8948-1_31,
© Springer Science+Business Media New York 2015

Introduction

Oncologic patients comprise a consistent if not significant portion of surgical patients. Many of these patients will have undergone perioperative treatment for their diseases by means of chemotherapy, radiation therapy, or a combination of the two. With regard to the chemotherapeutic agents, specific preoperative, intraoperative, and postoperative anesthetic considerations must be taken when providing care to this special subset of surgical patients.

Malignant cells are best eradicated by treatment with chemotherapy. In order for chemotherapy to be effective, there must be a complete destruction of all cancer cells within the body so that recurrence of the malignant process does not occur. In recognition of the need for total cell kill in oncologic patients, the chemotherapy drugs are often used in combination, utilizing their different mechanisms of action and different toxicity profiles. Chemotherapy agents are also administered over short time periods with specific time intervals instead of continuous therapy. This is due to the fact that nonmalignant cells show greater and faster recovery from pulsed chemotherapy than do the malignant cells.

Drug Class and Mechanism of Action

Many chemotherapeutic drugs can be defined by the portion of the cell cycle they affect. There are four phases of the cell cycle that all cells undergo during the process of cell division. In basic terms, the cycles are G1 (synthesis of cellular components needed for DNA synthesis), S (representing DNA synthesis and DNA genome replication), G2 (synthesis of cellular components for mitosis), and M (representing mitosis or actual cellular division and replication). Figure 31.1 illustrates this concept [3]. The activity of certain chemotherapeutic agents is described specifically to the portion of the cell cycle they disrupt, and these drugs are referred to as cell cycle-specific agents [7]. Other chemotherapy drugs are described as cell cycle-nonspecific agents [7].

Antimetabolites (S-Phase)

Antimetabolite drugs are also referred to as nucleic acid synthesis inhibitors [10]. They include folate analogs, pyrimidine analogs, and purine analogs. Their particular usefulness is in destroying cells during the S-phase (synthesis phase) of the cell cycle.

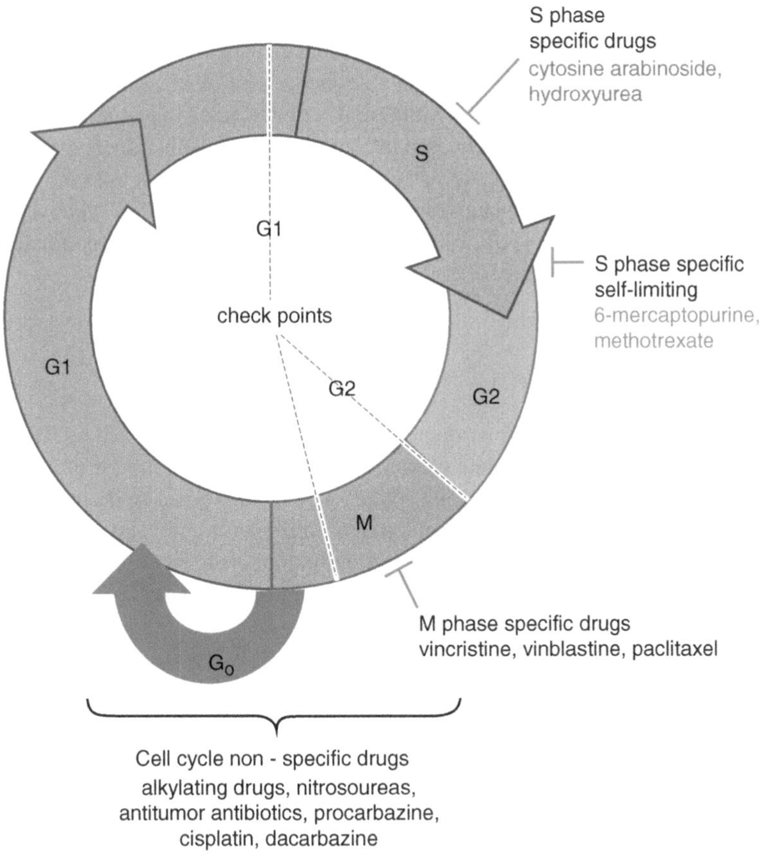

Fig. 31.1 Four phases of cell division (Source: Brunton et al. [3]. Copyright © McGraw Hill Companies, Inc)

Folate Analogs: Methotrexate and Pemetrexed

Methotrexate

Methotrexate is transferred into cells via a reduced folate carrier, and it inhibits dihydrofolate reductase (DHFR) which is the enzyme that uses reduced folate as a methyl donor in the synthesis of both purines and pyrimidines. The disruption of DHFR interferes with the synthesis of tetrahydrofolate, causing an intracellular folate deficiency. The end result of this folate deficiency is that the 1-carbon transfer reactions necessary for the synthesis of DNA, RNA, and key cellular proteins cease. Methotrexate can be administered intravenously, intrathecally, and by oral route, but oral bioavailability is erratic at doses greater than 25 mg/m^2. It is eliminated mainly through renal excretion which is a reflection of glomerular filtration and tubular secretion. Elimination may be impaired in renal insufficiency. Around 50 % of the drug is found unchanged in the urine, suggesting that significant metabolism of methotrexate does not occur. Leucovorin (5-formyltetra-hydrofolate) is used as rescue therapy for normal cells subjected to undue toxicity from methotrexate. Methotrexate is widely used in combination with other drugs in treatment of malignant disorders and also in some nonmalignant diseases. It is used in the treatment of acute lymphoblastic leukemia in children but not adults and is effective as the sole agent in choriocarcinoma [10]. Psoriasis and rheumatoid arthritis are nonmalignant disease processes that also show benefit with treatment by methotrexate.

Pemetrexed

Like methotrexate, pemetrexed works to inhibit the S-phase of the cell cycle, and it is transported into cells via a folate carrier. Its main target is to inhibit thymidylate synthase, but it also targets DHFR and other enzymes involved in de novo purine nucleotide biosynthesis [7, 10]. Supplementation with folate and vitamin B12 appears to reduce the toxicity of pemetrexed without altering its clinical efficacy. In combination with cisplatin, it is used for the treatment of non-small cell lung cancer and also mesothelioma.

Pyrimidine Analogs: Fluorouracil, Capecitabine, Cytarabine, and Gemcitabine

Pyrimidine analogs prevent the biosynthesis of pyrimidine nucleotides (cytosine, thymine, uracil), or they mimic these nucleotides to the extent that they interfere with vital cellular activities such as synthesis and nucleic acid function.

5-Fluorouracil

5-Fluorouracil (5-FU) requires activation via several enzymatic reactions in which it ultimately prevents the de novo synthesis of thymidylate preventing DNA synthesis. It is also converted into another form which gets inserted into RNA and interferes with mRNA translation and RNA processing. Therefore, 5-FU's cytotoxic effect works by means of both DNA and RNA inhibitory effects. 5-FU is the mainstay agent in the treatment of colorectal cancer, as both adjuvant therapy and therapy for advanced disease. It is also effective against a variety of other solid tumors. Its half-life is only 10–15 min, and therefore it is often administered as a continuous infusion over bolus dose schedules. Eighty to 85 % of the drug is metabolized by dihydropyrimidine dehydrogenase (DPD), which of note roughly 5 % of cancer patients are deficient in this enzyme [10]. DPD-deficient patients manifest severe toxic effects of myelosuppression, nausea and vomiting, diarrhea, and neurotoxicity.

Capecitabine

This fluoropyrimidine carbamate drug has 70–80 % oral bioavailability, and it functions as a prodrug. After extensive metabolism in the liver, it is eventually hydrolyzed by thymidine phosphorylase to 5-FU directly within the tumor [10]. Thymidine phosphorylase expression is found to be significantly higher in the tissue cells of tumors when compared to normal tissue. Capecitabine is used in the treatment of metastatic breast cancer as well as metastatic colorectal cancer. In certain regimens (as illustrated by the Table 31.1 in the following section), it replaces 5-FU therapy as an oral agent.

Cytarabine

Cytarabine (ara-C) is an antimetabolite drug specific to the S-phase of the cell cycle. It is converted to the monophosphate form by deoxycytidine kinase and further to the triphosphate metabolite, ara-TMP, which is the main cytotoxic agent. Ara-TMP blocks DNA synthesis and repair by competitively inhibiting DNA polymerase-α and DNA polymerase-β. The drug is rapidly cleared and must be administered by continuous infusion for a 5–7-day period. It is used primarily for hematologic malignancies and is ineffective against solid tumors [7, 10].

Gemcitabine

Gemcitabine is also metabolized initially by deoxycytidine kinase to the monophosphate and eventually triphosphate nucleotide form. Its cytotoxic effects are mediated by multiple pathways. Like cytarabine, it inhibits DNA polymerase-α and DNA polymerase-β and blocks DNA synthesis and repair. It also inhibits ribonucleotide reductase which decreases the amount of deoxyribonucleoside triphosphates required for DNA synthesis. The third antitumor mechanism occurs when the triphosphate form of gemcitabine is incorporated into DNA, resulting in chain termination. Gemcitabine is used for a wide variety of malignancies including non-small cell lung cancer, bladder cancer, ovarian cancer, soft tissue sarcoma, and non-Hodgkin's lymphoma [7]. Its original approval was for the treatment of pancreatic cancer [7].

Purine Analogs: 6-Mercaptopurine, Thioguanine, and Hydroxyurea

Purine analogs, like the aforementioned group of pyrimidine analogs, prevent or interfere with the biosynthesis of DNA structures by mimicking the purine nucleotides (purine and adenine).

Table 31.1 An overview of malignancies categorized by organ system affected [9]

	Site and/or type of malignancy	Treatment modalities	Chemotherapy agents used	Perioperative clinical considerations
Head and neck cancer	Lip	Primary en bloc surgical resection when possible. Radiation and chemotherapy as adjunct or primary treatment if resection not possible or contraindicated	Adjunct/induction *Cisplatin* alone *Cisplatin +5-FU*	Postradiation and surgical changes to head and neck anatomy in relation to airway management
	Oropharynx Nasopharynx oral cavity larynx		Advanced disease (incurable) *Cisplatin* or *carboplatin +5-FU + cetuximab* (non-nasopharyngeal)	Neurotoxic and peripheral neuropathy occurring with taxanes and platinum agents and perioperative pain management
	Ethmoid sinus Maxillary sinus		*Cisplatin* or *carboplatin + paclitaxel* or *docetaxel*	
	Ethmoid sinus Maxillary sinus			
	Salivary gland			
Breast cancer	Invasive or noninvasive	Surgical treatment ranging from lumpectomy to radical mastectomy	AC (doxorubicin/Adriamycin + cyclophosphamide) + paclitaxel weekly or biweekly	Doxorubicin- and daunorubicin-associated cardiomyopathy; a preoperative assessment of cardiac function is prudent
	Ductal or lobular Inflammatory Phyllodes (soft tissue sarcoma)	Radiation and chemotherapy as adjunct therapy depending on staging	TC (docetaxel + cyclophosphamide)	

Hematologic malignancies	Acute lymphoblastic leukemia (ALL)	Leukemias typically are treated by chemotherapy alone classified as regimens (induction, maintenance, etc.)	ALL induction therapy *TKI (tyrosine kinase inhibitor) + hyper-CVAD (imatinib or dasatinib + cyclophosphamide, vincristine, doxorubicin/adriamycin, and dexamethasone)*	Consider long-term consequences of induction chemotherapy agents when caring for surgical patients – i.e., cardiomyopathy
	Acute myeloid leukemia (AML)	Lymphomas often require tissue diagnosis (this can be a surgical procedure) and then are treated with chemotherapy +/– radiation therapy	Maintenance therapy *Methotrexate, 6-mercaptopurine*	Pediatric patients requiring anesthesia for maintenance therapy (often intrathecal chemotherapy) may have increased requirements for agents primarily cleared or metabolized in the liver due to induction of the P450 enzyme system
			AML induction therapy *ATRA (all trans retinoic acid) + daunorubicin + cytarabine*	In patients with the diagnosis of lymphoma, it is imperative to know the details of patients' disease process, for these patients can present with sizeable mediastinal masses which can cause hemodynamic compromise and airway compression that is positional in nature. Induction of general anesthesia in these patients can result in devastating outcomes if appropriate preoperative risk assessment is not performed
	Chronic myelogenous leukemia (CML)		CML treatment *TKI (imatinib)*	
	Hodgkin's lymphoma		Hodgkin's lymphoma *ABVD (adriamycin + bleomycin + vinblastine + dexamethasone)*	
	Non-Hodgkin's lymphoma		Non-Hodgkin's lymphoma *CHOP (cyclophosphamide + hydroxydaunorubicin + vincristine/"Oncovin" = trade name + prednisone)*	

(continued)

Table 31.1 (continued)

Site and/or type of malignancy	Treatment modalities	Chemotherapy agents used	Perioperative clinical considerations
Gastrointestinal cancers			
Colon cancer	In disease that is not metastatic, surgical resection occurs for most gastrointestinal cancers. Patients receive adjuvant or neoadjuvant chemotherapy and/or radiation therapy	Colorectal cancer *FOLFOX* (folinic acid/leucovorin + 5-FU + oxaliplatin) or *FOLFIRI* (folinic acid/leucovorin + 5-FU + irinotecan) or *CapeOX* (capecitabine + oxaliplatin)	Neurotoxic and peripheral neuropathy occurring with taxanes and platinum agents and perioperative pain management
Rectal cancer		Gastric cancer *Paclitaxel + carboplatin or cisplatin + 5-FU or capecitabine*	Many of these patients may have undergone chemotherapy and radiation treatment prior to oncologic surgery
Gastric cancer		Esophageal cancer *Paclitaxel + carboplatin or cisplatin +5-FU or capecitabine*	
Esophageal cancer			
Lung cancers			
Non-small cell lung cancers (NSCLC)	In appropriate candidates, surgical resection in combination with radiation therapy a typical treatment of NSCLC. Neoadjuvant and adjuvant chemotherapies are also used, according to staging	NSCLC *Cisplatin + gemcitabine* or in combination with another agent of the following: *etoposide, paclitaxel, docetaxel, vinorelbine*	Paraneoplastic syndromes can occur with small cell lung cancers including but not limited to Eaton-Lambert syndrome, carcinoid syndrome, syndrome of inappropriate antidiuretic hormone production, superior vena cava syndrome, and/or mediastinal lymphadenopathy that can cause similar hemodynamic or respiratory changes to mediastinal masses found with lymphoma [6]
Small cell lung cancers (SCLC)		SCLC *Cisplatin + etoposide or cisplatin + irinotecan*	

Genitourinary cancers	Prostate cancer	Depending on staging, surgical resection of primary tumor +/− with radiation chemotherapy depending on cancer type and staging	Prostate cancer Antiandrogen therapy + *paclitaxel or docetaxel*	Considerations are to be taken for patients exposed to agents that cause pulmonary toxicity such as bleomycin, where administration of high inspired oxygen fraction can worsen pulmonary disease and function [5]
	Testicular cancer		Testicular cancer *BEP* (bleomycin + etoposide + cisplatin) or *VIP* (etoposide + ifosfamide + cisplatin)	Neurotoxicity and peripheral neuropathy occurring with taxanes and platinum agents and perioperative pain management
	Ovarian cancer		Ovarian cancer *Paclitaxel + carboplatin or docetaxel + carboplatin*	
	Uterine cancer		Uterine cancer *Cisplatin + doxorubicin + paclitaxel*	
	Cervical cancer		Cervical cancer *Cisplatin*/*carboplatin + paclitaxel or cisplatin + topotecan*	
	Renal cancer		Renal cancer Clinical trial recommended or *temsirolimus*	
	Bladder cancer		Bladder cancer *DDMVAC* (dose-dense methotrexate + vinblastine + doxorubicin + cisplatin) *or gemcitabine + cisplatin or CMV* (cisplatin + methotrexate + vinblastine)	

(continued)

Table 31.1 (continued)

Site and/or type of malignancy		Treatment modalities	Chemotherapy agents used	Perioperative clinical considerations
Central nervous system cancers	Astrocytoma/oligodendroglioma	Surgical resection of tumors when appropriate, otherwise surgical biopsy as diagnostic procedure	Astrocytoma/oligodendroglioma *Temozolomide* and/or *PCV* (lomustine + procarbazine + vincristine)	The side effect profile of the chemotherapeutic agents can overlap with the symptoms caused by intracranial masses and the disease process
	Anaplastic gliomas and glioblastomas	Targeted radiotherapy and adjuvant chemotherapy	Anaplastic gliomas/glioblastoma *Temozolomide* or *PCV*	Peripheral neuropathy occurring as side effect of vinca alkaloids
	Primary CNS lymphoma		CNS lymphoma *Methotrexate + vincristine + cytarabine*	
	Meningioma		Meningioma *Hydroxyurea* or interferon alpha or somatostatin analog	
	Primary spinal cord tumors		Primary spinal cord tumors *Insufficient evidence for specific recommendations, salvage therapy if necessary*	
Soft tissue and bone cancers	Soft tissue sarcomas (i.e., rhabdomyosarcoma)	Treatment is often surgical excision if possible. Ewing's sarcoma class of tumors often receives neoadjuvant chemotherapy and/or radiation therapy	Rhabdomyosarcoma *Vincristine + dactinomycin + cyclophosphamide or vincristine + doxorubicin + cyclophosphamide*	Consider doxorubicin-associated cardiomyopathy; a preoperative assessment of cardiac function is prudent
	Chondrosarcoma		Chondrosarcomas/Ewing's sarcoma *VAC/IE* (vincristine + doxorubicin + cyclophosphamide/ifosfamide + etoposide) *or VAdriaC* (vincristine + doxorubicin + cyclophosphamide)	Surgical excision of certain soft tissue sarcomas run the risk of significant blood loss due to their location and size; prepare for adequate IV access and invasive hemodynamic monitoring if necessary [1]
	Ewing's sarcoma		Giant cell tumor of the bone *Denosumab, interferon alpha, peginterferon*	
	Giant cell tumor of the bone		Osteosarcoma *Cisplatin and doxorubicin or MAP* (high-dose methotrexate, cisplatin, doxorubicin)	
	Osteosarcoma			

6-Mercaptopurine (6-MP)

6-Mercaptopurine (6-MP) is one of the first thiopurine analogs to be found effective in cancer therapy. 6-MP must be metabolized by hypoxanthine-guanine phosphoribosyltransferase (HGPRT) in order for it to be made into its active monophosphate and eventual triphosphate form. The monophosphate form inhibits de novo synthesis of purine nucleotides, and the triphosphate form gets incorporated into RNA or DNA strands which either causes DNA damage or prevents further strand synthesis. 6-MP is also metabolized by the enzyme xanthine oxidase. Allopurinol, which inhibits xanthine oxidase, can be given with 6-MP which results in an increase in exposure of the cells to 6-MP. The dose of 6-MP is reduced 50–70 % when given in conjunction with allopurinol; otherwise, excessive toxicity would ensue [7, 10]. The drug can be given orally with good absorption and minimal damage to gastrointestinal epithelium, and it is used most commonly in the treatment of acute leukemia in children.

6-Thioguanine

Like 6-MP, thioguanine is effective in inhibiting several enzymes in the de novo purine nucleotide synthetic pathway. Thioguanine, unlike 6-MP, can be given concurrently with allopurinol without decreasing its dose as deamination is not part of its metabolic deactivation [7]. This drug is particularly useful as a co-treatment agent with cytarabine for adult acute leukemia.

Hydroxyurea

Hydroxyurea interferes with DNA synthesis by acting on the ribonucleoside diphosphate reductase enzyme. It has high oral bioavailability and can be given PO or IV, and its primary use is for treatment of chronic granulocytic leukemia [10].

DNA-Altering Drugs

A large group of antitumor agents that effectively prevent cells from undergoing replication are ones that change the structure of the cells' DNA. These drugs are classified as cell cycle-nonspecific agents and are largely comprised of alkylating agents and platinum analog agents. Both of these types of drugs induce physical changes by causing cross-links to inter- and intra-strand DNA structure, resulting in inhibition of DNA synthesis and function.

Alkylating Agents: Nitrogen Mustards

Cyclophosphamide, Mechlorethamine, Melphalan, and Chlorambucil

Of the nitrogen mustard alkylating agent subclassification, cyclophosphamide is the most clinically relevant and widely used much in part due to its good oral bioavailability and its efficacy against a wide variety of cancers and inflammatory diseases. It can also be administered effectively intravenously. The liver activates cyclophosphamide to aldophosphamide which is later converted to highly cytotoxic compounds by the targeted cells. This drug is excreted in part by the kidneys where a portion can be found unchanged in the urine. Mesna is utilized to protect the bladder from cyclophosphamide-induced hemorrhagic cystitis without interfering with the chemotherapeutic effect [4]. Beyond therapy for malignancies, cyclophosphamide is used to treat non-neoplastic conditions such as Wegener's granulomatosis and Rheumatoid arthritis due to its immunosuppressive characteristics.

Alkylating Agents: Nitrosoureas

Carmustine, Lomustine, Semustine, and Streptozocin

These agents undergo nonenzymatic decomposition which results in metabolites with alkylating and carbamoylating properties. They are highly lipid soluble and effectively cross the blood-brain barrier, making them effective in the treatment of brain malignancies. Of the above-listed agents, carmustine is the most widely used of the nitrosoureas. Like bleomycin, carmustine can cause interstitial pneumonitis and fibrosis with cumulative dose being the major risk factor of this occurrence [3, 10]. At doses above the range of 1,200–1,500 mg/m^2, 50 % of patients exhibit pulmonary toxicity. Streptozocin, out of all the nitrosoureas, causes minimal bone marrow toxicity, and it is used specifically for the treatment of insulin-secreting islet cell carcinoma of the pancreas and malignant carcinoid tumors.

Alkylating Agents: Alkyl Sulfonates

Busulfan

Busulfan is a good oral agent with high absorption, and it can also be administered intravenously. It is a very effective drug for the treatment of chronic myelogenous leukemia, resulting in 90 % rate of remission. In up to 4 % of patients, it produces progressive pulmonary fibrosis and is also associated with skin pigmentation and adrenal insufficiency [7].

Alkylating Agents: Triazenes

Dacarbazine and Temozolomide

The triazene types of alkylating agents transfer methyl groups to DNA structures. Dacarbazine is given intravenously, and it requires metabolic activation by the liver. It is a potent vesicant so care needs to be taken to avoid extravasation [7]. Temozolomide undergoes spontaneous breakdown to its alkylating intermediate and is effective in treating gliomas. Temozolomide can be given intravenously or orally [3].

Alkylating Agents: Bioreductive

Mitomycin-C

Mitomycin is an antibiotic that after undergoing metabolic activation becomes an alkylating agent effective in cross-linking DNA. It is most effective against hypoxic tumor cells where the environment is favorable toward reduction reactions [7]. Its toxic effects are active in all phases of the cell cycle, and it is used often in combination with radiation therapy. Mitomycin, along with 5-FU and radiation, is the mainstay treatment for squamous cell cancer of the anus. It is also used as a somewhat topical treatment for superficial bladder cancer where it is given as a vesicular infusion with little to no systemic absorption.

Platinum Analogs

Cisplatin, Carboplatin, and Oxaliplatin

The platinum analog group of chemotherapeutic drugs works in a similar fashion as alkylating agents with regard to their cytotoxic effects. They bind DNA causing intra- and interstrand cross-links, preventing DNA synthesis and function. Platinum cross-links work synergistically with other chemotherapeutic agents such as alkylating agents and others. Cisplatin is effective in treating a broad variety of solid tumors, and it must be given intravenously due to the fact that it has no oral bioavailability. Carboplatin is a second-generation platinum agent whose mechanism of action and efficacy are identical to cisplatin. Carboplatin has mostly replaced cisplatin use due to the fact that carboplatin carries less risk of renal and gastrointestinal toxicity. A third-generation platinum analog, oxaliplatin, also shares its mechanism of action with cisplatin and carboplatin. However, cancers that are resistant to carboplatin and cisplatin are still sensitive to oxaliplatin. Oxaliplatin has become one of the mainstay agents in the treatment of GI cancers, and its main toxicity side effect involves neurotoxicity, which will be further detailed later in this chapter.

Antitumor Antibiotics (G2-M Phase)

Many of the antitumor antibiotics used in clinical practice are also classified as naturally occurring products. The first antibiotic identified and used as chemotherapy is dactinomycin (actinomycin D), a cell cycle-nonspecific agent similar to mitomycin. It is still a relevant agent used in the treatment of a few different solid tumors, it is minimally metabolized with excretion via urine and bile, and it does not cross the blood-brain barrier. Some of its more recognizable clinical uses are for the treatment of Wilms tumor and rhabdomyosarcoma in children and for choriocarcinoma in adult women.

Anthracyclines

Doxorubicin (Adriamycin), Daunorubicin, and Idarubicin

The anthracycline class of antibiotics is derived from *Streptomyces peucetius* var. *caesius*. These antibiotic agents exert their cytotoxic effects via four mechanisms: (1) binding of DNA that disrupts synthesis of DNA and RNA, (2) inhibition of topoisomerase II, (3) binding to cellular membranes altering fluidity and ion transport, and (4) generation of free radicals through iron-dependent, enzyme-mediated reductive reactions [3]. While not every mechanism of cytotoxicity is completely understood, it has been established that the cardiotoxicity caused by the anthracycline class of chemotherapy agents is due to the free radical formation. Oncologists often will utilize a drug called dexrazoxane, which helps minimize cardiotoxicity. Doxorubicin and daunorubicin are among the first and most relevant agents in this class, while several analogs of these drugs exist such as idarubicin, epirubicin, and mitoxantrone.

Bleomycin

Bleomycin is a cell cycle-specific agent that works at the G2 phase. It is an antibiotic that was isolated from *Streptomyces verticillus* in 1966. It inhibits DNA synthesis by binding to DNA causing single- and double-strand breaks, as well as free radical production. It can be given intravenously, intramuscularly, and subcutaneously, and it is dependent on renal excretion. It is used for a variety of tumors including head and neck cancers and squamous cell cancer of the skin, vulva, and cervix, and it is one the agents used in the treatment of Hodgkin's and non-Hodgkin's lymphoma [10]. The side effect of pulmonary toxicity is dose limited and frequently presents as pneumonitis. A more detailed explanation of this side effect can be read later in this chapter.

Antimitotic Drugs (M Phase)

The antimitotic drugs disrupt the function of cell division which ultimately leads to cell death. The mechanism of action of these agents works at different points of mitosis, mostly acting against or disrupting microtubule function and/or formation.

Vinblastine and Vincristine

The vinca alkaloids are naturally occurring class of antitumor agents derived from the periwinkle plant *Vinca rosea* [3, 7, 10]. These agents work at the mitotic phase by disrupting microtubule formation which is an important component of the mitotic spindle. Vincristine and vinblastine are both derivatives of *V. rosea*, and their mechanism of action is identical. Their uses however do differ. Vinblastine is effective in Hodgkin's and non-Hodgkin's lymphoma, breast cancer, and germ cell cancer. While vincristine shares some of the treatment profile for the aforementioned lymphomas, it is also effective for acute lymphoblastic leukemia, multiple myeloma, and a variety of pediatric tumors. Vincristine is not effective against solid tumors in the adult population. The main side effect and dose-limiting toxicity is neurotoxicity, which is often manifested as a peripheral sensory neuropathy.

Paclitaxel and Docetaxel

The taxane group of chemotherapeutic agents is derived from the evergreen tree Pacific or European yew (*Taxus brevifolia*, *Taxus baccata*). Both paclitaxel and docetaxel work as mitotic spindle poisons by binding to microtubules and enhancing tubulin polymerization, promoting microtubule assembly [10]. However, this microtubule formation facilitated by the taxane drugs occurs without a key component (guanosine triphosphate), rendering division impossible and leading to mitotic arrest and cell death. High dosing of taxanes, like the vinca alkaloids, is restricted due to the incidence of severe neurotoxicity. The peripheral neuropathy pattern that occurs follows a glove and stocking distribution.

Monoclonal Antibodies

Monoclonal antibodies (mAbs) are a class of drugs that are target directed. They bind to specific cell surface receptors or antigens, and in doing so they recruit immune cells and complement to their newly created antigen-antibody complex [2, 8]. Currently, there is a large amount of research focusing on mAb therapy for numerous diseases, including rheumatoid arthritis, multiple sclerosis, and different types of cancer. MAb therapy can be used to destroy malignant tumor cells as well as inhibit tumor growth by blocking specific cell receptors. Several of the cytotoxic monoclonal antibody agents are directed against epidermal growth factor receptor (EGFR), which belongs to the family of transmembrane tyrosine kinase receptors. Cetuximab will be the agent to serve as the example for discussion.

Cetuximab works as a growth factor receptor inhibitor, and it targets EGFR which is overexpressed in a number of solid tumors. The EGFR pathway is responsible for key events in cellular growth such as proliferation, invasion, metastasis, and angiogenesis. Cetuximab is used in combination with irinotecan for metastatic colon cancer, it is given on a biweekly basis, and it is well tolerated with the main adverse effects being an acneiform skin rash, hypomagnesemia, and hypersensitivity infusion reaction.

In addition to cetuximab, the current "big 5" therapeutic agents on the market are used to treat malignancies, autoimmune disease, or both. Bevacizumab and trastuzumab are used to treat malignancies. Adalimumab and infliximab are used to help manage autoimmune disorders, and rituximab is used in both oncology and autoimmune disorders [2, 7].

Tyrosine Kinase Inhibitors

Gefitinib and Imatinib

Like the monoclonal antibodies, these agents are also target-directed cytotoxic agents. However, they enter the cell and inhibit enzymatic function – specifically the tyrosine kinase function of EGFR [7].

Indications/Clinical Pearls

Table 31.1 is an overview of malignancies categorized by organ system affected. Agents and treatment modalities are abridged and provide a brief summary of the some of the more common and recognizable drugs used for each type of cancer. By no means is Table 31.1 complete or detailed as to the staging and exact treatment course of each malignancy. Comprehensive guidelines are available at the website NCCN.org (National Comprehensive Cancer Network). Chemotherapeutics can greatly inhibit the capacity of the patient to fight off infection making it significantly important that they be administered timely and appropriate antimicrobial agents and ongoing antibacterial, antifungal, and antiviral agents. Patients on long-term steroids can lack the capacity to generate a response to surgical stress and may need a stress dose of steroids.

Unique Side Effects/Adverse Outcomes/Clinical Pearls

Doxorubicin and Daunorubicin

Doxorubicin and daunorubicin are associated with a cardiomyopathy that is a dose-related phenomenon and can be irreversible. Less than 3 % of patients receiving a cumulative dose of <400 mg/m^2 develop congestive heart failure (CHF), while the incidence of CHF can be as high as 18 % in patients who receive a cumulative dose of >700 mg/m^2. There are two types of cardiomyopathies that may occur, an acute form that occurs in 10 % of patients that tends to resolve within 1–2 months after discontinuation of therapy. This form occurs at all dosing levels, and it is characterized by nonspecific ST-T changes and decreased QRS voltage by ECG, premature ventricular contractions, supraventricular tachydysrhythmias, and cardiac conduction abnormalities. A more severe form occurs in 2 % of patients that has a mortality rate as high as 60 % within 3 weeks of symptom onset [10]. It presents with symptoms of progressive heart failure that is unresponsive to inotropic treatments or mechanical assist device therapy.

Bleomycin

Bleomycin is associated with a dose-related pulmonary toxicity [10]. Generally speaking, a dose of greater than 450 mg puts a patient at risk for pulmonary damage. Bleomycin is inactivated by hydrolase enzyme, an enzyme that is relatively deficient in the lung tissues. Bleomycin therefore tends to accumulate in the lung tissue producing pulmonary capillary endothelial damage, alveolar epithelial injury, necrosis of type 1 alveolar cells, and proliferation of type II alveolar cells. There have been case reports of early postoperative respiratory failure and acute respiratory distress syndrome after general anesthesia in patients who have received bleomycin therapy. It is thought that high inspired oxygen content and excessive crystalloid administration contribute to the risk of pulmonary complications, and animal studies show that hyperoxia immediately after bleomycin exposure increases pulmonary damage [5]. While there is inconclusive evidence as to exactly what time period after bleomycin treatment the risk of high oxygen exposure diminishes, it is prudent to limit inspired oxygen concentrations to less than 30 % when caring for these patients.

Busulfan

Like bleomycin, busulfan can cause pulmonary toxicity in the form of pulmonary fibrosis. This occurs in up to 4 % of patients receiving busulfan [3, 7]; however, it is not influenced by high inspired oxygen concentration. Busulfan is also associated with skin pigmentation and adrenal insufficiency.

Cyclophosphamide

Cyclophosphamide is a commonly used chemotherapy agent. Large doses of cyclophosphamide can cause pericarditis and pericardial effusion, which has been reported to progress to cardiac tamponade in some cases [4]. Interstitial cystitis and bladder cancer are associated with cyclophosphamide administration. These side effects are attributed to the effects of the toxic metabolite called acrolein. Preventive measures that can be taken to avoid bladder toxicity include adequate hydration, pulse dosing (versus continuous), and also the coadministration of 2-mercaptoethanesulfonate, which conjugates acrolein in the urine.

Neurotoxicity

Several chemotherapeutic agents have neurotoxic side effects that manifest as peripheral neuropathy [6]. Platinum-containing agents, taxanes, and the certain drugs that belong to the class of vinca alkaloids such as vincristine can all cause neurotoxicity in the form of peripheral neuropathy. Oxaliplatin can cause an acute form of peripheral neuropathy of the upper and lower extremities, mouth, and throat. Paresthesias or dysesthesias are often triggered by exposure to cold. A more chronic form of peripheral neuropathy encompassing both sensory and motor functions occurs with cisplatin. Paclitaxel causes a sometimes disabling sensory peripheral neuropathy in a glove and stocking distribution, which can be more severe in patients with preexisting diabetic peripheral neuropathy. Vincristine causes a sensory peripheral neuropathy, but also autonomic dysfunction can occur as well, with reports of ileus, constipation, orthostasis, and urinary retention.

Dosing Options

The dosing and choice of the different chemotherapeutic regimens are specific to patient circumstances as well as to disease process. Different combinations exist for each specific cancer; often times the drug choice can be tailored to the individual based on comorbidities as well as side effect profile. A comprehensive description of the regimens for chemotherapy by cancer type can be found on the National Comprehensive Cancer Network (NCCN) website – at www.nccn.org. A detailed discussion of dosing options for chemotherapy is beyond the scope of this review.

Side Effects/Black Box Warnings

Normal rapidly dividing cells within the body are most affected by chemotherapeutic drugs. These organ systems within our bodies include bone marrow, gastrointestinal mucosa, skin, and hair follicles. Thus, it is consistent that the shared side effect profile of the majority of chemotherapeutic agents includes myelosuppression, nausea and vomiting, mucositis, and alopecia. Nausea and vomiting are due to both the local gastrointestinal effects and central chemoreceptor activation within the CNS [10]. Serotonin antagonists as antiemetics have been effective in the treatment of chemotherapy-induced nausea. Myelosuppression resulting in neutropenia, thrombocytopenia, or anemia can be a dose-limiting factor for chemotherapeutic regimens prompting temporary or permanent withdrawal of therapy.

Summary

Be familiar with surgical patients that have recently received either neoadjuvant chemotherapy or radiation for their current oncologic issue for which they are being operated on. As a consulting physician, it is prudent to learn and to familiarize one-self with both the short- and long-term side effects of certain chemotherapy agents for patients and how they may affect your perioperative management.

Additional preoperative testing may be appropriate in patients who have received chemotherapy to either rule in or rule out underlying pathology that accompanies side effect profiles of whichever chemotherapeutic agents the patient has received. Meticulous concern with even minor details will alert the anesthesiologist to provide appropriate care and to minimize the risk for potential morbidity and mortality.

Chemical Structures

Chemical Structure 31.1 Methotrexate (MTX)

Chemical Structure 31.2 Vincristine

Chemical Structure 31.3 Fluorouracil

Chemical Structure 31.4 Mercaptopurine

Chemical Structure 31.5 Cisplatin

Chemical Structure 31.6 Bleomycin

References

1. Anderson MR, et al. Anesthesia for patients undergoing orthopedic oncologic surgeries. J Clin Anesth. 2010;22:565–72.
2. Beck A, Wurch T, Bailly C, Corvaia N. Strategies and challenges for the next generation of therapeutic antibodies. Nat Rev Immunol. 2010;10(5):345–52. doi:10.1038/nri2747. PMID 20414207.
3. Brunton LL, et al. Goodman & Gilman's pharmacologic basis of therapeutics. 12th ed. New York: McGraw Hill Companies; 2011.
4. Clowse MB, Stone JH. General toxicity of cyclophosphamide and chlorambucil in inflammatory diseases. UptoDate. 2013.
5. Hay JG, Haslam PL, Dewar A, et al. Development of acute lung injury after the combination of intravenous bleomycin and exposure to hyperoxia in rats. Thorax. 1987;42:374–82.

6. Hines RL, Marschall KE. Stoelting's anesthesia and co-existing disease. 5th ed. Philadelphia: Churchill Livingstone; 2008.

7. Katsung BG, Masters SB, Trevor AJ. Basic and clinical pharmacology. 11th ed. New York: McGraw Hill Medical; 2009.

8. Murillo O, et al. Potentiation of therapeutic immune responses against malignancies with monoclonal antibodies. Clin Cancer Res. 2003;9:5454–64.

9. NCCN Clinical Practice Guidelines in Oncology. NCCN.org: Version 1.2012 – Head and Neck Cancers; Version 1.2013 – Breast Cancer; Version 2.2012 – Acute lymphoblastic Leukemia; Version 1.2013 – Acute Myeloid Leukemia; Version 3.2013 – Chronic Myelogenous Leukemia; Version 3.2013 – Colon Cancer; Version 2.2012 – Esophageal Cancer; Version 2.2012 – Gastric Cancer; Version 4.2014 – Rectal Cancer; Version 2.2013 – Small Cell Lung Cancer; Version 2.2013 – Non-Small Cell Lung Cancer; Version 1.2012 – Testicular Cancer; Version 1.2013 – Prostate Cancer; Version 1.2013 – Ovarian Cancer, Including Fallopian Tube Cancer and Primary Peritoneal Cancer; Version 3.2012 – Uterine Neoplasms; Version 2.2012 – Cervical Cancer; Version 1.2013 – Kidney Cancer; Version 1.2013 – Central Nervous System Cancers; Version 3.2012 – Soft Tissue Sarcoma; Version 2.2013 – Bone Cancer.

10. Stoelting RK, Hillier SC. Pharmacology and physiology in anesthetic practice. 4th ed. Baltimore: Lippincott Williams & Wilkins; 2006. p. 551–68.

Chapter 32
Antimicrobial Agents

Rebecca Johnson, Richard Lancaster, and Timothy Ku

Contents

R. Johnson, MD • R. Lancaster, MD (✉) • T. Ku, MD
Department of Anesthesiology, Tulane Medical Center, New Orleans, LA, USA
e-mail: rjohns3@tulane.edu; rlancast@tulane.edu; tku@tulane.edu

A.D. Kaye et al. (eds.), *Essentials of Pharmacology for Anesthesia,*
Pain Medicine, and Critical Care, DOI 10.1007/978-1-4614-8948-1_32,
© Springer Science+Business Media New York 2015

Introduction

An antimicrobial is an agent which kills microorganisms or inhibits their growth. Antimicrobials which kill microbes are known as microbicidal, and those which inhibit their growth are known as microbiostatic. Disinfectants such as bleach are nonselective antimicrobials.

Perioperative Antibiotic Prophylaxis

Patients are constantly at risk of acquiring an infection during the perioperative period. In an effort to minimize perioperative infections, patients are given surgical antibiotic prophylaxis for most surgical procedures and some minimally invasive procedures. The antibiotic selection is based upon potential pathogens associated with the specific procedure. Cephalosporins are the most commonly used antibiotic class for surgical prophylaxis due to their broad antimicrobial spectrum and low incidence of associated allergic reactions. Current recommendations state that surgical antimicrobial prophylaxis should be administered within 1 h prior to incision of the surgery and no more than 2 h prior to incision for patients receiving vancomycin or a fluoroquinolone due to the long infusion time [2, 13].

In addition to surgical infection risks, patients are also at risk of developing nosocomial infections of the respiratory tract, urinary tract, and the bloodstream as a result of the use of ventilators, Foley catheters, and central venous catheters, respectively. Healthcare workers should minimize the use of unnecessary indwelling catheters as well as use proper hand hygiene, barrier precautions, and antibiotic stewardship to lower the incidence and risk for the spread of infection.

Antibiotic Selection

After establishment of an infection, antimicrobial selection should consider the spectrum of action of the antimicrobial against the suspected pathogens, the penetrance of the antimicrobial at the site of infection, and the dose necessary to achieve therapeutic concentrations while minimizing adverse reactions and toxicity. Identification of the causative organism in a blood or urine culture allows the most appropriate selection of antibiotics. A sensitivity profile may also be performed for the particular pathogen isolated that reveals what antibiotics are likely to be most effective. The culture and sensitivity may take a few days for identification, and during this initial time period, a broad-spectrum antibiotic regimen may be used until antibiotics may later be narrowed, especially during life-threatening infections seen frequently in critical care.

Special Considerations

If there is an infected foreign body or prosthesis, antibiotics will be more effective after removal of the source of infection. Many antibiotics are unable to cross the blood-brain barrier, and specific antibiotics may need to be chosen to treat CNS infections. The placenta allows select drugs to be transferred to the fetus similar to the blood-brain barrier in the CNS. It is affected by lipid solubility, molecular weight, and protein binding of the drugs. Antimicrobial administration during pregnancy may place the fetus at risk for certain teratogenic effects, although most antibiotics are safe during pregnancy. However, it should be noted that tetracyclines, quinolones, and trimethoprim are contraindicated in pregnancy.

The elderly have a progressive decrease in muscle mass, decrease in total body water, and increase in body fat. The result is a smaller volume of distribution for water-soluble drugs and a larger volume of distribution for lipid-soluble drugs. This can lead to increased plasma concentrations for water-soluble drugs and decreased plasma concentrations for lipid-soluble drugs. Additionally, there is decreased plasma albumin, which affects protein-bound drugs, decreased hepatic metabolism due to decreased hepatic blood flow, and decreased renal excretion due to decreased glomerular filtration rate. Administration of aminoglycosides, vancomycin, and piperacillin-tazobactam may require dosing adjustments and monitoring of renal function.

Penicillins

Mechanism of Action
Inhibits cell wall mucopeptide synthesis

Indications
First gen: syphilis, group A strep, rheumatic fever prophylaxis, meningitis (meningococcal), septicemia (meningococcal), anthrax. Second gen: sinusitis (acute bacterial), otitis media (acute), *H. pylori* infection, endocarditis prophylaxis, dental abscess, Lyme disease, cervicitis/urethritis (chlamydial), meningitis (bacterial), typhoid fever, GBS prophylaxis intrapartum. Third gen: UTI, prostatitis. Fourth gen: urinary tract (complicated), community-acquired pneumonia, acute cholangitis, moderate to severe infections, uncomplicated gonorrhea, pseudomonas; none are effective for *S. aureus*.

Dosing Options
PO, IM, IV

Drug Interactions
BCG vaccine live, demeclocycline, doxycycline, lymecycline, minocycline, myco-phenolate, oxytetracycline, probenecid, tetracycline, typhoid vaccine live

Side Effects
Common: rash, urticaria, fever, pruritus, fatigue, headache, nausea, vomiting, diar-rhea. Serious: anaphylaxis (0.004–0.15 %), hypersensitivity reaction – immediate or delayed (up to 10 % of patients) – serum sickness, exfoliative dermatitis, Stevens-Johnson syndrome, superinfection, *Clostridium* difficile-associated diarrhea, hemo-lytic anemia, neutropenia, interstitial nephritis, renal tubular necrosis

Summary
The key structural feature of the penicillins is the four-membered beta-lactam ring. These drugs are classified according to their structure, beta-lactamase susceptibility, and spectrum of activity. Penicillins interfere with the synthesis of peptidoglycan, a structural component of the constantly remodeling bacterial cell wall, and are bac-tericidal against gram-positive cell walls. They are less effective against gram-negative bacteria due to a difference in the cell wall not allowing access to the peptidoglycan site of synthesis.

Bacteria develop resistance by producing beta-lactamase enzymes that hydro-lyze the beta-lactam ring of penicillins. Methicillin, oxacillin, nafcillin, cloxacil-lin, and dicloxacillin are considered beta-lactamase-resistant penicillins because they are not susceptible to the staphylococcal beta-lactamases. Other penicillins are paired with beta-lactamase inhibitors such as clavulanic acid, sulbactam, and tazo-bactam. These compounds irreversibly bind and inhibit beta-lactamase produced by many bacteria. Commonly used combinations include clavulanic acid with amoxicillin, sulbactam with ampicillin, and tazobactam with piperacillin. Allergic cross-reactivity between penicillins and cephalosporins remains controversial. Reported probability of an allergic reaction due to cephalosporins in patients with a known penicillin allergy is 8 % [9]. The third-generation cephalosporins are less likely than the first-generation cephalosporins to result in cross-allergic reactions with penicillin. If a patient reports an allergic reaction with penicillin, the physician must determine the likelihood of an immediate type I hypersensitivity reaction. If there is concern for a type I reaction, then a cephalosporin should not be adminis-tered [3].

Cephalosporins

Mechanism of Action
Inhibits cell wall mucopeptide synthesis

Indication

First gen: surgical antimicrobial prophylaxis, endocarditis prophylaxis. Second gen: surgical antimicrobial prophylaxis, infections (uncomplicated gonococcal), PID. Third gen: meningitis (bacterial), infections (gonococcal), PID, surgical antimicrobial prophylaxis, epididymitis. Fourth gen: febrile neutropenia, UTI, infections (bacterial), pneumonia

Dosing Options

IM, IV

Drug Interactions

BCG vaccine live

Common Side Effects

Include diarrhea, rash, vomiting, nausea, abdominal pain, anorexia, urticaria, and thrombophlebitis. Serious side effects include neutropenia, thrombocytopenia, anaphylaxis, Stevens-Johnson syndrome, nephrotoxicity, seizures, and *Clostridium* difficile-associated diarrhea.

Summary

The first-generation cephalosporins are predominantly effective against gram-positive organisms, and the following generations have increased activity against gram negatives. The first-generation cephalosporins, such as cefazolin, are inexpensive and exhibit low toxicity. For these reasons, cefazolin is the most common first-line drug used for routine surgical antimicrobial prophylaxis. Cefoxitin is a commonly used second-generation cephalosporin, which is resistant to beta-lactamase produced by gram-negative bacteria. Because of the increased gram-negative coverage, cefoxitin is the preferred drug for surgical antimicrobial prophylaxis for colon resection or any case with the potential for gastrointestinal contamination of the surgical field. Cefuroxime, another second-generation cephalosporin, can cross the blood-brain barrier and be used to treat meningitis. The third-generation cephalosporins (e.g., cefotaxime and ceftriaxone) have further increased activity against gram-negative organisms and increased resistance to beta-lactamases and are very useful in CNS infections. Cefotaxime is effective against most gram-negative bacteria with the exception of pseudomonas. Ceftriaxone is commonly used for the treatment of community-acquired pneumonia, meningitis, and gonorrhea. The fourth-generation cephalosporins, such as cefepime, exhibit activity similar to third generation with greater resistance to beta-lactamases and are used against pseudomonas. Cefepime is frequently used for febrile neutropenia.

Carbapenems

Mechanism of Action

Inhibits cell wall mucopeptide synthesis

Indication
Anaerobes, aerobes, gram-positive and many gram-negative bacteria

Dosing Options
IV

Drug Interactions
Decreases levels of valproic acid [17]

Side Effects
Imipenem has a rare seizure association.

Summary
Carbapenems are a class of beta-lactam antibiotics and have a structure that makes them highly resistant to most beta-lactamases. Examples of carbapenems include imipenem and meropenem. Imipenem has a very broad spectrum of activity against aerobic and anaerobic, gram-positive, and gram-negative bacteria. Imipenem is metabolized in the renal tubules and is coadministered with cilastatin to prevent this inactivation. Meropenem also has a very broad spectrum of activity including *Pseudomonas* and is used frequently for febrile neutropenia [12].

Vancomycin

Mechanism of Action
Impairs cell wall synthesis of gram-positive bacteria

Indication
Severe *Staphylococcus* and *Streptococcus* infections, drug of choice for methicillin-resistant *Staphylococcus aureus*, and can treat CSF shunt-related infections due to coagulase-negative staphylococci [7]

Dosing Options
IV; PO for the treatment of staphylococcal enterocolitis and antimicrobial-associated pseudomembranous enterocolitis; determination of drug levels is important to guide dosing.

Drug Interactions
Aminoglycosides, BCG, bile acid sequestrants, colistimethate, neuromuscular blocking agents, NSAIDS, sodium picosulfate, typhoid vaccine

Side Effects
Drug-induced histamine release, hypotension, possible cardiac arrest with rapid infusion (<30 min), red man syndrome even with slow administration, anaphylactoid

allergic reactions (hypotension, erythema, bronchospasm), ototoxicity with high plasma levels (>30 mcg/ml), and possible nephrotoxicity when administered with aminoglycosides [5, 10, 14]

Aminoglycosides

Some common aminoglycosides include streptomycin, gentamicin, tobramycin, amikacin, and neomycin.

Mechanism of Action
Several proposed mechanisms of action, most of which involve inhibiting bacterial protein synthesis

Indication
Aerobic, gram-negative bacterial infections

Dosing Options
Usually IV/IM, sometimes topically, PO for GI contamination

Drug Interactions
Second- to fourth-generation cephalosporins, cyclosporin, loop diuretics, neuromuscular blocking agents, penicillins, vancomycin

Side Effects
Nephrotoxicity, ototoxicity, skeletal muscle weakness, and potentiation of nondepolarizing neuromuscular blocking drugs [7]

Fluoroquinolones

Fluoroquinolones include ciprofloxacin, norfloxacin, ofloxacin, and lomefloxacin.

Mechanism of Action
Direct inhibitors of bacterial DNA synthesis

Indication
Most enteric gram-negative bacilli; most commonly used to treat complicated urinary tract infections and bacterial gastroenteritis [8]

Dosing Options
PO, IV. Decreased dosing is required in patients with renal failure.

Drug Interactions

Each agent has multiple specific interactions; most notably as a class, may potentiate QT prolongation with amiodarone, possibly leading to torsades de pointes.

Side Effects

GI upset and central nervous system disturbances such as dizziness and insomnia; black box warning of potential tendonitis or tendon rupture [21]. Avoidance in patients with known history of myasthenia gravis is advised due to risk of fluoroquinolone-associated myasthenia gravis exacerbation.

Tetracyclines

Some commonly used tetracyclines include tetracycline, doxycycline, and demeclocycline.

Mechanism of Action

Reversibly bind to 30S ribosomal subunit and inhibit bacterial protein synthesis

Indication

Treatment of choice for certain infections caused by mycoplasma, chlamydia, rickettsia, and spirochete pathogens; can treat severe cystic acne, rosacea, anthrax, and bubonic plague; off-label use of demeclocycline for the treatment of hyponatremia caused by the syndrome of inappropriate antidiuretic hormone

Dosing Options

PO, IV, topical for eye or skin infections

Drug Interactions

Reduced activity with concomitant calcium, decreased methotrexate levels

Side Effects

Should not be given to children and pregnant or nursing women as they can interfere with bone development and may permanently discolor teeth; can also cause phototoxicity and catabolic response

Lincosamides

The most commonly administered lincosamide is clindamycin. Lincomycin is also a lincosamide.

Mechanism of Action
Inhibits bacterial protein synthesis

Indication
Gram-positive bacteria and anaerobes, particularly in the GI and female genital tract

Dosing Options
PO, IV, IM

Drug Interactions
BCG, erythromycin, kaolin, neuromuscular blocking agents, sodium picosulfate, typhoid vaccine

Side Effects
Pseudomembranous colitis, diarrhea, skin rashes, and potentiation of the neuromuscular blockade even in the absence of nondepolarizing neuromuscular blocking drugs [1]

Macrolides

The most commonly administered macrolides include erythromycin, azithromycin, and clarithromycin.

Mechanism of Action
Inhibit bacterial protein synthesis

Indication
Most gram-positive bacteria, community-acquired respiratory infections; erythromycin also demonstrates prokinetic properties and has been used to achieve gastric emptying prior to endoscopy procedures [11].

Dosing Options
PO (all), IV (erythromycin and azithromycin only)

Drug Interactions
Erythromycin is extensively metabolized by cytochrome P450 3A, so the use with other strong inhibitors of this cytochrome is not recommended.

Side Effects
GI intolerance common with erythromycin; tinnitus, hearing loss, and thrombophlebitis can occur with prolonged IV administration; erythromycin can also prolong the QT interval and lead to torsades de pointes [19].

Oxazolidinones

Linezolid is in the class of oxazolidinones.

Mechanism of Action
Inhibits the function of the initiation complex required for ribosomal function, effectively inhibiting protein synthesis [6]

Indication
Bacteriostatic against *Staphylococcus* and *Enterococcus*, including methicillin-resistant *Staphylococcus aureus* and vancomycin-resistant *Enterococcus*; bactericidal against most streptococcal strains [18]

Dosing Options
IV, PO

Drug Interactions
Reversible inhibitor of monoamine oxidase, so patients may have exaggerated hypertensive responses to sympathomimetic drugs; also advisable to avoid decongestants and food and drink high in tyramine content

Side Effects
Include nausea and vomiting, headache, and rarely reversible bone marrow suppression (thrombocytopenia, anemia, leukopenia); black box warning in patients taking serotonergic antidepressants as this can lead to serotonin

Other Antimicrobials

See Table 32.1.

Monobactams

The most common in this class is aztreonam.

Mechanism of Action
Inhibits cell wall mucopeptide synthesis

Table 32.1 Other antibiotics

Drug	Mechanism	Indication	Dosing options	Drug interactions	Side effects
Monobactam (aztreonam)	Inhibition of cell wall mucopeptide synthesis	Strong activity against gram-negative bacteria; may be substituted for penicillins or cephalosporin	IV, IM	Few reported	Rash, GI upset, rarely toxic epidermal necrolysis
Streptogramin (quinupristin dalfopristin)	Inhibition of protein synthesis through binding to ribosomal subunits	Vancomycin-resistant infections	IV	Increased plasma concentration of drugs metabolized by CYP3A4 (includes fentanyl) [7]	Phlebitis with peripheral intravenous administration, arthralgias, myalgias, and increased levels of bilirubin
Polymyxins (polymyxin B polymyxin E)	Altered bacterial cytoplasmic membrane permeability through phospholipid binding	Specific gram-negative bacilli including *E. coli*, *Klebsiella*, and *Pseudomonas aeruginosa*; useful in treatment of severe urinary tract infections and sensitive strains of *P. aeruginosa* for patients with cystic fibrosis, neutropenia, and/or immune compromise	IV, IM, and topical for infections of the skin, mucous membranes, eyes, and ears	Few reported	Pain with IM injection, skeletal muscle weakness, potentiation of nondepolarizing muscle relaxants, and nephrotoxicity
Nitrofurantoin	Inhibition of bacterial enzymes and possibly cell wall synthesis	Uncomplicated mild urinary tract infections	PO	Probenecid decreases renal clearance	GI upset, rarely pneumonitis, neuropathies, chronic active hepatitis
Metronidazole	Deactivates bacterial enzymes	Most anaerobic gram-negative bacilli and clostridium species	PO, IV	Disulfiram-like reaction with concurrent alcohol ingestion	Dry mouth, metallic taste, nausea, and rarely pancreatitis and neuropathy

Indication
Strong activity against gram-negative bacteria; may be used for penicillin or cephalosporin allergic patients due to lack of cross-reactivity

Dosing Options
IV, IM

Drug Interactions
Few reported

Side Effects
Rash, GI upset, rarely toxic epidermal necrolysis

Streptogramins

Quinupristin and dalfopristin are in the class of streptogramins.

Mechanism of Action
Bind to bacterial ribosomal subunits and inhibit protein synthesis

Indication
Vancomycin-resistant infections

Dosing Options
 IV

Drug Interactions
Increase plasma concentrations of drugs such as fentanyl that depend on CYP3A4 for hepatic metabolism [7]

Side Effects
Phlebitis with peripheral intravenous administration, arthralgias, myalgias, and increased levels of bilirubin

Polymyxins

This class includes both polymyxin B and polymyxin E (colistimethate).

Mechanism of Action
Bind to phospholipids, altering their permeability and damaging the bacterial cytoplasmic membrane

Indication
Certain gram-negative bacilli including *E. coli*, *Klebsiella*, and *Pseudomonas aeruginosa*; useful in treatment of severe urinary tract infections and sensitive strains of *P. aeruginosa*, which are a significant problem for patients with cystic fibrosis, neutropenia, and/or immune system compromise

Dosing Options
IV, IM; topical for infections of the skin, mucous membranes, eyes, and ears

Drug Interactions
Few reported

Side Effects
Pain with IM injection, skeletal muscle weakness, potentiation of nondepolarizing muscle relaxants, and nephrotoxicity

Sulfonamides

Clinically useful sulfonamides include sulfisoxazole, sulfamethoxazole, sulfasalazine, sulfacetamide, trimethoprim, and trimethoprim-sulfamethoxazole.

Mechanism of Action
Competitive inhibitors of the bacterial enzyme responsible for the incorporation of para-aminobenzoic acid into the immediate precursor of folic acid; trimethoprim prevents the reduction of dihydrofolate to tetrahydrofolate by selectively inhibiting dihydrofolate reductase.

Indication
Uncomplicated urinary tract infections and *H. influenza* otitis media in children

Dosing Options
PO, IV

Drug Interactions
May increase the effect of oral anticoagulants, methotrexate, sulfonylurea, hypoglycemic drugs, and thiazide diuretics; indomethacin, probenecid, and salicylates may displace sulfonamides from plasma albumin and increase the concentrations of free drug in the plasma.

Side Effects
Allergic reactions ranging from skin rash to anaphylaxis, drug fever, hepatotoxicity (<0.1 %), acute hemolytic anemia, and agranulocytosis; hemolytic anemia may occur in patients with glucose-6-phosphate deficiency syndrome.

Nitrofurantoin

Mechanism of Action
Inhibits bacterial enzymes, possibly cell wall synthesis

Indication
Uncomplicated mild urinary tract infections

Dosing Options
PO

Drug Interactions
Probenecid decreases renal clearance.

Side Effect
GI upset, rarely pneumonitis, neuropathies, chronic active hepatitis

Metronidazole

Mechanism of Action
Deactivates bacterial enzymes

Indication
Most anaerobic gram-negative bacilli and *Clostridium* species

Dosing Options
PO, IV

Drug Interactions
Disulfiram-like reaction with concurrent alcohol ingestion

Side Effects
Dry mouth, metallic taste, nausea, and rarely pancreatitis and neuropathy

Antifungals

See Table 32.2.

Table 32.2 Antifungals

Drug	Administration	Indications	Side effects	Notes
Nystatin	PO, vaginal tablets, topical	Candida	Rare	Candidal infections are common in immunosuppressed
Amphotericin B	IV	*Cryptococcus*, histoplasmosis, coccidioidomycosis, blastomycosis, disseminated candidiasis	Renal impairment possibly permanent, hypokalemia, hypomagnesemia, fever, chills, dyspnea during infusion, anemia, thrombocytopenia, seizures, allergic reactions	Does not penetrate CSF or vitreous humor; intrathecal injection may be needed; decrease dose when Cr >3.5
Flucytosine	PO	In combination with amphotericin B	Transaminitis and hepatomegaly	Rapid resistance; clearance dependent on renal function
Griseofulvin	PO	Fungal infections of skin, hair, nails	Headache in up to 15 % (can be severe), peripheral neuritis, fatigue, blurred vision, syncope, hepatotoxicity	Decreases activity of warfarin-like anticoagulants

Antituberculous Drugs

Due to varying mechanisms and the possibility of antimicrobial resistance, a multidrug regimen is required for patients with active tuberculosis without known drug sensitivities. During the initial 2 months of treatment, a combination of daily isoniazid, rifampin, pyrazinamide, and either ethambutol or streptomycin is employed, after which only isoniazid and rifampin are needed assuming the organism is drug sensitive. The goal of treatment is an additional 4 months of treatment or 3 months of negative sputum cultures. Active pulmonary tuberculosis with positive sputum cultures, on the other hand, must be treated in a negative pressure isolation room until three consecutive sputum cultures from separate days are negative [22].

Isoniazid

Mechanism of Action
Unknown, possible inhibition of cell wall synthesis

Indication
Part of multidrug regimen for active TB, monotherapy for latent TB, prevention of TB

Dosing Options
PO, IV, IM

Drug Interactions
Increases defluorination of volatile anesthetics [15], decreases levels of ketoconazole, increases levels of some anticonvulsants and barbiturates

Side Effects
Hepatotoxicity, increases clearance of pyridoxine (can lead to anemia and peripheral neuropathy)

Rifamycins

Mechanism of Action
Inhibits RNA synthesis

Indication
Multidrug therapy for active TB (resistance develops quickly); prophylaxis for household contacts of meningococcal-infected patients

Dosing Options
PO, IV

Drug Interactions
Inducer of CYP450 enzymes which decreases levels of warfarin, oral contraceptives, opioids, anti-HIV therapy (especially rifampin), and methadone

Side Effects
Hepatic dysfunction can occur in elderly patients with preexisting liver disease. Dosages need to be adjusted in patients with hepatic dysfunction.

Ethambutol

Mechanism of Action
Likely inhibits cell wall synthesis

Indication
Multidrug therapy for active TB

Dosing Options
PO

Drug Interactions
Aluminum hydroxide may decrease absorption.

Side Effects
Optic neuritis, decreased visual acuity, inability to see the color green

Pyrazinamide

Mechanism of Action
Exact mechanism unknown

Indication
Multidrug therapy for active TB

Dosing Options
PO

Drug Interactions
May increase levels of cyclosporine

Side Effects
Hepatitis, rash, arthralgias, hyperuricemia, abdominal distention

Antiviral Drugs

Viruses are intracellular organisms which use the host cells to carry out their necessary functions. They are comprised of a nucleic acid core enveloped by a protein-containing outer coat. They are classified as DNA or RNA viruses based on what type of genetic material they carry. Development of antiviral medications is hindered by their potential toxicity to host cells. See Table 32.3.

Antiretroviral Drugs for HIV/AIDS-Infected Patients

Current guidelines for multidrug antiretroviral therapy, also known as HAART (highly active antiretroviral therapy), are to initiate treatment for the following: patients with AIDS-defining illnesses, patients with CD4 counts <350 cells/mm^3 (though evidence is mounting that patients with higher CD4 counts may still have long-term benefit of initiating therapy), patients with HIV-associated nephropathy, patients with coinfection with hepatitis B or C viruses, and pregnant patients. Intrapartum patients with high viral loads (>400 HIV RNA copies per

Table 32.3 Antivirals

Drug	Administration	Indications	Side effects	Notes
Acyclovir	PO, IV, topical	Prophylactic, initial or recurrent genital herpes, varicella	Headache, thrombophlebitis, elevated BUN, and Cr following rapid IV administration	Recent studies suggest acyclovir may delay progression of HIV-1
Ganciclovir	PO, IV, ophthalmic	CMV treatment and prophylaxis, CMV retinitis	Bone marrow suppression, azoospermia	G-CSF, GM-CSF can prevent granulocytopenia
Amantadine	PO	Influenza A, prophylaxis for sick contacts of influenza A	Seizures, coma, CNS toxicity	Accumulates in renal dysfunction
Interferon (various)	IV, intranasal	Notably chronic hepatitis B, rhinovirus	Flulike symptoms, bone marrow suppression, immune system disorders, CNS disturbances	Generic term for glycoproteins produced during viral infections
Lamivudine	PO	HIV, chronic hepatitis B	Return of hepatitis B upon discontinuation	May bridge to liver transplant; NRTI used in HIV therapy

ml) or unknown levels should receive IV zidovudine during labor as prophylaxis for perinatal transmission. Current guidelines also recommend neonates born to HIV-infected mothers receive 6 weeks of zidovudine prophylaxis initiated as close to delivery as possible. Other medications may be added based on the mother's prenatal regimen (or lack thereof) and viral load [23].

Multidrug therapy classically consists of three or more drugs of different classes to suppress viral replication and prevent drug resistance, which would otherwise develop rapidly. After initiation of treatment, HIV RNA levels are checked every 4 weeks until levels are <50 copies/ml, after which monitoring is extended to every 3 months [23].

Nucleoside Reverse Transcriptase Inhibitors

Mechanism of Action
Structural analogues of human nucleosides, when incorporated into viral DNA, terminate chain elongation.

Indication
Multidrug therapy for AIDS; zidovudine (AZT), shown to slow progression of AIDS, decreases maternal-fetal transmission.

Dosing Options
PO, some available IV

Drug Interactions
Concomitant probenecid decreases metabolism and excretion of AZT.

Side Effects
Class associated: lactic acidosis (1–2 % of patients reaching life-threatening levels) and lipoatrophy. Drug specific: notably, abacavir hypersensitivity syndrome (fever, rash, cough, oral lesions, nausea) which may be life-threatening; didanosine-induced pancreatitis [4]

Nonnucleoside Reverse Transcriptase Inhibitors

Mechanism of Action
Inhibit function of viral reverse transcriptase enzyme

Indication
Multidrug regimen for AIDS

Dosing Options
PO

Drug Interactions
Protease inhibitors, statins, warfarin, phenytoin, phenobarbital, antidepressants

Side Effects
Class associated: Stevens-Johnson syndrome. Drug specific: notably, nevirapine-associated hepatotoxicity [4]

Protease Inhibitors

Mechanism of Action
Prevent normal cleaving of viral protein precursors

Indication
Multidrug therapy for AIDS

Dosing Options
PO

Drug Interactions
Inhibitors of the cytochrome P450 enzymes, with ritonavir being the most potent, leading to higher than expected plasma levels of drugs that are dependent on this system for metabolism, including anticoagulants, anticonvulsants, calcium channel blockers, analgesics, lidocaine, antimicrobials, corticosteroids, antiemetics, and neuroleptics such as droperidol. Ritonavir may also be responsible for decreased bioavailability of oral hypoglycemic, phenytoin, and NSAIDs.

Side Effects
Glucose intolerance (with up to 25 % of patients experiencing abnormal glucose tolerance testing) and hypercholesterolemia, sometimes requiring treatment with pravastatin (which has the least drug interaction profile) though the long-term cardiovascular risk is unknown; ritonavir can cause elevations in triglycerides, which may also need treatment [4, 16].

Clinical Pearls

- Obtain a good history of antibiotic allergy during preoperative evaluation.
- Vancomycin, delivered too rapidly, will result in red man syndrome which can cause hypotension. It can also cause anaphylaxis. Whenever administering this antibiotic, use an infusion pump to ensure it is not delivered too rapidly.

Chemical Structures

Chemical Structure
32.1 Penicillin V

Chemical Structure
32.2 Vancomycin

Chemical Structure
32.3 Gentamicin

Chemical Structure

32.4 Ciprofloxacin

Chemical Structure

32.5 Isoniazid

References

1. Ahdal OA, Bevan DR. Clindamycin-induced neuromuscular blockade. Can J Anaesth. 1995; 42:614–7.
2. Bratzler DW, Dellinger EP, Olsen KM, Perl TM, Auwaerter PG, Bolon MK, et al. Clinical practice guidelines for antimicrobial prophylaxis in surgery. Am J Health Syst Pharm. 2013;70(3):195–283. doi:10.2146/ajhp120568.
3. Bryson EO, Frost EA, Rosenblatt MA. Management of the patient reporting an allergy to penicillin. Middle East J Anesthesiol. 2007;19(3):495–512. Review.
4. Carr A, Cooper DA. Adverse effects of antiretroviral therapy. Lancet. 2000;356:1423–8.
5. Davis RL, Smith AL, Koup JR. The "red-man's syndrome" and slow infusion of vancomycin. N Engl J Med. 1985;313:756–7.
6. Diekema DJ, Jones RN. Oxazolidinone antibiotics. Lancet. 2001;358:77–8.
7. Hines RL, Marschall KE. Stoelting's anesthesia and co-existing diseases. 6th ed. Pennsylvania: Elsevier Inc.; 2012.
8. Hooper DC, Wolfson JS. Fluoroquinolone antimicrobial agents. N Engl J Med. 1991;324: 384–94.
9. Kelkar PS, Li JT. Cephalosporin allergy. N Engl J Med. 2001;345:804–8.
10. Levy JH, Kettlekamp N, Goertz P, et al. Histamine release by vancomycin. A mechanism for hypotension in man. Anesthesiology. 1987;67:122–5.
11. Lin HC, Sanders SL, Gu YG, et al. Erythromycin accelerates solid emptying at the expense of gastric sieving. Dig Dis Sci. 1994;39:124–8.
12. Linden P. Safety profile of meropenem: an updated review of over 6,000 patients treated with meropenem. Drug Saf. 2007;30(8):657–68.
13. Mangram AJ, Horan TC, Pearson ML, Silver LC, Jarvis WR. Guideline for prevention of surgical site infection, 1999. Hospital Infection Control Practices Advisory Committee. Infect Control Hosp Epidemiol. 1999;20(4):250–78; quiz 279–80.
14. Mayhew JF, Deutsch S. Cardiac arrest following administration of vancomycin. Can Anaesth Soc J. 1985;32:65–6.
15. Mazze RI, Woodruff RE, Heerdt ME. Isoniazid-induced enflurane defluorination in humans. Anesthesiology. 1982;57:5–8.

16. Morgan Jr GE, Mikhail MS, Murray MJ. Clinical anesthesiology. 4th ed. New York: McGraw-Hill Companies, Inc; 2006. Glucose intolerance.

17. Mori H, Takahashi K, Mizutani T. Interaction between valproic acid and carbapenem antibiotics. Drug Metab Rev. 2007;39(4):647–57.

18. Muto CA, Jernigan JA, Ostrowsky BE, Richet HM, Jarvis WR, Boyce JM, Farr BM. SHEA guideline for preventing nosocomial transmission of multidrug-resistant strains of Staphylococcus aureus and enterococcus. Infect Control Hosp Epidemiol. 2003;24(5):362–86.

19. Ray WA, Murray KT, Meredith S, Narasimhulu SS, Hall K, Stein CM. Oral erythromycin and the risk of sudden death from cardiac causes. N Engl J Med. 2004;351:1089–96.

20. Spellberg B, Bartlett JG, Gilbert DN. The future of antibiotics and resistance. N Engl J Med. 2013;368(4):299–302.

21. Tanne JH. FDA adds "black box" warning to fluoroquinolone antibiotics. BMJ. 2008;337:a816.

22. US Department of Health and Human Services. Initial therapy for tuberculosis in the era of multidrug resistance: recommendations of the Advisory Council for the Elimination of Tuberculosis. MMWR Morb Mortal Wkly Rep. 1993;42:1–7.

23. US Department of Health and Human Services. Panel on antiretroviral guidelines for adults and adolescents. Available at http://aidsinfo.nih.gov/ContentFiles/AdultandAdolescentGL.pdf. Section accessed 16 Mar 2013.

Chapter 33
Herbal Medications and Vitamin Supplements

Philip Gregory, Andrew Abe, and Darren Hein

Contents

Introduction

The Dietary Supplement Health and Education Act (DSHEA) of 1994 established the current regulatory framework for dietary supplements. This act opened the door for the explosion of dietary supplements to come to market with limited regulatory oversight by the US Food and Drug Administration (FDA). The Act defines dietary supplements as any products taken by mouth which contain a dietary ingredient intended to supplement the diet. A dietary ingredient can include vitamins, minerals, amino acids, enzymes or metabolites, and herbs or other botanical products. Dietary supplements may come in a variety of formulations (e.g., capsules, liquids, extracts), so long as the label on such products does not represent the supplement as a conventional food item [1]. The popularity of

P. Gregory, PharmD (✉) • D. Hein, PharmD
University of Kansas & Evidence-Based Practice,
Creighton University, Omaha, NE, USA
e-mail: pgregory@creighton.edu; darrenhein@creighton.edu

A. Abe, PharmD
Drug Information Center,
University of Kansas, Lawrence, KS, USA
e-mail: andrewabe@ku.edu

A.D. Kaye et al. (eds.), *Essentials of Pharmacology for Anesthesia,*
Pain Medicine, and Critical Care, DOI 10.1007/978-1-4614-8948-1_33,
© Springer Science+Business Media New York 2015

supplement use has grown considerably over the past two decades as evidenced by the multibillion dollar supplement industry [2]. Over 55 million US adults report using supplements in their lifetime, and a recent national survey found that nearly 18 % of the US adults use non-vitamin, non-mineral supplements each month [3, 4]. People most commonly report taking supplements because they are "good for you." Additionally, many seek supplementation to prevent osteoporosis, improve memory, prevent colds and influenza, boost immunity, and increase energy among many other uses [5]. Unlike drugs, safety and effectiveness of dietary supplements are not required to be proven before marketing. However, some safety-focused regulations do apply to dietary supplements. As of 2006, post-marketing adverse event reports related to dietary supplements must be reported by manufacturers to the FDA [6]. This post-marketing surveillance has greatly increased the number of reports to the FDA, but the overall number is still relatively low.

The specific safety concerns of dietary supplement use in anesthesia, critical care, and pain management will be discussed in this chapter.

Commonly Used Dietary Supplements

Vitamins and minerals are the most commonly used supplements. This is true in the general population and the hospitalized and preoperative population [7–9]. The use of herbal and other dietary supplements is also common in the hospitalized and preoperative population [8–10]. The use of dietary supplements in hospitalized or perioperative patients is a significant concern due to potential interactions and other safety concerns. As many as 70 % of these patients do not disclose their use of these supplements if they are not specifically asked [11]. This is likely due to the perception that supplements are natural and therefore safe.

The most commonly used vitamins and minerals in the hospitalized or preoperative population include multiple vitamins, B vitamins, and vitamins C, E, and D [8]. The most common herbs used in this population include valerian, chamomile, garlic, ginkgo, St. John's wort, soy, aloe, and echinacea (Tables 33.1, 33.2, and 33.3) [7, 8]. Most of these dietary supplements have a good safety record and are well tolerated by most patients. However, in many cases, evidence of clinically meaningful benefit is absent or contradictory. For several supplements, there are concerns about potential interactions or other safety concerns related to the use in the perioperative period. In these cases, the risk of using the supplement may significantly outweigh any known benefit of continuing to use the supplement.

Potential Drug-Supplement Interactions and Complications

Supplements interact with drugs through the same mechanisms as drugs interact with other drugs. These interactions can be categorized as either *pharmacodynamic* or *pharmacokinetic*. Pharmacodynamic interactions can often be predicted based on

Table 33.1 Commonly used vitamins and minerals

Supplement	Typical usage	Pharmacology
Vitamin A	Cataracts Glaucoma Improving vision Skin conditions	Fat-soluble vitamin which supports cell growth and immune function [12]
B vitamins	Fatigue Cognitive function Weight loss	Supports various bodily functions (i.e., energy production, growth and development, blood cell production) [13]
Vitamin C	Common cold	A water-soluble vitamin with antioxidant effects [14]
Vitamin D	Osteoporosis	Primarily regulates calcium and phosphorus levels and bone homeostasis. It may also play a role in immune function, inflammation, and cell growth [15]
Vitamin E	Cardiovascular disease	Fat-soluble vitamin with antioxidant properties. May also increase nitric oxide and superoxide in platelets which reduce platelet aggregation [16]
Vitamin K	Osteoporosis	Functions as a coenzyme involved in blood coagulation, as well as a cofactor which enables bone proteins to have a higher calcium binding effect [17]
Calcium	Osteoporosis	Supports essential body functions such as bone maintenance, nerve transmission, muscle contractions, and blood coagulation [18]
Chromium	Diabetes Weight loss	Trace element which increases the action of insulin. It is a component of glucose tolerance factor [19]
Iron	Anemia	Mainly found in red blood cells and muscle cells as it is essential for the oxygen carbon dioxide exchange. It is also a cofactor in the synthesis of neurotransmitters (i.e., dopamine and serotonin) [20]
Magnesium	Cardiovascular health Pain Headache	Supports essential body functions (i.e., bone structure, regulate blood sugar, blood pressure) [21]

a supplement's pharmacology. These types of interactions involve either additive or oppositional pharmacological effects. A pharmacodynamic interaction occurs, for example, when two or more substances are taken together that have similar pharmacological effects, resulting in additive or synergistic effects.

An important example of pharmacodynamic interactions related to supplements involves those supplements that affect blood clotting (Table 33.4). Over 90 supplements have the potential to affect platelet aggregation and blood clotting [13].

Glucosamine is one of the most commonly used dietary supplements on the market. It is typically used for symptoms of osteoarthritis. In 2008, it was recognized that glucosamine taken as a single ingredient or combined with chondroitin has the potential to affect platelet aggregation and interact with antiplatelet or anticoagulant drugs. The first report of this interaction was in 2004 [50]. However, in this instance, doubling the typical therapeutic dose of glucosamine combined with chondroitin was used, resulting in an increased international normalized ratio (INR) in a patient

Table 33.2 Commonly used herbs

Supplement	Typical usage	Pharmacology
Aloe	Laxative	Aloe gel – may inhibit bradykinin, histamine, inflammation, as well as thromboxane A2 (vasoconstrictor)
	Psoriasis Sunburn Wound healing	Aloe latex – increases mucus secretions and peristalsis in colon [22]
Black cohosh	Menopause PMS	Exhibits anti-inflammatory and estrogen-like effects. While it does not appear to bind directly to estrogen receptors, it may induce estrogen-dependent genes [23]
Blueberry	Eye health	Contains antioxidants [24]
Chamomile	Colic Dyspepsia Insomnia	May have an anti-inflammatory and antihistamine effect [25]. Conflicting evidence suggests that it may also bind to GABA receptors [26]
Cranberry	UTI	Prevents adhesion of bacteria to urinary tract. Juice may contain salicylic acid (active metabolite of aspirin), which has anti-inflammatory and antiplatelet effects [27, 28]
Echinacea	Upper respiratory tract infections	Antiviral, anti-inflammatory, antifungal, and various immunostimulatory effects [29]
Evening primrose oil	Eczema PMS	Has an anti-inflammatory effect and may also inhibit platelet inhibition [30]
Garlic	Dyslipidemia	Thought to produce antihyperlipidemic, antihypertensive, and antifungal effects. May have antiplatelet, antithrombotic, and pro-fibrinolytic activity [31]
Ginkgo	Cognitive function Dementia Memory impairment	Thought to have antioxidant effects, reduced oxidative stress/damage, anti-inflammatory effects, and decreased platelet aggregation (inhibits platelet-activating factor binding, platelet thromboxane A2, and thromboxane B2) [32]
Ginseng (American)	Diabetes Erectile dysfunction Vitality Stress	Thought to promote an increase in both insulin sensitivity and insulin release, immunomodulating activity, and may affect acetylcholine in CNS [33, 34]
Ginseng (*Panax*)	Cognitive function Depression Erectile dysfunction Fever Stimulant Stress	*Panax* ginsenosides affect blood pressure and CNS stimulation, decrease platelet aggregation and coagulation, have immunomodulating activity, and may lower triglycerides [35, 36]
St. John's wort	Depression	Inhibits reuptake of serotonin, dopamine, and norepinephrine similar to conventional antidepressants [37]
Soy	Dyslipidemia Cardiovascular disease Menopausal symptoms	May decrease bile acid secretion and also increase LDL reuptake [38]. Soy isoflavones have selective estrogen-modulating (SERM) effects [13]

Table 33.2 (continued)

Supplement	Typical usage	Pharmacology
Valerian	Insomnia	May decrease breakdown of GABA, leading to decreased CNS activity [39]
Yohimbe	Erectile dysfunction Sexual dysfunction Weight loss	Yohimbine, derived from yohimbe bark, is thought to dilate blood vessels and block monoamine oxidase (MAO), calcium channels, and serotonin receptors peripherally. It also penetrates the CNS and blocks alpha 2-adrenergic receptors [40, 41]

Table 33.3 Commonly used non-botanical supplements

Supplement	Typical usage	Pharmacology
Coenzyme Q10	Statin-induced myopathy Migraine headache	Primarily acts as an antioxidant and cofactor in multiple metabolic pathways such as the production of adenosine triphosphate (ATP) [42, 43]
Fish oil	Hypertriglyceridemia Cardiovascular disease	Reduces triglycerides [44]. Also has anti-inflammatory and antithrombotic action through inhibition of thromboxane A2 and arachidonic acid [45]
Glucosamine	Osteoarthritis	Glycosaminoglycan which is an essential building block of cartilage and synovial fluid [46]
Probiotics (i.e., *Lactobacillus*)	Diarrhea Irritable bowel syndrome General health	Adheres and colonizes in the gut, inhibiting the growth of pathogenic bacteria which may cause diarrhea [47]
SAMe	Depression Osteoarthritis	Increased dopamine and norepinephrine levels with increased serotonin turnover. May increase membrane fluidity, which increases signal transduction across neuronal membranes. Also acts as a methyl donor to catechol-O-methyltransferase, degrading L-dopa [48, 49]

Table 33.4 Selected supplements with antiplatelet or anticoagulant effects[a] [13]

Andrographis	Fish oil	Horse chestnut
Black tea	Garlic	Policosanol
Boldo	Ginger	Resveratrol
Chondroitin	Ginkgo	Saw palmetto
Danshen	Glucosamine	Turmeric
Dong quai	Green tea	Vitamin E
Fenugreek	Guarana	Willow bark

[a]Note: not a complete list

taking warfarin. Later reports described several cases of increased INR, bruising, and bleeding events in patients taking typical amounts of glucosamine alone or in combination with chondroitin [51, 52]. Chondroitin is a small component of a heparinoid compound with modest anticoagulant effects. How glucosamine might affect bleeding is a bit unclear. However, some animal model research suggests that it might have antiplatelet activity [13, 52].

Ginkgo is a common herbal supplement that has been linked with bleeding risk. Gingko is typically used to improve memory in otherwise healthy adults and for treating symptoms of dementia. Concerns about bleeding risk with ginkgo resulted from a multitude of case reports describing bleeding events, often in the perioperative period, in patients taking the supplement [53–58]. However, more recent evidence suggests that ginkgo might not have a meaningful effect on bleeding risk. Some clinical trials show no effect on platelet aggregation or on bleeding time [59]. Studies also show no effect of single doses of ginkgo on bleeding time when combined with clopidogrel (*Plavix*) or ticlopidine (*Ticlid*) [60, 61].

The case of ginkgo illustrates an important point to keep in mind when evaluating potential interactions between drugs and supplements. Roughly 30 % of potential interactions between supplements and drugs are based on in vitro or animal model research or case reports. By definition, this is preliminary and weak evidence. Even though this level of evidence raises important concerns about potential interactions, more reliable evidence is often needed to better understand the clinical significance of potential interactions.

In addition to potentially interacting with other antiplatelet or anticoagulant drugs, supplements that affect platelet aggregation may also present risk during the perioperative period. Some supplements such as gingko and saw palmetto have been linked to reports of perioperative bleeding events [13, 62]. Table 33.4 provides a list of selected supplements that have been shown to have antiplatelet or anticoagulant effects. These supplements have the potential to interact with other antiplatelet or anticoagulant drugs as well as adversely affect patients in the perioperative period.

Several supplements have the potential to cause central nervous system (CNS) depression (Table 33.5). Many of these are used as "sleepy time" teas such as chamomile, lavender, and lemon balm. Although there is often little to no evidence documenting sedative effects with these products, they clearly have a mild sedative effect in those who use them.

Other products have clearly documented sedative effects. *Valerian* is one of the most commonly used herbal supplements with sedative effects. Constituents in valerian seem to have benzodiazepine-like effects [13, 39]. Theoretically, combining valerian with other sedatives, especially benzodiazepines, might result in additive

Table 33.5 Selected supplements with CNS depressant effects[a] [13]

Chamomile	Lavender	Skullcap
Hops	Lemon balm	Theanine
Kava	Melatonin	Valerian
L-tryptophan	Passionflower	

[a]Note: not a complete list

Table 33.6 Selected supplements with hypoglycemic effects[a] [13]

Agaricus mushroom	Cinnamon	Panax ginseng
Alpha-lipoic acid	Chromium	Prickly pear cactus
American ginseng	Fenugreek	Vanadium
Banaba	Glucomannan	
Bitter melon	Gymnema	

[a]Note: not a complete list

Table 33.7 Selected supplements with blood pressure effects[a] [13]

Andrographis	Horny goat weed	Licorice
Casein peptides	Garlic	Pycnogenol
Coenzyme Q10	L-arginine	Theanine

[a]Note: not a complete list

Table 33.8 Selected supplements with stimulant effects[a] [13]

Bitter orange (synephrine)	Ephedra (ephedra alkaloids)	Raspberry ketone
Dimethylamylamine (DMAA)	Higenamine	Yohimbe

[a]Note: not a complete list

sedation. Valerian has also been shown to increase levels of alprazolam by 19 %. This is probably due to valerian inhibition of cytochrome P450 3A4 metabolism of alprazolam [63].

Similar to CNS depressant supplements, those with hypoglycemic effects have the potential to interact with other hypoglycemic agents and adversely affect patient outcomes during the perioperative period (Table 33.6). Several supplements have direct insulin-like or insulin-stimulating effects. These are the most likely supplements to result in hypoglycemic effects and adverse outcomes. Supplements with these effects include banaba, bitter melon, fenugreek, and gymnema [13]. Other supplements affect blood glucose levels through an insulin-sensitizing effect. Some of these include cinnamon, chromium, prickly pear cactus, and vanadium. Although these can still lower blood glucose levels, they are less likely to result in serious hypoglycemia [13, 62].

Several dietary supplements have blood pressure-lowering effects (Table 33.7). Most of these provide a modest effect on blood pressure which is likely to be clinically insignificant in many cases. There are no reports of perioperative complications in patients taking these supplements.

Dietary supplements with stimulant effects can increase both heart rate and blood pressure. Examples of these include ephedra, bitter orange which contains synephrine, and dimethylamylamine (DMAA), among others (Table 33.8). While ephedra and bitter orange have not been linked to serious complications during anesthesia, the products have been implicated in other serious spontaneous adverse events including stroke, myocardial infarction, QT interval prolongation, and arrhythmia [13].

A number of supplements have the potential to impact neurotransmitters such as serotonin. Because of this, blood pressure and vascular activity may be affected in patients taking these products [62]. *St. John's wort*, for example, has been linked to cardiovascular collapse during anesthesia induction [64]. Additionally, the use of

Table 33.9 Selected supplements with serotonergic effects[a] [13]

5-HTP	Phosphatidylserine	St. John's wort
L-tryptophan	SAMe	Theanine

[a]Note: not a complete list

Table 33.10 Selected supplements that affect cytochrome P450 [13]

Supplement[a]	CYP1A2	CYP2C19	CYP2C9	CYP2E1	CYP2D6	CYP3A4
Cat's claw						X
Chamomile	X					X
Danshen						X
Devil's claw		X	X			X
Evodia	O					X
Feverfew		X	X			X
Garlic				X		O
Ginkgo[b]	X	O	X		X	X/O
Goldenseal					X	X
Grapefruit	X	X	X			X
Hu Zhang						X
Indole-3-carbinol	O					
Ipriflavone	X		X			
Kava	X	X	X	X	X	X
Quercetin			X		X	X
Red clover	X	X	X			X
St. John's wort	O	O	O			O
Schisandra[b]			O			X/O
Siberian ginseng	X		X		X	X
Valerian						X

X enzyme inhibition, O enzyme induction

[a]Note: not a complete list

[b]Conflicting evidence regarding CYP3A4 induction or inhibition

St. John's wort in combination with meperidine has led to serotonergic crisis according to anecdotal reports [65]. Other dietary supplements with serotonergic properties include SAMe, 5-HTP, and L-tryptophan (Table 33.9). The use of these products in combination with other serotonergic drugs may increase the risk of serotonergic side effects and serotonin syndrome. These products should be avoided in the perioperative period if possible [62].

In addition to the pharmacodynamic interactions listed previously, it is important to consider *pharmacokinetic* interactions between dietary supplements and drugs when assessing the safety of supplement use in anesthesia, critical care, and pain management. Pharmacokinetic interactions are those which impact the means by which the body absorbs, distributes, metabolizes, and excretes drugs or dietary supplements. The most common pharmacokinetic interactions are metabolic interactions involving the cytochrome P450 (CYP450) system (Table 33.10). Because many of the drugs utilized in anesthesia, critical care, and pain management are metabolized by this system, it is important to identify which supplements can lead to changes in metabolism of these drugs. Concomitant use of supplements which *inhibit* CYP450 isozymes can increase the plasma levels and duration of effect of drugs metabolized by these enzymes. Conversely, concomitant use of supplements which *induce* CYP450 isozymes can decrease the levels and duration of effect of drugs metabolized by these isozymes.

More than 50 % of all marketed drugs are metabolized to some degree by CYP450 isozyme 3A4 (CYP3A4). Thus, supplements which inhibit or induce CYP3A4 are of particular concern [66]. *St. John's wort*, for example, is a potent inducer of this isozyme. A number of case reports show a pharmacokinetic interaction between cyclosporine and St. John's wort in organ transplant patients. The supplement has been shown to reduce plasma cyclosporine levels by up to 70 %, leading to subtherapeutic drug levels and, ultimately, acute organ rejection [67–69]. St John's wort has a large potential for drug interactions, and thus determining safe yet effective doses of drugs which interact with this supplement can be difficult [70].

In addition to St. John's wort, some *garlic* preparations have been shown to induce CYP3A4, while other formulations have not [71]. Furthermore, clinical evidence suggests garlic may reduce the activity of CYP2E1 by up to 40 % [70]. Because anesthetics such as enflurane, halothane, isoflurane, and methoxyflurane are metabolized by this isozyme, patients taking garlic supplements may require smaller doses of the aforementioned drugs [13].

Kava impacts CYP2E1 in a similar fashion to garlic and thus may prolong the effects of certain anesthetics [72]. Additionally, both kava and *valerian* inhibit CYP3A4. Because of this, they can potentially increase plasma concentrations of drugs metabolized by CYP3A4. Examples of these include alfentanil, alprazolam, amlodipine, clarithromycin, ketoconazole, lidocaine, midazolam, verapamil, and serotonin receptor antagonists, among many others. It should be noted, however, that the interaction potential of both kava and valerian with drugs metabolized by CYP3A4 is based on in vitro data. This is weaker evidence than that supporting the St. John's wort and garlic interactions [11, 13].

Other Safety Concerns

One of the biggest problems plaguing the dietary supplement industry is the issue of adulteration and contamination. Adulteration occurs if a dietary supplement contains an ingredient which is present in sufficient quantities to be poisonous or harmful to human health. Contamination on the other hand can be defined as any foreign substance which would make a product tainted. Therefore, a contamination is a form of adulteration [73]. When the FDA or Health Canada recognizes a risk with a dietary supplement, such as adulteration, they post an alert to the public on their website. According to the authors' research (unpublished data, April 2013), from 2005 to 2012, a total of 1,356 dietary supplement alerts were posted through either the FDA or Health Canada. The most common reason for these alerts was a contaminant, and the most common contaminant reported was a pharmaceutical product (65 %)

Table 33.11 Supplement quality programs

US Pharmacopeia (USP) Dietary Supplement Verification Program	Voluntary program; supplements are verified to contain what is stated on the label, comply with good manufacturing practices, and are not adulterated. Their logo is printed on each dietary supplement reviewed. Similar in scope to the NSF program
National Sanitation Foundation (NSF)	Voluntary program; supplements are verified to contain what is stated on the label, comply with good manufacturing practices, and are not adulterated. Their logo is printed on each dietary supplement reviewed. Similar in scope to the USP program
ConsumerLab.com	Voluntary program; supplements are tested at a snapshot in time. Less rigorous testing program compared to USP or NSF. Unlike USP or NSF, ConsumerLab.com operates on a subscription-based service

followed by a heavy metal contaminant (9 %), bacterial contaminant (5 %), and fungal contaminant (1 %). Of the pharmaceutical contaminants identified, the most common group of compounds that was noted was phosphodiesterase-5 inhibitors (e.g., sildenafil, tadalafil) which accounted for approximately 53 % of all pharmaceutical contaminants. The second most common pharmaceutical contaminant noted was sibutramine which accounted for 32 % of all pharmaceutical contaminants. Overall, dietary supplements marketed for weight loss and sexual enhancement accounted for over a half of all dietary supplement alerts from 2005 to 2012 and suggest that these types of products warrant the most concern for patient safety.

Supplement quality programs such as the US Pharmacopeia (USP) review dietary supplements to ensure that products contain what is stated on the label to help to quality control dietary supplements. Participation in these programs is voluntary. To date, relatively few manufacturers participate in these quality assurance programs. Table 33.11 describes three well-known supplement quality programs.

Guidelines

Most patients do not voluntarily disclose their use of dietary supplements to their physician or any other health professional. This is why it is extraordinarily important that dietary supplements are mentioned by name upon hospital admittance and/or in the preoperative patient interview. Patients should be asked to use specific terminology about the use of "dietary supplements," "food supplements," "nutritional supplements," "herbal products," "herbal teas," "vitamins," etc. Using these different terms will help patients recognize the kinds of products you are asking about. Additionally, patients should be encouraged to bring in the containers of the supplements they are taking in order to generate a reliable, comprehensive list of products and their ingredients [66, 74].

Since many dietary supplements have meaningful pharmacological effects, there is potential for them to interact with anesthesia or other medications used in an acute care setting and potentially result in harm to the patient. For most supplements, there is little or no harm in discontinuing them temporarily. Therefore, discontinuation prior to hospital admission or a surgical procedure is often considered the most reasonable approach [13]. The American Society of Anesthesiologists currently recommends that all dietary supplements be discontinued 2 weeks prior to an elective surgical procedure [66, 74].

Nonetheless, in emergency situations, discontinuation may not be a possibility. In these cases, obtaining an accurate history is critically important so that any potential complications can be anticipated and addressed [74].

Summary

The use of dietary supplements continues to grow, and thus the challenge of managing anesthesia, critical care, and pain in patients taking these supplements remains. The first step in meeting this challenge requires gathering an accurate list of the supplements each patient is taking. For this to happen, an open line of communication must exist between patient and practitioner. Once supplements are identified, a decision to continue the supplements, discontinue the supplements, and/or modify drug therapy should be made. Understanding which supplements can impact coagulation, blood pressure, blood glucose, and the central nervous system will help with these decisions. Identifying the dietary supplements which can lead to increased or decreased levels of certain drugs via pharmacokinetic interactions is also very important. A general rule of thumb is to have patients discontinue nonessential dietary supplements at least 2 weeks prior to any surgical procedures they have scheduled.

Chemical Structures

Chemical structure
33.1 Glucosamine

References

1. Significant amendments to the FD&C Act: Dietary Supplement Health and Education Act of 1994. U.S. Food and Drug Administration website. Available at: http://www.fda.gov/RegulatoryInformation/Legislation/FederalFoodDrugandCosmeticActFDCAct/SignificantAmendmentstotheFDCAct/ucm148003.htm. Accessed 28 Mar 2013.

2. Consumer Union of US Inc. Dangerous supplements: what you don't know about these 12 ingredients could hurt you. September 2010. Available at: http://www.consumerreports.org/cro/2012/05/dangerous-supplements/index.htm. Accessed 19 Jan 2013.

3. Wu CH, Wang CC, Kennedy J. Changes in herb and dietary supplement use in the US adult population: a comparison of the 2002 and 2007 National Health Interview Surveys. Clin Ther. 2011;33(11):1749–58.

4. Barnes PM, Bloom B. Complementary and alternative medicine use among adults and children: United States, 2007. Natl Health Stat Report. 2008;12:1–23.

5. Kaufman DW, Kelly JP, Rosenberg L, Anderson TE, Mitchell AA. Recent patterns of medication use in the ambulatory adult population of the United States: the Slone survey. JAMA. 2002;287(3):337–44.

6. Significant Amendments to the FD&C Act: Dietary Supplement and Nonprescription Drug Consumer Protection Act. U.S. Food and Drug Administration Web site. http://www.fda.gov/RegulatoryInformation/Legislation/FederalFoodDrugandCosmeticActFDCAct/SignificantAmendmentstotheFDCAct/ucm148035.htm. Accessed 3 Apr 2013.

7. Kaye AD, Clarke RC, Sabar R, Vig S, et al. Herbal medicines: current trends in anesthesiology practice – a hospital survey. J Clin Anesth. 2000;12:468–71.

8. Grauer RP, Thomas RD, Tronson MD, Heard GC, Diacon M. Preoperative use of herbal medicines and vitamin supplements. Anaesth Intensive Care. 2004;32:173–7.

9. Norred CL. Complementary and alternative medicine use by surgical patients. AORN J. 2002;76:1013–21.

10. Lucenterforte E, Gallo E, Pugi A, Giommoni F, et al. Complementary and alternative drugs use among preoperative patients: a cross-sectional study in Italy. Evid Based Complement Alternat Med. 2012;2012:527238.

11. Ang-Lee MK, Moss J, Yuan CS. Herbal medicines and perioperative care. JAMA. 2001;286: 208–16.

12. Denke MA. Dietary retinol–a double-edged sword. JAMA. 2002;287(1):102–4.

13. Jellin JM, Gregory PJ, eds. Natural Medicines Comprehensive Database. Therapeutic Research Center: Stockton, 2013. Available at: www.naturaldatabase.com. Accessed 28 Mar 2013.

14. Pohanka M, Pejchal J, Snopkova S, et al. Ascorbic acid: an old player with a broad impact on body physiology including oxidative stress suppression and immunomodulation: a review. Mini Rev Med Chem. 2012;12(1):35–43.

15. Herr C, Greulich T, Koczulla RA, et al. The role of vitamin D in pulmonary disease: COPD, asthma, infection, and cancer. Respir Res. 2011;12:31.

16. Liu M, Wallmon A, Olsson-Mortlock C, Wallin R, Saldeen T. Mixed tocopherols inhibit platelet aggregation in humans: potential mechanisms. Am J Clin Nutr. 2003;77(3):700–6.

17. Vermeer C, Schurgers LJ. A comprehensive review of vitamin K and vitamin K antagonists. Hematol Oncol Clin North Am. 2000;14:339–53.

18. Power ML, Heaney RP, Kalkwarf HJ, et al. The role of calcium in health and disease. Am J Obstet Gynecol. 1999;181(6):1560–9.

19. Vincent JB. The biochemistry of chromium. J Nutr. 2000;130:715–8.

20. Dallman PR. Biochemical basis for the manifestations of iron deficiency. Annu Rev Nutr. 1986;6:13–40.

21. Saris NE, Mervaala E, Karppanen H, Khawaja JA, Lewenstam A. Magnesium: an update on physiological, clinical, and analytical aspects. Clin Chim Acta. 2000;294:1–26.

22. Klein AD, Penneys NS. Aloe vera. J Am Acad Dermatol. 1988;18:714–20.

23. Wuttke W, Gorkow C, Seidlova-Wuttke D. Effects of black cohosh (Cimicifuga racemosa) on bone turnover, vaginal mucosa, and various blood parameters in postmenopausal women: a double-blind, placebo-controlled, and conjugated estrogens-controlled study. Menopause. 2006; 13:185–96.

24. Giacalone M, Di Sacco F, Traupe I, Topini R, Forfori F, Giunta F. Antioxidant and neuroprotective properties of blueberry polyphenols: a critical review. Nutr Neurosci. 2011;14(3):119–25.

25. Wang Y, Tang H, Nicholson JK, et al. A metabonomic strategy for the detection of the metabolic effects of chamomile (Matricaria recutita L.) ingestion. J Agric Food Chem. 2005;53:191–6.

26. Avallone R, Zanoli P, Puia G, et al. Pharmacological profile of apigenin, a flavonoid isolated from Matricaria chamomilla. Biochem Pharmacol. 2000;59:1387–94.
27. Lee YL, Owens J, Thrupp L, Cesario TC. Does cranberry juice have antibacterial activity? JAMA. 2000;283:1691.
28. Duthie GG, Kyle JA, Jenkinson AM, et al. Increased salicylate concentrations in urine of human volunteers after consumption of cranberry juice. J Agric Food Chem. 2005;53: 2897–900.
29. Barrett B. Medicinal properties of Echinacea: a critical review. Phytomedicine. 2003;10: 66–86.
30. Guivernau M, Meza N, Barja P, Roman O. Clinical and experimental study on the long-term effect of dietary gamma-linolenic acid on plasma lipids, platelet aggregation, thromboxane formation, and prostacyclin production. Prostaglandins Leukot Essent Fatty Acids. 1994;51:311–6.
31. Ali M, Thomson M, Afzal M. Garlic and onions: their effect on eicosanoid metabolism and its clinical relevance. Prostaglandins Leukot Essent Fatty Acids. 2000;62:55–73.
32. Kudolo G. Ingestion of Ginkgo biloba extract significantly inhibits collagen-induced platelet aggregation and thromboxane A2 synthesis. Altern Ther. 2001;7:105.
33. McElhaney JE, Gravenstein S, Cole SK, et al. A placebo-controlled trial of a proprietary extract of North American ginseng (CVT-E002) to prevent acute respiratory illness in institutionalized older adults. J Am Geriatr Soc. 2004;52:13–9.
34. Vuksan V, Stavro MP, Sievenpiper JL, et al. Similar postprandial glycemic reductions with escalation of dose and administration time of American ginseng in type 2 diabetes. Diabetes Care. 2000;23:1221–6.
35. Park HJ, Lee JH, Song YB, Park KH. Effects of dietary supplementation of lipophilic fraction from Panax ginseng on cGMP and cAMP in rat platelets and on blood coagulation. Biol Pharm Bull. 1996;19:1434–9.
36. Sievenpiper JL, Arnason JT, Leiter LA, Vuksan V. Decreasing, null and increasing effects of eight popular types of ginseng on acute postprandial glycemic indices in healthy humans: the role of ginsenosides. J Am Coll Nutr. 2004;23:248–58.
37. Calapai G, Crupi A, Firenzuoli F, et al. Serotonin, norepinephrine and dopamine involvement in the antidepressant action of hypericum perforatum. Pharmacopsychiatry. 2001;34:45–9.
38. Normen L, Dutta P, Lia A, et al. Soy sterol esters and B-sitostanol ester as inhibitors of cholesterol absorption in human small bowel. Am J Clin Nutr. 2000;71:908–13.
39. Houghton PJ. The scientific basis for the reputed activity of Valerian. J Pharm Pharmacol. 1999;51:505–12.
40. Montorsi F, Strambi LF, Guazzoni G, et al. Effect of yohimbine-trazodone on psychogenic impotence: a randomized, double-blind, placebo-controlled study. Urology. 1994;44:732–6.
41. Ernst E, Pittler MH. Yohimbine for erectile dysfunction: a systematic review and meta-analysis of randomized clinical trials. J Urol. 1998;159:433–6.
42. Thompson PD, Clarkson P, Karas RH. Statin-associated myopathy. JAMA. 2003;289:1681–90.
43. Turunen M, Olsson J, Dallner G. Metabolism and function of coenzyme Q. Biochim Biophys Acta. 2004;1660:171–99.
44. Nestel PJ. Fish oil and cardiovascular disease: lipids and arterial function (abstract). Am J Clin Nutr. 2000;71:228S–31.
45. Calder PC. N-3 polyunsaturated fatty acids, inflammation and immunity: pouring oil on troubled waters or another fishy tale? Nutr Res. 2001;21:309–41.
46. Sherman AL, Ojeda-Correal G, Mena J. Use of glucosamine and chondroitin in persons with osteoarthritis. PM R. 2012;4(5 Suppl):S110–6.
47. Gupta V, Garg R. Probiotics. Indian J Med Microbiol. 2009;27:202–9.
48. Rosenbaum JF, Fava M, Falk WE, et al. The antidepressant potential of oral S-adenosyl-l-methionine. Acta Psychiatr Scand. 1990;81:432–6.
49. Bottiglieri T. S-Adenosyl-L-methionine (SAMe): from the bench to the bedside–molecular basis of a pleiotrophic molecule. Am J Clin Nutr. 2002;76:1151S–7.
50. Rozenfeld V, Crain JL, Callahan AK. Possible augmentation of warfarin effect by glucosamine-chondroitin. Am J Health Syst Pharm. 2004;61:306–7.

51. Knudsen J, Sokol GH. Potential glucosamine-warfarin interaction resulting in increased international normalized ratio: case report and review of the literature and MedWatch database. Pharmacotherapy. 2008;28:540–8.

52. Yue QY, Strandell J, Myrberg O. Concomitant use of glucosamine may potential the effect of warfarin. The Uppsala Monitoring Centre. Available at: www.who-umc.org/graphics/9722. pdf. Accessed 28 Apr 2008.

53. Benjamin J, Muir T, Briggs K, Pentland B. A case of cerebral haemorrhage-can Ginkgo biloba be implicated? Postgrad Med J. 2001;77:112–3.

54. Rowin J, Lewis SL. Spontaneous bilateral subdural hematomas with chronic Gingko biloba ingestion. Neurology. 1996;46:1775–6.

55. Miller LG, Freeman B. Possible subdural hematoma associated with Ginkgo biloba. J Herb Pharmacother. 2002;2:57–63.

56. Bent S, Goldberg H, Padula A, Avins AL. Spontaneous bleeding associated with Ginkgo biloba: a case report and systematic review of the literature. J Gen Intern Med. 2005;20:657–61.

57. Meisel C, Johne A, Roots I. Fatal intracerebral mass bleeding associated with Ginkgo biloba and ibuprofen. Atherosclerosis. 2003;167:367.

58. Vale S. Subarachnoid haemorrhage associated with Ginkgo biloba. Lancet. 1998;352:36.

59. Kellermann AJ, Kloft C. Is there a risk of bleeding associated with standardized ginkgo biloba extract therapy? A systematic review and meta-analysis. Pharmacotherapy. 2011;31:490–502.

60. Aruna D, Naidu MU. Pharmacodynamic interaction studies of Ginkgo biloba with cilostazol and clopidogrel in healthy human subjects. Br J Clin Pharmacol. 2007;63:333–8.

61. Kim BH, Kim KP, Lim KS, et al. Influence of Ginkgo biloba extract on the pharmacodynamic effects and pharmacokinetic properties of ticlopidine: an open-label, randomized, two-period, two-treatment, two-sequence, single-dose crossover study in healthy Korean male volunteers. Clin Ther. 2010;32:380–90.

62. Gregory PJ. The perioperative use of natural medicines. Therapeutic Research Center: Stockton, 2012. Available at: www.naturaldatabase.com. Accessed 28 Mar 2013.

63. Donovan JL, DeVane CL, Chavin KD, et al. Multiple night-time doses of valerian (Valeriana officinalis) had minimal effects on CYP3A4 activity and no effect on CYP2D6 activity in healthy volunteers. Drug Metab Dispos. 2004;32:1333–6.

64. Irefin S, Sprung J. A possible cause of cardiovascular collapse during anesthesia: long-term use of St. John's wort. J Clin Anesth. 2000;12:498–9.

65. Kaye AD, Baluch A, Kaye AM. Mineral, vitamin, and herbal supplements. In: Fleisher LA, editor. Anesthesia and uncommon diseases. 6th ed. Philadelphia: Elsevier; 2012. p. 477.

66. Kaye AD, Baluch A, Kaye AJ, Frass M, Hofbauer R. Pharmacology of herbals and their impact in anesthesia. Curr Opin Anaesthesiol. 2007;20:294–9.

67. Bauer S, Stormer E, Johne A, et al. Alterations in cyclosporin A pharmacokinetics and metabolism during treatment with St. John's wort in renal transplant patients. Br J Clin Pharmacol. 2003;55:203–11.

68. Mandelbaum A, Pertzborn F, martin-Facklam M, Wiesel M. Unexplained decrease of cyclosporine trough levels in a compliant renal transplant patient. Nephrol Dial Transplant. 2000;15:1473–4.

69. Morschella C, Jaber BL. Interaction between cyclosporine and Hypericum perforatum (St. John's wort) after organ transplantation. Am J Kidney Dis. 2001;38:1105–7.

70. Gurley BJ, Gardner SF, Hubbard MA, et al. Cytochrome P450 phenotypic ratios for predicting herb-drug interactions in humans. Clin Pharmacol Ther. 2002;72:276–87.

71. Piscitelli SC, Burstein AH, Welden N, et al. The effect of garlic supplements on the pharmacokinetics of saquinavir. Clin Infect Dis. 2002;34:234–8.

72. Gurley BJ, Gardner SF, Hubbard MA, et al. In vivo effects of goldenseal, kava kava, black cohosh, and valerian on human cytochrome P450 1A2, 2D6, 2E1, and 3A4/5 phenotypes. Clin Pharmacol Ther. 2005;77:415–26.

73. Cole MR, Fetrow CW. Adulteration of dietary supplements. Am J Health Syst Pharm. 2003;60(15):1576–80.

74. Kaye AD, Kucera L, Sabar R. Perioperative anesthesia clinical considerations of alternative medicine. Anesthesiol Clin N Am. 2004;22:125–39.

Chapter 34
Minerals and Electrolytes

Amit Prabhakar, Alan David Kaye, and Amir Baluch

Contents

A. Prabhakar, MD, MS
Department of Anesthesiology, Louisiana State University
Health Sciences Center, New Orleans, LA, USA
e-mail: aprab1@lsuhsc.edu

A.D. Kaye, MD, PhD (✉)
Department of Anesthesiology, Tulane Medical Center, New Orleans, LA, USA

Department of Anesthesiology, Louisiana State University
Health Sciences Center, New Orleans, LA, USA
e-mail: alankaye44@hotmail.com

A. Baluch, MD
Metropolitan Anesthesia Consultants, Dallas, TX, USA
e-mail: abaluchmd@yahoo.com

A.D. Kaye et al. (eds.), *Essentials of Pharmacology for Anesthesia,*
Pain Medicine, and Critical Care, DOI 10.1007/978-1-4614-8948-1_34,
© Springer Science+Business Media New York 2015

Introduction

Thorough knowledge and understanding of minerals and electrolytes is essential for physicians of all specialties, including anesthesiology. The use of supplements such as minerals and electrolytes has dramatically increased in recent years. There are numerous reasons for this increase, including anecdotal reports of efficacy, abundance of advertisements, lower cost compared to prescription medications, and ease of access to these supplements. As patients continue to look to alternative means for their medical care, it is imperative for the physician to be cognizant of the physiological mechanisms and metabolism of the most common minerals and electrolytes. This topic is of top priority for anesthesiologists who must be aware of potential adverse interactions with both prescription drugs and over-the-counter medications. Anesthesiologists will inevitably encounter patients with various mineral and electrolyte abnormalities preoperatively and must be able to accommodate accordingly during the perioperative and postoperative phases of patient care.

Iron

Iron deficiency is the most common nutrient deficiency in the world. It is estimated that over 700 million people worldwide have iron deficiency anemia [1]. Iron is a key component of hemoglobin and myoglobin and is associated with hundreds of enzymes and protein structures. Therapeutic uses of iron supplementation vary extensively, ranging from treatment of anemia to restless leg syndrome.

The human body contains approximately 3–5 g of iron with about 60–70 % of that amount being utilized within hemoglobin [2]. The average Western diet contains approximately 15 mg of iron, of which only 1–2 mg is absorbed [2]. Absorption primarily occurs via specialized epithelial cells in the duodenum [2]. Dietary iron intake acts to compensate for normal nonspecific iron losses such as cell desquamation in the skin, intestinal loss, and menstruation in women [2]. Because mammals do not possess any specific mechanisms for iron excretion, levels are primarily regulated by the amount of absorption [3, 4]. Absorption is regulated by three signals including dietary intake, iron store regulators, and an erythropoietic regulator [2, 5]. Iron overload can be due to primary causes such as genetic disorders or secondary causes such as repeat blood transfusions. High iron levels are related to worsening of neuronal injury secondary to cerebral ischemia, cardiomyopathies, and even preterm delivery [6, 7].

Iron may inhibit absorption of many drugs including levodopa, methyldopa, carbidopa, penicillamine, thyroid hormone, captopril, and antibiotics in both the quinolone and tetracycline families [8–12]. There are also drugs which may decrease the amount of iron absorbed. These drugs include antacids, histamine (H2) blockers, proton pump inhibitors, and cholestyramine [13, 14]. Because of these interactions, iron should not be given within 2 h of other pharmaceuticals to avoid alterations in drug or mineral absorption [15].

Calcium

Calcium deficiency is a common problem in both the developed and nondeveloped worlds. Patients may utilize calcium supplementation for a variety of medical ailments including osteoporosis, premenstrual syndrome, and parathyroid problems. Normal calcium levels range from 8.7 to 10.4 mg/dL [16]. When evaluating calcium levels in a clinical setting, it is important to take albumin levels into consideration. Approximately 40 % of calcium is bound to protein, mainly albumin. Thus low serum albumin levels can give falsely low calcium levels, and high albumin levels can result in falsely high serum calcium levels [16]. Serum calcium levels are regulated by the action of three hormones: parathyroid hormone, 1, 25-dihydroxyvitamin D (calcitriol), and calcitonin [16].

Hypercalcemia is defined as levels above 10.5 and is further broken down into mild, moderate, and severe hypercalcemia. Severe hypercalcemia, defined as levels greater than 14 mg/dL, accounts for more than 3 % of hospital admissions from the ED [16]. In the United States, more than 90 % of cases are due to either primary hyperparathyroidism or malignancy. Symptoms range from renal stones, bone pain, impaired concentration, confusion, fatigue, and muscle weakness [16]. Treatment depends on the primary cause and includes the use of bisphosphonates, IV fluids, calcitonin, and hemodialysis.

Calcium may interfere with a variety of commonly used drugs, specifically those used for the management of hypertension and other cardiac problems. The effects of calcium channel blockers may be affected by calcium supplementation, as calcium has been shown to antagonize the effects of verapamil [17]. Calcium has recently been used in the successful management of calcium channel overdose [18]. Beta-blocker levels may also be decreased with calcium supplementation, leading to a greater inotropic and chronotropic presentation that is anticipated [15].

Thiazide diuretics have been shown to increase serum calcium concentration, which can subsequently result in hypercalcemia due to increased calcium resorption in the kidneys. Dysrhythmias may occur in patients taking digitalis and calcium together. Medications such as tetracyclines, quinolones, bisphosphonates, and levothyroxine may all be decreased by calcium supplementation and should not be taken within 2 h of calcium intake [13, 14].

Chromium

Chromium is a very commonly used supplement, with an estimated ten million people in the United States taking it in 1996 [19]. It is an essential nutrient involved in the metabolism of carbohydrates, proteins, and lipids. Research has shown that chromium is a cofactor for insulin function, a number of insulin receptors, and facilitation of insulin receptor phosphorylation. This results in enhanced glucose transport into the liver, muscle, and adipose tissue [20–25]. Dietary sources of chromium include brewer's yeast, beer, whole grains, meat, liver, and cheese [26, 27]. A recent study found that adults in the United States consume far less than the minimum estimated safe and adequate daily dietary intake of chromium of 50–200 mcg/day [28–30]. Patients may be inclined to add chromium supplementation because of consumer belief that it may improve glucose tolerance in diabetics, improve lipid profiles, and subsequently improve overall body habitus. Clinical implications of chromium use are of particular importance as over 20 million Americans have diabetes [31–33].

A recent article reviewed 15 studies and analyzed the efficacy of chromium supplementation in diabetic patients [20]. All 15 reviewed studies showed benefits in at least one parameter of diabetes management, including reduced HbA1c measurements, improved lipid profiles, and reduced need of insulin and other oral hypoglycemic drugs [20]. However these benefits were not observed in nonobese and nondiabetic patients [19]. In fact, chromium supplementation in 31 patients with normal glycemic control actually resulted in a paradoxical decrease in insulin sensitivity [19]. Because evidence of chromium supplementation benefits remains controversial, caution should be used by the clinician before encouraging use.

Chromium is generally well tolerated; however, some patients may experience nervous system symptoms, such as perceptual, cognitive, and motor dysfunction even with low doses. Toxicity has also been reported in patients taking various doses of chromium. Toxicity is manifested as anemia, thrombocytopenia, hemolysis, weight loss, and liver and renal toxicity. These side effects resolved with discontinuation of chromium use [34].

Magnesium

Magnesium is the fourth most common mineral salt in the human body [35]. It plays many important roles in structure, function, and metabolism and is involved in numerous essential physiological reactions. Dietary sources of magnesium include cocoa powder, chocolate, almonds, peanuts, vegetables, and seafood [35]. Most individuals consume the recommended amount of 250–350 mg in their diet [36]. It is concentrated mainly in the bone (60 %), muscle (20 %), and soft tissues (20 %) [35]. Absorption and loss of magnesium are primarily driven by the gastrointestinal and renal systems. Hypomagnesemia is defined as a plasma concentration below 0.7 mmol/L and is manifested clinically by anorexia, weakness, positive Trousseau and Chvostek signs, hypokalemia, and hypocalcemia [37]. Hypermagnesemia is manifested as reduced deep tendon reflexes, flushing, nausea, vomiting, and possible respiratory depression [38].

Magnesium has many uses clinically. Magnesium is commonly used in obstetrical patients with both preeclampsia and eclampsia. High magnesium doses can produce a tocolytic and hypotensive effect in these patients via an inhibitory effect on NMDA receptors. Magnesium also plays a key role in the management of cardiac arrhythmias, most notably torsades de pointes [39].

However, the effect of magnesium on cellular physiology is especially relevant to the anesthesiologist when considering its effect on muscle relaxants. Magnesium has been found to potentiate the effects of nondepolarizing skeletal muscle relaxants such as tubocurarine. This prolongation of neuromuscular blockade is the result of (i) a reduction in the amount of acetylcholine released from motor nerve terminals, (ii) a decrease in the depolarizing action of acetylcholine at the endplate, and (iii) depression of muscle fiber membrane excitability [35, 40]. Therefore patients taking magnesium should be advised to withhold use prior to surgical procedures [13]. Subtherapeutic serum magnesium levels may affect the duration of action of relaxant anesthetics such as mivacurium [41].

The absorption of certain drugs such as antibiotics, ACE inhibitors, phenytoin, and H2 blockers may also be affected by magnesium intake. Because of this, it is recommended to not take magnesium within 2 h of other medications. The mineral may also potentiate the action of oral hypoglycemics such as sulfonylureas, thus increasing the risk of hypoglycemic episodes [42].

Selenium

Selenium is an essential trace element that functions in a variety of enzyme-dependent pathways. Selenium is vital to various antioxidant pathways, particularly in the active site of glutathione peroxidase. As dietary selenium levels decrease, glutathione levels also subsequently decrease [43]. Patients primarily utilize this supplement in an attempt to improve immune function although data remain inconclusive [15].

Toxicity with selenium supplementation begins at intake greater than 750 mcg/day. Manifestations of toxicity vary widely and range from loss of hair and fingernails, garlic-like breath, gastrointestinal issues, or central nervous system changes [44, 45]. Of note, few interactions with other medications have been found [13].

Zinc

The recognition of zinc deficiency is relatively new when compared to other mineral and electrolyte deficiencies. It was first described when it was found to be associated with adolescent dwarfism in 1961 in patients in the Middle East [46]. In the United States, the Food and Nutrition Board of the National Academy of Sciences declared zinc an essential nutrient in 1974 [47]. Zinc is ubiquitous in cellular metabolism, being associated with almost every enzymatic process in the body [47, 48]. Zinc has been shown to be an essential component in gene expression and both cellular growth and differentiation [47]. While severe zinc deficiency is rare in the developed world, clinical manifestations are wide ranging and can affect the epidermal, gastrointestinal, immune, central nervous, and reproductive systems [49].

Patients today may commonly utilize zinc supplementation to alleviate symptoms associated with the common cold. While rare, patients may inadvertently overmedicate themselves. Zinc toxicity can be manifested as anemia, neutropenia, dyslipidemia, decreased immune function, pancreatitis, and copper deficiency [50, 51]. Zinc supplements may also interfere with absorption of tetracyclines, fluoroquinolones, and penicillins and should not be ingested within 2 h of administration of these drugs [14, 50].

Phosphate

Phosphorus is an essential component for numerous biological processes in the human body. About 80 % of phosphorus is found in the bone, while approximately 9 % is stored in the skeletal muscle where it acts as the major intracellular anion opposite to the cation potassium [52]. Phosphorus is also known to be essential for maintaining cellular structural integrity and both anabolic and catabolic cellular processes [52]. It is critical for energy and fuel storage as it is an essential component of adenosine triphosphate. The normal adult ingests approximately 1 g of phosphorus daily; however, this number varies with diet. Metabolism is primarily influenced by renal, gastrointestinal, and endocrine mechanisms [52]. Normal serum levels range between 2.4 and 4.1 mg/dL.

A true phosphate deficiency is rare due to its abundance in diet. However there are certain clinical situations in which the healthcare provider needs to be aware of. These include chronic alcohol abuse, diabetic ketoacidosis, and refeeding syndrome in cachectic patients [52, 53]. The manifestation of phosphate disturbances can vary widely and is often associated with other electrolyte disturbances. Deficiencies in phosphorus have been linked to dysfunction of red blood cells, leukocytes, platelets, and the central nervous system [54]. CNS symptoms are compatible with a metabolic encephalopathy and include excessive irritability, confusion, numbness, seizures, and possibly even coma [55].

Sodium

Sodium is the major cation of the extracellular space. It is tightly regulated by numerous body processes to preserve a relative constant concentration in both body fluids and total body content [56]. Normal sodium levels range between 135 and 140 mEq/L and can be used as barometer of extracellular fluid volume. Homeostasis is primarily maintained by the kidneys, specifically at the proximal tubule and loop of Henle. Hormones that increase sodium reabsorption are renin, angiotensin II, aldosterone, and ADH. A hormone that influences the excretion of sodium is atrial natriuretic peptide, or ANP. The release of these hormones is governed by osmoreceptors in the hypothalamus, baroreceptors in the carotid bodies, and the renal glomerulus [57].

Hyponatremia is due to the imbalance of water to salt in the body and can be divided into three main etiologies: (1) euvolemic, (2) hypervolemic, or (3) hypovolemic [16]. Euvolemic hyponatremia is defined as an increase in total body water without a corresponding increase in sodium. This can be caused by a glucocorticoid deficiency, hypothyroidism, SIADH, or drugs. Hypervolemic hyponatremia is defined as an increase in both sodium and water but with greater water gain. Causes of this state include acute or chronic renal failure, nephritic syndrome, or cirrhosis. Lastly, hypovolemic hyponatremia occurs when both sodium and water are lost from the body but with greater sodium loss. Etiologies of this state can be further subdivided into renal and extrarenal.

Hypernatremia is the result of either excess salt intake or inadequate water intake. This state is intimately tied with hypertension. Sodium restriction has been well documented to be an effective method of blood pressure control either by itself or in conjunction with antihypertensive medications. Sodium restriction can maximize the hypotension produced by therapeutic agents such as beta-blockers, angiotensin-converting enzyme inhibitors, diuretics, and other vasodilators [58].

The correction of either hypernatremia or hyponatremia is dependent on the acuity of the disturbance and the presence or absence of symptoms. Caution must be used by healthcare workers when correcting sodium abnormalities as rapid correction can result in neurological sequelae such as central pontine myelinolysis [59].

Potassium

In contrast to sodium, potassium is the most prevalent cation intracellularly. This fact is dependent on active transport through the cell membrane by a sodium-potassium pump which maintains an intracellular cation ratio of 1:10 [60]. Normal serum levels of potassium are between 3.6 and 5.0 mmol/L. The daily minimum intake is considered to be approximately 1,600–2,000 mg [60]. Potassium is found in a variety of foods including various fruits, vegetables, and nuts [61]. Potassium levels are primarily regulated by the kidneys but are also influenced by such factors as insulin and adrenaline and physiological pH [62].

It has been estimated that over 20 % of hospitalized patients have hypokalemia and approximately 40 % of outpatients on diuretic therapy will have it [63]. Clinical manifestations of hypokalemia include generalized muscle weakness, paralytic ileus, and various cardiac arrhythmias. Electrocardiographic changes can include flat or inverted T waves, ST-segment depression, and prominent U waves [60, 64]. Several clinical and epidemiological studies have also implicated hypokalemia in the maintenance of essential hypertension. These studies showed that potassium replenishment had an antihypertensive effect [65].

Conclusion

Healthcare workers need to have a comprehensive knowledge of the clinical implications of electrolyte and mineral abnormalities. The anesthesiologist is tasked with
the job to regulate the patient's physiological functions and appreciate the effect of
these electrolytes as it relates to various surgical procedures. These agents, in addition to all other medications taken by the patient, should be screened by all healthcare workers, in particular anesthesiologists, as many of these substances may
interact with anesthetic agents.

Chemical Structures

Chemical   Structure
34.1 Ferrous sulfate

Chemical   Structure
34.2 Zinc sulfate

Chemical Structure
34.3 Calcium carbonate

References

1. Shils ME, Olson JA, Shike M. Modern nutrition in health and disease. 9th ed. Baltimore: Williams and Wilkins; 1999. p. 210–860, 1422, 1424, 1772.
2. Papanikolaou G, Pantopoulos K. Iron metabolism and toxicity. Toxicol Appl Pharmacol. 2005;202:199–211.
3. Andrews NC. Disorders of iron metabolism. N Engl J Med. 1999;341:1986–95.
4. Finch C. Regulators of iron balance in humans. Blood. 1994;84:1697–702.
5. Roy CN, Enns CA. Iron homeostasis: new tales from the crypt. Blood. 2000;96:4020–7.
6. Davolos A, Castillo J, Marrugat J, et al. Body iron stores and early neurologic deterioration in acute cerebral infarction. Neurology. 2000;54:1568–74.
7. Lao TT, Tam K, Chan LY. Third trimester iron status and pregnancy outcome in non-anemic women: pregnancy unfavorably affected by maternal iron excess. Hum Reprod. 2000;15:1843–8.
8. Lehto P, Kivisto KT, Neuvonen PJ. The effect of ferrous sulphate on the absorption of nor-floxacin, ciprofloxacin, and ofloxacin. Br J Clin Pharmacol. 1994;37:82–5.

9. Campbell NR, Hasinoff BB. Iron supplements: a common cause of drug interactions. Br J Clin Pharmacol. 1991;31:251–5.

10. Heinrich HC, Oppitz KH, Gabbe EE. Inhibition of iron absorption in man by tetracycline [German]. Klin Wochenschr. 1974;52:493–8.

11. Osman MA, Patel RB, Schuna A, et al. Reduction in oral penicillamine absorption by food, antacid, and ferrous sulphate. Clin Pharmacol Ther. 1983;33:465–70.

12. Campbell NR, Hasinoff BB, Stalts H, et al. Ferrous sulphate reduces thyroxine efficacy in patients with hypothyroidism. Ann Intern Med. 1992;117:1010–3.

13. Hendler SS, Rorvik DR, editors. PDR for nutritional supplements. Montvale: Medical Exonomics, Inc; 2001.

14. Minerals. Drug facts and comparisons. St. Louis: Facts and Comparisons. p. 27–30.

15. Supplements and anesthesiology. In: Kelly Anne M, Kaye AD, Baluch A, Hoover J, editors. Nutrient-drug interactions. Chapter 7. CRC Press; 2006. p 209–36.

16. AlZahrani A, Sinnert R, Gernsheimer J. Acute kidney injury, sodium disorders, and hypercalcemia in the aging kidney. Clin Geriatr Med. 2013;29:275–319.

17. Bar-Or D, Gasiel Y. Calcium and calciferol antagonize effect of verapamil in atrial fibrillation. Br Med J (Clin Res Ed). 1981;282:1585–6.

18. Durward A, Guerguerian AM, Lefebvre M, Shemie SD. Massive diltiazem overdose treated with extracorporeal membrane oxygenation. [Case Reports. Journal Article]. Pediatr Crit Care Med. 2003;4(3):372–6.

19. Masharani U, Gjerde C, McCoy S, Maddux BA, Hessler D, Goldfine ID, Youngren JF. Chromium supplementation in non-obese non diabetic subjects is associated with a decline in insulin sensitivity. BMC Endocr Disord. 2012;12:31.

20. Broadhurst CL, Domenico P. Clinical studies on chromium picolinate supplementation in diabetes mellitus. Diabetes Technol Ther. 2006;8:677–87.

21. Anderson RA. Chromium, glucose intolerance, and diabetes. J Am Coll Nutr. 1998;17:548–55.

22. Vincent JB. The biochemistry of chromium. J Nutr. 2000;130:715–8.

23. Anderson RA. Chromium, glucose tolerance, diabetes and lipid metabolism. J Adv Med. 1995;8:37–50.

24. Cefalu WT, Hu FB. Role of chromium in human health and diabetes. Diabetes Care. 2004;27:2741–51.

25. Wang H, Kruszewski A, Brautigan DL. Cellular chromium enhances activation of insulin receptor kinase. Biochemistry. 2005;44:8167–75.

26. Anderson RA, Bryden NA, Polansky MM. Dietary chromium intake. Freely chosen diets, institutional diet, and individual foods. Biol Trace Elem Res. 1992;32:117–21.

27. Offenbacher EG, Pi-Sunyer FX, Stoecker BJ. Chromium. In: O'Dell BL, Sunde RA, editors. Handbook of nutritionally essential mineral elements. New York: Marcel Dekker; 1997. p. 389–411.

28. Anderson RA, Kozlovsky AS. Chromium intake, absorption and excretion of subjects consuming self selected diets. Am J Clin Nutr. 1985;41:1177–83.

29. Lukaski HC. Chromium as a supplement. Annu Rev Nutr. 1999;19:279–302.

30. Juturu V, Komorowski JR. Consumption of selected food sources of chromium in the diets of American adults [abstract]. FASEB J. 2003;17:A1129.

31. Centers for disease control and prevention: the 2005 National Diabetes Fact Sheet. 2005. www.cdc.gov/diabetes.

32. American Diabetes Association: diabetes statistics-total prevalence of diabetes & pre-diabetes. 2005. http://www.diabetes.org/diabetes-statistics/prevalence.jsp.

33. NIDDK: National Diabetes Statistics. NIH Publication Number 06-3892. 2005. http://diabetes.niddk.nih.gov/dm/pubs/statistics/index.htm.

34. Cerulli J, Grabe DW, Gauthier L, et al. Chromium picolinate toxicity. Ann Pharmacother. 1998;32:428–31.

35. Dube L, Granry JC. The therapeutic use of magnesium in anesthesiology, intensive care and emergency medicine: a review. Can J Anesth. 2003;50(7):732–46.

36. Fawcett WJ, Haxby EJ, Male DA. Magnesium: physiology and pharmacology. Br J Anaesth. 1999;83:302–30.

37. Kelepouris E, Agus ZS. Hypomagnesemia: renal magnesium handling. Semin Nephrol. 1998;18:58–73.
38. Morisaki H, Yamamoto S, Morita Y, Kotake Y, Ochiai R, Takeda J. Hypermagnesemia induced cardiopulmonary arrest before induction of anesthesia for emergency cesarean section. J Clin Anesth. 2000;12:224–6.
39. Han JU. About uses of magnesium during perioperative period. Korean J Anesthesiol. 2012;62:509–11.
40. Ghoneim MM, Long JP. The interaction between magnesium and other neuromuscular blocking agents. Anesthesiology. 1970;32:23–7.
41. Hodgson RE, Rout CC, Rocke DA, Louw NJ. Mivacurium for caesarean section in hypertensive parturients receiving magnesium sulphate therapy. Int J Obstet Anesth. 1998;7(1):12–7.
42. Kivisto KT, Neuvonem PJ. Effect of magnesium hydroxide on the absorption and efficacy of tolbutamide and chlorpropamide. Eur J Clin Pharmacol. 1992;42:675–9.
43. Ursini F, Heim S, Kiess M, et al. Dual function of the selenoprotein PHGPx during sperm maturation. Science. 1999;285(5432):1393–6.
44. Patterson BH, Levander OA. Naturally occurring selenium compounds in cancer chemoprevention trials: a workshop summary. Cancer Epidemiol Biomarkers Prev. 1997;6:63–9.
45. Fan AM, Kizer KW. Selenium: nutritional, toxicologic, and clinical aspects. West J Med. 1990;153:160–7.
46. Prasad AS, Halsted JA, Nadimi M. Syndrome of iron deficiency anemia, hepatosplenomegaly, hypogonadism, dwarfism, and geophagia. Am J Med. 1961;31:532–46.
47. Hambridge M. Human zinc deficiency. J Nutr. 2000;130:1344S–9.
48. Fierke C. Function and mechanism of zinc. J Nutr. 2000;130:1437S–46.
49. Hambridge KM, Walravens PA. Disorders of mineral metabolism. Clin Gastroenterol. 1982;11:87–118.
50. Bratman S, Girman AM. Handbook of herbs and supplements and their therapeutic uses. St Louis: Mosby, Inc.; 2003.
51. Mikszewski JS, Saunders HM, Hess RS. Zinc-associated pancreatitis in a dog. J Small Anim Pract. 2003;44(4):177–80.
52. Knochel JP. The pathophysiology and clinical characteristics of severe hypophosphatemia. Arch Intern Med. 1977;137:203–20.
53. Krebs H. Rate limiting factors in cell respiration. CIBA Foundation Symposium on Regulation of Cell Metabolism. Boston: Little Brown & Co; 1959, p. 1–10.
54. Territo MC, Tanaka KR. Hypophosphatemia in chronic alcoholism. Arch Intern Med. 1974;134:445–7.
55. Silvis SE, Paragas PD. Paresthesias, weakness, seizures and hypophosphatemia in patients receiving hyperalimentation. Gastroenterology. 1972;62:513–20.
56. Bennett WM. Drug interactions and consequences of sodium restrictions. Am J Clin Nutr. 1997;65:678S–81.
57. Ram CVS, Garret BN, Kaplan NM. Moderate sodium restriction and various diuretics in the treatment of hypertension. Arch Intern Med. 1981;141:1015–9.
58. Wasserstell-Smoller S, Oberman A, Blaufox MD, Davis B, Langford H. The trial of antihypertensive interventions and management study. Am J Hypertens. 1992;5:37–44.
59. King JD, Rosner MH. Osmotic demyelination syndrome. Am J Med Sci. 2010;339:561–7.
60. Cohn JN, Kowey PR, Whelton PK, Prisant M. New guidelines for potassium replacement in clinical practice. Arch Intern Med. 2000;160:2429–36.
61. Mandal AK. Hypokalemia and hyperkalemia. Med Clin North Am. 1997;81:611–39.
62. Tannen RL. Chap 3. Potassium disorders. In: Kokko JP, Tannen RL, editors. Fluid and electrolytes. 3rd ed. Philadelphia: WB Saunders; 1996.
63. Gennari FJ. Hypokalemia. N Engl J Med. 1998;339:451–8.
64. Santeusanio F, Knochel JP, Schlein EM, et al. Effect of acute hyperkalemia on plasma insulin and glucagon. J Lab Clin Med. 1973;81:809–17.
65. Krishna GG, Kapoor SC. Potassium depletion exacerbates essential hypertension. Ann Intern Med. 1991;115:77–83.

Chapter 35
Disinfection Agents and Antiseptics

Valeriy Kozmenko, Rudolph R. Gonzales Jr., James Riopelle, and Alan David Kaye

Contents

V. Kozmenko, MD (✉) • J. Riopelle, MD
Director of the Parry Center for Clinical Skills and Simulation,
University of South Dakota Sanford School of Medicine,
Sioux Falls, SD, USA
e-mail: val.kozmenko@usd.edu, vvkozmenko@gmail.com; jriope@lsuhsc.edu

R.R. Gonzales Jr., RN, MSN, CNOR, CRCST, CHL
Sterile Processing Services, North Texas Veterans Administration Health Care System,
Medical Center of Louisiana, Dallas, TX, USA
e-mail: rgonza3@lsuhsc.edu

A.D. Kaye, MD, PhD
Department of Anesthesiology, Louisiana State University Health Sciences Center,
New Orleans, LA, USA

Department of Anesthesiology, Tulane Medical Center, New Orleans, LA, USA
e-mail: alankaye44@hotmail.com

A.D. Kaye et al. (eds.), *Essentials of Pharmacology for Anesthesia,
Pain Medicine, and Critical Care*, DOI 10.1007/978-1-4614-8948-1_35,
© Springer Science+Business Media New York 2015

Introduction

Germicidal agents are nonspecific antimicrobial agents that are too toxic to be administered internally but are safe and effective when used topically. When applied to living tissue (e.g., the skin), they are termed *antiseptics*. When applied to inanimate objects (e.g., environmental surfaces or instruments used to perform medical procedures), they are termed *disinfectants*. All of these agents work at least by damaging microbial surfaces, often by alkylation, oxidation, or reaction with proteins. Products capable of destroying all forms of microbial life, including bacterial spores, are termed *sterilizing agents*.

Agents Used as Antiseptics

Alcohols

In 60–90 % solution in water, both ethyl alcohol and isopropyl alcohol are capable of killing vegetative (but not spore) forms of nearly all bacteria as well as fungi, and most viruses, most likely by denaturation of bacterial proteins. Long used for skin antisepsis, ethyl alcohol has more recently been combined with other agents to increase efficacy (iodine: DuraPrep®; chlorhexidine: ChloraPrep®). An important disadvantage is flammability; this happens only when the prep solution that is applied does not evaporate fully and when electrocautery is also employed. Alcoholic solutions should not be applied to mucosal surfaces and must be kept away from the eyes: even brief application may result in a requirement for corneal transplantation.

Polymer-Iodine Complex

Iodine's broad-spectrum antiseptic properties have been known since 1811. Postulated mechanisms of bactericidal action include (1) membrane destabilization, (2) inhibition of protein synthesis, (3) free electron transport inhibition, and (4) nucleic acid denaturation. Iodine's low solubility limited clinical use until Lugol combined iodine with potassium iodide salt. In 1952, Shalanski and Shalanski incorporated molecular iodine into the large polymer, polyvinylpyrrolidone to form a complex, povidone-iodine (Betadine®), that releases iodine into aqueous solution in three bactericidal forms: free molecular iodine, hypoiodous acid (HOI), and iodine cation (the most effective).

Povidone-iodine exerts its antimicrobial effects on bacteria, viruses, yeasts, fungi, and protozoa. The 10 % solution marketed for skin disinfection must be diluted before applying to the cornea or deep tissues such as open wounds.

To achieve cutaneous antisepsis prior to central venous cannulation, some studies suggest greater antibacterial efficacy if polymer-bound iodine dispersed in alcoholic solution is used, e.g., iodine acrylate copolymer (povacrylex; 0.7 % available iodine) in 74 % isopropyl alcohol (DuraPrep®). Iodophor solution from a single-use container is more reliably bacteria-free than the solution from a multidose container. A small percentage of patients will experience cutaneous reactions such as erythema, urticaria, or blistering.

Chlorhexidine Gluconate

Chlorhexidine (Chemical Structure 35.5 – see end of chapter) is a cationic bis-biguanide detergent-antiseptic that kills target organisms via membrane disruption and cytoplasmic precipitation. It is effective against all microbial organisms commonly associated with catheter-related infections and adheres to the stratum, prolonging protection after application for hours. A 4 % aqueous solution (Hibiclens®) is marketed for skin cleaning and preoperative surgical hand scrub. A 2 % solution in 70 % isopropyl alcohol (ChloraPrep®) has been approved by the US Food and Drug Administration (FDA) for preoperative skin prep. The use of a color-tinted solution can help ensure even coverage. Waiting for applied solution to dry prior to needle insertion is recommended.

Evaluations of available evidence have led task forces of several large, respected medical organizations to recommend 2 % alcoholic chlorhexidine as the best available skin prep solution prior to central venous cannulation [1] (except perhaps in neonates where povidone-iodine in alcohol may be preferred). The American Society of Regional Anesthesia accepts the use of alcoholic chlorhexidine solution prior to neuraxial blockade despite case reports and experimental evidence that clinically used concentrations are toxic when applied directly to neural tissue [1, 2]. A recent large retrospective study of its use prior to spinal anesthesia seems to confirm safety when used in this setting [3].

Agents and Techniques Used for Disinfection [4–8]

The extent of disinfection required prior to the use of medical equipment varies depending on the site of application: (1) *sterilization* if contacting deep tissues, (2) *high-level disinfection* (HLD; destruction of vegetative microbes but not spores) if contacting intact mucosa, and (3) *low-level disinfection* (LLD; destruction of most vegetative bacteria, some fungi, and some viruses in <10 min) if contacting intact skin. Standard and videolaryngoscopes and bronchoscopes are reusable anesthesia equipment most often requiring sterilization/disinfection. Anesthesia providers should also know how to perform LLD of the surfaces of an anesthesia workstation and how to decontaminate an environmental spill of blood or a disinfectant solution used in their facility. Because of the consequences of process failure (inoculation of a patient with a pathogenic organism), all HLD and sterilization processes require monitoring (usually both chemical and biological) to verify satisfactory completion.

High-Level Disinfection (HLD)

Inadequate HLD of laryngoscope blades has resulted in fatal bacterial outbreaks in neonatal intensive care units, and inadequate HLD of bronchoscopes has been proven to be the cause of many scores of reported cases of Mycobacterium and Pseudomonas infections [9, 10]. Such HLD failures require notification of patients' physicians, hospital offices of infection control and risk management, and sometimes state and federal authorities. All HLD methods described in this chapter have been approved by the US Food and Drug Administration (FDA). Not all techniques are compatible with every piece of medical equipment, however. Manufacturers of both equipment and disinfection agents are normally quite willing to make compatibility testing data and recommendations based on such data available on request, and it is often already published on the company website. All chemical solutions used for HLD are toxic if ingested or applied to the cornea. Some also require avoidance of inhalation.

Performance of HLD of a bronchoscope should typically include the following steps:

1. Immediately after use – to prevent drying of secretions which can affix and protect from cleaning a contaminated biofilm – rinsing the exterior scope and flushing suction channels with tap water, then wiping the exterior with an antiseptic-impregnated cloth or paper towel
2. Rapidly transferring the scope to a designated are where it can be leak checked, immersed in a detergent solution, and all surfaces and mechanically cleaned ports and suction channels using cylindrical brushes (very hot or hard water is not advised since excessive heat and contained minerals can inactivate enzymes, such as proteases, lipases, and amylases, often used to fortify medical-instrument-grade detergents.)
3. Disinfecting by immersion + flushing with an approved biocidal solution (glutaraldehyde, ortho-phthalaldehyde, peracetic acid/H_2O_2)
4. Rinsing with microfiltered or sterile water (failure of this step potentially later permitting residual disinfectant to contact and severely irritate airway mucosa)
5. Active drying using alcohol and/or forced air
6. Storing in a cabinet or other container that is physically separate from contaminated equipment and that permits any residual moisture to evaporate

Glutaraldehyde (Cidex®) and ortho-phthalaldehyde (Cidex OPA®) are alkylating agents, the former less expensive and the latter faster-acting and causing far less irritation to the eyes and mucous membranes. Both have excellent compatibility with most equipment and full efficacy at room temperature. Glutaraldehyde is sometimes sold in alcoholic solution. Disadvantages include (1) a tendency for these chemicals to coagulate blood and other proteins, causing them to stick to equipment surfaces, and (2) the need to frequently monitor solution strength using color test strips. Due to environmental toxicity, some state governments have classified both agents as toxic waste and prohibit their disposal into public sewer systems without preliminary neutralization, e.g., using glycine, Na bisulfite, or dilute Na hydroxide. Federal occupational safety statues mandate low exposure limits. Large spills of either agent may require handling by a hazardous material (hazmat) response team [11].

Two peroxide solutions – hydrogen peroxide and peracetic acid – are capable of achieving HLD at low temperature (<40 °C) by oxidation. Neither have important environmental toxicity since the former breaks down into water and oxygen and the latter to these two reactants (by generating H_2O_2 in solution) plus acetic acid. Hydrogen peroxide is marketed as a concentrated solution (e.g., Steris Revital-Ox Resert XL HLD accelerated H_2O_2) and peracetic acid/hydrogen peroxide solution as either a concentrate (e.g., Rapicide™) or as dry crystals (e.g., Steris Reliance DG®). Because they react with metals and glues, peroxide solutions should not be used with some bronchoscope models. Unlike the aldehydes, neither fixes protein to equipment surfaces. H_2O_2 vapor is nonirritating to mucosa. In contrast, peracetic acid is highly irritating and is therefore normally used within a sealed automated washing/disinfecting machine.

Sterilization

A sterilization process is not required for equipment contacting intact mucosa, but should be applied to a laryngoscope that was employed in a traumatic intubation or in a patient in whom disease has compromised mucosal integrity. Unlike surgical supplies, airway equipment used in anesthesia need *not* ordinarily be stored as sterile so that HLD techniques with extended immersion times but no provision for sterile packaging are usually appropriate.

Steam autoclaving (which kills by protein coagulation and oxidation) is widely employed for sturdy metal surgical equipment. Intolerance of batteries, light bulbs, and plastic components to moist heat ordinarily discourages use of this technique on laryngoscopes and bronchoscopes.

Ethylene oxide (EtO; C_4H_2O) is a relatively inexpensive gaseous cyclic ether that kills microbes by alkylation and has excellent material compatibility. It has long been the mainstay of low-temperature sterilization of delicate equipment. Disadvantages include (1) that it is a flammable, and potentially explosive, biotoxin (carcinogenic, mutagenic) with general anesthetic properties but a (deceptively) pleasing aroma, (2) that it must be destroyed rather than released into the environment, and (3) that it has the longest cycle time of any sterilizing agent (4 h for sterilization; 12 h for dilutional aeration).

Hydrogen peroxide vapor, unlike ETO gas, is an effective agent for sterilizing laryngoscope blades but cannot diffuse sufficient distances to penetrate the full length of bronchoscope channels. It can be used in two forms for low-temperature sterilization: (1) in high concentration (e.g., Amsco ®V-Pro™ 1 Plus) or (2) as sub-atmospheric pressurized ionized gas plasma (Sterrad®). The former kills by oxidation, the latter by oxidation-induced ultraviolet irradiation and by photodesorption (atom-by-atom erosion). Both have a relatively short cycle time, and neither emits toxic environmental waste. Polypropylene sterilization bags must be used as H_2O_2 adsorbs to paper.

Infrequently used (though approved) methods of sterilization include:

- Immersion in peracetic acid solution – limited because sterilized items are wet, and therefore, cannot be stored as sterile
- Dry heat in a convection oven – non-rusting, but limited by requirement for higher temperatures, longer cycle times, and more uneven penetration with a sealed package
- Gamma irradiation (often from ^{60}Co) – limited by need for expensive equipment, dangerous supplies (and so extensive regulatory supervision), and unreliable sterilization of surfaces lying behind thick or metallic portions of an irradiated item, thus mainly employed by manufacturers of disposable cloth or plastic surgical supplies and implants

Low-Level Disinfection (LLD)

Present recommendations are for performing LLD of the anesthesia work area and laryngoscope handle, i.e., killing such vegetative (nonspore) pathogens as Pseudomonas sp., methicillin-resistant *Staphylococcus aureus* (MRSA), vancomycin-resistant Enterococcus (VRE), many fungi, and hepatitis, immunodeficiency, and SARS coronaviruses within one to a few minutes. Surfaces should be wiped with an aqueous or alcoholic solution of one of several approved agents.

Quaternary ammonium solutions (active molecules being ammonium compounds in which there are four nitrogenous bonds to alkyl or heterocyclic radicals and a fifth to a halide, sulfate, or similar anion) have detergent as well as disinfectant properties. They are often supplied in squirt bottles or saturated disposable towelettes. Such is the active ingredient of Lysol®, Dettol®, Bactine®, and Sani-Wipes (0.0175 benzyl ammonium chloride + 5.5 % isopropyl alcohol). These compounds are inactivated by soaps, inhibited by calcium and magnesium ions and cotton, and ineffective against some strains of Pseudomonas and some non-enveloped viruses. These agents are *not* approved for HLD.

Aqueous ethyl and isopropyl alcohol 70–90 % solutions – both more rapidly dissipating than aqueous solutions used for LLD – are preferred agents when there is a possibility of the presence of Mycobacterium tuberculosis. These solutions, however, penetrate proteinaceous material poorly and have limited efficacy against a few hydrophilic viruses (notably polio and Coxsackie). Alcoholic solutions are not approved for HLD.

Sodium hypochlorite solution 5.25–6.15 % (household bleach) is a powerful oxidizing agent. In 1:10–1:100 dilution, it is an effective LLD agent and (at 1:10 dilution) may be the preferred agent to use to disinfect areas of blood spill after initial (gloved) cleaning because of its effectiveness against hepatitis viruses, HIV, and *Clostridium difficile*. It has long-term stability when stored away from light. Disadvantages include odor, eye irritation, corrosive effects on metals, bleaching effect on fabric, release of toxic fumes in the event of contact with ammonia or acid (e.g., vinegar), and greatly reduced effectiveness in the presence of organic material. Na hypochlorite is approved for HLD in Great Britain but not the USA.

Hydrogen peroxide 3–6 %, available as spray and wipes, is also a powerful oxidizing agent but decomposes to only oxygen and water (no environmental toxicity). HLD is achievable using H_2O_2 but only at high concentrations or together with peracetic acid (see above).

Summary

Recent recommendations for pre-procedural skin antisepsis favor alcoholic solutions of iodophors and chlorhexidine, but these should be allowed to dry before skin puncture, especially for neuraxial regional anesthesia. Approved agents and techniques for sterilization and high-level disinfection of medical devices have increased in number and complexity, but newer methods are more efficient and environmentally friendly.

Chemical Structures

Chemical Structure
35.1 Ethyl alcohol/ethanol

Chemical Structure 35.2 Povidone-iodine

Chemical Structure
35.3 Sodium hypochlorite

Chemical Structure
35.4 Hydrogen peroxide

Chemical Structure 35.5 Chlorhexidine

References

1. American Society of Anesthesiologists Task Force on Central Venous Access, Rupp SM, Apfelbaum JL, Blitt C, Caplan RA, Connis RT, Domino KB, Fleisher LA, Grant S, Mark JB, Morray JP, Nickinovich DG, Tung A. Practice guidelines for central venous access: a report by the American Society of Anesthesiologists Task Force on central venous access. Anesthesiology. 2012;116:539–73.
2. Hebl JR. The importance and implications of aseptic techniques during regional anesthesia. Reg Anesth Pain Med. 2006;31:311–23.
3. Sviggum HP, Jacob AK, Arendt KW, Mauermann ML, Horlocker TT, Hebl JR. Neurologic complications after chlorhexidine antisepsis for spinal anesthesia. Reg Anesth Pain Med. 2012;37:139–44.
4. Rutala WA (ed) Disinfection, sterilization and antisepsis: principles, practices, current issues, new research, and new technologies (2010 ed)—In: Proceedings of the Conference on. Washington DC: Association for Professionals in Infection Control and Epidemiology, Inc (APIC), 2010 (Proceedings of conference Ft. Lauderdale FL 2009-06-06).
5. Rutala WA, Weber DJ (2008) For the healthcare infection control practices advisory committee, Centers for Disease Control (CDC). Guideline for disinfection and sterilization in healthcare facilities. http://www.cdc.gov/hicpac/pdf/guidelines/disinfection_nov_2008.pdf
6. Lind N, Ninemeier JD, editors. Central service technical manual. 7th ed. Chicago: International Association of Healthcare Central Service Materiel Management; 2007.
7. FDA (approved sterilants and HDL agents) http://www.fda.gov/MedicalDevices/DeviceRegulationandGuidance/ReprocessingofSingle-UseDevices/ucm133514.htm. Accessed Jan 2013
8. CDC (summary of proper use of available sterilization & HLD techniques) http://www.cdc.gov/hicpac/pdf/guidelines/disinfection_nov_2008.pdf. Accessed Jan 2013
9. Call TR, Auerbach FJ, Riddell SW, Kiska DL, Thongrod SC, Tham SW, Nussmeier NA. Nosocomial contamination of laryngoscope handles: challenging current guidelines. Anesth Analg. 2009;109:479–83.
10. Muscarella LF. Reassessment of the risk of healthcare-acquired infection during rigid laryngoscopy. J Hosp Infect. 2008;68:101–7.
11. OSHA (glutaraldehyde) http://www.osha.gov/Publications/glutaraldehyde.pdf. Accessed Jan 2013

Chapter 36
Psychopharmacologic Agents and Psychiatric Drug Considerations

Charles Fox, Alan David Kaye, and Henry Liu

Contents

The clinical anesthesiologist should appreciate that mental illnesses, cognitive disorders, and mental health problems affect all walks of life. It is a fact that few families in America are untouched by mental illness [1]. An estimated 26.2 % of Americans aged 18 and older suffer from a diagnosable mental disorder in a given year. Mental disease interferes with life activity and ability to function and constitutes a pervasive and prevalent health problem among varied American

C. Fox, MD (✉)
Department of Anesthesiology, LSU Health Science Center Shreveport, Shreveport, LA, USA
e-mail: cfox1@lsuhsc.edu

A.D. Kaye, MD, PhD
Department of Anesthesiology, Tulane Medical Center, New Orleans, LA, USA

Department of Anesthesiology, Louisiana State University Health Sciences Center,
New Orleans, LA, USA
e-mail: alankaye44@hotmail.com

H. Liu, MD
Department of Anesthesiology, Tulane Medical Center, New Orleans, LA, USA
e-mail: henryliula@gmail.com

A.D. Kaye et al. (eds.), *Essentials of Pharmacology for Anesthesia,*
Pain Medicine, and Critical Care, DOI 10.1007/978-1-4614-8948-1_36,
© Springer Science+Business Media New York 2015

population subsets, including the young and the elderly [2]. The presence of mental disorders, associated symptoms, possible concomitant pathology, and prescribed medications is of significance to all health-care providers and not simply those in the field of mental health.

Mental disorders and their associated use of psychotropic medications, including antidepressants, anxiolytic drugs, major tranquilizers, anticonvulsants, and mood stabilizers, introduce neurochemical, behavioral, cognitive, and emotional factors that increase the complexity of medical or surgical tasks [3]. The use of psychotropic medications has increased significantly over the last several decades, with psychiatrists and family practice physicians prescribing tranquilizers, neuroleptics, and antidepressants, even among youth. In the case of depression alone, numerous complexities have been described in prescribing medications and understanding side effect and adverse effect profiles, as well as drug interactions with other medications prescribed for mental and physical problems [4].

In this framework, we will discuss psychopharmacologic medications used as treatment for mood disorders and nonaffective psychoses. Also, we will discuss the side effects, drug interactions, and mechanism of action for these medications. Lastly, we will outline issues and concerns that anesthesia care providers face in planning case management.

Pharmacologic Therapy for Mood Disorders

Selective Serotonin Reuptake Inhibitors

Selective serotonin reuptake inhibitors (SSRIs) are undoubtedly the most commonly prescribed antidepressant medications. Discoveries from psychopharmacologic research have altered depression treatment protocols, particularly over the past 20 years, and the use of antidepressants has increased threefold to fivefold from 1988 to 1994 among youth younger than 20 years of age [5]. In recent decades, primary care physicians have initiated more antidepressant pharmacotherapy than have psychiatrists. There is literature outlining the pharmacology of depression treatment and its medication, including side effects, adverse drug effects, and drug-drug interactions, as well as patient-specific factors such as gender, age, and other illnesses.

Mechanism of Action

Antidepressants do act on a multitude of receptors and induce various neurochemical modulating effects (Table 36.1, pharmacology of antidepressants) [6]. The SSRIs are the most frequently encountered antidepressants by practicing anesthesiologists. SSRIs selectively potentiate the transmission of central nervous impulses along serotonergic pathways while having little effect on other neuroendocrine pathways, such as those involving norepinephrine or acetylcholine. Thus, SSRIs lack many of the side effects associated with other classes of antidepressants.

Table 36.1 Commonly prescribed antidepressants and side effects

Class	Generic (trade) names	Common side effects and special points
SSRIs	Citalopram (Celexa, Cipram, Cipramil, Serostat)	SSRIs are safer when overdosed
	Escitalopram (Lexapro)	GI: nausea, diarrhea, headache
	Fluvoxamine (Dumirox, Faverin, Floxyfral, Luvox)	GU: loss of libido, ED, fail to reach orgasm
	Fluoxetine (Prozac, Sarafem)	Increase of suicidal ideation, hyponatremia
	Paroxetine (Paxil)	Serotonergic syndrome
	Sertraline (Zoloft)	
TCAs	Amitriptyline (Elavil, Endep, Entrofen)	Cardiac: increase heart rate and/or blood pressure
	Amoxapine (Asendin)	Dry mouth, blurred vision, drowsiness, dizziness, skin rash, weight gain or loss
	Clomipramine (Anafranil)	Sexual problems
	Desipramine (Norpramin, Pertofran)	
	Doxepin (Adapin, Sinequan)	
	Imipramine (Norfranil, Tofranil, Tipramine)	
	Maprotiline (Ludiomil)	
	Nortriptyline (Aventyl, Noratren, Pamelor)	
	Protriptyline (Vivactil)	
	Trimipramine (Surmontil)	
MAOIs	Deprenyl (Eldepryl)	Heart attack, liver inflammation, stroke, seizure
	Phenelzine (Nardil)	Severe hypertension if taken together with certain food or beverage rich in tyramine
	Selegiline (Emsam)	Weight gain, constipation, dry mouth, dizziness, headache, drowsiness, insomnia, and sexual side effects
	Tranylcypromine (Parnate)	
RIMA	Moclobemide (Aurorix)	Urticaria, angioedema, asthma, insomnia, anxiety, agitation, vertigo, headache, seizure, nausea, diarrhea, hypertension
NARI	Reboxetine (Edronax, Vestra)	Dry mouth, constipation, headache, drowsiness, dizziness, sweating, insomnia, hypertension
NDRI	Bupropion (Wellbutrin, Wellbutrin SR)	Restlessness, insomnia, headache, worsening of migraine conditions, tremor, dry mouth, agitation, confusion, rapid heartbeat, dizziness, nausea, constipation, menstrual complaints, and rash
SNRI	Venlafaxine (Effexor)	Nervousness, agitation, headache, insomnia, seizure, nausea, diarrhea, rash, sexual side effects (problems with arousal or satisfaction)
	Duloxetine (Cymbalta)	
CRIRB	Nefazodone (Dutonin, Serzone)	Drowsiness, nausea/vomiting, headache, and dry mouth. Rare cases of liver failure leading to transplant and/or death in patients have been reported with nefazodone
	Trazodone (Desyrel, Trazon, Trialodine)	

(continued)

Table 36.1 (continued)

Class	Generic (trade) names	Common side effects and special points
NSSA	Mirtazapine (Remeron)	Dizziness, blurred vision, sedation, somnolence, malaise/lassitude, increased appetite and weight gain, dry mouth, constipation, enhanced libido and sexual function, and vivid, bizarre, lucid dreams or nightmares
Herbal	Gingko biloba remedies	Gingko: nausea, diarrhea, dizziness, headache, bleeding, weakness, seizure, headache
	Ginseng	Ginseng: nervousness, excitability, headache, euphoria, bleeding
	Hypericum perforatum (St. John's wort)	St John's wort: GI symptoms, dizziness, confusion, tiredness, sedation

Data from www.clinical-depression.co.uk/dlp/treating-depression/side-effects-of-antidepressants

Abbreviations: CRIRB (combined reuptake inhibitors and receptor blockers), *ED* erectile dysfunction, *GI* gastrointestinal, *GU* genitourological, *MAOI* monoamine oxidase inhibitors, *NARI* noradrenaline reuptake inhibitors, *NaSSa* noradrenergic and specific serotonergic antidepressants, *NDRI* norepinephrine and dopamine reuptake inhibitors, *NSSA* noradrenergic and specific serotonergic antidepressants, *RIMA* (reversible inhibitors of monoamine oxidase type), *SNRI* serotonin and noradrenaline reuptake inhibitors, *SSRIs* selective serotonin reuptake inhibitors, TCAs tricyclic antidepressant drugs, *GI* gastrointestinal, *SIADH* syndrome of inappropriate secretion of antidiuretic hormone (vasopressin)

Side Effects and Drug Interactions

However, SSRIs may cause nausea, diarrhea, headache, sexual dysfunction, agitation, and insomnia aside from some mild sedative effects. Specifically, escitalopram is possibly associated with hyponatremia. Fluoxetine is a potent inhibitor of the cytochrome P450 2D6 isoenzyme [7]. The inhibition of this enzyme leads to a rise in the plasma concentration of drugs that depend on hepatic metabolism for clearance (such as β-blockers, benzodiazepines, and some cardiac anti-dysrhythmic drugs). The most obvious results of this inhibition derive from the treatment of the patients' depression itself, because patients may be treated with several antidepressants from different classes. Concomitant treatment of depressed patients with both fluoxetine and a tricyclic drug may result in substantial rises in plasma concentrations of the latter. A small subgroup of depressed patients may have an increased rate of suicide when treated with SSRIs [8, 9].

Combining SSRIs with monoamine oxidase inhibitors (MAOIs) may precipitate *serotonin syndrome*, which is similar to neuroleptic malignant syndrome both in its presentation and its mortality and is marked by flushing, restlessness, anxiety, chills, ataxia, insomnia, and hemodynamic instability. Combination of fluoxetine with the mood stabilizers carbamazepine or lithium may also precipitate this syndrome.

Warnings: The use of selective serotonin reuptake inhibitors (SSRIs) has been linked to an increased risk of bleeding due to possible SSRI-induced increase in gastric acid secretion or SSRI-related effects on platelet reactivity. Recently the

Food and Drug Administration (FDA) warning cautioned that citalopram dosages exceeding 40 mg/day could expose patients to an increased risk of abnormal heart rhythms – QT interval prolongation, including torsades de pointes.

Clinical Pearls

For anesthetic management, SSRIs do not pose too much challenge. SSRIs have little effect on seizure threshold. Some seizures in patients using *SSRIs* may be caused by hyponatremia or in patients on other medications that also produce these effects including diuretics. Some attention should be paid to drug combinations and the effects of drugs taken by patients on the cytochrome system if the patient has been taking barbiturates, benzodiazepines, and certain neuromuscular-blocking drugs.

Tricyclic Antidepressants

Mechanism of Action

The tricyclic antidepressants (TCAs) were the most widely used drugs to treat clinical depression prior to the SSRIs after imipramine (Tofranil) was shown to be effective for treating depression in the 1950s. TCAs primarily work by increasing the level of norepinephrine in the brain and, to a lesser extent, serotonin levels. Some TCAs also are antihistamines (which block the action of histamine) or anticholinergic (which blocks the action of acetylcholine, a neurotransmitter). These additional actions allow for uses of TCAs other than for treating depression as well as introduce additional side effects.

Side Effects and Drug Interactions

A TCA's chemical structure is composed of three conjoined rings. If the nitrogen atom on the center ring is a tertiary amine, the drug belongs to the first-generation TCAs; most side effects associated with TCAs are more pronounced with first-generation TCAs. If it is a secondary amine, the drug is a second-generation tricyclic. TCAs may inhibit the antihypertensive effect of clonidine (Catapres). Therefore, combining TCAs with clonidine may lead to dangerous elevations in blood pressure. TCAs may affect the heart's electrical conduction system. Combining TCAs with drugs that also affect the heart's conduction system (disopyramide, pimozide, procainamide) may increase the frequency and severity of an abnormal heart rate and rhythm [10]. Combining TCAs with carbamazepine (Tegretol) may result in lower TCA blood levels because carbamazepine increases the breakdown of TCAs, potentially reducing the effect of TCAs. TCAs may increase the blood pressure-elevating effect of epinephrine, norepinephrine, dopamine, phenylephrine, and dobutamine.

It is generally believed that the TCAs are equally potent with regard to treatment of depression. On the other hand, all of the TCAs cause some anticholinergic symptoms, orthostatic hypotension, cardiac dysrhythmia, and sedation. However, they do so in varying degrees when compared with their efficacy as antidepressants. This differing side effect profile serves as the basis for much of the strategy employed by practitioners prescribing these drugs. For example, a drug that causes a greater degree of sedation might be chosen preferentially for patients experiencing insomnia as part of their symptomatology. Similarly, practitioners might avoid drugs that have greater anticholinergic activity in patients who have glaucoma or reflux disease, for example. The degree of cardiac dysrhythmia potential is essentially the same for TCAs, and they should be avoided in patients with known cardiac conduction abnormalities such as second-degree or higher atrioventricular blocks. It has been shown that despite their potential for causing cardiac dysrhythmias, they may paradoxically show some anti-dysrhythmic activity. Also of note is the fact that despite the electrocardiographic (ECG) changes that occur with these drugs, the changes tend to dissipate with ongoing treatment, implying some sort of tolerance on the part of the cardiac conduction system to these effects.

Commonly, seizure activity associated with antidepressant therapy is seen after an acute overdose. Dose-dependent seizure activity has been traditionally reported with imipramine, amitriptyline, clomipramine, and maprotiline. Bupropion, while not a TCA, is well known for its risk of seizures – especially in higher doses or in patients with predisposing factors like family history.

Clinical Pearls

Anesthetic management of patients who are on TCAs revolves around the side effects of these medications and their interactions with other drugs. The mechanism of the antidepressant effects of TCAs involves enhancement of serotonergic and noradrenergic activity. TCAs' inhibition of histaminergic, cholinergic, and α_1-adrenergic activity is responsible for many of their side effects. The main concerns for these patients being treated with a TCA center around the cardiovascular system and the interaction of the drug with a specific neurotransmitter, such as norepinephrine. Since the administration of TCAs causes an increase of this neurotransmitter to be stored in noradrenergic nerve terminals, the administration of indirect-acting vasopressors such as ephedrine may cause an exaggerated release of epinephrine. This effect is most pronounced with acute treatment and gradually dissipates after the first 2–3 weeks. Caution is therefore advised with regard to using drugs with sympathomimetic effects on patients receiving TCAs. TCAs' anticholinergic effects can potentially cause a problem to anesthesiologists, because many drugs used by anesthesiologists are anticholinergics or have anticholinergic effects. Preoperatively, some anesthesiologists employ scopolamine for its sedative, anxiolytic, and antisialagogic properties. Intraoperatively, glycopyrrolate and atropine are both used for their anticholinergic properties. Pancuronium, which has significant anticholinergic effects, is still used for procedures requiring a long period of muscle relaxation, especially cardiac surgery. Atropine and glycopyrrolate have been noted to have increased muscarinic activity in the presence of TCAs, and the administration of pancuronium has been documented to precipitate tachydysrhythmias in a sample of patients studied. Furthermore, there is the possibility that preoperative treatment with scopolamine may increase the incidence of emergence delirium, although there are no formal studies that support this suspicion.

Monoamine Oxidase Inhibitors

Mechanism of Action

MAOIs were the first class of antidepressants to be developed. MAOIs elevate the levels of norepinephrine, serotonin, and dopamine by inhibiting an enzyme called monoamine oxidase. Monoamine oxidase breaks down norepinephrine, serotonin, and dopamine. When monoamine oxidase is inhibited, norepinephrine, serotonin, and dopamine are metabolized significantly less, increasing the concentration of all three neurotransmitters in the brain. As a consequence, they act to extend the effect of norepinephrine at the nerve terminals. MAOIs fell out of favor because of concerns about interactions with certain foods and numerous drug interactions and the introduction of newer and safer antidepressants. MAOIs are still available and reserved primarily for the treatment of patients who have failed treatment with other antidepressants.

Side Effects and Drug Interactions

The MAOIs are devoid of many side effects of other classes of antidepressants. Their principal side effect is the possibility to precipitate profound hypertension crisis, as well as serotonin syndrome when foods are consumed that contain the substance tyramine (most commonly wines or cheeses) or when combined with drugs with intrinsic sympathomimetic effects such as meperidine and certain β-blockers. Tyramine and sympathomimetic drugs stimulate the release of norepinephrine from noradrenergic nerve terminals, and owing to the mechanism of the drug, the α-adrenergic effects of the neurotransmitter become pronounced. Other side effects of the drug include orthostatic hypotension, sedation, blurry vision, and peripheral neuropathy.

Clinical Pearls

It was suggested that MAOIs be discontinued 2–3 weeks before any elective procedure involving general anesthesia. This precaution is no longer encouraged or practical for many procedures, because discontinuation of the drug may acutely place patients at greater risk for suicide [11]. MAOIs can also significantly increase the MAC. Furthermore, serum cholinesterase activity may be impaired, requiring the dose of succinylcholine to be reduced [12]. Liver function indices may become elevated during treatment with MAOIs. As with TCAs, indirect-acting vasopressors as well as epinephrine-containing local anesthetics should be avoided because of their potential to cause severe hypertension. Finally, because MAOIs are known to interact with opioids, their use should be limited by necessity. Meperidine is the most commonly involved of the narcotics, but, with the exception of fentanyl, they all have the possibility of precipitating a hyperpyrexic response that can be confused with malignant hyperthermia and carry a similar potential for mortality. Postoperative pain control can be achieved with minimal use of opioids and employment of alternatives such as NSAIDs, and regional anesthesia is preferred whenever possible [13].

Lithium Carbonate

Mechanism of Action

Lithium carbonate was the first and is still the most important antimanic agent. While the mechanism of action of lithium is still not precisely understood, lithium is widely distributed throughout the CNS, where it is believed to have a variety of effects. It is known that lithium interacts with many neurotransmitter systems, increasing the synthesis of serotonin while decreasing norepinephrine release, and these effects are thought to be responsible for its clinical effect.

Side Effects

Lithium has a very narrow therapeutic level, so monitoring for toxicity must continually occur. Lithium toxicity is evidenced by weakness, sedation, ataxia, and widening of the QRS complex on the electrocardiogram. These symptoms in patients receiving lithium demand drug withdrawal and testing of serum lithium levels, because with greater toxicity, atrioventricular blockade, cardiovascular instability, seizures, and death may result.

Besides the possibility of toxicity, lithium also has long-term effects that require periodic monitoring. Lithium is known to inhibit the release of thyroid hormones, resulting in hypothyroidism in as many as 5 % of patients receiving the drug. It may also cause nephrogenic diabetes insipidus that does not respond to treatment with vasopressin. In a small percentage of patients, leukocytosis may develop, noted as a white blood cell count between 10,000 and 14,000 cells/mm. All of these effects resolve with withdrawal of the drug but mandate periodic testing of patients' thyroid levels, urine osmolality, and white blood cell count. In patients with known sinus nodal dysfunction, it may be prudent first to place a permanent pacemaker secondary to possible disturbances of the cardiac conduction system by lithium treatment [3].

Clinical Pearls and Drug Interactions

Lithium is the most commonly prescribed drug for bipolar disorder, and lithium interacts with several classes of anesthetic agents. Firstly, lithium prolongs the duration of several nondepolarizing neuromuscular relaxants because of lithium's ability to replace sodium in the propagation of action potentials [14]. So clinicians need to adjust the dosing and selecting the appropriate nondepolarizing muscle relaxants. Secondly, due to the blocking effects of lithium on the release of epinephrine and norepinephrine from the brainstem, the MAC of many volatile agents is reduced in patients receiving lithium. Thus, a patient's emergence from general anesthesia may potentially be affected [15].

Pharmacology for Nonaffective Psychosis

Mechanism of Action

The method of action of all antipsychotics is direct interference with the centrally located dopaminergic neurotransmitter system. Older antipsychotics such as haloperidol have been largely replaced in clinical practice with atypical antipsychotics (Tables 36.2, 36.3, and 36.4). Furthermore, they have been shown to stimulate the parasympathetic and to block the effects of the α-adrenergic stimulation of the sympathetic nervous system.

Black Box Warnings: Ziprasidone
This medicine should not be administered to patients who have a known history of or demonstrated QT prolongation, with a recent acute myocardial infarction, or with uncompensated heart failure (www.fda.gov).

Side effects are numerous, and some of the concerns beyond black box warnings listed above can be accentuated intraoperatively and postoperatively related to hypovolemia during general or regional anesthesia including hypotension, tachycardia, ventricular fibrillation, and torsades de pointes.

Most antipsychotics are metabolized by the cytochrome P450 enzyme system.

The incidence of extrapyramidal side effects is higher with older, more potent agents such as haloperidol. With the advent of clozapine, the incidence of these side effects has decreased markedly. However, they still occur and can be life-threatening. One such reaction that is seen rarely is laryngospasm, requiring treatment with an anticholinergic medication or diphenhydramine. Nearly every neuroleptic medication may cause tardive dyskinesia, with clozapne posing the least risk.

Black Box Warnings

(www.fda.gov) for clozapine include:

- Agranulocytosis, which can be life-threatening and therefore baseline, intratreatment periods, and 4 weeks after discontinuation, white blood cell counts and absolute neutrophil counts should be performed.
- Seizure (higher dose further increases the risk)
- Myocarditis
- Suicidal behavior with discontinuation

  Additional side effects include:

- Orthostatic hypotension, with or without syncope
- Respiratory and/or cardiac arrest
- Increased adverse effects noted with concomitant use of benzodiazepines or any other psychotropic drug

Nonaffective Psychoses Medications *(Tables 36.2, 36.3, and 36.4)*

Clinical Pearls

Perhaps the most feared complication of treatment with antipsychotics is neuroleptic malignant syndrome (NMS). NMS is very similar to malignant hypothermia (MH) and may share a similar etiologic mechanism. This syndrome most often occurs within the first several weeks of treatment with or a significant dosage increase of antipsychotic medications. It manifests as increased body temperature, skeletal muscle rigidity, and sympathetic nervous system instability (blood pressure fluctuations, diaphoresis, and tachydysrhythmias). If these concerns become significant, muscle relaxation with a nondepolarizing neuromuscular blocking drug and subsequent mechanical ventilation of the lungs may become necessary [16]. The treatment of this disorder requires withdrawal of the offending agent and initiation of bromocriptine or dantrolene therapy. Of these two therapies, dantrolene is preferred by some practitioners because of bromocriptine potentially precipitating hypotension. Additional treatments are supportive and include antipyretics, intravenous hydration, and dialysis, in addition to those measures just described. Mortality in untreated cases can be as high as 20 %. If the patient survives, further treatment with antipsychotics is usually not suggested secondary to the possibility of recurrence. In these patients, alternative therapies like lithium or ECT are advocated.

Physicians are more acutely aware of mood disorders and nonaffective psychoses than in previous times. As a result, there has been a dramatic increase in the number of pharmacologic options for these patients. Because of this, there has been a substantial increase in the number of patients presenting to the hospital for surgery

Table 36.2 Typical neuroleptics

Structure	Generic name	Proprietary name	Route	PO dosage (mg/d)
Phenothiazine (aliphatic)	Chlorpromazine	Thorazine	PO, IM	20–800
Phenothiazine (piperidine)	Thioridazine	Mellaril	PO	105–800
Phenothiazine (piperazine)	Fluphenazine	Prolixin	PO, IM, SC	1–20
Phenothiazine (piperazine)	Perphenazine	Trilafon	PO, IM	12–64
Phenothiazine (piperazine)	Trifluoperazine	Stelazine	PO, IM	4–20
Thioxanthene	Thiothixene	Navane	PO	6–60
Butyrophenone	Haloperidol	Haldol	PO, IM	1–20
Diphenylbutylpiperidine	Pimozide	Orap	PO	1–10
Dibenzoxazepine	Loxapine	Loxitane	PO	20–250
Dihydroindolone	Molindone	Moban	PO	50–225

Parenteral doses are generally twice as potent as oral doses, *PO* oral, *IM* intramuscular, *SC* subcutaneous
[a]Dosage information taken from Tarascon Pocket Pharmacopoeia mg/d: milligrams per day

Table 36.3 Atypical neuroleptics

Structure	Generic name	Proprietary name	Route	PO dosage (mg/d)
Benzisoxazole	Risperidone	Risperdal	PO, IM	1–16
Dibenzodiazepine	Clozapine	Clozaril	PO	12.5–900
Thienobenzodiazepine	Olanzapine	Zyprexa	PO, IM	5–20
Dibenzothiazepine	Quetiapine	Seroquel	PO	50–800
Indole	Ziprasidone	Geodon	PO, IM	40–160

Parenteral doses are generally twice as potent as oral doses, *PO* oral, *IM* intramuscular, *SC* subcutaneous
[a]Dosage information taken from Tarascon Pocket Pharmacopoeia; mg/d: milligrams per day

Table 36.4 Recently approved FDA atypical neuroleptics

Structure	Generic name	Proprietary name	Route	Usual dosage range (mg/day)
Piperidinyl-benzisoxazole	Paliperidone	Invega	PO	3–12 mg/day
		Invega Sustenna	IM	39–234 mg/month
Dibenzo-oxepino pyrroles	Asenapine	Saphris	SL	10–20 mg/day
Piperidinyl-benzisoxazole	Iloperidone	Fanapt	PO	2–24 mg/day
Piperidinyl-benzisothiazole	Latuda	Lurasidone	PO	40–120 mg/day

Pertinent side effects of these medications: acute- and late-onset (tardive) extrapyramidal side effects, agranulocytosis, anticholinergic effects, disturbances of cardiac rhythm, dry mouth, dysregulation of temperature, hypersalivation, orthostatic hypotension, sedation, seizures, thromboembolism, tremors, and withdrawal symptoms

who are being treated with one or more of the above medications. Some of these medications can cause dramatic issues for the patient if the caregiver involved is unaware of their mechanism of action or possible side effects. The clinical anesthesiologist should appreciate the pharmacologic effects and side effects and drug interactions of these agents. On a positive note, newer psychiatric drugs are improved in terms of efficacy and side effects/drug interactions from those in the past. Regular review of evolving newer classes of psychiatric drugs is warranted, regardless of specialty or subspecialty.

Chemical Structures

Chemical Structure 36.1 Citalopram

Chemical Structure 36.2 Escitalopram

Chemical Structure 36.3 Glycopyrrolate

Chemical Structure 36.4 Haloperidol

Chemical Structure 36.5 Ziprasidone

Chemical Structure 36.6 Chlorpromazine

References

1. SG-Report:http://www.surgeongeneral.gov/library/mentalhealth/chapter2/sec2_1.html#epidemiology.
2. Kessler RC, Chiu WT, Demler O, Walters EE. Prevalence, severity, and comorbidity of twelve-month DSM-IV disorders in the National Comorbidity Survey Replication (NCS-R). Arch Gen Psychiatry. 2005;62(6):617–27.
3. Derrer SA, Helfaer MA. Evaluation of the psychiatric patient. In: Rogers MC, Tinker JH, Covino BG, Longnecker DE, editors. Principles and practice of anesthesiology. St. Louis: Mosby-Year Book; 1993. p. 567–74.

4. Barkin RL, Schwer WA, Barkin SJ. Recognition and management of depression in primary care: a focus on the elderly: a pharmacotherapeutic overview of the selection process among the traditional and new antidepressants. Am J Ther. 1999;7:205–26.
5. Zito JM, Safer DJ, dosReis S, et al. Rising prevalence of antidepressants among US youth. Pediatrics. 2002;109:721–7.
6. Haddox JD, Chapkowski SL. Neuropsychiatric drug use in pain management. In: Raj PP, Abrams BM, Benzon HT, et al., editors. Practical management of pain. 3rd ed. St. Louis: Mosby; 2000. p. 489–512.
7. Stevens JC, Wrighton SA. Interaction of the enantiomers of fluoxetine and norfluoxetine with human liver cytochrome P450. J Pharmacol Exp Ther. 1993;266:964–71.
8. Kaizar EE, Greenhouse JB, Seltman H, Kelleher K. Do antidepressants cause suicidality in children? A Bayesian meta-analysis. Clin Trials. 2006;3(2):73–90; discussion 91–8.
9. Gibbons RD, Brown CH, Hur K, Marcus SM, Bhaumik DK, Mann JJ. Relationship between antidepressants and suicide attempts: an analysis of the Veterans Health Administration data sets. Am J Psychiatry. 2007;164(7):1044–9.
10. Veith RC, Raskind MA, Caldwell JH, et al. Cardiovascular effects of tricyclic antidepressants in depressed patients with chronic heart disease. N Engl J Med. 1982;306:954–9.
11. El-Ganzouri AR, Ivankovich AD, Braverman B, et al. Monoamine oxidase inhibitors: should they be discontinued preoperatively? Anesth Analg. 1985;64:592–6.
12. Wong KC. Preoperative discontinuation of monoamine oxidase inhibitor therapy: an old wives' tale. Semin Anesthesiol. 1986;5:145–8.
13. Browne B, Linter S. Monoamine oxidase inhibitors and narcotic analgesics: a critical review of the implications for treatment. Br J Psychiatry. 1987;151:210–2.
14. Hill GE, Wong KC, Hodges MR. Lithium carbonate and neuromuscular blocking agents. Anesthesiology. 1977;46:122–6.
15. Lichtor JL. Anesthesia for ambulatory surgery. In: Barash PG, Cullen BF, Stoelting RK, editors. Clinical anesthesia. 4th ed. Philadelphia: Lippincott Williams & Wilkins; 2001. p. 1217–38.
16. Geiduschek J, Cohen SA, Khan A, Cullen BF. Repeated anesthesia for a patient with neuroleptic malignant syndrome. Anesthesiology. 1988;68:134–7.

Chapter 37
Cocaine, Methamphetamine, MDMA, and Heroin

Ethan O. Bryson

Contents

E.O. Bryson, MD
Departments of Anesthesiology and Psychiatry,
The Mount Sinai School of Medicine, New York, NY, USA
e-mail: ethan.bryson@mountsinai.org

A.D. Kaye et al. (eds.), *Essentials of Pharmacology for Anesthesia,*
Pain Medicine, and Critical Care, DOI 10.1007/978-1-4614-8948-1_37,
© Springer Science+Business Media New York 2015

Introduction

Though not as frequently as alcohol, cannabis, or tobacco, patients do present for surgery either under the influence of or having recently used drugs such as cocaine, methamphetamine, MDMA, and illicit opioids like heroin. The pharmacology of these drugs is not as well established as the anesthetic agents and other medications that have been developed for legitimate use, but since many of these drugs were once used licitly, the information is available. An understanding of the pharmacology of the drugs of abuse as well as the potential for drug-drug or drug-enzyme interaction is essential information for the perioperative health-care professional tasked with the management of the substance-abusing patient.

Cocaine

Cocaine (benzoylmethylecgonine), Chemical Structure 37.1 (see end of chapter), is a natural alkaloid with pharmacologically diverse properties derived from the Erythroxylon coca plant. It acts as a central nervous system stimulant and has significant sympathomimetic properties. First used by the Andean people to treat high-altitude fatigue in South America, cocaine has also been used as a topical local anesthetic, as a spinal anesthetic, and as a dilator of the pupil for cataract surgery [1]. In 1914, the Harrison Narcotic Act limited its medical use in the United States, though recreational use continues to increase. As recently as 2008, some 0.7 % of all adults reported using cocaine regularly in the United States, with 1.7 % of adults aged 18–25 using cocaine more than once per month [2]. Trauma patients requiring surgery are surprisingly likely to be recent users of cocaine, with one study reporting 38 % of patients had a serum or urine test positive for cocaine [3].

Mechanism of Action

Cocaine is lipophilic and readily diffuses across the blood-brain barrier where it acts centrally by inhibiting the action of monoamine transport proteins on presynaptic nerve terminals. Cocaine blocks the reuptake of the sympathomimetic neurotransmitters dopamine, norepinephrine, and serotonin prolonging adrenergic stimulation, primarily in the synaptic terminal and ventral basal nuclei of dopamine neurons. It inhibits the dopamine transporter, decreasing dopamine uptake from the synaptic cleft, and it is this amplified concentration of synaptic dopamine which is responsible for the euphoria experienced by users of this drug. Physiologic tolerance develops immediately, resulting in tachyphylaxis of subjective effects, and the need for increasingly larger doses of cocaine to achieve the same degree of euphoria is universally observed. In addition to the inhibition of the active reuptake of endogenously released norepinephrine from adrenergic nerve fibers [4], cocaine also blocks catecholamine-binding sites, increasing free norepinephrine levels which stimulate the cardiovascular system peripherally [5]. Sympathetic stimulation secondary to increased plasma levels of norepinephrine results in an increase in systolic, diastolic, and mean arterial blood pressure; heart rate; and core body temperature.

Cocaine blocks slow sodium channels and fast potassium channels in neuronal cell membranes to halt propagation of nerve impulses making it an effective local anesthetic. These effects vary according to concentration and can produce a wide spectrum of possible dysrhythmias and electrocardiographic findings [6]. At low concentrations, cocaine delays ventricular recovery, and at high concentrations, it speeds recovery. Cocaine has been implicated in prolongation of the QT interval by prolongation of the action potential duration [7]. Sodium and potassium channel blockade results in QRS and QTc prolongation and may be the mechanism for the induction of ventricular arrhythmias such as torsades de pointes, monomorphic ventricular tachycardia, accelerated idioventricular rhythms, or Brugada syndrome [8]. Various types of bundle branch blocks, supraventricular tachycardia, asystole, and ventricular fibrillation have also been reported [9].

Adverse Effects

The acute adverse effects of cocaine ingestion are primarily related to vasoconstriction and hypertension. These effects are immediate and result from the inhibition of catecholamine reuptake and decreased production of the vasodilator nitric oxide. Arrhythmias, systemic and pulmonary hypertension, tachycardia, coronary vasoconstriction, and cardiac ischemia have all been reported. The risk of developing flash pulmonary edema, myocardial infarction, dissection of any artery including the coronaries and aorta, and sudden death is increased in at-risk patients. Interestingly, the risk of coronary artery vasospasm resulting in ischemia-induced cardiac arrhythmias is high immediately after ingestion but remains elevated even after the level of sympathetic stimulation returns to pre-ingestion baseline [10]. This is probably due to chronic changes such as myocardial hypertrophy, hypertrophic cardiomyopathy, and accelerated atherosclerosis and possibly the development of a prothrombotic state [11]. Delayed vasoconstriction occurs secondary to the production of active metabolites. Over time, the chronic cocaine user develops pathology related to the compensatory mechanisms of the organs exposed to chronically elevated blood pressure.

Methamphetamine

Methamphetamine (Chemical Structure 37.2 – see end of chapter) is a synthetic derivative of amphetamine with limited medical use and high abuse potential. It is a schedule II drug and currently available only through a prescription that cannot be refilled. Once ingested, this non-catecholamine exerts its effects through sympathetic nervous system activation in a manner similar to that of cocaine with both increased release of and decreased reuptake of endogenous catecholamines [12]. As with cocaine, heart rate and blood pressure are increased and appetite and fatigue are suppressed. Time of onset and effects of the drug vary, depending on the route of administration, but the typical half-life is about 12 h.

Mechanism of Action

Methamphetamine acts directly to release an initial surge of dopamine from presynaptic nerve terminals. In the process these nerve terminals, as well as adjacent serotonin-releasing nerve terminals, are damaged [13]. Subsequent methamphetamine use does not produce the same subjective effects experienced by the user due to a permanent structural change in brain chemistry, and imaging studies performed on the brains of human methamphetamine addicts have shown alterations in the activity of the dopamine system [14].

Adverse Effects

Chronically increased levels of circulating catecholamines result in vasoconstriction, and the chronic methamphetamine abuser will behave physiologically as a chronic, poorly controlled hypertensive; blood pressure may be labile and difficult to control [15]. Long-term exposure to methamphetamine can lead to left ventricular hypertrophy and a propensity for arrhythmias similar to that seen in chronic cocaine users. Decreased cardiac compliance, diastolic dysfunction, and heart failure are common [16]. The extreme weight loss associated with long-term abuse can significantly decrease levels of albumin and affect both protein binding and metabolism of many common anesthetic agents. Severe dental problems are common, including chronic infections, loose teeth, and oral abscesses that may present a significant issue with airway management.

Damage to the smaller cerebral arteries can lead to areas of focal ischemia in the brainstem resulting in persistent stereotyped and uncontrolled movements. These physical alterations in the biochemical structure of the brain have been associated with reduced motor skills and impaired verbal learning and may also be responsible for the emotional lability commonly seen in chronic methamphetamine abusers.

Acutely, the development of anxiety, confusion, insomnia, mood disturbances, and violent behavior is common. Chronic methamphetamine use may result in psychotic features such as paranoia; visual, auditory, and tactile hallucinations; and delusions.

MDMA

MDMA (3,4-methylenedioxymethamphetamine or Ecstasy, Chemical Structure 37.3 at the end of the chapter) was first patented in 1914 by Merck Pharmaceuticals as an appetite suppressant [17, 18], subsequently used as a psychotherapeutic drug [19, 20], and given its high abuse potential, eventually classified by the Drug Enforcement Administration (DEA) as a Schedule I drug in the 1980s. MDMA is usually taken orally as a small pill or capsule although it can be crushed and snorted or dissolved for injection [21]. No commercial preparations are available, so the drug is now produced illegally with variable purity and little quality control [22]. MDMA is structurally similar to both the hallucinogen mescaline and the stimulant amphetamine. It is a psychostimulant drug that produces effects similar to other stimulants such as methamphetamine and other psychedelics such as mescaline, as well as a number of distinctive effects. Most users report experiencing euphoria, happiness stimulation, and a general sense of well-being. Effects related to cardio-vascular stimulation and autonomic effects such as dry mouth, sweating, restless-ness, tremor, jaw clenching, and restlessness are less common but do occur in a number of patients [23].

Mechanism of Action

MDMA increases the release and decreases reuptake of serotonin, dopamine, and norepinephrine from presynaptic nerve terminals in the mammalian brain [24, 25] through direct interaction of the drug with the membrane transporters involved with the uptake and storage of these neurotransmitters [26]. The drug has been shown to have both direct agonist properties at serotonergic and dopaminergic receptors as well as mild inhibition of monoamine oxidase (MAO) [27].

Adverse Effects

Serotonergic overload in the hypothalamic thermoregulatory center has led to hyper-thermia [28–30], with temperatures as high as 42 °C recorded [31], and sustained muscular activity with a disregard for normal body signals such as thirst is thought to compound central effects [32, 33]. Hyponatremia secondary to inappropriate antidiuretic hormone release (SIADH) and excessive water intake is less common but has been reported as well as acute fulminant liver failure secondary to hepatic necrosis [34].

Anesthetic Considerations for Patients Who Abuse Stimulant-Type Drugs

Patients may report recent illicit stimulant use during the preanesthetic interview, which begs the question: should an elective case be postponed under these circumstances? Since most deaths related to stimulant abuse are not due to overdose but to pathophysiology developed from long-term use, it would seem the risk would not decline significantly by delaying the case. Most now believe that asymptomatic patients with a normal blood pressure, heart rate, ECG, and temperature may have elective surgeries performed without increased risk of complications [35]. It is reasonable, however, to view chronic stimulant abuse as a risk factor for the physiologic consequences of long-term use much in the way that chronic hypertension due to some other mechanism increases the risk for end-organ damage. These patients should have a preoperative workup of specific organ-system complaints before elective cases.

Heroin

Opioids are either naturally occurring compounds extracted from the poppy plant (*Papaver somniferum*) or synthetic and semisynthetic derivatives designed as agonists to the same receptor(s). Forms of these drugs have been available for recreational and medicinal use for thousands of years and can be taken orally, nasally, subcutaneously, or intravenously to produce analgesia, euphoria, or both [36]. Heroin (Chemical Structure 37.4 – see end of chapter) is a semisynthetic derivative of naturally occurring opioids. The increasing availability of this highly addictive drug in increasing purity and decreasing cost has resulted in a new generation of addicts who primarily use the drug nasally instead of intravenously [37]. The epidemic of prescription drug addicts who no longer fit the classic image of the "dropout" who uses heroin on the edge of society is increasingly turning to heroin as tighter controls are placed on controlled prescription opioids [38].

Mechanism of Action

Heroin, regardless of the route of administration, is enzymatically converted to morphine and produces euphoria and other alterations in mood by stimulating the release of dopamine from specific nerves originating from the ventral tegmental area of the mammalian brain. Even a small dose induces positive signal changes visible on functional magnetic resonance imaging (fMRI) studies of reward structures such as the nucleus accumbens, amygdala, cortex, and hippocampus [39]. Dopamine released from neurons of the presynaptic ventral tegmental area into the nucleus accumbens causes euphoria, reinforces behavior, and is responsible for the generation of craving and the psychological aspects of withdrawal. The mesocortical dopamine circuit includes projections from the ventral tegmental area to the cortex and anterior cingulate allowing for conscious experience of effects including drug craving and compulsion to take more [40].

There are three opioid receptor types (μ, δ, and k), and each is coupled to the Gi/o protein present in the nucleus accumbens [41]. Agonists selective for the μ- and δ-receptors produce reward, while selective κ-receptor agonists produce aversive effects [42]. Activation of the μ, δ, and k receptor inhibits adenylate cyclase, reducing intracellular cyclic adenosine monophosphate (AMP) levels; decreases cAMP-dependent protein kinase A activity; and reduces phosphorylation of cytoplasmic and nuclear targets [43]. Neuronal transmission is reduced through inhibition of the voltage-gated Ca^{2+} channel and activation of the inwardly rectifying K^+ channels [44].

The locus ceruleus is thought to play a critical role in feelings of alarm, panic, fear, and anxiety, and it contains high concentrations of noradrenergic neurons and opioid receptors. Agonist activity at μ-receptors in this area results in inhibition of neural activity and is likely responsible for generating feelings of calm and anxiolysis [45].

Adverse Effects

Heroin carries an extremely high risk for abuse and the development of addiction. Characteristics such as rapid onset and intensity of effect increase this potential [46]. Genetic factors also influence the metabolism of drugs and may make some people more prone to developing addiction when exposed. For example, CYP2D6 partial activity occurs in approximately 5–10 % of whites, 1 % of Asians, 20 % of African-Americans, and 3 % of Mexican Americans, and a deficiency in CYP2D6 gene results in the inability to enzymatically convert codeine to morphine, preventing codeine abuse [47].

The development of tolerance and hypersensitivity after repeated exposure is common. Several mechanisms to explain the development of tolerance which have been proposed include the uncoupling of G proteins from receptors such that they are still expressed on the surface of cells but are less responsive (desensitization) and the internalization of activated opioid receptors (downregulation) through endocytosis such that the actual number of receptors expressed on the cell surface is reduced [48]. Hypersensitivity to opioids is characterized by dramatically increased sensitivity to painful stimuli and is thought to develop through spinal sensitization to glutamate and substance P [49]. Allodynia (pain is elicited by a normally non-painful stimulus) may occur secondary to NMDA receptor agonist action and as NMDA antagonists have been shown to be an effective treatment [50].

Anesthetic Considerations for Patients Who Abuse Heroin

The chronic use of heroin is associated with the development of tolerance to other opioids and related drugs, and such patients will require a greater amount of opioid anesthetics per weight than the opioid-naive patient [37]. As well, patients who have developed opiate hyperalgesia or hyperesthesia may have become hypersensitive to surgical and other stimuli and may require even higher doses of anesthetic agents than would be expected from tolerance alone. Agents such as ketamine should be considered in refractory cases. The wide range of cutting agents used to reduce the purity of heroin (sugar, starch, acetaminophen, procaine, benzocaine, quinine, steroids, clenbuterol, or even fentanyl [51–53]) may cause any number of unanticipated problems encountered in the heroin-abusing patient. The recent availability of higher-purity heroin has allowed a larger percentage of users to either snort or smoke heroin, reducing but not eliminating the prevalence of syringe-borne diseases, such as HIV and hepatitis [54, 55].

Summary

The management of the substance-abusing patient can present a significant challenge during the perioperative period. The perioperative health-care professional needs to be aware of the basic pharmacologic properties of the drugs of abuse and maintain a high index of suspicion regarding illicit use. The acutely intoxicated patient and the chronic abuser in withdrawal can present in ways that can mimic other organic processes and may, in fact, obscure the presentation of concurrent medical issues. Often these drugs contain contaminants which can react with licit medications in unexpected ways. Inhibition or enhancement of expected activity has been reported and is often not possible to predict. Careful evaluation and supportive management is key, keeping an eye out for unsuspected reactions. The perioperative health-care professional can and should play an important role in the identification of the substance-abusing patient and encourage subsequent referral for detoxification and treatment.

Chemical Structures

Chemical Structure
37.1 Cocaine
(benzoylmethylecgonine)

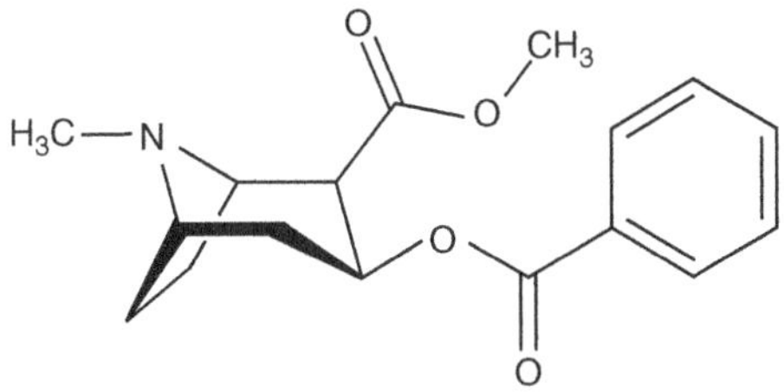

Chemical Structure
37.2 Methamphetamine
(*N*-methylamphetamine)

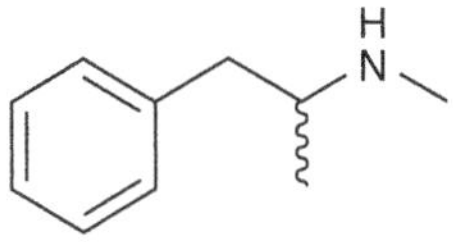

Chemical Structure
37.3 MDMA
(3,4-methylenedioxy-*N*-
methylamphetamine)

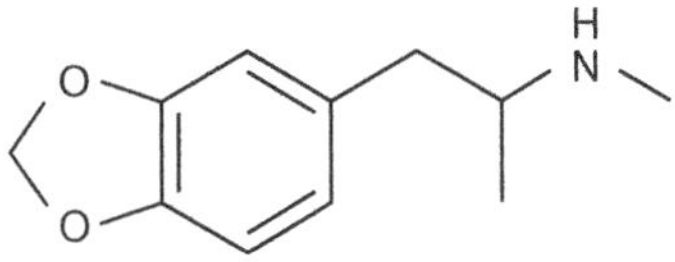

Chemical Structure
37.4 Heroin
(diacetylmorphine or
morphine diacetate)

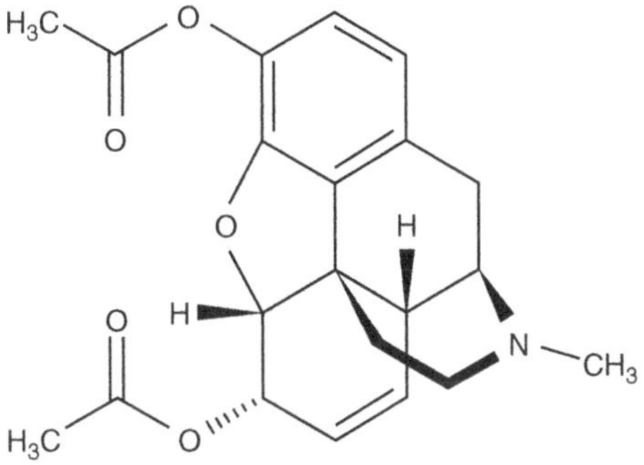

References

1. Katzung BG. "Drugs of abuse". Basic and clinical pharmacology. 10th ed. New York: McGraw-Hill companies; 2007. p. 518–23.
2. US Department of Health and Human Services. National survey on drug use and health. Washington, DC: US Department of Health and Human Services; 2008.
3. Brookoff D, Campbell EA, Shaw LM. The underreporting of cocaine-related trauma: drug abuse warning network reports vs hospital toxicology tests. Am J Public Health. 1993;83(3):369–71.
4. Jatlow PI. Drug of abuse profile: cocaine. Clin Chem. 1987;33:66B–71.
5. Hertting G, Axelrod J, Whitby LG. Effect of drugs on the uptake and metabolism of H3-norepinephrine. J Pharmacol Exp Ther. 1961;134:146–53.

6. Kaye AD, Weinkauf JL. The cocaine addicted patient. In: Bryson EO, Frost EAM, editors. Perioperative addiction. New York: Springer Science and Business Media; 2011.
7. Wang Z, Fermini B, Nattel S. Mechanism of flecainide's rate-dependent actions on action potential duration in canine atrial tissue. J Pharmacol Exp Ther. 1993;267:575–81.
8. Bauman JL, Grawe JJ, Winecoff AP, Hariman RJ. Cocaine-related sudden cardiac death: a hypothesis correlating basic science and clinical observations. J Clin Pharmacol. 1994;34:902–11.
9. Afonso L, Mohammad T, Thatai D. Crack whips the heart: a review of the cardiovascular toxicity of cocaine. Am J Cardiol. 2007;100(6):1040–3.
10. Lucena J, Blanco M, Jurado C, Rico A, Salguero M, Vazquez R, Thiene G, Basso C. Cocaine-related sudden death: a prospective investigation in south-west Spain. Eur Heart J. 2010;31(3):318–29.
11. Heesch CM, Negus BH, Steiner M. Effects of in vivo cocaine administration on human platelet aggregation. Am J Cardiol. 1996;78:237–9.
12. Yu Q, Montes S, Larson D, Watson RR. Effects of chronic methamphetamine exposure on heart function in uninfected and retrovirus-infected mice. Life Sci. 1995;75:29–43.
13. National Institute on Drug Abuse. Methamphetamine abuse and addiction: what is methamphetamine? Bethesda: National Institute of Health; 1998. NIDA research report series, NIH publication 98-4210.
14. Volkow ND, Chang L, Wang GJ, et al. Association of dopamine transporter reduction with psychomotor impairment in methamphetamine abusers. Am J Psychiatry. 2001;158(3):377–82.
15. Bryson EO. Spotlight on methamphetamine. In: Bryson EO, Frost EAM, editors. Perioperative addiction. New York: Springer Science and Business Media; 2011.
16. Karch SB, Stephens BG, Ho CH. Methamphetamine related deaths in San Francisco; demographic, pathologic and toxicologic profiles. J Forensic Sci. 1999;44:359–68.
17. Suarez RV, Riemersma R. "Ecstasy" and sudden cardiac death. Am J Forensic Med Pathol. 1988;9:339–41.
18. Shulgin AT. The background and chemistry of MDMA. J Psychoactive Drugs. 1986;18:291–304.
19. Greer GR, Tolbert R. A method of conducting therapeutic sessions with MDMA. J Psychoactive Drugs. 1998;30(4):371–9.
20. Greer G, Tolbert R. Subjective reports of the effects of MDMA in a clinical setting. J Psychoactive Drugs. 1986;18:319–27.
21. DeMaria Jr S. Club drugs: methylenedioxymethamphetamine, flunitrazepam, ketamine hydrochloride, and gamma-hydroxybutyrate. In: Bryson EO, Frost EAM, editors. Perioperative addiction. New York: Springer Science and Business Media; 2011.
22. Wolff K, Hay AWM, Sherlock K, Conner M. Contents of "ecstasy". Lancet. 1995;346:1100–1.
23. De la Torre R, Farre M, Roset PN, Pizarro N, Abanades S, Segura M. Human pharmacology of MDMA: pharmacokinetics, metabolism, and disposition. Ther Drug Monit. 2004;26:137–44.
24. Morgan MJ. Ecstasy (MDMA): a review of its possible persistent psychological effects. Psychopharmacology (Berl). 2000;152:230–48.
25. Morton J. Ecstasy: pharmacology and neurotoxicity. Curr Opin Pharmacol. 2005;5:79–86.
26. De la Torre R, Yubero-Lahoz S, Pardo-Lozano R, Farre M. MDMA, methamphetamine, and CYP2D6 pharmacogenetics: what is clinically relevant? Front Genet. 2012;3:235, 1–8.
27. Battaglia G, Yeh SY, De Souza EB. MDMA-induced neurotoxicity: parameters of degeneration and recovery of brain serotonin neurons. Pharmacol Biochem Behav. 1988;29(2):269–74.
28. Hall AP. "Ecstasy" and the anaesthetist. Br J Anaesth. 1997;79:697–8.
29. Milroy CM, Clark JC, Forrest ARW. Pathology of deaths associated with "Ecstasy" and "Eve" misuse. J Clin Pathol. 1996;49:149–53.
30. Schmidt CJ, Black CK, Abbate GM, Taylor VL. MDMA induced hyperthermia and neurotoxicity are independently mediated by 5-HT2 receptors. Brain Res. 1990;529:85–90.

31. Logan ASC, Stickle B, O'Keefe N, Hewitson H. Survival following 'Ecstasy' ingestion with a peak temperature of 42°C. Anaesthesia. 1993;48:1017–8.
32. Nimmo SM, Kennedy BW, Tullett WM, Blyth AS, Dougall JR. Drug-induced hyperthermia. Anaesthesia. 1993;48(10):892–5.
33. Benowitz NL. Amphetamines. In: Olson KR, editor. Poisoning and drug overdose. 3rd ed. Stamford: Appleton & Lange; 1999. p. 68–70.
34. Henry JA, Hill IR. Fatal interaction between ritonavir and MDMA. Lancet. 1998;352:1751–2.
35. Hill GE, Ogunnaike BO, Johnson ER. General anaesthesia for the cocaine abusing patient: is it safe? Br J Anaesth. 2006;97:654–7.
36. Gutstein Howard B, Akil Huda. Chapter 21: Opioid analgesics. In: Brunton LL, Lazo JS, Parker KL, editors. The pharmacological basis of therapeutics. 11th ed. New York: Goodman & Gilman's; Accessed online 24 Nov 2012.
37. Bryson EO. The anesthetic implications of illicit opioid abuse. Int Anesthesiol Clin. 2011;49(1):67–78.
38. Substance Abuse and Mental Health Services Administration. Results from the 2008 National Survey on Drug Use and Health: National Findings (Office of Applied Studies, NSDUH Series H-36, HHS Publication No. SMA 09-4434). Rockville; 2009. http://www.oas.samhsa.gov/nsduh/2k8nsduh/2k8Results.pdf. Accessed 24 Nov 2012.
39. Becerra L, Harter K, Gonzalez RG, Borsook D. Functional magnetic resonance imaging measures of the effects of morphine on central nervous system circuitry in opioid-naive healthy volunteers. Anesth Analg. 2006;103:208–16.
40. Lewis M, Souki F. The anesthetic implications of acute opioid intoxication and dependence. In: Bryson EO, Frost EAM, editors. Perioperative addiction. New York: Springer Science and Business Media; 2011.
41. Trescot A, Datta S, Lee M, Hansen H. Opioid pharmacology. Pain Phys. 2008;11:S133–53.
42. Stoelting RK. Opioids agonists and antagonists. In: Stoelting RK, Hillier S, editors. Pharmacology & physiology in anesthetic practice. 4th ed. Baltimore: Lippincott Williams & Wilkins; 2006. p. 87–126.
43. Nestler EJ. Molecular neurobiology of addiction. Am J Addict. 2001;10:201–17.
44. Fukuda K. Intravenous opioid anesthetics. In: Miller RD, editor. Miller's anesthesia. 6th ed. Philadelphia: Elsevier; 2005.
45. Camí J, Farré M. Drug addiction. N Engl J Med. 2003;349:975–86.
46. Roset P, Farre M, de la Torre R, et al. Modulation of rate of onset and intensity of drug effects reduces abuse potential in healthy males. Drug Alcohol Depend. 2001;64:285–98.
47. Kathiramalainathan K, Kaplan HL, Romach MK, et al. Inhibition of cytochrome P450 2D6 modifies codeine abuse liability. J Clin Psychopharmacol. 2000;20:435–44.
48. Joseph EK, Reichling DB, Levine JD. Shared mechanisms for opioid tolerance and a transition to chronic pain. J Neurosci. 2010;30(13):4660–6.
49. Angst MS, Clark JD. Opioid-induced hyperalgesia: a qualitative systematic review. Anesthesiology. 2006;104:570–87.
50. Mizoguchi H, Watanabe C, Yonezawa A, Sakurada S. New therapy for neuropathic pain. Int Rev Neurobiol. 2009;85:249–60.
51. Koushesh HR, Afshari R. A new illicit opioid dependence outbreak, evidence for a combination of opioids and steroids. Drug Chem Toxicol. 2009;32(2):114–9.
52. Wingert WE, Mundy LA, Nelson L, Wong SC, Curtis J. Detection of clenbuterol in heroin users in twelve postmortem cases at the Philadelphia medical examiner's office. J Anal Toxicol. 2008;32(7):522–8.
53. Ojanperä I, Gergov M, Rasanen I, Lunetta P, Toivonen S, Tiainen E, Vuori E. Blood levels of 3-methylfentanyl in 3 fatal poisoning cases. Am J Forensic Med Pathol. 2006;27(4):328–31.
54. Office of Applied Studies, Substance Abuse and Mental Health Services Administration, 2007. http://www.samhsa.gov/data/2k7/heroinTX/heroinTX.pdf. Accessed 1 Jun 2014.
55. Broz D, Ouellet LJ. Prevalence and correlates of former injection drug use among young non-injecting heroin users in Chicago. Subst Use Misuse. 2010;45(12):2000–25.

Part III
Clinical Subspecialties

Chapter 38
Cardiac Surgery

Henry Liu, Hong Yan, Ming Chen, Mingbing Chen,
Charles Fox, and Alan David Kaye

Contents

H. Liu, MD (✉) • M. Chen, MD
Department of Anesthesiology, Tulane University Medical Center,
New Orleans, LA 70112, USA
e-mail: henryliula1@gmail.com

H. Yan, MD
Department of Anesthesiology, Wuhan Central Hospital, Wuhan, China

M. Chen, MD
Department of Anesthesiology, Hubei Women and Children's Hospital, Wuhan, China

C. Fox, MD
Department of Anesthesiology, LSU Health Science Center Shreveport,
Shreveport, LA, USA
e-mail: cfox1@lsuhsc.edu

A.D. Kaye, MD, PhD
Department of Anesthesiology, Louisiana State University Health Sciences Center,
New Orleans, LA 70112, USA

A.D. Kaye et al. (eds.), *Essentials of Pharmacology for Anesthesia,*
Pain Medicine, and Critical Care, DOI 10.1007/978-1-4614-8948-1_38,
© Springer Science+Business Media New York 2015

Basic Cardiac Anatomy and Physiology

1. Cardiac function relies on its normal electric initiation and conduction, myocardial contractility, and all four valves ensuring the blood flowing in normal direction. To maintain this function, adequate coronary blood/oxygen supply to the heart is critical. In basic cardiac electric system, the rhythmic cardiac contraction originates spontaneously in the sinoatrial node (SA) located in the wall of RA adjacent to superior jugular vein (SVC) opening; electric impulse is conducted to the atrioventricular node (AV) located at the lower part of atrial septum immediately above the attachment of septal cusp of tricuspid valve; then the electric signal travels to the bundle of His (or AV bundle) and continues to the right bundle branch and left bundle branch and finally extends into the small Purkinje fibers. In cardiac cycle, after RA and LA receive systemic venous return and pulmonary blood return, respectively, atrial contractions move blood into RV and LV, respectively; this is the diastole. Then LV contracts to propel blood into aorta and then systemic circulation, and RV contracts to force blood into pulmonary artery; thus, deoxygenated blood gets oxygenation in the lungs. This phase is called systole.

2. Excitation-Contraction Coupling: During systole, there is a 50-fold increase in intracellular calcium concentrations. The cardiac action potential is responsible for the increase in intracellular calcium in two ways: Calcium ions enter the cell from the extracellular space during the plateau phase of action potential, and the spike of the action potential triggers the release of calcium from the intracellular stores within the sarcoplasmic reticulum [1]. This coupling is the physiological process of converting an electric stimulus (action potential) to a mechanical response (myocardial contraction). An action potential arrives to depolarize the cell membrane resulting in an increase in cytosolic calcium level. The cytoplasmic calcium binds to troponin C, moving the troponin complex off the actin binding site allowing the myosin head to bind to the actin filament. By hydrolyzing ATP, myosin can now cycle through attached and detached states to actin. The attached states are known as "cross bridges" between the actin and myosin filaments. Activation of this cross-bridge cycling may induce sarcomere shortening and of the muscle as a whole.

3. Blood Supply to the Heart: The coronary arteries supply oxygenated blood to the heart. Both left coronary artery and right coronary artery (RCA) originate from the root of ascending aorta just above aortic valve. Left coronary artery extends into left anterior descending artery (LAD) and left circumflex coronary artery (LCCA). Most of the blood flow to the LV occurs in diastole when aortic blood pressure exceeds the LV chamber pressure, but coronary blood flow to the RA, LA, and RV occurs throughout the cardiac cycle because both systolic and diastolic aortic blood pressures are greater than the pressure within these cardiac chambers [2].

4. Left Ventricular Preload and Afterload: LV afterload is the aortic blood pressure. LV preload is the end-diastolic LV volume (EDLVV), not EDLVP, which is often

misunderstood as the LV preload. Currently, we have been using EDLVP as an alternative LV preload parameter because EDLVV is not easy to measure in clinical practice with current technology.

5. Starling's Law: The more myocardial fibers are stretched (or greater the diastolic volume of the heart) within the physiological limits, the greater the energy of the ensuing contraction. Beyond these limits, the energy of contraction falls off.

Drugs Commonly Used in Cardiac Anesthesiology

Anesthetic management for cardiac surgical procedures involves many different categories of drugs. The commonly used drugs in cardiac anesthesia will be discussed in this chapter.

Anticoagulation and Blood-Preserving Drugs

Heparin

(a) Introduction: Heparin is the most commonly used anticoagulant in clinical use for many decades. It physiologically exists in the mast cells. Heparin in current medical practice is extracted from either bovine lungs or porcine intestine, with molecular weights ranging from 3,000 to 40,000 Da.

(b) Drug Class: Highly sulfated and negatively charged glycosaminoglycan polymer.
Mechanism of Action: Heparin works by binding to antithrombin III (AT III) and potentiates AT-III's effect by 1,000-folds, thus inhibiting thrombin and Factor Xa.

(c) Indications: Used for the systemic anticoagulation during cardiopulmonary bypass for cardiac procedures, vascular procedures, and other scenarios in which systemic or regional anticoagulation is necessary.
Clinical Pearls:
When loading dose of heparin is given, sometimes it can induce hypotension due to the histamine effect because heparin is extracted from mast cells, which contain high concentration of histamine. So some commercial product might contain small amount of histamine. In this situation, a small dose of phenylephrine will prevent or treat the hypotension induced by heparin.

(d) Dosing Options: The traditional dosing strategy is giving 30,000 units to initiate systemic anticoagulation. Now the heparin dose is calculated by perfusionists or anesthesia providers. For other vascular procedures, usually we give 5,000 units to prevent thrombosis. Activated clotting time (ACT) is currently used to monitor the effect of heparin.

(e) Drug Interactions:

- Oral anticoagulants: Heparin may prolong the one-stage prothrombin time (PT). Therefore, when heparin sodium is given with warfarin sodium, a period of at least 5 h after the last intravenous dose should elapse before the blood is drawn if a valid PT is to be obtained.
- Platelet inhibitors: Drugs such as acetylsalicylic acid, dextran, phenylbutazone, ibuprofen, indomethacin, dipyridamole, hydroxychloroquine, and others that interfere with platelet aggregation reactions may induce bleeding and should be used with caution in patients receiving heparin sodium.
- Other Interactions: Tetracyclines, digitalis, nicotine, antihistamines, or nitroglycerin may partially counteract the anticoagulant action of heparin sodium.
- Drug/Laboratory Test Interactions: In patients with hyperaminotransferasemia, significant elevations of aminotransferase (SGOT [S-AST] and SGPT [SALT]) levels have occurred in a high percentage of patients (and healthy subjects) who have received heparin. Since aminotransferase determinations are important in the differential diagnosis of myocardial infarction, liver disease, and pulmonary emboli, rises that might be caused by drugs (like heparin) should be interpreted with caution.

(f) Side Effects: Hemorrhage, allergic reaction, thrombocytopenia, altered protein binding, decreased MAP, decreased antithrombin III level, etc.

Argatroban

(a) Introduction: Argatroban is used for patients with heparin-induced thrombocytopenia (HIT). Argatroban is given intravenously, and its half-life is 50 min. It is monitored with activated partial thromboplastin time (aPTT) or ACT. It is metabolized in the liver. It can be used in patients with renal insufficiency, different from lepirudin, which is better avoided in renal patient.

(b) Drug Class: Small-molecule direct thrombin inhibitor.
Mechanism of Action: Argatroban exerts its anticoagulant effects by inhibiting thrombin-catalyzed or thrombin-induced reactions, including fibrin formation; activation of coagulation Factors V, VIII, and XIII; activation of protein C; and platelet aggregation. Argatroban does not require the cofactor antithrombin III for antithrombotic activity.

(c) Indications/Clinical Pearls:

- Prophylaxis or treatment of thrombosis in patients with HIT or at risk for HIT
- Percutaneous coronary interventions in patients with HIT
- Systemic anticoagulation for cardiac surgery in patients with HIT

(d) Dosing Options: Initially infusion at 2 µg/kg/min.

(e) Drug Interactions:

- Heparin: If argatroban is to be initiated after cessation of heparin therapy, allow sufficient time for heparin's effect on the aPTT to decrease prior to initiation of argatroban therapy.
- Oral anticoagulant agents: Pharmacokinetic drug-drug interactions between argatroban and warfarin (7.5 mg single oral dose) have not been demonstrated. However, the concomitant use of argatroban and warfarin (5–7.5 mg initial oral dose, followed by 2.5–6 mg/day orally for 6–10 days) results in PT prolongation.
- Glycoprotein IIb/IIIa antagonists: The safety and effectiveness of argatroban with glycoprotein IIb/IIIa antagonists have not been established.

(f) Side Effects: Major or minor bleeding, hives; difficulty breathing; swelling of your face, lips, tongue, or throat.

Bivalirudin (Trade Name Is Angiomax), Recombinant Hirudin (Lepirudin, Desirudin)

(a) Introduction: Hirudin is derived from the leech. Recombinant hirudin includes lepirudin, desirudin. Bivalirudin is a synthetic 20 amino acid peptide based on hirudin [3].

(b) Drug Class: A specific and reversible direct thrombin inhibitor.
Mechanism of Action: Bivalirudin binds both to the catalytic site and to the anion-binding exosite of circulating and clot-bound thrombin.

(c) Indications:

- Use as an anticoagulant in patients with unstable angina undergoing percutaneous transluminal coronary angioplasty (PTCA).
- Use as an anticoagulant with glycoprotein II/IIIa inhibitor in patients with unstable angina undergoing PTCA. Bivalirudin is intended for use with aspirin and has been only studied in patients receiving concomitant aspirin (325 mg daily).
- Bivalirudin has been used for patients with HIT and undergoing open heart surgery with cardiopulmonary bypass and systemic anticoagulation.

Clinical Pearls: The clearance of bivalirudin is decreased in renal insufficiency patients, reduced by 20 % in moderate renal insufficiency and 80 % in dialysis-dependent patient. Thus, for renal patient, argatroban may be a better option than bivalirudin.

(d) Dosing Options: Bolus dose is 0.75 mg/kg, followed by an infusion of 1.75 mg/kg/h for the duration of the procedure. ACT should be performed 5 min after bolus dose, and an additional bolus of 0.3 mg/kg can be given if necessary.

(e) Drug Interactions: There is an increased risk of bleeding if used in combination with heparin, warfarin, or thrombolytics.

(f) Side Effects: Bleeding, hypotension, thrombocytopenia, nausea, angina pectoris, headache, allergic reactions, etc.

Antithrombin III (Trade Name Is Thrombate)

(a) Introduction: Thrombate is a lyophilized preparation of purified human anti-thrombin III. It is used for patients with antithrombin III deficiency.
(b) Drug Class: Purified human antithrombin III.
Mechanism of Action: Thrombate inactivates coagulation system enzymes/factors including Factors II, VII, IX, X, and XI.
(c) Indications: Hereditary antithrombin III deficiency when patients undergo surgical or obstetric procedures, or they have thromboembolic problems.
Clinical Pearls:

- Hereditary antithrombin III deficiency is an under recognized congenital disease.
- The response to Thrombate is highly variable; check AT-III level regularly.
- Aseptic technique is strictly required during reconstitution.

(d) Dosing Options: Thrombate dose is determined by pre-use plasma AT-III level. To achieve 100 % AT-III level, Thrombate dose is calculated with this formula:

$$\text{Thrombate dose}\left(\text{IU}\right) = \left[\text{desired AT - III level - baseline AT - III level}\right] \times \text{Body weight}\left(\text{kg}\right)/1.4$$

Because the AT-III level recovery varies, thus 20 min after infusion of initial dose, recheck AT-III level and recalculate the additional dose necessary to correct AT-III deficiency. Then it is recommended to measure AT-III level every 12 h and maintain AT-III level greater than 80 %. The whole calculated dose should be infused over 10–20 min [4].
(e) Drug Interactions:
In the presence of heparin, the rate of antithrombin-thrombin inactivation is increased to 1.5 to 4×10^7/M/s; the reaction is accelerated 2,000–4,000-folds. Factor IXa inhibition is increased by 500–1,000-folds.
(f) Side Effects: Dizziness, chest tightness, chest, shortness of breath, nausea, foul taste in mouth, chills, cramps, hives, fever, and light-headedness.

Protamine

(a) Introduction: Clinically, protamine is used to antagonize the anticoagulant effects of heparin. Protamine itself is a weak anticoagulant.
(b) Drug Class: Heparin antagonist.
Mechanism of Action: Protamine binds to heparin to form a stable ion pair.
(c) Indications:

- Reversal of heparin.

Clinical Pearls:

- There is a large individual variation in response to protamine infusion; it is better to start with slow infusion, get a sense of patient's response to protamine, and then set the rate of infusion.

- If patient has very unfavorable response to protamine, some alternative strategies may be considered:

  - Allow heparin effects to dissipate
  - Intravenous platelet concentrates
  - Methylene blue
  - Hexadimethrine

(d) Dosing Options: IV 1–2 mg per 100 unit of heparin.
(e) Drug Interactions:
    Protamine is not compatible with many antibiotics (the cephalosporins, penicillins).
(f) Side Effects:

  - Anaphylaxis
  - Hypotension and bradycardia
  - Pulmonary hypertension and dyspnea
  - Flushing and feeling warm

Tranexamic Acid (Cyklokapron)

(a) Introduction: Tranexamic acid is an intravenous antifibrinolytic agent used in cardiac surgical procedures. It is ten times as potent as aminocaproic acid (Amicar).
(b) Drug Class: Synthetic amino acids.
    Mechanism of Action:

  - Competitive inhibitor of plasminogen activator
  - Noncompetitive inhibitor of plasmin at higher concentrations

(c) Indications:

  - Cardiac surgery for reducing blood loss
  - Hemophilia for short-term use (2–8 days)

  Clinical Pearls:

  - Tranexamic acid solution cannot be mixed with blood.
  - Dose in renal patients needs to be reduced.

(d) Dosing Options: 10–20 mg/kg loading dose bolus; then 1–2 mg/kg/h continuous infusion. Tranexamic acid should be started before CPB.
(e) Drug Interactions:

  - Tranexamic acid increases the effects of Factor IX by pharmacological synergism. Thus, it may increase the risk of thrombosis.
  - Tranexamic acid and mestranol increase each other's effects by pharmacological synergism, thus increasing the risk of thromboembolic event.

(f) Side Effects: Nausea, vomiting, diarrhea, hypotension, thromboembolic events, pulmonary embolism, and cerebral thrombosis.

Aminocaproic Acid (Amicar)

(a) Introduction: An intravenous antifibrinolytic agent.
(b) Drug Class: Synthetic amino acid.
    Mechanism of Action: Fibrinolysis-inhibitory effects by inhibition of plasminogen activator and antiplasmin activity.
(c) Indications: Cardiac or other surgical procedures to reduce blood loss when fibrinolysis is contributing to bleeding.
    Clinical Pearls: Infusion before CPB; may have higher plasma level in renal patients.
(d) Dosing Options: 100–150 mg/kg bolus and then 10–15 mg/kg/h continuous infusion. Or intravenous bolus 5 g and then infuse 1 g per hour.
(e) Drug Interactions:

   • Ethinyl estradiol: Concomitant use of aminocaproic acid with ethinyl estradiol may lead to additive hypercoagulability.
   • Mestranol: Mestranol decrease effects of aminocaproic acid by pharmacological antagonism.

(f) Side Effects:

   • Allergic reaction
   • Edema, headache, and malaise
   • Cardiovascular: bradycardia, hypotension, and thrombosis
   • Nausea, vomiting, diarrhea, and abdominal pain
   • Dyspnea and pulmonary embolism
   • Myalgia, pruritus, and tinnitus,

Desmopressin Acetate (DDAVP)

(a) Introduction: DDAVP is a synthetic analog of the pituitary hormone 8-arginine vasopressin (ADH) which is an antidiuretic hormone.
(b) Drug Class: Synthetic hormone like ADH.
    Mechanism of Action: DDAVP increases water permeability in renal tubular cells, thus decreasing urine volume and increasing urine osmolality.
(c) Indications:

   • Von Willebrand's disease and hemophilia: Facilitate the release of platelets from bone marrow
   • Central diabetes insipidus: For the temporary management of polyuria or polydipsia after head trauma or surgery
   • Nocturnal enuresis
   • Renal impairment
   • Thrombocytopenia

Clinical Pearls: DDAVP is usually given intravenously over 10 min.

(d) Dosing Options: 0.3 mcg/kg intravenously over 15–30 min.
Intranasal Dosing: 5–40 mcg/day divided to every 8–12 h.

(e) Drug Interactions:
The concomitant administration of some drugs (e.g., tricyclic antidepressants, selective serotonin reuptake inhibitors, chlorpromazine, opiate analgesics, NSAIDs, lamotrigine, and carbamazepine) with DDAVP may increase the risk of water intoxication with hyponatremia.

(f) Side Effects: Transient headache, nausea, flushing, and mild abdominal cramps.

Recombinant Coagulation Factor VIIa (NovoSeven)

(a) Introduction: Though NovoSeven is not a pharmacological agent, it is often used in cardiac and other surgical procedures.

(b) Drug Class: Recombinant coagulation Factor VIIa.
Mechanism of Action: NovoSeven is used to activate the extrinsic coagulation pathway to facilitate hemostasis.

(c) Indications:

- Congenital Factor VII deficiency: Prevention and treatment of bleeding.
- Hemophilia A or B patients with inhibitors to Factor VIII or IX.

Clinical Pearls:

- NovoSeven is one of the vitamin K-dependent coagulation factors.
- NovoSeven is provided with a bottle of dissolvent for its reconstitution.

(d) Dosing Options: 90 mcg/kg intravenously every 2 h.

(e) Drug Interactions:

- Hemorrhage
- Hypertension, hypotension, and angina pectoris
- Pain and fever
- Headache, cerebral infarct, and cerebral ischemia
- Nausea and vomiting
- Arthralgia and hemarthrosis

(f) Side Effects: Thrombotic event, pyrexia, hemorrhage, injection site reactions, headache, hypertension, hypotension, pain, edema, and nausea.

Amnesic Sedatives

Midazolam, Lorazepam, and Diazepam

(a) Introduction: Midazolam (Versed), lorazepam (Ativan), and diazepam (Valium) are very commonly used as perioperative anxiolytics, intraoperative amnesics, and other sedation purposes. Almost no invasive anesthetic/surgical procedure should be performed without any sedation. There are evidences that preoperative anxiety is associated with poor postoperative outcome for cardiac surgery patients, especially in elderly patients [5]. Tully et al. found that anxiety, stress, and depression are risk factors for postoperative atrial fibrillation [6].

(b) Drug Class: Benzodiazepine.

Mechanism of Action: All benzodiazepines work by binding to stereospecific benzodiazepine receptors on the postsynaptic GABA neuron, thus activating the inhibitory GABAa receptor complex. GABA is one of the principal inhibitory neurotransmitters in the central nervous system.

(c) Indications:

- Perioperative anxiolysis
- Intravenous sedation
- Amnesic use

Clinical Pearls:

- Midazolam provides more rapid onset amnesia and sedation effects than diazepam.
- Midazolam is so widely used in anesthesia practice, and only in few scenarios is midazolam not used.

(d) Dosing Options:

- Midazolam: IV 1–3 mg for adults, 0.05 mg/kg for pediatric patients; 0.4–1 mg/kg PO for preoperative sedation
- Lorazepam: IV 1–3 mg for adults
- Diazepam: IV 5 mg for adults
- Preoperative anxiolysis for pediatric patients: Midazolam: 0.5–0.7 mg/kg orally

(e) Drug Interactions:

- Midazolam and other anesthetic agents like volatile agents (reduce MAC) and opioids potentiate each other.
- All drugs which inhibit P450 may prolong the sedative effect of benzodiazepines. These drugs include cimetidine, erythromycin, diltiazem, verapamil, ketoconazole, itraconazole, etc.

(f) Side Effects:

- Oversedation, agitation, dystonia, amnesia, diplopia, ataxia, weakness, dysarthria, *and* euphoria
- Nausea, vomiting, and hiccups
- Injection site pain
- Hypotension, rash, cardiac arrest, bradycardia, tachycardia, and syncope
- Respiratory depression, apnea, paradoxical CNS stimulation, bronchospasm, and anaphylaxis/anaphylactoid reaction

Dexmedetomidine

(a) Introduction: Dexmedetomidine offers sedation without respiratory depression.
(b) Drug Class: α_2-Adrenergic agonist.
   Mechanism of Action: Selective α_2-adrenergic agonist with sedative properties.
(c) Indications:

   - Procedural sedation: Dexmedetomidine can be used to sedate patient for endoscopy and radiological and other procedures.
   - ICU sedation: Dexmedetomidine can also be used in ICU sedation for intubated patient or for weaning from ventilation.

   Clinical Pearls:

   - Dexmedetomidine can lower BP in some patients; it may not be indicated for hypotensive patients.
   - Individual variation in response to dexmedetomidine may necessitate dose adjustments to achieve desired clinical outcome.
   - Elderly patients (>65 years old) and patients with liver dysfunction need dose reduction.

(d) Dosing Options: Loading dose 0.2–1 mcg/kg over 10 min. Maintenance infusion dose at 0.2–0.7 mcg/kg/h.
(e) Drug Interactions:
   Dexmedetomidine and anesthetics, opioids, and sedatives likely have synergistic effects.
(f) Side Effects: Hypotension, hypertension, nausea/vomiting, and bradycardia are common side effects.

Opioids: Fentanyl, Morphine, Sufentanil, and Remifentanil

(a) Introduction: Opioids are very commonly used in cardiac anesthesia, especially fentanyl and sufentanil, for preoperative sedation, blocking responses to endotracheal intubation, and intra- and postoperative analgesia.
(b) Drug Class: Opioids.
   Mechanism of Action: Working on central opioid receptors.
(c) Indications:

   - Preoperative sedation
   - Intraoperative and postoperative analgesic agents

   Clinical Pearls:

   - There is a trend to decrease the total dosage of opioids during cardiac surgery over the last two decades.
   - For elderly cardiac surgery patients, opioid dose should be decreased, especially initially to test the patient's response to opioids.

- Meperidine is not indicated for postoperative analgesia now. Meperidine is only indicated for postoperative shivering.

(d) Dosing Options:

- Fentanyl: Bolus 1–3 mcg/kg. Infusion at 0.1–4 mcg/kg/h
- Sufentanil: Bolus 1–2 mcg/kg. Infusion at 0.3–1.5 mcg/kg/h
- Alfentanil: Bolus 20–50 mcg/kg. Infusion at 0.5–3 mcg/kg/min
- Remifentanil: Bolus 1–3 mcg/kg over 1 min. Infusion at 0.05–2 mcg/kg/min
- Morphine: Bolus 1–4 mg IV
- Meperidine: Bolus 25–75 mg IV. For postoperative shivering 12.5–25 mg IV

(e) Drug Interactions:

- Opioids have synergistic effects with other intravenous anesthetic agents. Other CNS depressants may potentiate the effects of opioids also.
- An extremely important drug interaction is the combination of meperidine with MAOI that can cause significant blood pressure change, CNS symptoms, respiratory arrest, and hyperpyrexia.

(f) Side Effects:

- Sedation and dizziness
- Nausea, vomiting, constipation, and delayed gastric emptying
- Physical dependence, tolerance, and hyperalgesia
- Respiratory depression
- Immunologic and hormonal dysfunction
- Muscle rigidity, chest tightness, and myoclonus

Induction Agents

Etomidate

(a) Introduction: Etomidate is an intravenous anesthetic agent used for patient who has decreased cardiac function. A well-known side effect of etomidate is its suppression of adrenal gland function. This suppression can even occur after single induction dose [7].
(b) Class: Carboxylated imidazole
Mechanism of Action: Acts through potentiating GABAa-mediated chloride channels.
Etomidate is very commonly used for induction of general anesthesia in cardiac surgery. Etomidate has less myocardial depressive effects than other induction agents (propofol, thiopental etc.).
(c) Indication: Induction of general anesthesia or intravenous sedation.
(d) Dosing:
Anesthesia IV Induction: Children >10 years and adults: initial 0.2–0.6 mg/kg over 30–60 s and total intravenous maintenance of anesthesia 10–20 mcg/kg/ min.

Patients scheduled for cardiac surgery are likely in the situation needing smaller dose of intravenous induction agents, and many times a less cardiodepressive induction agent is chosen. That is the reason that etomidate is often the choice of induction agent for cardiac surgery.

(e) Drug Interactions: Fentanyl increases its plasma level and prolongs its elimination half-life. Opioids may decrease etomidate-induced myoclonus during induction.

(f) Side Effects: Adrenal gland suppression, nausea, vomiting, injection site pain, transient myoclonus, averting movements, apnea, arrhythmias, bradycardia, tachycardia, decreased cortisol synthesis (shock), hyper-/hypotension, and laryngospasm.

Propofol

(a) Currently, the most commonly used intravenous anesthetic agent.

(b) Class: Isopropylphenol.

Mechanism of Action: Propofol causes global central nervous system (CNS) depression through the potentiation of the chloride current mediated through the $GABA_A$ receptor complex. It may also cause reduced glutamatergic activity through NMDA receptor blockade.

(c) Indication:

- Induction of general anesthesia.
- Intravenous sedation.
- Neurosurgical procedures: Propofol produces a decrease in both $CMRO_2$ and cerebral blood flow (CBF), thus decreasing ICP. Propofol also critically depresses cerebral perfusion pressure (CPP) due to a decrease in both CBF and MAP as a result of systemic peripheral vasodilatation.
- Burst suppression: Propofol can produce burst suppression on an EEG which is an endpoint that has been used for the administration of IV anesthetics for neuroprotection.

(d) Dosing: Bolus 2–2.5 mg/kg. Continuous infusion at 50–200 mcg/kg/min.

(e) Drug Interactions:

- Propofol potentiates non-depolarizing neuromuscular blockers.
- Fentanyl and alfentanil plasma concentrations may be increased with administration of propofol.

(f) Side Effects:

- Pain at injection site
- Hypotension, bradycardia, and asystole
- Involuntary muscle movements and seizures
- Respiratory acidosis during weaning, pulmonary edema, hyperlipidemia, rash, pruritus, and anaphylaxis/anaphylactoid reaction
- Propofol infusion syndrome
- Pancreatitis, phlebitis, and thrombosis
- Renal tubular toxicity

Ketamine

(a) Introduction: Ketamine is a very commonly used induction agent in pediatric anesthesia. It is also used for uncooperative patients by giving intramuscularly.
(b) Class: Phencyclidine.
   Mechanism of Action: Noncompetitive NMDA receptor antagonist that blocks glutamate. Ketamine produces a cataleptic-like state by direct action on the cortex and limbic system. Ketamine also has some analgesic property.
(c) Indications:

- Pediatric anesthesia induction.
- Induction of anesthesia in adult patients with asthma or other reactive airway.
- Ketamine given intramuscularly for patients who are combative or uncooperative.
- Ketamine can also be used for animal anesthesia.
- Neurosurgical procedures: Unlike other IV anesthetics, ketamine is a cerebral vasodilator with resultant increases in CBF, CMRO2, and ICP. It is not administered if patients have known intracranial disease due to the risk in increasing ICP.

Clinical Pearls:

- Ketamine is very useful for induction of general anesthesia in trauma patients.
- Ketamine is relatively contraindicated in coronary artery patient because its potential increase of heart rate.

(d) Dosing: Bolus 0.5–2 mg/kg. Continuous infusion at 0.1–0.5 mg/min. Pediatric bolus dose 0.5–1 mg/kg/dose IV. Continuous IV infusion: 5–20 mcg/kg/min.
(e) Drug Interactions:

- Ketamine potentiates non-depolarizing neuromuscular-blocking drugs.
- Combination with theophylline may predispose patient to seizures.
- Diazepam attenuates its cardiostimulatory effects and prolongs its elimination half-life. Sympathetic antagonists may unmask its direct myocardial depressant effects.
- Lithium may prolong its actions.

(f) Side Effects: Sialorrhea, anorexia, nausea, vomiting, hypertension, tachycardia, arrhythmias, diplopia, nystagmus, fasciculations, depressed reflexes, hallucinations, bradycardia, hypotension, cystitis, respiratory depression, laryngospasm, increased intraocular pressure, emergence delirium, tonic-clonic movements, and anaphylaxis.

Muscle Relaxants

This section may be well covered by other book chapters.

Rocuronium

(a) Introduction: Rocuronium is often used during induction and intubation because of its fast onset and moderate duration, especially in some patients who may not tolerate well to succinylcholine. Pancuronium is often used for the maintenance of muscle relaxation due to its long-acting effect.

(b) Drug Class: Monoquaternary aminosteroid non-depolarizing neuromuscular blocker.

Mechanism of Action:

(c) Indications:

- Facilitating endotracheal intubation
- Maintenance of muscular paralysis during surgery or other clinical scenarios
- Substitute to succinylcholine for rapid sequence induction (RSI)
- Paralysis of intubated patients in ICU setting

Clinical Pearls:

- Its fast onset is only second to succinylcholine.
- Currently, rocuronium is very commonly used in clinical anesthesia, for both intubation and maintenance of paralysis.

(d) Dosing Options: 0.6 mg/kg for intubation and 1.2 mg/kg for RSI.

(e) Drug Interactions:

- Anticonvulsants: Carbamazepine and phenytoin decrease the duration and intensity of rocuronium-induced muscle relaxation.
- Antibiotics: Aminoglycosides, vancomycin, tetracycline, bacitracin, polymyxins, colistin, and other antibiotics can enhance the neuromuscular blocking effects.
- Lithium can increase the duration of rocuronium.
- Local anesthetic agents can increase the duration of rocuronium.
- Inhalational agents: Many inhalational anesthetic agents (isoflurane, enflurane) can enhance the neuromuscular block effects of rocuronium.

(f) Side Effects:

- Transient hypotension or hypertension
- Allergic reaction, especially in patients with asthma
- Cardiac dysrhythmia

Pancuronium (Pavulon)

(a) Introduction: Pancuronium is the most commonly used long-acting muscle relaxant.

(b) Drug Class: Non-depolarizing neuromuscular blocker.

(c) Indications: Maintenance of muscular paralysis for long surgical procedures, especially for those procedures in which patients will usually be maintained intubated at the end of surgery.

Clinical Pearls: Since pancuronium is very long acting, it is rarely used in surgery with short or moderate duration. Since it is long acting, even if reversal agents are given, patients may still develop "recurarization" in recovery; patients with renal dysfunction may have even longer duration of pancuronium.

(d) Dosing Options: Intubating dose is 0.08–0.12 mg/kg, and maintenance dose is 0.01–0.015 mg/kg.

(e) Drug Interactions:

- Prior succinylcholine use will enhance the neuromuscular blocking effect of pancuronium.
- Volatile agents usually also enhance the neuromuscular blocking effect of pancuronium.
- Some antibiotics (neomycin, streptomycin, kanamycin, gentamicin, etc.) may enhance the neuromuscular blocking effect of pancuronium.

(f) Side Effects:

- Prolonged muscle paralysis and muscle weakness
- Salivation and skin rash
- Hypotension and tachycardia

Inotropic Agents

Endogenous Catecholamines: Epinephrine, Norepinephrine, and Dopamine

Epinephrine

(a) Introduction: Epinephrine is widely used in many clinical scenarios. Epinephrine normally exists in human body and is one of the natural endogenous hormones.

(b) Drug Class: Synthetic sympathomimetic catecholamine.

Mechanism of Action: Epinephrine works by activating on both α- and β-adrenergic receptors.

(c) Indications:

- Cardiac arrest
- Severe cardiac bradycardia
- Severe hypotension
- Severe bronchospasm
- Anaphylaxis
- Induction of mydriasis for intraocular surgery

Clinical Pearls:

- For those patients not in life-threatening situation, try to start with less than 1 mg IV to avoid overshooting hypertension and tachycardia, especially for those patients with coronary artery disease.
- Epinephrine comes with many different intravenous forms. There are some easily injectable epinephrine syringes readily usable in battlefield by injured soldiers.
- Epinephrine should not be used to treat circulatory collapse or hypotension caused by phenothiazines, which serves as a reversal of the pressor effects of epinephrine and may result in further lowering of blood pressure.

(d) Dosing Options:
Bolus injection: Adult: 0.05–1 mg IV, children: 0.01 mg/kg IV
Continuous infusion: 0.01–0.3 mcg/kg/min

(e) Drug Interactions:

- Epinephrine and halogenated volatile agents (halothane) induce cardiac dysrhythmia.
- Epinephrine and MAOI induce hypertensive crisis.
- Beta-blockers may antagonize the effects of epinephrine.
- Ergot alkaloids may reverse the pressor effects of epinephrine.

(f) Side Effects:

- Tachycardia
- Hypertension
- Cardiac dysrhythmia
- Anxiety, apprehensiveness, restlessness, tremor, sweating, and palpitations
- Weakness, dizziness pallor, nausea, and vomiting
- Headache and respiratory difficulties

Norepinephrine

(a) Introduction: Norepinephrine is often used in patients with low systemic vascular resistance (SVR) and mildly decreased myocardial contractility. It is used to treat septic patients with hypotension.
(b) Drug Class: Synthetic sympathomimetic catecholamine.
Mechanism of Action: Norepinephrine activates both α- and β-adrenergic receptors.
(c) Indications:

- Mild to moderate heart failure with hypotension
- Septic shock and sepsis
- Severe low SVR status
- Adjunct for cardiac arrest

Clinical Pearls:

- For those patients with mild heart failure and hypotension, norepinephrine is a great drug to increase SVR and improve cardiac contractility.
- Long-term use may cause peripheral/extremity ischemia ("Levophed toes").

(d) Dosing Options:
Continuous infusion: 0.5–30 mcg/min. Start with small dose and titrate to effects.
(e) Drug Interactions:

- Norepinephrine and halogenated volatile agents (halothane) will likely induce cardiac/ventricular dysrhythmia.
- Norepinephrine and MAOI may induce hypertensive crisis.
- Beta-blockers may antagonize some of the norepinephrine effects.

(f) Side Effects:

- Tachycardia or bradycardia
- Hypertension
- Cardiac dysrhythmia
- Anxiety, apprehensiveness, restlessness, tremor, sweating, and palpitations
- Weakness, dizziness pallor, and nausea and vomiting
- Headache and respiratory difficulties

Dopamine

(a) Introduction: In perioperative setting, dopamine is more often used to improve cardiac output, treat hypotension in shock syndrome, or preserve kidney arterial blood flow to maintain renal function.
(b) Drug Class: Synthetic catecholamine precursor.
Mechanism of Action: α_1-, β_1-, β_2-adrenergic and dopaminergic receptor agonist.
(c) Indications:

- Low cardiac output status: Dopamine increases cardiac output via its direct inotropic effects on myocardium and increase in HR.
- Situations potentially compromise renal perfusion.
- Mild to moderate hypotension.

Clinical Pearls:

- For those clinical procedures like abdominal aortic aneurysm repair which may potentially compromise renal blood flow, dopamine use is debatable in terms of preserving renal arterial flow.
- For hypotension management, dopamine is more suitable for mild to moderate hypotension; for severe hypotension, dopamine won't be potent enough in restoring blood pressure as other more potent agents like norepinephrine or epinephrine.

(d) Dosing Options:

- Continuous infusion: 2–20 mcg/kg/min, IV.
- 2–5 mcg/kg/min: The traditionally believed "renal dose," inhibit aldosterone and redistribute blood to the kidneys
- 5–10 mcg/kg/min: β_1 effects more than α effects. So dopamine improves cardiac output.
- 10–15 mcg/kg/min: Both α effects and β_1 effects.
- >15 mcg/kg/min: α effects predominate.

(e) Drug Interactions:

- Dopamine and halogenated volatile agents (halothane) may induce cardiac dysrhythmia.
- Dopamine and MAOI induce hypertensive crisis.
- Dopamine and diuretics may have additive or synergistic effects on the urine output.
- Butyrophenones (haloperidol) and phenothiazines can suppress the dopaminergic renal and mesenteric vasodilatation.
- Dopamine with vasopressors, vasoconstricting agents (ergonovine), and some oxytocic drugs may lead to severe hypertension.
- Dopamine and phenytoin may lead to hypotension and bradycardia.

(f) Side Effects:

- Tachycardia or bradycardia
- Hypertension
- Ventricular dysrhythmia
- Dyspnea, nausea, and vomiting
- Headache, anxiety, and piloerection

Dobutamine

(a) Introduction: Dobutamine is very commonly used in cardiac surgery or other low cardiac output status. It is also used for patients with pulmonary hypertension with right heart failure.
(b) Drug Class: Synthetic sympathomimetic agent
Mechanism of action: β_1 and minimal β_2 effects. Increase cardiac output, decreases SVR and PVR.
(c) Indications:

- Cardiac decomposition due to organic heart diseases or cardiac surgery;

Clinical Pearls:

- Dobutamine's β_2 effect may sometimes cause peripheral vasodilatation and lower blood pressure.
- Dobutamine can cause significant tachycardia.

(d) Dosing Options: Start with 0.5–1 mcg/kg/min, then titrate to effects.
(e) Drug Interactions:
Dobutamine may work synergistically with nitroprusside in increasing cardiac output and lowering pulmonary wedge pressure.
(f) Side Effects:

- Tachycardia and other dysrhythmia and palpitation
- Hypertension or hypotension
- Injection site reactions
- Shortness of breath, nausea, and headache

Nesiritide (Natrecor)

(a) Introduction: Nesiritide is a relatively newer inotropic agent for patient with heart failure. Nesiritide can reduce pulmonary capillary wedge pressure and improved short-term (3 h) symptoms of dyspnea [8].
(b) Drug Class: Synthetic analog of B-type natriuretic peptide (BNP).
Mechanism of action: Nesiritide binds to the particulate guanylate cyclase receptor of vascular smooth muscle and endothelial cells, then leading to increased intracellular concentrations of guanosine $3'5'$-cyclic monophosphate (cGMP) and smooth muscle cell relaxation. Nesiritide dilates both veins and arteries.
(c) Indications:
Nesiritide is used in acutely decompensated heart failure, patient has dyspnea at rest or with minimal activity.
(d) Dosing Options:
IV bolus 2 mcg/kg and then continuous infusion at 0.01 mcg/kg/min.
(e) Drug Interactions:
If used with vasodilators or ACEI, nesiritide may cause increase in symptomatic hypotension.
(f) Side Effects:

- Hypotension
- Headache and dizziness
- Injection site reactions
- Allergic reactions and nausea
- Back pain, pruritus, and rash

Phosphodiesterase III Inhibitors: Milrinone, Amrinone

(a) Introduction: Phosphodiesterase inhibitors are considered inodilators which increase myocardial contractility and cause vasodilatation leading to decreased PVR and SVR.

(b) Drug Class: Phosphodiesterase inhibitor
Mechanism of action: Inhibition of phosphodiesterase leads to increased intracellular cAMP and ionized calcium level, thus increasing myocardial contractility and improving ventricular relaxation. In vascular smooth muscle cells, increased cAMP leads to vascular relaxation.

(c) Indications:

- Acute decompensated heart failure
- Pulmonary hypertension with right heart failure

Clinical Pearls:
Milrinone is significantly more popular than amrinone because of its lack of thrombocytopenic effect.

(d) Dosing Options:

- Milrinone: Loading dose is 50 mcg/kg IV, infusion at 0.25–0.75 mcg/kg/min
- Amrinone: Loading dose is 0.75–1.5 mg/kg IV (use 1.5 mg/kg when just weaning off CPB), infusion at 5–20 mcg/kg/min

(e) Drug Interactions
Phosphodiesterase inhibitors work synergistically with β-adrenergic receptor agonists.

(f) Side Effects

- Ventricular dysrhythmia
- Hypotension
- Headache, hypokalemia, tremor, and thrombocytopenia
- Anaphylaxis
- Thrombocytopenia (amrinone)

Digoxin

(a) Introduction: Digitalis is the oldest category of inotropes. It has been used clinically over 100 years.

(b) Drug Class: Digitalis, inotrope
Mechanism of action: Inhibition of Na-K ATPase leads to increased intracellular calcium level. Also digoxin has vagomimetic effects.

(c) Indications:

- Mild to moderate heart failure
- Atrial fibrillation

Clinical Pearls:

- There is a significant individual variation in response of patients to digoxin.
- Digoxin has a very narrow therapeutic range. It is easy to have side effects from digoxin.
- Digoxin has multiple drug interactions.

(d) Dosing Options: 10–15 mcg/kg in divided intravenous doses, usually 0.25–0.5 mg as initial dose, 0.25 mg every 4 h.

(e) Drug Interactions

- Potassium-losing diuretics are a major contributing factor to digitalis toxicity.
- Calcium, especially intravenous calcium administration, may produce serious arrhythmias in patients taking digoxin.
- Drugs increase plasma digoxin level: amiodarone, quinidine, verapamil, propafenone, indomethacin, itraconazole, alprazolam, and spironolactone (reduction in clearance and/or in volume of distribution of the drug); erythromycin, tetracycline, clarithromycin, propantheline, and diphenoxylate (increase digoxin absorption); and carvedilol
- Drugs lower digoxin plasma level: Antacids, kaolin-pectin, sulfasalazine, neomycin, cholestyramine, certain anticancer drugs, and metoclopramide (interfere with intestinal digoxin absorption); rifampin (by increasing the non-renal clearance of digoxin).
- Thyroid hormone administration to a digitalized, hypothyroid patient may increase the dose requirement of digoxin. Concomitant use of digoxin.
- Sympathomimetics increases the risk of cardiac arrhythmias.
- Succinylcholine may cause a sudden extrusion of potassium from muscle cells and may thereby cause arrhythmias in digitalized patients.
- Calcium channel blockers, β-blockers, and digoxin may cause advanced or complete heart block.

(f) Side Effects

- Cardiovascular:
- Atrioventricular block, AV dissociation, or cardiac arrest
  Ventricular dysrhythmia even ventricular fibrillation

- CNS: Visual disturbances, headache, weakness, dizziness, and mental disturbances
- Gastroenterological: Nausea, vomiting, anorexia, diarrhea, and abdominal pain
- Others: Gynecomastia, thrombocytopenia, and rash

Levosimendan (Simdax) [9]

(a) Introduction: Levosimendan is a new kind of inotropes. It works by sensitizing intracellular calcium and opening potassium channels. Levosimendan did better than dobutamine in patients with history of congestive heart failure (CHF) and patients taking β-blockers when they are hospitalized with acute decompensated heart failure [10, 11]. Since levosimendan achieved approval in Sweden in 2000, about 40 other countries worldwide have approved the drug, but it remains unlicensed in the USA. Orion withdrew their application from the USA, but Orion entered an agreement with Abbott to market the product worldwide.

(b) Drug Class: Calcium sensitizer
Mechanism of action:

- Calcium sensitization
- Potassium channel opening

(c) Indications:
Acutely decompensated heart failure
Clinical Pearls: This is a relatively new drug; read the insert material before giving to the patient.
(d) Dosing Options: Loading dose of 6 or 12 μg/kg in 10-min, followed by continuous infusion at 0.1 or 0.2 μg/kg/min for 24 h.
(e) Drug Interactions: No information yet.
(f) Side Effects

- Headache, dizziness, and insomnia
- Hypotension, ventricular tachycardia, atrial fibrillation, tachycardia, ventricular extrasystoles, myocardial ischemia, and extrasystoles
- Nausea, vomiting, constipation, and diarrhea
- Decreased hemoglobin and hypokalemia

Omecamtiv Mecarbil

(a) Introduction: This is one of the inotropes under development but close to clinical availability.
(b) Drug Class: Cardiac myosin activator
Mechanism of Action: Omecamtiv mecarbil increases the rate of phosphate release. This allows for the power stroke of the actin-myosin bridge to occur and more power strokes are occurring at once.
(c) Indications: Heat failure management.
(d) Dosing Options: Loading dose 0.125–1 mg/kg/h, maintenance infusion at 0.0625–0.5 mg/kg/h.

Antidysrhythmic Agents

Amiodarone

(a) Introduction: Amiodarone has been used as an antidysrhythmic drug for over three decades. Currently it is gaining popularity in the treatment of ventricular dysrhythmia.
(b) Drug Class: Antidysrhythmic agent, predominantly Class III effects.
Mechanism of Action:

- Inhibit adrenergic stimulation
- Decrease atrioventricular conduction and sinus node function

- Produce α- and β-adrenergic blocking effects
- Prolong PR, QRS, and QT intervals

(c) Indications

- Ventricular fibrillation
- Recurrent hemodynamically unstable ventricular tachycardia

Clinical Pearls: Amiodarone may induce life-threatening side effects, so it is imperative to monitor the patient very closely.

(d) Dosing Options:
Loading dose 150–300 mg IV over 10 min.
Maintenance infusion at 1 mg/min for 6 h, 0.5 mg/h for 18 h, with a total dose approximately 1 g/day.

(e) Drug Interactions:
Amiodarone may increase the effects of oral anticoagulants, phenytoin, diltiazem, digoxin, and quinine.

(f) Side Effects

- Negative inotropic effect and vasodilating effect may lead to hypotension.
- Prolong QT interval.
- Sinus bradycardia, even atrioventricular block.
- Long-term oral use may cause pulmonary fibrosis, hepatitis, cirrhosis, and hypothyroidism.

Esmolol

(a) Introduction: Esmolol is the most commonly used short-acting selective β_1-blocker.
(b) Drug Class: β-blocker
Mechanism of Action: Blocks β-adrenergic receptor.
(c) Indications:

- Supraventricular tachycardia
- Perioperative tachycardia

Clinical Pearls:
For perioperative transient known cause tachycardia, bolus dose may be enough. Because esmolol is very short-acting, for sustaining tachycardia, continuous infusion of esmolol may be needed.

(d) Dosing Options:
For transient control of heart rate, give 10 mg IV bolus and may repeat till heart rate is controlled.
For maintenance infusion at 50–200 mcg/kg/min for up to 48 h.

(e) Drug Interactions

- Esmolol increases digoxin blood level by 10–20 %.
- Esmolol prolongs the duration of succinylcholine and mivacurium.

- Esmolol may increase the risk of clonidine, guanfacine, and moxonidine withdrawal rebound hypertension.
- Esmolol may be antagonized by concomitant use of sympathomimetics.

(f) Side Effects/Black Box Warnings (If Any)
  - Hypotension
  - Nausea
  - Dizziness and somnolence
  - Injection site reactions

Labetalol

(a) Introduction: Labetalol is a commonly used long-acting nonselective β-blocker with some selective α_1-adrenergic blocking effects.
(b) Drug Class: Nonselective β- adrenergic blocker and selective α_1-adrenergic blocker.
  Mechanism of Action: Blocks β-adrenergic and α_1-adrenergic receptors.
(c) Indications:

  - Tachycardia
  - Hypertension: Labetalol either used alone or in combination with other antihypertensive medications to lower high blood pressure.

  Clinical Pearls:

  - Labetalol is a long-acting β-blocker; it should be cautious to give labetalol intraoperatively because labetalol may interfere catecholamine effects. Blood pressure fluctuation is a common phenomena intraoperatively, when blood pressure becomes very low and catecholamine is used to increase blood pressure, its blood pressure increasing effects may be antagonized by labetalol.
- Patients with therapeutic plasma level of labetalol may be hard to be resuscitated if somehow they develop cardiac arrest. This is because both catecholamine and labetalol work on β_1-receptors. If β_1-receptors are blocked by labetalol, epinephrine will be significantly less effective in resuscitating the heart.

(d) Dosing Options: IV bolus dose 5–10 mg increments, with 5 min interval. Continuous infusion at 2–8 mcg/min.
(e) Drug Interactions:

  - Labetolol with tricyclic antidepressant: Patient may experience tremor.
  - Labetalol may augment nitroglycerin's PB-lowering effects and blocks its reflex tachycardia.
  - Labetolol may increase the dosing requirement of bronchodilating β-agonists.
  - Cimetidine may increase the bioavailability of labetalol;
  - Labetalol may increase the risk of bradycardia if combined with digitalis.

(f) Side Effects: Fatigue, nausea, dizziness, nasal stuffiness, ejaculation problem in man, dyspnea, postural hypotension, and vertigo.

Adenosine

(a) Introduction: Adenosine is an endogenous nucleoside existing in all cells. Adenosine slows AV node conduction and prevent reentry pathway; thus it is used to treat PSVT and PSVT with WPW syndrome and induce cardiac arrest. Its effect is not blocked by atropine.

(b) Drug Class: Endogenous nucleoside
Mechanism of Action: Slows down AV node conduction

(c) Indications:

- PSVT: Adenosine may convert PSVT, with WPW syndrome or without, to sinus rhythm.
- Decrease heart rate in some scenarios in cardiac surgery or other clinical applications.
- Induce short episode or cardiac arrest for intra-aortic endovascular stent placement.

Clinical Pearls:

- Adenosine has to be given rapidly through the IV port closest to the heart, followed with saline flush immediately after injection.
- Adenosine does not convert atrial fibrillation, atrial flutter, or ventricular dysrhythmia.
- Atropine does not block adenosine effects.

(d) Dosing Options: Initially 6 mg IV push, may repeat with 12 mg in 1–2 min. Pediatric dosing: 0.05–0.1 mg/kg initially, may repeat with incremental 0.05–0.1 mg/kg. Max bolus dose is 0.3 mg/kg.

(e) Drug Interactions:

- Methylxanthines (caffeine, theophylline) may block adenosine effects.
- Dipyridamole (nucleoside transporter) may potentiate adenosine effects.

(f) Side Effects:

- Headache, sweating, and facial flushing
- Nausea
- Chest pain, palpitation, and hypotension
- Light-headedness, dizziness, blurred vision, and neck and back pain
- Dyspnea, chest pressure, and hyperventilation

Magnesium

(a) Introduction: Magnesium is the second most plentiful cation in intracellular fluid. Magnesium sulfate as a medicine has been in clinical utilization for many years.

(b) Drug Class: Electrolyte

Mechanism of Action: Inhibition of acetylcholine release at neuromuscular junction, CNS depressant, and anticonvulsant

(c) Indications:

- Hypomagnesemia (used for treatment or prevention)
- Convulsion
- Uterine tetanus
- Cardiac dysrhythmia: Torsades de Pointes

Clinical Pearls:
Monitoring magnesium level is very important. Normal plasma level is 1.5–2.2 mEq/L; therapeutic level for preeclampsia is 4–5 mEq/L.

(d) Dosing Options:
Hypomagnesemia: IV 4–8 g in 10–20 % solution given over 8 h
Preeclampsia/eclampsia: IV bolus 2–4 g in 10–20 % solution over 5 min then infusion at 1–2.5 g/h.
Torsades de Pointes: IV 1–2 g, infusion at 0.5–1 g/h.

(e) Drug Interaction: No information yet.

(f) Side Effects

- Hypotension
- Hypothermia
- Stupor, respiratory depression
- Flushing

Lidocaine

(a) Introduction: Lidocaine is a sodium channel blocker used most commonly in regional nerve block and surgical wound infiltrations.

(b) Drug Class: Sodium channel blocker
Mechanism of Action: Inhibition of ionic influxes through the neuronal membrane; thus lidocaine blocks the action potential initiation and its conduction through the nerve fibers.

(c) Indications:

- Regional nerve blocks
- Wound infiltration
- Cardiac ventricular dysrhythmia

Clinical Pearls
Lidocaine can be used after ventricular dysrhythmia being converted to normal cardiac rhythm.

(d) Dosing Options: 1–1.5 mg/kg IV bolus, may repeat up to 3 mg/kg. Continuous infusion at the rate of 1–4 mg/min. 30–50 mcg/kg/min.

(e) Drug Interactions

- Phenothiazines and butyrophenones may reduce or even reverse the pressor effect of epinephrine.
- Lidocaine with vasopressors or ergot-type monitoring may potentiate MAOIs.

(f) Side Effects:

- Light-headedness; apprehension, euphoria, and dizziness
- Bradycardia and hypotension
- Allergic reaction
- Nausea
- Allergic reactions

Atropine

(a) Introduction: One of the most commonly used anticholinergic agents.
(b) Drug Class: Antimuscarinic (anticholinergic, antiparasympathetic)
  Mechanism of Action: Competitively blocking acetylcholine at muscarinic receptor
(c) Indications:

- Treatment or prevention of vagal response due to intra-abdominal or ocular stimulation.
- As an antisialogogue, atropine can decrease salivary secretions and decrease respiratory tract secretions.
- Bradycardia: Atropine can increase heart rate.
- Cardiac arrest: Atropine is used in ACLS.
- As an antidote for cholinergic agents or cholinesterase poisoning (organ phosphorus insecticides).
- Antidote for some mushroom poisoning (mushroom with alkaloid muscarine).

Clinical Pearls:

- Atropine is commonly used intraoperatively if HR falls to certain level. It is easy to have overshooting tachycardia if 1 mg IV is given. So for those with coronary artery disease, it might be better to give smaller dose initially to figure out patient's response, then adjust the dose accordingly.
- Atropine can be given endotracheal if no IV access in emergency situations.
- Children are more susceptible to atropine's toxic effect than adults.

(d) Dosing Options: 0.5–1 mg IV initially for most anticholinergic indications. For organophosphorus poisoning, atropine is given in much larger doses.
  Pediatric patients: 0.01–0.03 mg/kg IV.
(e) Drug Interactions:

- Atropine may worsen topiramate's effects of increased body temperature and decreased sweating.

- Atropine may also worsen zonisamide's effects of increased body temperature and decreased sweating.

(f) Side Effects:

- Tachycardia and palpitation
- Dilated pupils, blurred vision, and photophobia
- Dry mouth
- Anhidrosis
- Constipation and thirst
- Difficult micturition
- Delirium and restlessness

Vasoactive Drugs

Phenylephrine

(a) Introduction: It is one of the most commonly used vasoconstrictors during surgery.
(b) Drug Class: α-adrenergic receptor agonist.
  Mechanism of Action: Stimulation of α-adrenergic receptor.
(c) Indications:

- Hypotension with low SVR
- Nasal decongestant

  Clinical Pearls:

- Phenylephrine increases BP via α-adrenergic effect, but it does not have inotropic effect. For those patients with compromised myocardial contractility and hypotension, phenylephrine should not replace positive inotrope(s).
- This drug is used very commonly intraoperatively. It can be given as bolus dose or continuous intravenous infusion.

(d) Dosing Options: It can be given IV bolus at 50–200 mcg dependent upon the severity of hypotension. Intravenous continuous infusion rate is 20–100 mcg/min.
(e) Drug Interactions:

- If phenylephrine is used concomitantly with MAOI, significant hypertension may occur.
- The pressor effect of phenylephrine is also potentiated by tricyclic antidepressants.
- Phenylephrine may augment the cardiodepressant effect of volatile anesthetic agents.

(f) Side Effects:

- Hypertension
- Reflex bradycardia

Vasopressin

(a) Introduction: Vasopressin is a synthetic analog of arginine vasopressin. It has antidiuretic effects and also constricts visceral vasculatures.
(b) Drug Class: Antidiuretic hormone.
Mechanism of Action: Induce vascular smooth muscle constriction and increase reabsorption of water from kidneys.
(c) Indications:

- Severe hypotension
- Cardiac arrest
- Vasoplegic syndrome
- Postoperative abdominal distension
- Upper GI bleeding
- Diabetes insipidus

Clinical Pearls:

- For those patients on ACEI who suffer refractory hypotension, vasopressin is one of the choices.
- Vasopressin can be used for gastric irrigation to induce varicose vein constriction to minimize bleeding.

(d) Dosing Options:

- Continuous IV infusion at the rate of 0.01–0.04 units/kg.
- May be given bolus when used in ACLS; the dose is 40 units IV, IO, ET.

(e) Drug Interactions:
Carbamazepine, chlorpropamide, clofibrate, urea, fludrocortisone, and tricyclic antidepressant may potentiate the antidiuretic effects.
(f) Side Effects:

- Cardiac arrest
- Abdominal cramps and nausea/vomiting
- Hypertension
- Allergic reaction

Nicardipine

(a) Introduction: Nicardipine (Cardene) is a direct arterial dilating agent. It belongs to the dihydropyridine category.

(b) Drug Class: Calcium channel blocker
Mechanism of Action: Decrease of intracellular calcium level by blocking the transmembrane movement of calcium ions.

(c) Indications:

- Hypertensive crisis
- Hypertension associated with many different clinical pathological conditions
- Prevention of vascular graft spasm
- Treatment of vascular spasmatic contraction (Reynolds's syndrome)

Clinical Pearls:
Nicardipine is indicated more for severe hypertension; it is indicated for short-term control of hypertensions and hypertensive crisis. It can easily be converted to oral formulation.

(d) Dosing Options:
Continuous infusion started at 5 mg/h with an incremental dose of 2.5 mg/h, max dose is 15 mg/h.
Bolus dose is 0.3–0.5 mg/bolus.

(e) Drug Interactions:

- Cimetidine can increase nicardipine plasma level when nicardipine is taken orally.
- B-blocker: If premixed with nicardipine, be very cautious in patients with decreased cardiac contractility.
- Nicardipine can increase the plasma level of cyclosporine.

(f) Side Effects:

- Headache
- Hypotension, tachycardia, angina pectoris, and atrioventricular block
- Nausea/vomiting and dyspepsia

Clevidipine (Cleviprex)

(a) Introduction: Clevidipine is a newer generation of dihydropyridine L-type calcium channel blocker.

(b) Drug Class: Calcium channel blocker.
Mechanism of Action: Blocks transmembrane influx of calcium.

(c) Indications:
Control of hypertension when oral medication is not feasible.
Clinical Pearls: Clevidipine is especially good for patient who has renal insufficiency or liver disease because its clearance is not dependent upon renal or liver function.

(d) Dosing Options: Initially start at 1–2 mg/h, may double dose in 90 s initially, most patients achieve therapeutic range at 4–6 mg/h. Max dose is 32 mg/h.

(e) Drug Interactions:

- Clevidipine may increase the risk of bradycardia or AV block if patient is on dolasetron.
- Tizanidine may augment clevidipine's antihypertensive effects.

(f) Side Effects: Hypotension and reflex tachycardia

Nitroprusside (Nitropress)

(a) Introduction: Nitroprusside is a very old antihypertensive drug and also the gold standard in efficacy of hypotensive effect.
(b) Drug Class: Vasodilator
Mechanism of Action: Release nitric oxide and induce cGMP to cause vascular relaxation.
(c) Indications: Immediate control of hypertension in hypertensive crisis or urgency. It is also indicated for controlled hypotension.
Clinical Pearls:
Nitroprusside can develop tachyphylaxis.
Cyanide toxicity can be a serious side effect from nitroprusside.
Nitroprusside solution needs to be covered to avoid light exposure.
(d) Dosing Options: Start at 0.5–1 mcg/kg/min, titrate upward every 3–5 min till the desired blood pressure range. Max dose is 10 mcg/kg/min.
(e) Drug Interactions: All other antihypertensive drugs can potentially augment nitroprusside's hypotensive effect.
(f) Side Effects:

- Hypotension
- Cyanide toxicity and methemoglobinemia
- Abdominal pain, bradycardia, tachycardia, and hypothyroidism

Nitric Oxide

(a) Introduction: Nitric oxide is currently used mostly to lower pulmonary hypertension.
(b) Drug Class: Endogenous short-acting vasodilating substance.
Mechanism of Action: Binding to heme moiety of cyclic guanylate cyclase, thus activating guanylate cyclase and increase intracellular cGMP level.
(c) Indications:

- Pulmonary hypertension
- Neonate respiratory failure with pulmonary hypertension

Clinical Pearls: Nitric oxide has to be given via a special nitric oxide delivery system, which is connected to the inspiratory arm of breathing circuit.

(d) Dosing Options: Initially start with 20 PPM. The dose may increase to 60 PPM.

(e) Drug Interactions

- No formal drug interaction study data.
- Nitric oxide donor compounds like nitroprusside and nitroglycerin may have additive effects with nitric oxide, increasing the risk of methemoglobinemia.

(f) Side Effects:

- Intracranial hemorrhage.
- Seizure.
- Pulmonary hemorrhage.
- Gastrointestinal hemorrhage.
- Hypotension.
- Accidental exposure of medical staffs may cause chest discomfort, dizziness, dry throat, dyspnea, and headache.

Nitroglycerin

(a) Introduction: Nitroglycerin is a very commonly used coronary artery dilator.

(b) Drug Class: Vasodilator
Mechanism of Action: Vascular smooth muscle relaxation

(c) Indications:

- Acute coronary syndrome with chest pain
- Hypertension

Clinical Pearls
Although nitroglycerin is not contraindicated in most perioperative hypertensive patients, nitroglycerin is not well indicated for most perioperative hypertension because the hallmark of perioperative hypertension is hypovolemia and high peripheral vascular resistance due to elevated catecholamine level. Thus, direct arterial dilators are better than venous dilators to induce decrease venous return and lower cardiac output.

(d) Dosing Options: Starting dose is 0.2–0.4 mg/h, may increase to 0.8 mg/h.

(e) Drug Interactions
Nitroglycerin may be synergistic with many other vasodilators.

(f) Side Effects:

- Headache and light-headedness
- Hypotension
- Reflex tachycardia
- Syncope and rebound hypertension

Chemical Structures

Chemical Structure 38.1 Argatroban

Chemical Structure 38.2 Labetalol

Chemical Structure 38.3 Nicardipine

Chemical Structure 38.4 Dopamine

Chemical Structure
38.5 Adenosine

References

1. http://healthyheart-sundar.blogspot.com/2011_03_01_archive.html.
2. Kaplan JA, Reich DL, Savino JS. Cardiac physiology: the echo era. In: Kaplan, Reich, Konstadt, Savino, editors. Chapter 5, in 6th edition, Kaplan's cardiac anesthesia. by Saunders, an imprint of Elsevier Inc. St Louis, Missouri. 2011. ISBN: 9781437716177.
3. Kaplan JA, Reich DL, Savino JS. Transfusion Medicine and Coagulation Disorders. Edited by Kaplan, Reich, Konstadt and Savino. 2011 by Saunders, an imprint of Elsevier Inc. St Louis, Missouri. 2011-04-08, ISBN 9781437716177.
4. http://www.rxlist.com/angiomax-drug.htm.
5. http://www.rxlist.com/thrombate-drug.htm.
6. Williams JB, Alexander KP, Morin JF, Langlois Y, Noiseux N, Perrault LP, Smolderen K, Arnold SV, Eisenberg MJ, Pilote L, Monette J, Bergman H, Smith PK, Afilalo J. Preoperative anxiety as a predictor of mortality and major morbidity in patients aged >70 years undergoing cardiac surgery. Am J Cardiol. 2013;111(1):137–42. doi:10.1016/j.amjcard.2012.08.060. PMID: 23245838.
7. Tully PJ, Bennetts JS, Baker RA, McGavigan AD, Turnbull DA, Winefield HR. Anxiety, depression, and stress as risk factors for atrial fibrillation after cardiac surgery. Heart Lung. 2011;40(1):4–11. doi:10.1016/j.hrtlng.2009.12.010.
8. Archambault P, Dionne CE, Lortie G, LeBlanc F, Rioux A, Larouche G. Adrenal inhibition following a single dose of etomidate in intubated traumatic brain injury victims. CJEM. 2012;14(5):270–82.
9. Liu H, Fox CJ, Zhang S, Kaye AD. Cardiovascular pharmacology: an update. Anesthesiol Clin. 2010;28(4):723–38. doi:10.1016/j.anclin.2010.09.001. Review. PMID: 21074748.
10. Levosimendan: http://www.orion.fi/Documents/Publications%20and%20Media%20main%20file/Presentation%20materials%20PDF/Simdax%20Fact%20Sheet.pdf.
11. Mebazaa, et al. Eur J Heart Fail. 2009;11:304–11.

Chapter 39
The Intensive Care Unit

Brian O'Gara and Shahzad Shaefi

Contents

Introduction

Caring for patients in the intensive care unit demands constant, meticulous thought and consideration while implementing every aspect of their management. Among the many life-sustaining therapies provided for those in the intensive care unit (ICU), the use of an individually tailored pharmacologic regimen has the potential to dramatically improve the overall health of the patient as well as to do great harm.

B. O'Gara, MD • S. Shaefi, MD (✉)
Department of Anesthesia, Harvard Medical School, Boston, MA 02215, USA

Department of Anesthesia, Critical Care and Pain Medicine,
Beth Israel Deaconess Medical Center, Boston, MA, USA
e-mail: bpogara@bidmc.harvard.edu; sshaefi@bidmc.harvard.edu

A.D. Kaye et al. (eds.), *Essentials of Pharmacology for Anesthesia,*
Pain Medicine, and Critical Care, DOI 10.1007/978-1-4614-8948-1_39,
© Springer Science+Business Media New York 2015

Severe derangements in the physiologic responses and homeostatic mechanisms of critically ill patients often times result in challenges in constructing a durable therapeutic regimen. At times, these alterations in function can be difficult to detect, and their effects on the intended action of pharmacologic substances are often impossible to quantify. Knowledge of these specific disease processes, their potential effects on pharmacodynamics and pharmacokinetics, as well as an intimate familiarity with the pharmacologic agents most often used in the intensive care unit can lead to an optimized approach to improving the health of the critically ill patient.

Therapeutic Index and Intended Effect

As is always the case when providing any modality of therapy, one must decide whether the benefit of the intervention outweighs the risk that it may impose upon the patient. In the care of the critically ill, at times, the boundary between an acceptable risk and an unacceptable one can be obscured by the desire to provide life-saving or sustaining measures and the potential to create serious iatrogenic harm. Ideal pharmacologic regimens for these patients would then include drugs with a high therapeutic index (TI), defined as the ratio of therapeutic plasma levels to toxic plasma levels. In general, drugs with a favorable TI would exhibit an intended effect at a range of plasma levels far separated from a range in which the drug could cause potential harm. Often times, the critical nature of the patient's disease dictates the use of an agent with a more unfavorable risk profile, because of either a lack of alternatives or an unsustainable progression of disease without treatment. In these challenging cases, agents with lower therapeutic indices should be selected when their intended effect can either be readily observed with recognizable changes in the patient's vital signs and/or physical exam characteristics or directly measured with plasma concentrations.

Mode of Administration

Frequently, an agent's intended effect and therefore clinical benefit can be augmented by selecting a different mode of administration. For example, an agent may have a low therapeutic index or limited time periods of effective plasma concentrations when given via intermittent bolus. The same agent may display more stable and therefore easier to predict serum concentrations if given via continuous intravenous infusion. Ideal candidates for continuous infusion would be agents that have a short context-sensitive half-life and do not accumulate in tissues over time, which could lead to a more prolonged effect than is intended. Examples of medications in this category might include propofol, furosemide, and nitroglycerin. In certain cases, the intended plasma concentration may not be obtained rapidly via continuous infusion alone, and a loading dose may be necessary. Once the desired effect is observed, however, patients can be maintained on an appropriate dose without being subjected to the potentially harmful effects of labile plasma concentrations of agents with a low therapeutic index.

Bioavailability and Route of Administration

Bioavailability refers to the fraction of active drug that reaches the systemic circulation. Drugs given via an intravenous route are thought to be 100 % bioavailable. In general, drugs given via the enteral route are subjected to absorption via the intestinal tract into the portal venous system, where it then undergoes varying amounts of metabolism in the liver before it reaches the systemic circulation. This phenomenon is referred to as the first-pass effect. This effect may lead to decreased bioavailability of enterally administered agents, delays in achieving intended effects, as well as the production of possible harmful metabolites. In critically ill patients, the enteral route of administration may be inappropriate for these reasons as well as many others. Postsurgical or trauma patients may have severe alterations in either the continuity or function of their gastrointestinal tract. Many mechanically ventilated patients will be maintained on opioid infusions leading to ileus, prolonged intestinal transit time, and delayed entry of enterally absorbed medications into the portal system.

Many therapeutic agents can be given via alternative dosing routes. Due to predictable and sustained absorption when given via subcutaneous injection, this route has become the delivery method of choice for anticoagulants including both unfractionated and low molecular weight heparin. These medications are widely given to ICU patients to prevent venous thromboembolism, a common and often disastrous development in this patient group. Other delivery routes may be chosen to target a specific site of action. Inhaled nitric oxide and tobramycin are both incredibly selective for lung capillaries and distal alveoli, respectively, when given via the inhaled route. The same can be said for nebulized agents such as the beta-agonist albuterol and the anticholinergic ipratropium bromide. Finally, the sublingual or buccal route takes advantage of the rich capillary network seen within the oral cavity and has an additional advantage of its venous drainage bypassing the portal circulation via the superior vena cava. Substances available for this route of administration will then exhibit rapid uptake and near 100 % bioavailability. Examples include sublingual nitroglycerin, the fentanyl lollipop, and sublingual olanzapine.

Volume of Distribution

An agent's volume of distribution (Vd) can be thought of as the attempt to quantify the volume in the various compartments of the body that the agent can be found. This volume not only represents the circulating blood volume and the intended site of action but is also affected by many factors including protein binding, tissue binding, and lipid solubility of the drug in question. For these reasons, the Vd of most pharmacologic agents cannot be simply estimated by quantifying the extracellular fluid volume or lean body weight of the individual, and the resultant calculated volume tends to be a figure larger than the total body volume. The condition of critically ill patients tends to complicate matters even further. Patients may have dramatic alterations in their circulating volume, and the manner in which they were resuscitated can have implications for many pharmacologic agents. Patients receiving mainly crystalloid infusions will have a large volume of distribution for hydrophilic substances. Chronically ill patients will have conditions affecting their volume of distribution as well. Congestive heart failure may lead to fluid retention, increasing the Vd for hydrophilic agents. Chronic renal failure may lead to a similar increase in Vd via fluid retention, and conditions such as the nephrotic syndrome can lead to hypoalbuminemia, decreasing the Vd for highly protein-bound substances. Patients with hepatic failure and resultant productive protein deficits will also exhibit hypoalbuminemia as well as hypogammaglobulinemia, both essential binding sites for protein-bound drugs. Chronic or critical illness can have profound effects on the body's normal homeostatic mechanisms, often times leading to a hypercatabolic state. This can lead to muscle wasting and loss of lean body mass. This can have implications for substances that exhibit both protein binding and lipophilic peripheral tissue binding.

Lastly, critically ill patients can exhibit violations in normally contiguous boundaries between various bodily compartments which can have implications on both an agent's site of intended action and the possibility of acting upon an unintended compartment, which can lead to severe consequences. Examples of this include the diffuse capillary leak seen in sepsis, the localized pulmonary endothelial disruption seen in patients with the acute respiratory distress syndrome (ARDS), and disruptions of the blood-brain barrier by hemorrhage, tumor, or trauma. Prior knowledge of these disease states can have profound impact on an individualized pharmacologic regimen. For example, patients with elevated intracranial pressure may receive the osmotic diuretic mannitol in an attempt to draw interstitial fluid from the brain across the impermeable membrane of the blood-brain barrier. If this medication is given to a patient with elevated intracranial pressure with a disrupted blood-brain barrier, which can be the case with an intraparenchymal hemorrhage, the osmotic load will then be delivered to the brain parenchyma itself. This can lead to the disastrous consequence of localized tissue edema and an unintended increase in intracranial pressure.

Clearance

The body's metabolism and disposal of a drug can be drastically altered by critical illness. Disruptions in the major metabolic and excretory organs such as the liver and kidneys as well as alterations in both regional and systemic circulation can all affect the efficiency in which a drug is ultimately cleared.

Renal insufficiency, whether chronic or acute, can have multiple implications on drug clearance. Substances which are eliminated unchanged in the urine will remain in circulation and therefore have a prolonged half-life. This can be said about digoxin, insulin, and the aminoglycoside antibiotics. Some drugs are not metabolized directly by the kidneys but may rely on them for excretion of active metabolites. These metabolites, as in the case of morphine and its active metabolite morphine-6-glucuronide, can contribute to a prolonged effect when they are not efficiently cleared by the failing kidneys. Since renal clearance is dependent on glomerular filtration, often times the extent of impairment in renal clearance can be estimated with reasonable accuracy by the decrease in calculated creatinine clearance, which can be used to estimate glomerular filtration rate (GFR). Dosing adjustments for patients with lower GFR can then be made that result in either a decreased dose or increased dosing interval. For drugs with low therapeutic indices, this would ideally be done in conjunction with measurement of plasma levels. A major determinant of how much drug within the intravascular compartment reaches the processing and filtration sites within the kidney is systemic blood flow, as the kidneys normally receive about 25 % of the cardiac output. Patients with heart failure may fail to produce enough cardiac output to support the systemic circulation, and septic patients may exhibit profound decreases in peripheral vascular resistance. Either of these scenarios may result in decreased glomerular filtration and renal clearance. In the case of patients with fulminant renal failure requiring renal replacement therapy, the question often arises whether or not an administered drug will be filtered out into the dialysate. In general, agents that are highly water soluble, of low molecular weight, and with low Vd that do not display significant protein binding are thought to be susceptible to either hemodialysis or peritoneal dialysis. Other important factors to consider include the area and porosity of the dialyzing membrane.

In contrast to the relative predictability of renal insufficiency's effect on drug clearance, the patient with liver failure presents a challenge in the interpretation of to what extent their hepatic dysfunction may alter drug metabolism and elimination. The first level of complexity lies in the fact that for some substances, hepatic clearance is dependent not only on the inherent metabolic capability of the hepatocellular CYP450 system but on hepatic blood flow as well. Drugs with a high hepatic extraction ratio, meaning that they are efficiently metabolized and cleared by hepatocytes, are more affected by delivery via hepatic blood flow than metabolic capacity and are therefore classified as flow-limited. Critically ill patients may have multiple etiologies of decreased hepatic blood flow such as portal venous thrombosis, constriction of the splanchnic circulation from vasopressor therapy, or fibrosis of the liver from cirrhosis, therefore providing an intraparenchymal obstruction to hepatic blood flow. Substances which are less efficiently processed may rely more on the availability of hepatocytes for metabolism and are thought to be capacity limited.

Secondly, indices of hepatic dysfunction such as the Child score or MELD score do not readily correlate with the diseased liver's ability to conjugate and biotransform substances. The myriad of effects seen in patients with hepatic disease including the decreased production of albumin and gamma globulin and therefore reductions in drug protein binding can also have effects on clearance, mainly for drugs that are capacity limited. Finally, cirrhosis has been shown to have varying effects on different enzymes within the CYP450 system. While some enzymes' activity may be drastically reduced, others may not be affected or even show increased activity in cirrhosis.

Discussion of Commonly Used Agents

Sedatives, Analgesics, and Anxiolytics

Critical illness, as well as associated therapeutic measures, is often times characterized by severe discomfort, anxiety, or delirium. Each of these conditions has the potential to pose a significant barrier to both the intended outcome of a patient's care and also its implementation. Therefore, agents within this particular class are some of the most commonly prescribed to patients in the ICU, and knowledge of their action and potential side effects is paramount to their successful use.

Midazolam

Midazolam is a short-acting benzodiazepine used most commonly in the ICU as a continuous infusion for patients who are mechanically ventilated. A selective $GABA_A$ agonist, midazolam's intended effect is to produce sedation and anxiolysis, which may improve the patient's ability to tolerate the often times uncomfortable sensations that occur with mechanical ventilation. Its short elimination half-life observed in healthy individuals made it an ideal candidate for sedation provided by continuous infusion. However, critically ill patients have been observed to exhibit much more prolonged durations of sedation than their healthy counterparts [4]. In fact, some studies showed that patients were still fully sedated more than 10 h after the cessation of a midazolam infusion [3]. Suggestions for the etiology of this prolonged effect include an increased Vd or decrease in renal clearance seen in critically ill patients, the latter of which may also lead to an accumulation of active metabolites [2]. Prolonged, uninterrupted periods of sedation in critically ill patients may lead to an increased risk of delirium, a major predictive risk factor of overall ICU-related mortality, and can cause confusion in the interpretation of neurologic exam findings. For these reasons, midazolam may be slowly falling out of favor in its utility as a first-line medication for providing sedation in critically ill patients.

Propofol

Propofol is a short-acting, lipophilic diisopropylphenol used mainly for the induction and maintenance of general anesthesia. While its exact mechanism of action is unknown, the prevailing theory is that it acts to enhance the activity of $GABA_A$

receptors in the central nervous system [1]. The rapid emergence shown in patients in whom propofol has been administered has proven favorable in the sedation of critically ill patients. It exhibits a very low context-sensitive half-life, which means that even patients receiving prolonged continuous infusions will still display rapid emergence. Its rapid clearance is performed mainly via the liver with flow-limited characteristics, and little change in its elimination profile has been reported in patients with hepatic or renal disease. Recently, a specific potential for harm in patients receiving prolonged infusions of propofol has been described involving severe bradycardia leading to asystole, metabolic acidosis, and rhabdomyolysis. This particular grouping of symptoms in relation to a propofol infusion has been labeled the propofol infusion syndrome (PRIS), and as many as 38 fatalities have been reported. PRIS has been found to be associated with infusions of more than 4 mg kg^{-1} h^{-1} for over 48 h and is thought to be potentially due to propofol-induced mitochondrial dysfunction [5, 6]. Predisposing factors include young age and severe critical illness of the neurologic or respiratory system [7]. These findings have led to a revaluation of sedation protocols for critically ill patients who may require high doses of sedatives over a prolonged period. An additional area of concern for intensivists regards propofol's necessity for delivery in a lipid emulsion, which can contribute to a patient's dietary intake. The lipid emulsion can be thought of as similar to a 10 % parenteral lipid emulsion, amounting to 1.1 kcal/ml of fat [8]. In patients requiring large volumes of propofol to achieve adequate sedation, this can theoretically lead to overfeeding if other means of nutrition are not properly adjusted.

Fentanyl

Fentanyl is a synthetic opioid with a very rapid onset and limited duration of action. Its potency is thought to be 100 times more potent than morphine, and recovery from its analgesic and sedative effects is rapid. Fentanyl is most commonly used in the ICU as a continuous infusion for patients who may require both sedation and analgesia, such as most postsurgical patients who are mechanically ventilated. Recent observational data of human patients as well as experimental animal data suggest that fentanyl may play a significant role in causing acute opioid tolerance and opioid-induced hyperalgesia [9]. Authors of these studies therefore suggest that concurrent multimodal pain therapies, including the use of an NMDA antagonist such as ketamine, may mitigate the effects of opioid-induced hyperalgesia suggesting that NMDA excitation is a key component to hypersensitivity. The concept of fentanyl's role in perhaps creating a more painful response to normal stimuli may result in physician avoidance of its use in chronic pain patients who are cared for in the intensive care unit.

Dexmedetomidine

Dexmedetomidine is a selective alpha-2 adrenergic receptor agonist with anesthetic and sedative properties. It is used mainly in the form of a continuous infusion in the ICU. Due to its relative selectivity for the alpha-2 receptor, therapeutic doses may be accompanied by bradycardia and hypotension. At higher doses and with more rapid rate of infusion, the Alpha-1 effect can become more pronounced and hypertension can be seen. Dexmedetomidine has become more popular as a continuous sedative in mechanically ventilated patients because it does not have any negative impact on central respiratory drive, which can be seen with propofol and midazolam. Recent studies have shown that the use of dexmedetomidine as compared to midazolam in ventilated patients has been associated with fewer days spent on the ventilator and a decrease in delirium [10, 11]. The sympatholytic effects of dexmedetomidine have provided for an increased role in both the intraoperative and perioperative anesthetic and sedation regimens of cardiac surgery patients [12, 13]. Whereas this chemical sympathectomy may prove a desirable characteristic for the care of a critically ill patient with valvular heart disease or coronary artery disease, dexmedetomidine's propensity to cause hypotension and bradycardia may not be suitable for patients suffering from circulatory or septic shock who are reliant on cardiac output and therefore increases in heart rate to augment systemic perfusion.

Cardiovascular Agents

Supportive treatment of shock and maintenance of appropriate systemic and local perfusion to vital organs are of paramount importance in the management of critical illness and the prevention of secondary morbidity and mortality. The etiologies of shock and hypertension are numerous, and therefore, clinical pharmacology has evolved to provide a wide array of agents to correct these potentially life-threatening problems.

Vasopressors

Classically, vasopressors have been defined as agents that function mainly to augment peripheral vascular tone. Phenylephrine is probably the best known example of a true vasopressor. An alpha-1 adrenergic agonist, its main utility is direct arterial vasoconstriction. Due to its lack of beta-adrenergic activity, it tends to produce a reflex bradycardia in individuals with an intact baroreceptor response. This may be advantageous in certain patients where afterload and avoidance of tachycardia are at a premium as in the case of aortic stenosis. Circulatory shock is characterized by depletion of the body's natural endogenous catecholamines and vasoconstrictors. The mixed alpha- and beta-adrenergic agonist norepinephrine is regarded as a first-line vasopressor for the treatment of septic shock, as it is less likely than phenylephrine to reduce cardiac output [14]. A synthetic form of the naturally occurring vasopressin peptide exists that targets the V_1 receptor, resulting in direct vasoconstriction. Recent studies have suggested that the addition of low-dose vasopressin may reduce overall mortality in patients with less severe septic shock, and when used in combination with corticosteroid therapy may reduce mortality even further [15]. Unfortunately for certain groups of patients, such as those with high thoracic spinal cord injuries and resultant autonomic insufficiency, long-term vasopressor therapy may be necessary. In these cases, the oral alpha-1 agonist midodrine can be used. Midodrine is a prodrug of its active metabolite desglymidodrine and has a duration of 4–6 h. This may prove more convenient and cost-effective than prolonged continuous infusion in these patients.

Inotropes

Inotropes are agents that augment cardiac contractility and therefore increase cardiac output. Their main utility is in the treatment of cardiogenic shock and cases in which cardiac output needs to be maintained. The prototypical adrenergic agonist and perhaps the most powerful cardiac stimulant is epinephrine. With effects on both alpha- and beta-adrenergic receptors, epinephrine use results in activation of the abundance of beta-1 receptors found in the myocardium to increase cardiac contractility and heart rate. This effect comes at a price, however, as the heart's work is often less efficient and exhibits greatly increased myocardial oxygen demand. Furthermore, epinephrine use is often contraindicated in patients with a predisposition to dangerous tachyarrhythmias, which is often the case in the septic patient. This augmentation of beta-1 adrenergic activity has also resulted in the recommendation for avoidance of another naturally occurring catecholamine, dopamine, in the treatment of sepsis [14]. Critically ill patients with cardiogenic shock secondary to systolic heart failure require a different treatment strategy. Here, the augmentation of contractility is paramount, and even modest reductions in afterload will aid in the generation of cardiac output. Dobutamine is a mixed adrenergic agonist with activity mainly on the beta-1, beta-2, and alpha-1 receptor subsets. It therefore acts to augment cardiac contractility with minimal effects on systemic resistance. The selective PDE-3 inhibitor milrinone has more vasodilatory effects than dobutamine and, due to enhanced lusitropic effects, has been shown to be effective in the treatment of severe systolic heart failure when used in combination with beta blockade [16]. All inotropes exhibit to a lesser or greater degree bathmotropic, dromotropic, and chronotropic effects, and these often deleterious concomitant effects must be expected.

Antihypertensives

Treatment and prevention of extreme local and systemic hypertension in the ICU aims to prevent morbidity from an array of secondary adverse effects such as hemorrhagic stroke and myocardial ischemia. In these cases, often times the need for rapid onset and reliable titration to effect dictates the need for a continuous infusion. Some of the oldest and most reliable vasodilators are nitrates. Intravenous nitroglycerin is converted in vivo to nitric oxide (NO), which has a direct vasodilatory effect mainly on venous capacitance vessels. This serves to reduce cardiac preload and myocardial stretch, therefore reducing myocardial oxygen demand. Long-term use is complicated by tolerance, with patients often requiring escalating doses to achieve the desired effect.

Another nitrate, nitroprusside, is also converted to NO but has more effect on the arterial system than nitroglycerin. Its afterload reduction effects may be useful in patients suffering from systemic hypertension and systolic heart failure. Cyanide produced from the biotransformation of nitroprusside is converted to thiocyanate and then excreted by the kidneys. In patients with renal or hepatic failure, cyanide can accumulate and result in cyanide toxicity, impairing the utilization of oxygen by the cytochrome oxidase system. Long-term administration of any nitrate therapy can also result in methemoglobinemia resulting from the oxidation of hemoglobin by reactive NO species. The use of other arterial vasodilators such as the calcium channel blocker nicardipine may avert this problem. Nicardipine has the additional benefits of decreasing coronary vascular resistance, improving coronary blood flow, and reducing myocardial demand via negative inotropy. In certain cases, such as cerebral vasospasm after subarachnoid hemorrhage, patients may require higher systemic blood pressures and localized arterial relaxation. Nimodipine, a highly lipophilic calcium channel blocker, was developed to prevent cerebral vasospasm in these patients. Studies have shown that the use of nimodipine after subarachnoid hemorrhage can result in significant improvements in neurologic outcomes and reductions in mortality attributed to cerebral vasospasm [17]. Pulmonary vasodilators, most notably prostacyclin derivatives, phosphodiesterase type 5 inhibitors, and inhaled nitric oxide, are also within the intensivist's armamentarium largely for the treatment of acute right heart failure or pulmonary arterial hypertension.

Anticoagulants

Critical illness and the resultant stress response can result in the production of a hypercoagulable state. When combined with long periods of bed rest and physical inactivity, this can lead to the development of deep venous thrombosis (DVT). This condition when left untreated can lead to limb ischemia and the potential for fatal thromboembolism. The care of almost every single ICU patient involves some form of DVT prophylaxis, mainly in the form of injectable anticoagulants although newer oral anticoagulants have recently been introduced.

Heparin

Heparin is a glycosaminoglycan which is normally found in the secretory granules of mast cells. While it has no intrinsic anticoagulant activity, it exerts its effect by binding to and potentiating antithrombin, which works at various levels of the coagulation cascade to inhibit clot formation. Its main use in the ICU is subcutaneous injection for DVT prophylaxis, but it can also be given via continuous infusion to prevent catheter or device thrombosis in ECMO or venoarterial bypass or to treat coronary artery, pulmonary artery, or peripheral arterial clot formation. When used as a continuous infusion, its activity is monitored with laboratory analysis of the aPTT. Heparin's main adverse effect is bleeding, but approximately 0.3–0.5 % of ICU patients treated with unfractionated heparin may develop heparin-induced thrombocytopenia (HIT), characterized by platelet activation, thrombosis, and thrombocytopenia. HIT is thought to be caused by IgG antibodies against complexes of platelet factor 4 and heparin [17].

Heparin Derivatives and Newer Anticoagulants

Other forms of heparin which contain shorter glycan chains as in the low molecular weight heparins enoxaparin or fondaparinux have lesser incidence of HIT and may be used in the place of heparin in cases of suspected HIT. Recently, enoxaparin has become an attractive agent for DVT prophylaxis as it has been shown to be equally protective against DVT with similar incidence of bleeding as heparin, while needing fewer injections [18]. Although effective in preventing DVT and thromboembolism, a large multicenter trial recently found that enoxaparin use did not result in a reduction in overall mortality [19]. Newer anticoagulants such as the direct thrombin inhibitor dabigatran and the factor Xa inhibitor rivaroxaban have been developed and used for the prevention of venous thrombosis and primary prevention in atrial fibrillation. A particular benefit of these medications is that they are available orally and require little or no monitoring when dosed properly. Recent studies have shown that these medications have similar or even better reductions in rate of venous thrombosis when compared to enoxaparin, but their current use may be limited practically by their cost [20].

Corticosteroids

Critical illness and severe alterations in physiology induce a hormonal response which results in both the liberation of catecholamines and cortisol intended to aid the body's need for protein substrates and hemodynamic support and the possible reduced clearance of cortisol. Over time, this can result in a depletion of the body's normal steroid hormones. Pharmacologic therapies in sepsis, adrenal insufficiency, and other forms of critical illness have at times included the administration of exogenous corticosteroids, falling in and out of favor over the years. Steroids have also been used to reduce inflammation and swelling in the oropharynx, intracerebral vault, and spinal canal. A discussion of each class of steroid and their use is outside the scope of this chapter but select topics pertaining to ICU care will be included as follows.

Treatment of Septic Shock

Corticosteroid therapy in septic shock had been a mainstay of treatment for decades without clear evidence that it provided a mortality benefit. One study in 2002 showed that septic patients who failed a corticotropin stimulation test had a 10 % reduction in mortality when given supplemental corticosteroids [21]. This led to widespread adoption of steroid therapy, as time to shock reversal was also shown to decrease. Subsequent studies, however, have failed to reproduce this outcome. In fact, one large randomized study in 2008 failed to show any difference in 28-day mortality when steroid replacement was compared to placebo [22]. The reduction in time to shock reversal was again demonstrated, but the rates of superinfection and subsequent development of new sepsis and septic shock were higher in the treatment group. This recent development has led to recommendations from leading organizations to refrain from steroid therapy in septic shock in cases where adequate hemodynamic support can be achieved with fluid resuscitation and vasopressor therapy [14].

Intracerebral Hemorrhage and Traumatic Brain Injury

Corticosteroid therapy has been used for decades in the neurosurgical field and has proven to be beneficial in reducing the amount of vasogenic edema that occurs with intracranial tumors or in the postoperative setting [23, 24]. The exact mechanism for this effect however was poorly understood, but nevertheless, the benefit seen in these groups of patients led to the expansion of steroid therapy in treatment of other patients with neurologic catastrophes like intracerebral hemorrhage or traumatic brain injury. With the knowledge that steroid therapy can lead to adverse outcomes such as delayed wound healing, sepsis, hyperglycemia, and gastrointestinal bleeding, there has been a renewed effort to analyze the benefit of steroids in the treatment of acute hemorrhage and traumatic brain injury. A Cochrane Review published in 2006 analyzed 8 trials involving roughly 460 patients with either subarachnoid hemorrhage or primary intracerebral hemorrhage and found that steroid therapy did not provide any statistically meaningful reduction in mortality or poor neurologic outcome [25]. In 2005, a large randomized controlled trial was performed analyzing the effect of steroid therapy versus placebo in over 10,000 patients with traumatic brain injury. The results showed that steroid infusion for the first 48 h after injury resulted in a statistically significant increase in overall 6-month mortality [26]. This emerging data along with perhaps a better understanding of the different pathophysiologic mechanisms underlying cellular edema in hemorrhagic stroke and traumatic brain injury has led to a change in practice regarding the widespread use of steroid therapy in these patients.

Agents That Prevent and Treat Gastrointestinal Hemorrhage

Mucosal erosion and resultant gastrointestinal hemorrhage is a common and dreaded complication of critical illness if not properly prevented. The etiology of stress ulcer formation is complex, but may involve a combination of endogenous steroid inhibition of prostaglandin formation, decreased splanchnic blood flow and ischemia, and reperfusion injury. Patients most at risk for the development of stress ulcers and clinically significant bleeding include mechanically ventilated patients and those with coagulopathies [27]. Prevention of this occurrence with agents that raise gastric pH has proven to be easier than managing the complications of significant hemorrhage; therefore, the care of many ICU patients includes pharmacologic stress ulcer prophylaxis (SUP).

Antihistamines

Selective H_2 receptor antagonists such as ranitidine have the ability to reduce basal gastric parietal cell acid production by 70%. They have been clinically proven to reduce the rate of clinically significant gastrointestinal bleeding, but their benefit may be limited to patients who are not receiving enteral nutrition. Furthermore, antihistamine therapy in those patients receiving enteral nutrition may result in an increased risk of nosocomial pneumonia [28]. Other rare complications of H_2 receptor antagonists include confusion and delirium in the elderly, and several case reports have linked their use with the development of thrombocytopenia. Despite these concerns in limited subgroups of patients, antihistamine use continues to be a mainstay of stress ulcer prevention secondary to its effectiveness and relatively low cost compared with other agents such the other commonly used class of agents used for SUP such as proton pump inhibitors.

Proton Pump Inhibitors

By inhibiting the parietal cell H^+/K^+ ATPase, proton pump inhibitors (PPIs) such as omeprazole are the most potent inhibitors of both basal and stimulated gastric acid secretion. Their use can reduce gastric acid secretion by 80–95%. Despite this knowledge of the superior potency of proton pump inhibitors, available data regarding their superiority over antihistamines in SUP has been conflicting. A meta-analysis performed in 2008 of 7 clinical trials including over 900 patients failed to show any statistically significant difference between PPIs and H_2 in the prevention of stress-related upper gastrointestinal bleeding [29]. However, a more recent meta-analysis published in March of 2013 of 9 trials involving over 1,700 patients showed that PPI use resulted in a decreased rate of both clinically important and overt upper GI bleeding [30]. Despite this difference, this most recent analysis failed to show a mortality benefit from PPI use when compared with antihistamines.

Once upper gastrointestinal bleeding has occurred, the mainstay of pre-endoscopic pharmacotherapy has been the administration of proton pump inhibitors. Their use in this population for 24–48 h before endoscopy may reduce the appearance of stigmata of recent hemorrhage or need for endoscopic corrective procedures compared to controls including antihistamine therapy [31]. Prevailing theory over recent years regarding the dosing and mode of administration of PPI therapy of gastrointestinal bleeding suggested that a high-dose, continuous infusion would be the logical choice given the need for effective and continuous acid suppression. However, recent data suggests that neither high-dose nor continuous PPI infusions are needed to reduce the risk of rebleeding, need for surgery, or overall mortality in these patients as compared to lower, twice-daily dosing [32, 33].

Summary

Critically ill patients can present with severe derangements in physiology and homeostasis that can have varying effects on the pharmacokinetics and pharmacodynamics of the medications intended to treat them. Familiarity with these effects as well as knowledge of the commonly used drugs in the intensivist's armamentarium and the most relevant clinical data behind their use can aid in prescribing an individually tailored therapeutic regimen that has the potential to correct critical illness and lead the patient on a path to recovery and a meaningful quality of life.

References

1. Mihic SJ, Harris RA. Chapter 17: Hypnotics and sedatives. In: Brunton LL, Chabner BA, Knollmann BC, editors. Goodman & Gilman's The pharmacological basis of therapeutics. 12th ed. New York: McGraw-Hill; 2011.
2. Oldenhof H, et al. Clinical pharmacokinetics of midazolam in intensive care patients, a wide interpatient variability[quest]. Clin Pharmacol Ther. 1988;43(3):263–9.
3. Malacrida R, et al. Pharmacokinetics of midazolam administered by continuous intravenous infusion to intensive care patients. Crit Care Med. 1992;20(8):1123–6.
4. Shafer A. Complications of sedation with midazolam in the intensive care unit and a comparison with other sedative regimens. Crit Care Med. 1998;26(5):947–56.
5. Bray RJ. Propofol infusion syndrome in children. Pediatr Anesth. 1998;8(6):491–9.
6. Wolf A, et al. Impaired fatty acid oxidation in propofol infusion syndrome. Lancet. 2001;357(9256):606–7.
7. Kam PCA, Cardone D. Propofol infusion syndrome. Anaesthesia. 2007;62(7):690–701.
8. DeChicco R, et al. Contribution of calories from propofol to total energy intake. J Am Diet Assoc. 1995;95(9):A25.
9. Laulin J-P, et al. The role of ketamine in preventing fentanyl-induced hyperalgesia and subsequent acute morphine tolerance. Anesth Analg. 2002;94(5):1263–9.
10. Riker RR, Shehabi Y, Bokesch PM, et al. Dexmedetomidine vs midazolam for sedation of critically ill patients: a randomized trial. JAMA. 2009;301(5):489–99.
11. Jakob SM, Ruokonen E, Grounds RM, et al. Dexmedetomidine vs midazolam or propofol for sedation during prolonged mechanical ventilation: two randomized controlled trials. JAMA. 2012;307(11):1151–60.
12. Mukhtar AM, Obayah EM, Hassona AM. The use of dexmedetomidine in pediatric cardiac surgery. Anesth Analg. 2006;103(1):52–6.
13. Shehabi Y, et al. Prevalence of delirium with dexmedetomidine compared with morphine based therapy after cardiac surgery: a randomized controlled trial (DEXmedetomidine COmpared to Morphine-DEXCOM study). Anesthesiology. 2009;111(5):1075–84. doi:10.1097/ALN.0b013e3181b6a783.

14. Dellinger RP, et al. Surviving sepsis campaign: international guidelines for management of severe sepsis and septic shock, 2012. Intensive Care Med. 2013;39(2):165–228.
15. Russell JA, et al. Vasopressin versus norepinephrine infusion in patients with septic shock. N Engl J Med. 2008;358(9):877–87.
16. Zewail AM, et al. Intravenous milrinone in treatment of advanced congestive heart failure. Tex Heart Inst J. 2003;30(2):109–13.
17. Barker FG, Ogilvy CS. Efficacy of prophylactic nimodipine for delayed ischemic deficit after subarachnoid hemorrhage: a metaanalysis. J Neurosurg. 1996;84(3):405–14.
18. McGarry L, Stokes M, Thompson D. Outcomes of thromboprophylaxis with enoxaparin vs. unfractionated heparin in medical inpatients. Thromb J. 2006;4(1):17.
19. Kakkar AK, et al. Low-molecular-weight heparin and mortality in acutely ill medical patients. N Engl J Med. 2011;365(26):2463–72.
20. Yoshida Rde A, et al. Systematic review of randomized controlled trials of new anticoagulants for venous thromboembolism prophylaxis in major orthopedic surgeries, compared with enoxaparin. Ann Vasc Surg. 2013;27(3):355–69.
21. Annane D, et al. Effect of treatment with low doses of hydrocortisone and fludrocortisone on mortality in patients with septic shock. JAMA. 2002;288(7):862–71.
22. Sprung CL, et al. Hydrocortisone therapy for patients with septic shock. N Engl J Med. 2008;358(2):111–24.
23. Roth P, Wick W, Weller M. Steroids in neurooncology: actions, indications, side-effects. Curr Opin Neurol. 2010;23(6):597–602. doi:10.1097/WCO.0b013e32833e5a5d.
24. Bebawy JF. Perioperative steroids for peritumoral intracranial edema: a review of mechanisms, efficacy, and side effects. J Neurosurg Anesthesiol. 2012;24(3):173–7. doi:10.1097/ANA.0b013e3182578bb5.
25. Feigin VL, et al. Corticosteroids in patients with hemorrhagic stroke. Stroke. 2006;37(5):1344–5.
26. Collaborators CT. Final results of MRC CRASH, a randomised placebo-controlled trial of intravenous corticosteroid in adults with head injury? Outcomes at 6 months. Lancet. 2005;365(9475):1957–9.
27. Cook DJ, et al. Risk factors for gastrointestinal bleeding in critically ill patients. N Engl J Med. 1994;330(6):377–81.
28. Marik PE, et al. Stress ulcer prophylaxis in the new millennium: a systematic review and meta-analysis. Crit Care Med. 2010;38(11):2222–8. doi:10.1097/CCM.0b013e3181f17adf.
29. Lin PC, et al. The efficacy and safety of proton pump inhibitors vs histamine-2 receptor antagonists for stress ulcer bleeding prophylaxis among critical care patients: a meta-analysis. Crit Care Med. 2010;38(4):1197–205.
30. Alhazzani W, et al. Proton pump inhibitors versus histamine 2 receptor antagonists for stress ulcer prophylaxis in critically ill patients: a systematic review and meta-analysis*. Crit Care Med. 2013;41(3):693–705. doi:10.1097/CCM.0b013e3182758734.
31. Sreedharan A, et al. Proton pump inhibitor treatment initiated prior to endoscopic diagnosis in upper gastrointestinal bleeding. Cochrane Database Syst Rev. 2010;(7):CD005415.
32. Wang C, Ma MH, Chou HC, et al. High-dose vs non-high-dose proton pump inhibitors after endoscopic treatment in patients with bleeding peptic ulcer: a systematic review and meta-analysis of randomized controlled trials. Arch Intern Med. 2010;170(9):751–8.
33. Songür Y, et al. Comparison of infusion or low-dose proton pump inhibitor treatments in upper gastrointestinal system bleeding. Eur J Intern Med. 2011;22(2):200–4.

Chapter 40
Enteral and Parenteral Nutrition

Jillian Redgate and Sumit Singh

Contents

J. Redgate, RD, CNSC
Nutrition and Food Services, VA Greater Los Angeles Healthcare System,
Los Angeles, CA, USA
e-mail: jmredgate@gmail.com

S. Singh, MD, UCLA (✉)
Department of Anesthesiology, David Geffen School of Medicine at UCLA,
Los Angeles, CA, USA

Nutrition and Food Services, VA Greater Los Angeles Healthcare System,
Los Angeles, CA, USA
e-mail: spsingh@mednet.ucla.edu

A.D. Kaye et al. (eds.), *Essentials of Pharmacology for Anesthesia,*
Pain Medicine, and Critical Care, DOI 10.1007/978-1-4614-8948-1_40,
© Springer Science+Business Media New York 2015

Introduction

Critically ill patients have a multitude of stressors that cause disruption in homeostasis. Besides pathophysiologic changes resulting from critical illness, there are environmental, psychosocial, and nutritional stressors. These can lead to altered energy consumption and nutrient losses, resulting in faster depletion of body stores. Nutrition support is therefore an integral part of care of a critically ill patient. Lack of enteral nutrition (EN) can lead to a proinflammatory state resulting in increased oxidative stress, multiorgan failure, and a prolonged length of stay [1–3]. On the other hand, early and appropriate EN can decrease gut bacterial translocation, maintain gut-associated lymphoid tissue (GALT), and preserve upper respiratory tract immunity [1, 4, 5]. This translates to improved clinical outcomes and a decrease in costs, while reducing complication rates and length of stay [6]. Moreover, certain nutrients such as glutamine, arginine, and omega-3 (ω-3) fatty acids have been shown to have favorable clinical effects in critically ill patients [1, 7]. The dynamic interplay of pathophysiology and metabolism in critical illness suggests that we consider nutrition as a specific pharmacotherapeutic intervention by which an astute clinician can alter the disease process to achieve a favorable outcome.

In this chapter, we will provide an overview of nutrition support focusing on the critically ill patient. We will also discuss specific pharmaconutrients and their proposed mechanisms of action, along with a broad discussion of the interactions of nutrition with GI function, modulation of inflammation and immunity, and condition and disease-related indications for specialized nutrition support. We will also cover important drug-nutrient interactions as well as potential adverse effects associated with nutrition support.

Drug Class and Mechanism of Action

Enteral and Parenteral Nutrition

Artificial nutrition may be provided in the form of either EN or parenteral nutrition (PN). EN is defined by the American Society for Parenteral and Enteral Nutrition (ASPEN) as "nutrition provided through the gastrointestinal tract via a tube, catheter, or stoma that delivers nutrients distal to the oral cavity" [8]. EN is preferred over PN due to reduced cost and complications [8]. PN is defined as "nutrients provided intravenously" [9]. PN consists of a dextrose-amino acid solution including vitamins and minerals and an intravenous fat emulsion (IVFE) [9].

Pharmaconutrients

Specialized EN formulas containing pharmaconutrients may be beneficial for modulation of immune and inflammatory responses [1, 7, 10]. Researchers typically use commercial formulas in investigations; therefore, they have studied combinations rather than individual immune-modulating nutrients. This makes it difficult to determine precise individual dosing recommendations or to determine whether it is an individual nutrient or the synergistic effect of many pharmaconutrients that provide clinical benefit [7].

Arginine and glutamine are conditionally essential amino acids during acute periods of stress [7, 10]. Arginine is involved in many metabolic pathways, including conversion of ammonia to urea, protein and collagen synthesis, and release of anabolic hormones [10]. Arginine is required for the synthesis of polyamines which promote cell division and growth and may decrease production of proinflammatory cytokines and T cells [10]. Arginine is also involved in the production of nitric oxide [10]. Glutamine is a key substrate for gluconeogenesis and is an important fuel for rapid turnover cells, such as the small intestine epithelium and immune cells, including lymphocytes and macrophages [7, 10]. Additionally, it is involved in the regulation of T-cell proliferation, interleukin-2 production, and B-cell differentiation, as well as having a role in phagocytosis and superoxide production [10]. Parenteral supplementation has been shown to promote positive nitrogen balance and healing in postoperative patients and appears to support gut integrity in spite of its intravenous (IV) rather than enteral administration [1, 10].

Essential polyunsaturated ω-3 and omega-6 (ω-6) fatty acids are involved in cell membrane formation and production of prostaglandins and leukotrienes [10]. The less inflammatory derivatives of ω-3 fatty acids (such as 3-series prostaglandins and 5-series leukotrienes and D-series resolvins and protectins) compete with highly inflammatory ω-6 fatty acid derivatives (including 2-series prostaglandins and 4-series leukotrienes); therefore, a diet higher in ω-3 and lower in ω-6 fatty acids helps to modulate the inflammation and improve immune function [7, 10, 11].

Immune-modulating formulas may also contain increased amounts of nucleotides and antioxidants. Similar to arginine and glutamine, the need for dietary nucleotides is increased during periods of acute stress, since they are needed for synthesis of DNA and RNA and are vital for energy transfer and hormone function [7]. Nucleotide deficiency may worsen immune function and increase the risk of sepsis [12]. Antioxidant supplementation may be beneficial in critically ill (including septic) patients, those with acute respiratory distress, and those undergoing major surgery [1, 10, 13].

Indications and Clinical Pearls

The functions of artificial nutrition exceed provision of energy and nutrients in order to prevent or reverse malnutrition. Artificial nutrition can prevent loss of gut integrity and gut-associated immunity, modulate whole-body immune function and the inflammatory response, and improve clinical outcomes in many patient populations, including surgical, trauma, burn, and other critically ill patients.

Maintenance of Gut Integrity

The healthy gut acts as a physical barrier to antigens and contains specialized tissue that can trigger an immune response [4, 5]. During periods of acute stress such as critical illness, splanchnic hypoperfusion may cause injury to gut tissue within hours of injury [4, 5]. GALT, part of the mucosal-associated lymphoid tissue, is comprised of Peyer's patches, the appendix, epithelial cells, and a layer of the lamina propria [4]. Normally, antigens are detected and absorbed in small bowel Peyer's patches, where T and B cells are sensitized [4]. When nutrition support is held or provided with PN rather than EN or oral diet, levels of naïve T and B lymphocytes in Peyer's patches are significantly reduced [4]. Loss of GALT mass and function has been shown to reduce overall bodily immune function in both human and animal experiments [4, 5]. Provision of EN helps to maintain gut integrity by preventing loss of tight junction proteins, by maintaining GALT mass and function, and by improving blood flow to the bowel [1].

Modulation of the Inflammatory Response

Modification of essential fatty acid balance towards more ω-3 and fewer ω-6 fatty acids may improve clinical outcomes. High doses of oral ω-3-rich fish oil (1–7 g/day) have been shown to be beneficial for the treatment of rheumatoid arthritis and cardiovascular disease and possibly (though less conclusively) inflammatory bowel disease and asthma [11]. While animal models looking at the effects of fish oil supplementation have been promising, clinical research is less conclusive [11]. One area where the use of fish oil has clear clinical benefits is when proinflammatory IVFE is replaced with a fish oil IVFE [9, 11]. Unfortunately, the only IVFE available in the United States is made of soybean oil, which contains a relatively higher proportion of ω-6 fatty acids as compared to alternative formulations available in other countries, which contain other lipid sources, including medium chain triglycerides, olive oil, and/or fish oil [13].

Perioperative Nutrition Support

Provision of immunonutrition is beneficial when provided preoperatively, postoperatively, or perioperatively; however, positive effects, specifically decreased time of mechanical ventilation, decreased infectious morbidity, and decreased length of stay, are more prominent in patients who receive immunonutrition perioperatively [8]. ASPEN strongly recommends the use of immune-modulating formulas in patients undergoing major elective surgery with especially strong evidence for use in those undergoing major GI surgery [8, 14]. Further studies and meta-analyses after publication of ASPEN's recommendations continue to support the use of immune-modulating EN in surgical patients [15–17].

Respiratory Failure

Historically, formulas designed for use in those with acute lung injury (ALI) or acute respiratory distress syndrome (ARDS) were low in carbohydrate (CHO) and high in fat in order to decrease CO_2 production [18]. It was later discovered that excess energy is more detrimental than excess CHO provision [18]. Formulas designed to modulate inflammation and cellular oxidation associated with ALI/ARDS were developed more recently [17]. Current pulmonary formulas contain ω-3 fatty acids, borage oil (gamma-linolenic acid), and antioxidants with standard amounts of CHO and fat [17]. ASPEN's guidelines recommend these formulas for ALI/ARDS based on studies showing a reduction in mortality, ventilator days, length of stay, and organ failure [1]. The three studies this recommendation is based on, however, compared modern formulas to out-of-favor high-fat pulmonary formulas [19–21]. Since control formulas were high in total fat, they contained high levels of proinflammatory ω-6 fatty acids, which is a significant methodological flaw. When modern pulmonary formulas are compared to standard EN formulas, significant benefits are not observed [19]. Given the high cost of specialized formulas, clinicians should consider this recent evidence before using specialized pulmonary EN formulas.

Severe Acute Pancreatitis

Often the goal of therapy for acute pancreatitis is gut rest in order to minimize pancreatic stimulation. Unfortunately, this quickly leads to loss of gut integrity and bacterial overgrowth [22]. Consequently, there is increased inflammation and a blunted immune response due to downregulation of GALT, which can lead to or exacerbate existing systemic inflammation and worsen overall prognosis [22]. This can be prevented with early initiation of EN, ideally within 24–48 h, in patients with severe acute pancreatitis [26]. A polymeric formula is acceptable, although a semi-elemental formula may be considered if the standard formula is not tolerated [22]. Though feeding the small bowel past the ligament of Treitz has been recommended to minimize pancreatic stimulation, more recent studies have shown that gastric feeds may also be well tolerated [22, 23].

Other Critical Illness

Immunonutrition may also be beneficial in other critically ill patients, such as those with sepsis, trauma, burns, and traumatic brain injury [1, 10, 24–30]. The benefits for these patients, however, are less clear than for surgical patients, due to fewer available research studies [1, 10]. There is evidence that supports early EN (within

24–48 h of injury) in patients with severe burns [24–29] and traumatic brain injury [27]. Burn patients have extremely high protein-energy requirements and benefit from increased provisions of antioxidants, selenium, zinc, and copper for wound healing and prevention of cellular oxidation [28]. While there is evidence that immunonutrition may be beneficial in burn patients, more research is needed to confirm these benefits [26]. There is less available evidence regarding the use of immunonutrition in brain injury; however, animal studies have shown that gluta-mine supplementation may help maintain gut integrity and modulate inflammation in this patient population [29, 30].

Other Organ Failure

Patients with acute kidney injury should receive standard EN formulas unless elec-trolyte abnormalities occur. For these patients, specialized renal formulas should be considered [1]. Protein provision must be individualized based on other acute con-ditions, severity of renal failure, and blood urea nitrogen levels, keeping in mind that acute kidney injury is a hypermetabolic condition and that renal replacement therapy further increases protein needs [1, 31]. Otherwise healthy patients with chronic renal failure may require a renal, low-protein formula for preservation of renal function if not receiving dialysis. A renal, higher protein formula is indicated when receiving dialysis treatment [31].

Though specialized hepatic formulas high in branch-chained amino acids are available, these should be reserved for patients with refractory encephalopathy and should not be used routinely in those with hepatic failure [1]. As with most patient populations, EN is also the preferable form of artificial nutrition in those with hepatic dysfunction. However, PN is acceptable for those who cannot tolerate EN for more than 7 days, in spite of the potential hepatic side effects associated with PN therapy [32, 33]. In all cases of organ failure, nutrition assessment and determina-tion of appropriate nutrition support must be highly individualized, and clinicians should not rely on specialized formulas when choosing nutrition therapy.

Dosing Options

Estimating Protein-Energy Needs

Though indirect calorimetry is the gold standard for determination of estimated energy requirement (EER), it is often not available; therefore, predictive equations must be used [18, 34]. For healthy, normal-weight individuals, EER is around 25 kcal/kg of the actual body weight (ABW) [35]. Clinicians may also use the Mifflin St. Jeor equation using ABW, especially for overweight or obese individuals [34].

There are also a number of formulas for estimation of energy needs in the critically ill. The Academy of Nutrition and Dietetics recommends using the Penn State University 2003b equation [36] or the Penn State University 2010 equation for obese patients over the age of 65 [37].

While one may surmise that a critically ill patient has increased EER due to the severity of illness, EER in this population is actually around 23 kcal/kg [35]. Intake over 25 kcal/kg is associated with liver damage, especially when provided by PN [35]. Critically ill patients may, in fact, benefit from permissive underfeeding to 50–60 % of their EER during the first week after injury, especially if the patient is obese [1]. After 1 week, efforts should be made to avoid underfeeding, as it could result in decreased respiratory muscle strength, immunosuppression, worsened wound healing, and increased risk of infection [18]. Prevention of both underfeeding and overfeeding requires close monitoring and frequent adjustments to protein-energy provision in the critically ill population.

Protein intake may be of higher importance than energy provision in critically ill patients [35]. While normal protein requirements are around 0.8 g/kg ABW [38], critically ill patients require 1.2–2 g/kg ABW when their BMI is less than 30 or 2–2.5 g/kg ideal body weight or higher if the patient is obese [1]. Protein provision may need to be further modified in the setting of renal dysfunction [31].

Initiation and Advancement of Nutrition Support

In critically ill patients for whom an oral diet is not feasible, EN should be initiated within 24–48 h of injury to maximize benefits, including a decrease in infections, length of stay, and mortality [1]. Though ASPEN guidelines recommend a starting rate of 10–40 mL/h and advancing to goal rate by 10–20 mL/h every 8–12 h as tolerated [8], it should be noted that there is a lack of research regarding appropriate and safe initiation and advancement of EN support. For short-term nutrition support, a naso- or orogastric tube is preferred due to ease of placement [1]. Naso-jejunal tubes may be preferable in patients with a known risk of aspiration or those with a history of intolerance to gastric feeds [1, 8, 39]. If EN support will be required long term (more than 4 weeks, per ASPEN), placement of a long-term feeding device such as a gastrostomy or jejunostomy tube should be considered [8].

If a patient does not tolerate EN, it is preferable to withhold nutrition support for 7 days rather than to initiate early PN [1, 40]. For malnourished patients, however, PN should be considered earlier [7]. If EN is not achievable or sufficient for longer than 7 days, PN should be considered [1]. Due to the potentially proinflammatory effects of soy-based IVFE, ASPEN recommends withholding lipids for the first week of PN therapy [1]. In noncritically ill patients, there are no clear recommendations regarding when exactly EN or PN should be initiated. Clinicians need to consider many factors, including presence of malnutrition, inflammation, and expected duration of suboptimal oral intake.

Parenteral nutrition can be provided via a central venous catheter (CVC) or a peripheral vein [9]. Hypertonic PN formulas (those with an osmolarity greater than 900–1,100 mOsm/L) will not be well tolerated peripherally and should be provided via a CVC [9, 41]. Subclavian and jugular CVCs can be used when expected length of PN therapy is short term. However, a peripherally inserted central catheter (PICC) is preferable when PN is required for more than a few weeks in order to decrease the risk of infection and mechanical complication [9, 41]. Provision of PN via a femoral line is associated with increased infection risk and thrombosis and therefore should be avoided [9, 41]. Long-term PN (greater than 3 months) should be infused through a cuffed tunneled CVC or an implanted port, with a tunneled CVC being preferable [9, 41]. Catheters should have as few lumens as possible, with one lumen being reserved for infusion of PN only [41].

Drug Interactions

Interactions of EN formulations and medications can be complex and difficult to predict [42]. IV medications may be changed to an oral route in order to reduce costs, but run the risk of unreliable delivery or absorption due to their interaction with the feeding tube material or EN formula [42]. Following are some general principles that should be considered while administering drugs in patients receiving EN:

1. As some medications need alkaline or acidic medium for absorption, the location of the tip of the feeding tube (e.g., gastric, duodenal, or jejunal) can affect the absorption [42].
2. Tubes should be flushed with 15 ml of water before and after medication administration. Fifteen milliliters of water should also be used to flush tubes between administrations of different medications [8].
3. An elixir or liquid formulation should always be the preferred form of administration through feeding tubes. These should also be diluted with 30 ml of water before administration [43].
4. Solid medications can be crushed to a fine powder and mixed with water to form a slurry before administration. Gelatin capsules can be aspirated and contents dissolved in water [43].
5. In order to prevent EN contamination, medications should never be mixed with enteral feeds [8].
6. For enteral medication administration, gastric access is usually the preferred route, as gastric tubes have a larger lumen and are less prone to getting blocked. To prevent the clogging of smaller lumen feeding tubes (e.g., jejunostomy tubes), only liquid formulations should be administered through them [43].
7. Hypertonic medications are not well tolerated when delivered into the small intestine. The stomach can dilute hyperosmolar substances with gastric juices before transferring to the duodenum. When hypertonic medications are administered too quickly into the stomach, osmotic diarrhea may result from dumping of the stomach contents into the intestines [43].

Though many medications can be given concurrently with enteral feeds, some need tube feeds to be held before and after administration [44]. Others may require administration of a particular form to prevent degradation or drug-nutrient interaction [42]. Following are some specific drug and EN interactions:

Fluoroquinolones – Ciprofloxacin and ofloxacin absorption is decreased by EN; however, moxifloxacin absorption is not significantly affected [42, 45, 46]. Tablets are acceptable, while suspension is not [42]. EN should be withheld for 1 h before and 2 h after administration of ciprofloxacin tablets [42]. Since ciprofloxacin is mainly absorbed in the duodenum, administration through jejunostomy tubes should be avoided [42, 47].

Penicillin V – Bioavailability varies 30–80 % with concomitant administration of food [48]. EN should be withheld 1 h before and 2 h after administration, and higher doses may be considered [42].

Proton pump inhibitors – These are absorbed in the alkaline medium of the duodenum and are inactivated by gastric acid; therefore, formulations are made as enteric-coated delayed release granules or tablets [49]. Mixing delayed release capsules (omeprazole, lansoprazole) with acidic diluents (apple or orange juice) help to keeps the granules intact until they reach the duodenum [42]. Since there is a potential for occlusion by clumping of granules, especially through small-bore feeding tubes, another method of administration includes alkaline suspensions made by dissolving granules in a solution of 8.4 % sodium bicarbonate [42].

Theophylline – A greater than 30 % decrease of theophylline level has been reported with enteral feeding [50]. EN should be withheld for 1 h after administration of the medication [42].

Levothyroxine sodium – This may bind with EN feeding tubes, resulting in decreased drug efficacy [51]. When used for more than 1 week, EN should be withheld 1 h before and after administration, and thyroid function should be monitored weekly [42, 52].

Warfarin – Binding of warfarin with proteins in the EN can reduce bioavailability and decrease the anticoagulant effect [53]. Methods to overcome this problem include holding EN 1 h before and after administration, increasing warfarin dose, or changing to another anticoagulant such as heparin [54]. Once the patient is transitioned to an oral diet, a reduced warfarin dose may be necessary.

Carbamazepine – Adherence of carbamazepine to the walls of polyvinyl chloride (PVC) feeding tubes can occur, resulting in inadequate drug delivery. Therefore, serum concentration monitoring should be performed when the drug is being administered via a PVC tube [42].

Phenytoin – Absorption of phenytoin may be reduced by 70 % when administered concurrently with EN [55]. Possible causes of impaired absorption include adherence to the tube itself and binding to proteins and calcium salts [42]. EN should be withheld for 1 h before and after administration; otherwise, IV administration should be considered [42].

Sucralfate – Proteins in tube feeds can form insoluble complexes with sucralfate and result in clogging of the feeding tubes [56]. Additionally, the alkaline medium of EN may prevent activation of sucralfate. EN should be withheld for 1 h before and after administration [42].

Other EN-drug interactions may be more complex. Since all vasopressors decrease mesenteric perfusion and GI motility, administration of EN in hemodynamically unstable patients receiving vasopressors could cause nonobstructive bowel ischemia and EN intolerance [57]. This is not a contraindication to the provision of EN; in fact, hemodynamically unstable patients receiving multiple vasopressor medications may benefit most from early EN [58]. Therefore, EN should be administered early, but advanced cautiously with close monitoring to prevent complications [58]. If EN is not well tolerated, complete or supplemental PN should be considered [1]. Of note, as pure inotropes (milrinone, dobutamine, dopexamine) increase cardiac output and gut perfusion, EN should not cause the abovementioned complications.

Propofol does not interact with EN, but does provide additional kcal. It is a lipid solution that contains 1.1 kcal/ml and, when continuously administered at high rates (greater than 20 ml/h), in combination with full enteral feeding, may lead to overfeeding [59]. It is therefore recommended to closely monitor daily caloric intake and manipulate nutritional support accordingly [59].

Side Effects

Nutrition support is safe when administered by trained clinicians and tolerance is closely monitored. Safety is especially enhanced when facilities have a designated nutrition support team, including physicians, registered dietitians, pharmacists, and nurses [60–62]. Following are some potential side effects of EN and PN, as well as methods for prevention, and treatment recommendations.

Side Effects of Enteral Nutrition

Most studies have shown that immune-modulating EN formulas are safe for critically ill patients. There is some evidence that arginine supplementation may lead to increased mortality in septic patients based on three studies of poor design [1, 7]. Researchers theorized that increased nitric oxide production related to arginine metabolism may cause hemodynamic instability in severely critically ill patients [1, 7]. Many other studies and reports have not shown deleterious effects of arginine, but rather improved outcomes [1, 7]. Based on their review of the literature, ASPEN continues to recommend the use of arginine-containing enteral formulas in mild and moderate sepsis and cautions when used in severe sepsis [1].

The high protein content of most immune-modulating formulas in addition to the products of arginine and glutamine metabolism may increase blood urea nitrogen, which is of particular concern in patients with acute or chronic renal failure [7]. Unfortunately, if patients do require a lower protein or "renal formula," immune-enhancing enteral nutrition may not be possible since proper dosing of individual pharmaconutrients is unknown [7].

There is some evidence that EN delivered into the stomach may increase risk of esophageal reflux; therefore, naso-jejunal tubes may be preferable in patients with known risk of aspiration or those with a history of intolerance to gastric feeds [1, 8, 39]. In spite of the risk of reflux, there is insufficient evidence to support the routine placement of jejunal tubes over gastric tubes in critically ill patients [1, 39].

Side Effects of Parenteral Nutrition

The most common complication associated with PN is hyperglycemia. IV dextrose bypasses the enteroinsular axis, leading to a more pronounced hyperglycemia than would be expected with enteral CHO administration [63]. To prevent hyperglycemia, PN should be initiated and advanced slowly over days, while blood glucose is closely monitored and insulin administration is carefully titrated [9]. ASPEN also recommends that the CHO administration rate should not exceed 4–5 mg/kg/min for critically ill patients and those with diabetes mellitus [9].

Hypertriglyceridemia can occur due to dextrose overfeeding or overly rapid administration of IVFE [9]. This may increase the risk of pancreatitis and worsen pulmonary and immune function [9]. In order to prevent hyperlipidemia, the infusion rate of IVFE should be greater than 0.125 g/kg/h [9]. Those with hyperlipidemia may require cyclic IVFE infusion with at least a 12–24 h interruption and minimal IVFE volume [9].

The IVFE used for PN therapy contains an egg phospholipid emulsifier; therefore, those with an egg allergy may not tolerate IVFE [64]. Patients with a soy allergy also may not tolerate the IVFE since it is composed primarily of soybean and may contain trace soy proteins [64, 65]. In order to prevent an allergic reaction, IVFE should be initiated slowly in all patients in order to monitor tolerance before advancing to goal rate. Administration of IVFE should be avoided in those with known soy or egg allergies.

Perhaps the most severe side effect of PN is parenteral nutrition-associated liver disease (PNALD), which is a spectrum of issues including steatosis, cholestasis, and gallstones and may progress to cirrhosis if not managed appropriately [66]. The etiology of PNALD is complex, including hepatotoxic effects of PN, inappropriate PN management leading to overfeeding, and lack of enteral stimulation [63]. Management of PNALD includes prevention of CHO and/or lipid overfeeding, using EN or an oral diet to stimulate bile flow when possible, and cycling PN off for 8–10 h a day [66]. Clinicians should also consider other underlying etiologies, including small bowel bacterial overgrowth (which may be related to nutrition therapy), hepatotoxic medications, and infection as causes of hepatic dysfunction [66].

Parenteral nutrition increases risk of all infections, not just line infections. Patients receiving PN therapy have a higher prevalence of pneumonia and intra-abdominal abscess, in addition to line sepsis [67, 68]. There is also increased risk of mortality from line infections [67, 68]. The risk of infection can be decreased with the use of appropriate, dedicated ports only, proper catheter placement and care, and delaying initiation of PN or holding PN until infections have been adequately treated [62]. If line sepsis is suspected, the CVC should be removed and should not be replaced until the infection has been adequately treated [62].

Conclusion

The implications for artificial nutrition, especially with EN, far exceed simple nutrition support. Clinicians should be considering nutrition support as an integral part of their overall care plan, especially in critically ill patients and those undergoing major surgery. Provision of pharmaconutrients may improve patient outcomes and reduce cost of care by decreasing complications and length of stay. Safe administration of EN and PN requires closed monitoring by well-trained clinicians; therefore, a team approach is preferable to ensure patient safety and the best possible medical and nutritional outcomes in the critically ill population.

References

1. McClave SA, et al. Guidelines for the provision and assessment of nutrition support therapy in the adult critically ill patient: Society of Critical Care Medicine (SCCM) and American Society for Parenteral and Enteral Nutrition (A.S.P.E.N.). JPEN J Parenter Enteral Nutr. 2009;33(3):277–316.
2. Bengmark S. Gut microenvironment and immune function. Curr Opin Clin Nutr Metab Care. 1999;2(1):84–5.
3. Carrico CJ. The elusive pathophysiology of the multiple organ failure syndrome. Ann Surg. 1993;218(2):109–10.
4. Hermsen JL, Sano Y, Kudsk KA. Food fight!: parenteral nutrition, enteral stimulation and gut-derived mucosal immunity. Langenbecks Arch Surg. 2009;394(1):17–30.
5. Fukastu K, Kudsk KA. Nutrition and gut immunity. Surg Clin North Am. 2011;91(4):755–70.
6. Heyland DK. Nutritional support in the critically ill patient. A critical review of the evidence. Crit Care Clin. 1998;14(3):423–40.
7. Worthington ML, Cresci G. Immune-modulating formulas: who wins the meta-analysis race? Nutr Clin Pract. 2011;26(6):650–5.
8. Bankhead R, et al. Enteral nutrition practice recommendations. JPEN J Parenter Enteral Nutr. 2009;33(2):122–67.
9. Mirtallo J, et al. Safe practices for parenteral nutrition. JPEN J Parenter Enteral Nutr. 2004;28(6):S39–70.
10. Jayarajan S, Daly SM. The relationship of nutrients, routes of delivery, and immunocompetence. Surg Clin North Am. 2011;91(4):737–53.
11. Calder PC. The 2008 ESPEN Sir David Cuthbertson lecture: fatty acids and inflammation – from the membrane to the nucleus and from the laboratory bench to the clinic. Clin Nutr. 2010;29(1):5–12.
12. Kudsk KA. Immunonutrition in surgery and critical care. Annu Rev Nutr. 2006;26:463–79.

13. Vanek VW, et al. A.S.P.E.N. position paper: clinical role for alternative intravenous fat emulsions. Nutr Clin Pract. 2012;27(2):150–92.
14. Sánchez Álvarez C, Zabarte Martínez de Aguirre M, Bordejé Laguna L, Metabolism and Nutrition Working Group of the Spanish Society of Intensive Care Medicine and Coronary units. Guidelines for specialized nutritional and metabolic support in the critically-ill patient: update. Consensus SEMICYUC-SENPE: gastrointestinal surgery. Nutr Hosp. 2011;26 Suppl 2:41–5.
15. Klek S, et al. The immunomodulating enteral nutrition in malnourished surgical patients – a prospective, randomized, double-blind clinical trial. Clin Nutr. 2011;30(3):282–8.
16. Zhang Y, Gu Y, Guo T, Li Y, Cai H. Perioperative immunonutrition for gastrointestinal cancer: a systematic review of randomized controlled trials. Surg Oncol. 2012;21(2):e87–95.
17. Suzuki D, et al. Effects of perioperative immunonutrition on cell-mediated immunity, T helper type 1 (Th1)/Th2 differentiation, and Th17 response after pancreaticoduodenectomy. Surgery. 2010;148(3):573–81.
18. Krzak A, Pleva M, Napolitano LM. Nutrition therapy for ALI and ARDS. Crit Care Clin. 2011;27(3):647–59.
19. Gadek JE, et al. Effect of enteral feeding with eicosapentaenoic acid, gamma-linolenic acid, and antioxidants in patients with acute respiratory distress syndrome. Crit Care Med. 1999; 27:1409–20.
20. Singer P, et al. Benefit of an enteral diet enriched with eicosapentaenoic acid and gamma-linolenic acid in ventilated patients with acute lung injury. Crit Care Med. 2006;34:1033–8.
21. Pontes-Arruda A, Aragao AM, Albuquerque JD. Effects of enteral feeding with eicosapentaenoic acid, gamma-linolenic acid, and antioxidants in mechanically ventilated patients with severe sepsis and septic shock. Crit Care Med. 2006;34:2325–33.
22. Ong JP, Fock KM. Nutritional support in acute pancreatitis. J Dig Dis. 2012;13(9):445–52.
23. Petrov MS, Correia MI, Windsor JA. Nasogastric tube feeding in predicted severe acute pancreatitis. A systematic review of the literature to determine safety and tolerance. JOP. 2008;9(4):440–8.
24. Lu G, et al. Influence of early post-burn enteral nutrition on clinical outcomes of patients with extensive burns. J Clin Biochem Nutr. 2011;48(3):222–5.
25. Wasiak J, Cleland H, Jeffery R. Early versus late enteral nutritional support in adults with burn injury: a systematic review. J Hum Nutr Diet. 2007;20(2):75–83.
26. Kurmis R, Parker A, Greenwood J. The use of immunonutrition in burn injury care: where are we? J Burn Care Res. 2010;31(5):677–91.
27. Chiang YH, et al. Early enteral nutrition and clinical outcomes of severe traumatic brain injury patients in acute stage: a multi-center cohort study. J Neurotrauma. 2012;29(1):75–80.
28. Garcia de Lorenzo y Mateos A, Ortiz Leyba C, Sanchez SM, Metabolism and Nutrition Working Group of the Spanish Society of Intensive Care Medicine and Coronary Units. Guidelines for specialized nutritional and metabolic support in the critically-ill patient: update. Consensus SEMICYUC-SENPE: critically-ill burnt patient. Nutr Hosp. 2011;26 Suppl 2:59–62.
29. Chen G, Shi J, Qi M, Yin H, Hang C. Glutamine decreases intestinal nuclear factor kappa B activity and pro-inflammatory cytokine expression after traumatic brain injury in rats. Inflamm Res. 2008;57(2):57–64.
30. Feng D, et al. Influence of glutamine on intestinal inflammatory response, mucosa structure alterations and apoptosis following traumatic brain injury in rats. J Int Med Res. 2007;35(5):644–56.
31. Cano N, et al. ESPEN guidelines on enteral nutrition: adult renal failure. Clin Nutr. 2006;25(2): 295–310.
32. Plauth M, et al. ESPEN guidelines on enteral nutrition: liver disease. Clin Nutr. 2006;25(2): 285–94.
33. Plauth M, et al. ESPEN guidelines on parenteral nutrition: hepatology. Clin Nutr. 2009;28(4): 436–44.
34. Evidence-based nutrition practice guideline on adult weight management. Published May 2006 at http://andevidencelibrary.com/topic.cfm?cat=2798 and copyrighted by the Academy of Nutrition and Dietetics. Accessed 20 Mar 2013.

35. Grau T, Bonet A. Caloric intake and liver dysfunction in critically ill patients. Curr Opin Clin Nutr Metab Care. 2009;12(2):175–9.
36. Academy of Nutrition and Dietetics Evidence Analysis Library. If indirect calorimetry is unavailable or impractical, what is the best way to estimate resting metabolic rate (RMR) in non-obese adult critically ill patients? Academy of Nutrition and Dietetics. http://andevidencelibrary.com/conclusion.cfm?conclusion_statement_id=251361. Accessed 6 Mar 2013.
37. Academy of Nutrition and Dietetics Evidence Analysis Library. If indirect calorimetry is unavailable or impractical, what is the best way to estimate resting metabolic rate (RMR) in obese adult critically ill patients? Academy of Nutrition and Dietetics. http://andevidencelibrary.com/conclusion.cfm?conclusion_statement_id=251240. Accessed 6 Mar 2013.
38. World Health Organization. Protein and amino acid requirements in human nutrition: report of a Joint WHO/FAO/UNU expert consultation. WHO technical report series 935. 2007.
39. Lepelletier D, et al. Retrospective analysis of the risk factors and pathogens associated with early-onset ventilator-associated pneumonia in surgical-ICU head-trauma patients. J Neurosurg Anesthesiol. 2010;22(1):32–7.
40. Casaer MP, et al. Early versus late parenteral nutrition in critically ill adults. N Engl J Med. 2011;365(6):506–17.
41. Pittiruti M, Hamilton H, Biffi R, MacFie J, Pertkiewicz M, ESPEN. ESPEN guidelines on parenteral nutrition: central venous catheters (access, care, diagnosis and therapy of complications. Clin Nutr. 2009;28(4):365–77.
42. Wolht PD, et al. Recommendations for the use of medications with continuous enteral nutrition. Am J Health Syst Pharm. 2009;66(16):1458–67.
43. Williams NT. Medication administration through enteral feeding tubes. Am J Health-Syst Pharm. 2008;65(24):2347–57.
44. Belknap DC, Seifert CF, Petermann M. Administration of medications through enteral feeding catheters. Am J Crit Care. 1997;6:382–92.
45. Mueller BA, Brierton DG, Abel SR, et al. Effect of enteral feeding with Ensure on oral bioavailabilities of ofloxacin and ciprofloxacin. Antimicrob Agents Chemother. 1994;38(9):2101–5.
46. Wright DH, Pietz SL, Konstantinides FN, et al. Decreased in vitro fluoroquinolone concentrations after admixture with an enteral feeding formulation. JPEN J Parenter Enteral Nutr. 2000;24:42–8.
47. Nyffeler MS. Ciprofloxacin use in the enterally fed patient. Nutr Clin Pract. 1999;14:73–7.
48. McCarthy CG, Finland M. Absorption and excretion of 4 penicillins: penicillin G, penicillin V, phenethicillin and phenylmercaptomethylpenicillin. N Engl J Med. 1960;263:315.
49. Howden CW. Review article: immediate-release proton-pump inhibitor therapy–potential advantages. Aliment Pharmacol Ther. 2005;22 Suppl 3:25–30.
50. Gal P, Layson R. Interference with oral theophylline absorption by continuous nasogastric feedings. Ther Drug Monit. 1986;8:421–3.
51. Manessis A, Lascher S, Bukberg P, et al. Quantifying amount of adsorption of levothyroxine by percutaneous endoscopic gastrostomy tubes. JPEN J Parenter Enteral Nutr. 2008;32:197–200.
52. Smyrniotis V, et al. Severe hypothyroidism in patients dependent on prolonged thyroxine infusion through a jejunostomy. Clin Nutr. 2000;19(1):65–7.
53. Penrod LE, Allen JB, Cabacungan LR. Warfarin resistance and enteral feedings: 2 case reports and a supporting in vitro study. Arch Phys Med Rehabil. 2001;82:1270–3.
54. Dickerson RN, Garmon WM, Kuhl DA, et al. Vitamin K-independent warfarin resistance after concurrent administration of warfarin and continuous enteral nutrition. Pharmacotherapy. 2008;28:308–13.
55. Gilbert S, Hatton J, Magnuson B. How to minimize interaction between phenytoin and enteral feedings: two approaches. Nutr Clin Pract. 1996;11:28–31.
56. Giesing DH, Bighley LD, Iles HL. Effect of food and antacid on binding of sucralfate to normal and ulcerated gastric and duodenal mucosa in rats. J Clin Gastroenterol. 1981;3 suppl 2:111–6.
57. Wells DL. Provision of enteral nutrition during vasopressor therapy for hemodynamic instability: an evidence based review. Nutr Clin Pract. 2012;27(4):521–6.

58. Khalid I, Doshi P, DiGiovine B. Early enteral nutrition and outcome of critically ill patients treated with vasopressors and mechanical ventilation. Am J Crit Care. 2010;19(3):261–8.
59. Lowrey TS, Dunlap AW, Brown RO, Dickerson RN, Kudsk KA. Pharmacologic influence on nutrition support therapy: use of propofol in a patient receiving combined enteral and parenteral nutrition support. Nutr Clin Pract. 1996;11(4):147–9.
60. Kennedy JF, Nightingale JMD. Cost savings of an adult hospital nutrition support team. Nutrition. 2005;21:1127–33.
61. Schneider PJ. Nutrition support teams: an evidence based practice. Nutr Clin Pract. 2006; 21(1):62–7.
62. O'Grady NP, et al. Guidelines for the prevention of intravascular catheter related infections. Am J Infect Control. 2011;39(4 Suppl 1):S1–34.
63. Ranganath LR. The entero-insular axis; implications for human metabolism. Clin Chem Lab Med. 2008;46(1):43–56.
64. Buchman AL, Ament ME. Comparative hypersensitivity in intravenous lipid emulsions. JPEN J Parenter Enteral Nutr. 1991;15(3):345–6.
65. Weidmann B, Lepique C, Heider A, Schmitz A, Niederle N. Hypersensitivity reactions to parenteral lipid solutions. Support Care Cancer. 1997;5(6):504–5.
66. Kumpf VJ. Parenteral nutrition-associated liver disease in adult and pediatric patients. Nutr Clin Pract. 2006;21:279–90.
67. Kudsk KA, Croce MA, Fabian TC, et al. Enteral versus parenteral feeding: effects on septic morbidity after blunt and penetrating abdominal trauma. Ann Surg. 1992;215:503–11.
68. Pittet D, Wenzel RP. Nosocomial bloodstream infections: secular trends in rates, mortality, and contribution to total hospital deaths. Arch Intern Med. 1995;155:1177–84.

Chapter 41
Obstetrics

Laura Mayer, Richard Hong, and Jeff Bernstein

Contents

L. Mayer, MD (✉)
Department of Anesthesiology, Organization Ronald Reagan UCLA Medical Center,
Los Angeles, CA, USA
e-mail: lmayer@temple.edu

R. Hong
Department of Anesthesiology, Ronald Reagan UCLA Medical Center,
Los Angeles, CA, USA
e-mail: rhong@mednet.ucla.edu

J. Bernstein
Department of Anesthesiology, Montefiore Medical Center, Albert Einstein
College of Medicine, Bronx, NY, USA
e-mail: jbernste@montefiore.org

A.D. Kaye et al. (eds.), *Essentials of Pharmacology for Anesthesia,*
Pain Medicine, and Critical Care, DOI 10.1007/978-1-4614-8948-1_41,
© Springer Science+Business Media New York 2015

Introduction

Labor and delivery of a child can be very gratifying and a joyous occasion for all but may be both an intensely emotional and potentially uncomfortable experience for the mother. An anesthesiologist's role is to provide a pleasant and safe environment for both the mother and child in the peripartum period while considering the changes of pregnancy that can alter anesthetic pharmacology and pharmacokinetics of drugs affecting the baby and mother.

Since some medications have the ability to cross the placenta, systemic effects on the fetus are possible (see Table 41.1). The placenta, like the blood-brain barrier, features a semipermeable lipid bilayer. Factors that limit placental transfer include ionization, hydrophilicity, low maternal plasma concentration, and increased molecular size (>1,000 Da) [2]. Low fetal protein-binding capacity results in higher relative drug concentrations in the fetal circulation. In addition, there are many physiologic changes and known risks of pregnancy which also may affect the mother and child. All of these factors may affect the anesthetic plan for an obstetric patient.

This chapter will also discuss many pharmacologic therapies for the pregnant patient. Local anesthetics and opioids are the foundation of most neuraxial techniques used for labor analgesia and cesarean delivery. Pharmacologic induction and maintenance of general anesthesia is another anesthetic option for cesarean sections or non-obstetric surgeries. Tocolytic medications can stop unwanted uterine contractions (e.g., in the management of preterm labor patients). Uterotonic medications can be used to induce labor, augment uterine contractions, or to treat uterine atony. Teratogenic medications will also be reviewed as they may have possible deleterious consequences on the fetus.

Table 41.1 Drugs that do not cross the placenta or have minimal fetal effects after maternal administration [1]

Glycopyrrolate
Heparin
Insulin
Nondepolarizing neuromuscular blocker
Succinylcholine

Local Anesthetics for Neuraxial Anesthesia

Local Anesthetics

Introduction

Local anesthetics are used in different regional anesthetic techniques. Single-shot spinal injections are fast in onset but limited in duration. An epidural delivers medications using a catheter to administer a continuous titratable infusion or a bolus to the patient. These neuraxial techniques are central to obstetric anesthesia practice, but local anesthetics can also be administered in other ways (e.g., local infiltration, paracervical or pudendal blockade) to provide analgesia.

Drug Class and Mechanism of Action

The main role of local anesthetics in neuraxial anesthesia is to target the nerve root emerging from the spinal cord. (See Chap. 8.)

Indications/Clinical Pearls

During labor and delivery, visceral and somatic stimulation triggers different pain pathways. Primarily using local anesthetic and/or opioid medications, anesthesiologists temporarily block these pathways through epidural and/or spinal techniques.

Three percent 2-chloroprocaine should be considered in emergent cesarean sections for patients with in situ epidurals. The onset is fast because of the high concentration, but 3 % 2-chloroprocaine is relatively safe because of its rapid maternal and fetal metabolism [3].

Spinal doses for cesarean section vary widely between providers (see dosing options below) and are often adjusted based on patient factors and anticipated surgical duration. One starting point is the ED95 of intrathecal bupivacaine combined with commonly used adjuncts fentanyl and morphine. Consider 11.2 mg of hyperbaric bupivacaine with 10 mcg of fentanyl and 200 mcg of morphine or 13 mg of isobaric bupivacaine with 10 mcg of fentanyl and 200 mcg of morphine [4, 5].

Spinal doses for labor analgesia, usually by way of a combined spinal-epidural technique, vary greatly and the optimal doses are an active area of study. In an informal survey of practices, bupivacaine doses range from 0 to 3 mg in this application. An opioid, with or without isobaric bupivacaine, is commonly employed.

The addition of epinephrine (1:200,000) to epidural solutions can help reduce vascular absorption of local anesthetics by inducing vasoconstriction and decreasing vascular uptake. This adjunct can prolong the epidural block. The addition of sodium bicarbonate 8.4 % (e.g., 1–10 ml of lidocaine) to epidural solutions can

Table 41.2 Epidural doses for cesarean delivery [7]

Local anesthetic	Concentration (%)	Max dose (mg)	Onset (min)	Duration	Common adjuncts
Bupivacaine (Marcaine)	0.5	175–200	15–20	2–5 h	Epinephrine Fentanyl
Chloroprocaine (Nesacaine)	3	800–1,000	5–10	30–60 min	Meperidine Morphine
Lidocaine (Xylocaine)	2	350–500	5–15	60–120 min	Sufentanil Sodium bicarbonate
Ropivacaine (Naropin)	1	200–250	15–20	2–4 h	

Table 41.3 Spinal doses for cesarean delivery [7]

Local anesthetic	Concentration (%)	Dose (mg)	Onset	Duration (min)	Common adjuncts
Bupivacaine (Marcaine)	0.5–0.75	0.75–15	Fast	60–120	Epinephrine Fentanyl
Lidocaine (Xylocaine)	2–5	40–100	Fast	45–60	Meperidine
Tetracaine (Pontocaine)	0.2–0.5	5–10	Fast	75–150	Morphine Sufentanil
Ropivacaine (Naropin)	0.05–1	15–22.5	Fast	75–150	

speed the onset of local anesthetics by decreasing its ionization which makes it conducive for nerve penetration [6]. These adjuncts are commonly added to lidocaine epidural mixtures for cesarean delivery.

Dosing Options

For cesarean patients, there are many neuraxial anesthetic options (see Tables 41.2 and 41.3). The dosing requirement for epidural and spinal local anesthetics is approximately 30 % less in pregnancy due to the following: (a) engorgement of the epidural veins which decreases the CSF and epidural volumes in the vertebral column; (b) elevation in progesterone levels which may cause the neuron to be more sensitive to the local anesthetic; and (c) increases in CSF and epidural space pressures secondary to the progression of labor [8].

Labor epidural practices and pump settings also differ greatly across individual practices. In the United States, the most commonly used epidural solutions rely upon bupivacaine or ropivacaine as these local anesthetics provide a favorable differential blockade between motor and sensory effects. So-called "low-dose" epidurals for labor include bupivacaine concentrations less than or equal to 0.125 %. These concentrations are well studied for their efficacy and safety, and a lipophilic opiate (e.g., fentanyl, sufentanil) is frequently combined for its dose-sparing effect on the amount of local anesthetic needed. Ropivacaine has a higher minimum local analgesic concentration compared to bupivacaine, with a 0.6 potency ratio in parturients [9].

Drug Interactions

Chloroprocaine can decrease the efficacy and duration of epidural morphine [10].

Side Effects

The sympathetic fibers that innervate the heart and vasculature pass through the thoracic and lumbar regions of the spinal cord. The local anesthetic can block these fibers and cause a sympathectomy leading to hypotension if the block ascends high enough. This may be further complicated by supine aortocaval compression. Untreated or prolonged hypotension can cause uteroplacental hypoperfusion and subsequent fetal distress.

Sympathetic blockade also affects gut motility by allowing the parasympathetics to be unopposed. This causes increases in peristalsis, gut contraction, and sphincter relaxation.

The motor nerve fibers are affected by the local anesthetic concentration and can result in temporary muscular weakness and even paralysis. Efforts to communicate these possible effects to the mother should be made as paralysis can be disconcerting to the uninformed, awake patient. Muscle relaxation may impede the ability to ambulate during labor and to push during vaginal deliveries. Urinary retention is common as patients lose both the micturition reflex and the sensation of bladder fullness. Pregnant patients with neuraxial blocks often receive urinary catheters because of these effects and their inability to easily ambulate to bathroom because of motor blockade. A full bladder may hinder delivery efforts [11].

A thoracic blockade can affect the patient's perception of breathing and use of accessory muscles. A cervical level may cause diaphragmatic paralysis and respiratory distress.

Around the time of delivery, shivering is common and may be multifactorial but neuraxial techniques seem to potentiate a nonthermoregulatory etiology [12].

Neuraxial local anesthetics lower maternal blood pressure which can cause uterine hypoperfusion. This has potentially deleterious effects on oxygen delivery to the fetus [13]. In addition, there is possible fetal "ion trapping" that could subject the fetus to increased concentrations of local anesthetics. Fetal distress increases this risk as local anesthetics ionize and accumulate in the more acidic fetal circulation [14].

The antepartum patient is more susceptible to intravascular injections of local anesthetics due to venous distension of epidural veins. This increases risk of systemic exposure to local anesthetics which can result in serious cardiac and neurological complications. Cardiac toxicity can induce ventricular arrhythmias and cardiac arrest. Bupivacaine, a commonly used anesthetic for labor analgesia, binds to the heart avidly, raising the risk for cardiotoxicity. Serious neurological consequences include altered mental status, respiratory depression, loss of consciousness, and seizures. Spinal doses are unlikely to cause toxicity. However, there is an associated complication known as transient neurological symptoms that manifests as back, buttock, and lower extremity pain. It is most commonly described after 5 % hyperbaric lidocaine [15].

Summary

Local anesthetics are frequently used for labor and delivery to reduce the patient's pain and, in higher doses, they can be used for surgical anesthesia.

Opioids

Introduction

Opioids can provide analgesia for labor and delivery by several routes. Anesthesiologists frequently utilize opioids, usually with local anesthetics, in neuraxial techniques. Neuraxial opioids target the nerve roots and dorsal horn. In the usual neuraxial doses, the systemic uptake will not produce sufficient plasma concentrations to provide significant analgesia.

Indications/Clinical Pearls

Neuraxial opioids can improve block density and the duration of postoperative analgesia. The addition causes synergistic analgesia and has a dose-sparing effect on the amount of local anesthetics needed. Parenteral and enteral opioids are frequently offered as an alternative to neuraxial labor analgesia and for postdelivery pain relief.

Parenteral meperidine is commonly used around the world to treat early labor pain. An intramuscular dose (e.g., 100 mg) will provide pain relief for several hours [16].

Nalbuphine is a mixed agonist and partial antagonist of opiate receptors. It offers analgesia in early labor (e.g., 10 mg/70 kg IM, IV, or SC) and relief of opioid-induced pruritus (e.g., 2.5–5 mg IV) [17].

Dosing Options

For neuraxial opioid administration, drugs are chosen based on the pharmacologic properties best suited for their specific role, most notably lipid solubility.

Lipophilic agents will penetrate neuronal membranes and the dural sac quickly. Fentanyl and sufentanil are highly lipophilic with fast onset times (5–10 min) but relatively short durations (2–4 h). They are frequently used when the need for analgesia is immediate and/or brief. As an adjunct to local anesthetics, intrathecal dosing for fentanyl is 10–25 ug [18] and sufentanil is 2.5–7.5 ug [19]. The epidural dose for fentanyl is 50–100 ug and sufentanil 10–20 ug [1].

Conversely, agents like morphine and hydromorphone are less lipid soluble and therefore their onset and duration times are prolonged as they remain in the CSF/epidural space longer. Morphine has an onset time of 30–60 min and has an analgesic effect lasting up to 24 h, making it popular for postoperative pain relief. For this application, the morphine dose for spinals is 0.1–0.2 mg and the dose for epidurals is 3–4 ug [1]. A morphine sulfate extended-release liposome injection is also available and extends the duration of epidural analgesia beyond 24 h [20].

Drug Interactions

Neuraxial opioid doses are unlikely to precipitate adverse drug interactions.

Side Effects

Opioids cause pruritus especially when given neuraxially. Other maternal effects include decreased bowel motility, increased nausea and vomiting, sedation, urinary retention, and respiratory depression [21].

The fetus is unlikely to be directly affected by the relatively small opioid doses associated with neuraxial techniques. However, fetal bradycardia has been associated with increasing intrathecal doses of lipophilic opioids for labor analgesia [22–24].

Summary

Opioids have a wide range of uses in obstetrics and play a significant role in neuraxial techniques.

General Anesthetics and the OB Patient

Introduction

In the United States, rates of cesarean delivery are on the rise but few are performed under general anesthesia. Pregnant women may also present for non-obstetric surgeries requiring general anesthesia.

Indications/Clinical Pearls

General anesthesia during pregnancy is typically reserved for patients with contraindications to regional anesthesia, for situations where the benefit of quickly estab-
lishing surgical anesthesia outweighs the risks or for surgeries necessitating general
anesthesia. Pregnant women have greater associated morbidity, largely related to
the increased risk for aspiration and difficult airway. Therefore, the anesthetics
should be carefully chosen.

Nitrous oxide has analgesic properties which have been exploited for labor analgesia. In some countries, a 50/50 mixture of oxygen and nitrous oxide is self-
 administered by laboring women [25].
General anesthesia may be employed in situations where uterine relaxation is
 desired, such as uterine inversion.
Pregnant patients undergoing cesarean section have a greater risk for intraoperative
 awareness [26]. Postdelivery treatment with an amnestic agent like a benzodiazepine can help minimize recall until other maintenance anesthetics can be delivered in sufficient amounts.

Dosing Options

For rapid induction of general anesthesia, there are several options including etomidate (0.2–0.3 mg/kg), ketamine (1–2 mg/kg), increasingly popular propofol (2 mg/kg),
and now rarely used thiopental (3–4 mg/kg) [1].

Succinylcholine (1–1.5 mg/kg) can quickly provide adequate intubating conditions. Its speed relative to other paralytics makes it an optimal choice for intubation
of obstetric patients given risks of aspiration, the challenges of airway management,
and the urgency of delivering the fetus under these circumstances [27]. Serum cholinesterase levels decrease during pregnancy; however, obstetric patients do not
experience a significant clinical effect on neuromuscular blockade [28].

Inhalational agents are primarily used for maintenance anesthesia. The parturient
requires lower alveolar concentrations to achieve surgical anesthesia. Nitrous oxide
is often given to minimize the requirements of halogenated inhalational agents such
as sevoflurane and desflurane. Consider delivering sevoflurane or desflurane in
doses of 0.5 MAC or less (see side effects below) [1].

Drug Interactions

See Chaps. 3, 4, and 9.

Side Effects

Induction agents can enter fetal circulation with adverse effects for the neonate. Maternal hypotension after thiopental and propofol can potentially decrease utero-placental blood flow.

Nitrous oxide has minimal cardiovascular and uterine effects.

Halogenated agents can increase the risk of uteroplacental insufficiency through vasodilatory and cardiac depressive effects. These gases also attenuate uterine tone in a dose-dependent fashion, increasing the concern for uterine atony and hemorrhage. In addition, their small molecular size and lipophilicity allows them to cross the placenta and possibly cause the same depressive and sedative effects on the neonate [1, 29].

Summary

General anesthesia involves the use of induction, paralytic, and inhalational agents and deserves special pharmacologic considerations when employed in the obstetric population.

Aspiration Prevention

The traditional beliefs that pregnancy leads to increased gastric acid production, decreased gastric pH, decreased gastric emptying, and increased gastroesophageal reflex have been challenged and controversial over the years. The belief that rapid sequence intubation (RSI) is necessary in all pregnant patients undergoing general anesthesia after their first trimester of pregnancy has also been challenged. As always, the anesthetic goal with any pregnant woman is to avoid general anesthesia. General anesthesia is inevitable in some instances though, and therefore, precautions should be taken to avoid possible aspiration including proper ASA guidelines for preoperative fasting, RSI, and medications to help decrease gastric acidity and improve gastric motility.

The medications used to achieve the above results are H2 antagonists, non-particulate antacids such as sodium citrate, and metoclopramide. There is no evidence to support the link between these medications used to increase gastric pH and gastric motility and a decreased risk of pulmonary aspiration of gastric secretions [30]. ASA practice guidelines state, "the literature suggests that H2 receptor antagonists are effective in decreasing gastric acidity in obstetric patients and supports the efficacy of metoclopramide in reducing peripartum nausea and vomiting." They also agree that non-particulate antacid before operative procedures reduces maternal complications. H2 antagonist medications should be given 60–90 min before induction of general anesthesia, as this is the time taken for them to have their maximum effect on the patient. Non-particulate antacids should be taken 20 min prior to procedure. Particulate antacids must be avoided as their aspiration can lead to serious respiratory complications.

Non-opioid Analgesics

Opioid medications used to treat pain are an important tool in the postoperative care of our patients. The multimodal approach to treating pain has been emphasized in the literature for many years. Using non-opioid analgesics such as ketorolac and acetaminophen has been proven to decrease opioid consumption and overall patient satisfaction with regard to pain control.

Acetaminophen is available in intravenous form. Dosing of the medication is 1 g IV for those > 50 kg or 15 mg/kg for those <50 kg. The medication should be dosed every 6 h with a maximum intake of 4 g daily to avoid adverse side effects. It should be avoided in those with severe hepatic impairment. The IV form of the medication helps to avoid first-pass metabolism, which aids in its increased safety profile. The mechanism of acetaminophen is unknown, but it is thought to act by inhibiting synthesis of prostaglandins in the CNS and by blocking pain impulse generation in the periphery. The added benefits of no gastric irritation, platelet inhibition, respiratory depression, and overall decreased opioid intake in individuals make it an ideal drug for the obstetric population [31].

Ketorolac is the only intravenous nonsteroidal antiinflammatory medication widely available in the United States for obstetric use. It has been shown to reduce pain and narcotic use in the obstetric population [32]. The dosing of the medication is 30 mg intravenous and can be given every 6 h. It should be used with caution in patients with platelet dysfunction, renal disease, and severe asthma or hypersensitivity to NSAIDs.

Preeclampsia

Introduction

Preeclampsia is characterized by new-onset hypertension occurring after 20 weeks' gestation and can predispose the mother to organ failure, seizure, and stroke. Diagnosis includes two separate blood pressure readings greater than 140/90 as well as a 24-h urine sample with 300 mg of protein or more [33, 34]. Severe preeclampsia is suspected when blood pressures exceeds 160/110, proteinuria worsens to 5 g in 24 h, and/or when additional symptoms are present. HELLP syndrome is a variant of severe preeclampsia, with the acronym HELLP referencing the clinical triad of hemolysis, elevated liver enzymes, and low platelets [35]. Common treatment options for blood pressure management include magnesium, hydralazine, labetalol, methyldopa, and nifedipine. The drugs administered to preeclamptic patients only mitigate symptoms until the cure, fetal delivery, takes place.

Drug Class and Mechanism of Action

Magnesium sulfate inhibits calcium influx causing decreased smooth muscle contractility and vasodilation (see tocolytic section below), and it plays an important role in eclamptic seizure prophylaxis through multiple potential mechanisms.

Hydralazine directly targets the arterioles and arterial vasculature to increase substrate levels involved in vasodilation.

Labetalol is a long-acting alpha-1 and beta-adrenergic receptor antagonist which lowers the blood pressure by blocking smooth muscle vasculature and decreasing heart rate.

Methyldopa is metabolized to an α_2-adrenergic agonist that enters the CNS to decrease sympathetic output which lowers arterial blood pressure.

Nifedipine blocks calcium channels in the vasculature leading to vasodilation.

Indications/Clinical Pearls

Magnesium sulfate is used in preeclamptics to prevent seizure and in eclamptics to treat seizure [36].
Antihypertensives are used to prevent end-organ damage from rising maternal blood pressure.
Failure of these medication therapies puts the mother at great risk and is usually an indication for immediate delivery [34].

Dosing Options

Magnesium is given prophylactically with a loading dose of 4–6 g intravenously over 20 min followed by an infusion of 1–2 g/h for 24 h with serial serum magnesium levels assessed [34]. (See also magnesium discussion under tocolytics.)

Labetalol can be given 10–20 mg IV, then 20–80 mg every 20–30 min with a maximum dose of 300 mg.

Hydralazine can be bolused at 5 mg IV or IM, then 5–10 mg every 20–40 min.

Methyldopa 500–3,000 mg orally per 24 h in two divided doses.

Nifedipine can be given 10–30 mg orally and repeated every 45 min as needed [37].

Drug Interactions

Magnesium potentiates the blockading effect of nondepolarizing agents [38].

Magnesium used with another calcium channel blocker (e.g., nifedipine) can enhance cardiac depression, increase peripheral vasodilation, and/or cause significant muscular weakness [39, 40].

Side Effects

(See also magnesium discussion under tocolytics.)

Hydralazine can induce fetal thrombocytopenia, tachycardia, maternal headache or palpitations [37], and neonatal or maternal lupus-like syndromes [41].

Labetalol can lead to fetal hypoglycemia and growth restriction (if used in earlier trimesters) [37] and may exacerbate maternal asthma or congestive heart failure.

Methyldopa can cause sedation, increase the risk of maternal psychological depression, and elevate liver enzymes [33].

Nifedipine may cause flushing, diarrhea, headache, and nausea [42].

Summary

Various therapeutics are administered to preeclamptic women to limit harm as the disease progresses, but only delivery of the fetus is curative.

Conditions Associated with Tocolysis: Tocolytics

Preterm labor is defined as labor beginning before 37 weeks of gestation [43]. Chestnut states that 12–13 % of pregnancies in the United States result in preterm delivery with a significant morbidity and mortality associated with it [1]. Medications are available to help prevent preterm labor and give the obstetrician the opportunity to treat the unborn fetus in regard to lung maturity, risk for infection, and other associated conditions that may contribute to poor outcomes for the child.

Major causes of preterm labor such as placental abruption or infection must be ruled out before initiation of tocolytic therapy. Tocolytic therapy has only been shown to prolong preterm labor from 2 to 7 days [44]. Criteria for the use of tocolytic include gestational age between 20 and 34 weeks, reassuring fetal status, and no clinical signs of infection [45]. Assuming all criteria are met, four classes of drugs including beta- adrenergic agonists, calcium channel blockers, magnesium sulfate, and nonsteroidal antiinflammatory drugs can be used for tocolysis. Studies have shown that all of these drugs prolong labor to a degree, but no evidence has been found linking them to decreased morbidity or mortality in the fetus [46].

Calcium channel blockers are a mainstay in preventing preterm delivery. Nifedipine is the most commonly used for uterine relaxation. The mechanism of action is the block of voltage-dependent calcium cell membrane channels that decrease actin-myosin interaction resulting in the relaxation of the uterine smooth muscle. Initial dose of nifedipine is 30 mg by mouth or sublingual followed by 10–20 mg every 4–6 h [1]. Side effects include hypotension, headache, flushing, and dizziness.

Cyclooxygenase inhibitors used include indomethacin and ketorolac. The mechanisms of action by which these cause uterine relaxation are the inhibition of cyclo-oxygenase and thus prevention of the synthesis of prostaglandins from the precursor, arachidonic acid. Prostaglandins E2 and F2α play an important role in the stimulation of uterine contractions by increasing intracellular calcium and activation of myosin light chain kinases. Initial doses include indomethacin 50–100 mg by mouth or per rectum followed by 25–50 mg every 4 h or ketorolac 60 mg IM followed by 30 mg every 6 h [1]. ASRA guidelines state that patients on these medications can still receive neuraxial anesthesia safely as cyclooxygenase inhibition of platelets is only transient [47]. Side effects are minimal.

Beta-adrenergic agonists interact with beta-2 receptor sites on the outer membrane of uterine myometrial cells, activating the enzyme adenyl cyclase leading to enzymatic conversion of ATP to cAMP. This causes a rise in the intracellular concentration of cAMP and uterine relaxation. Terbutaline and in the past ritodrine (this drug has been removed from the US market) were commonly used as tocolytics. They have a greater affinity for the beta-2 receptor and work primarily here. Cardiac arrhythmias must be monitored for along with the side effects of hypotension, tachycardia, hyperglycemia, and hypokalemia and the possibility of pulmonary edema.

Magnesium sulfate functions as a competitive antagonist of calcium either at the motor end plate or cell membrane reducing calcium influx into the myocyte and leading to uterine muscle relaxation. Magnesium levels must be constantly monitored to avoid the side effects of respiratory depression and cardiovascular collapse. The level of 4–8 mEq/L is the therapeutic dose. Magnesium causes loss of deep tendon reflexes above 10 mEq/L, respiratory depression above 15 mEq/L, and cardiovascular collapse over 20 mEq/L in serum [48]. It should also be noted that patients receiving magnesium will have a decreased mean alveolar concentration for inhaled anesthetics and be more sensitive to the affects of neuromuscular blocking agents [49]. Alpha-adrenergic drugs such as phenylephrine, which is commonly used to support low blood pressures in patients, may also have a decreased effect.

Drugs Used in Postpartum Hemorrhage

Postpartum hemorrhage (PPH) is a major cause of morbidity and mortality in pregnant women in the United States and worldwide. It is estimated that the prevalence of postpartum hemorrhage is 4–6 % [50]. Postpartum hemorrhage can be defined as the loss of more than 500 mL of blood following vaginal delivery or greater than 1,000 mL of blood following cesarean section [1].

Communication between the anesthesiologist and obstetrician is key in recognizing and treating significant blood loss. Volume resuscitation either by crystalloid, colloid, or blood products may be necessary to stabilize the patient, but medications are also available to aid in the treatment of postpartum hemorrhage. Causes of PPH include uterine atony (most commonly), retained products of conception, uterine rupture, coagulopathies, placental abnormalities, and lacerations and tears [51].

Uterine atony is the disease process that is most receptive to treatment by uterotonic medications. Risk factors that predispose a patient to uterine atony include multiple gestation, macrosomia, polyhydramnios, increased parity, prolonged labor, necessity for general anesthesia and inhaled volatile anesthetic, chorioamnionitis, and the use of tocolytic agents [1]. Multiple medications exist for the treatment of uterine atony and PPH, but oxytocin is first line for the prevention and treatment of atony [52].

Oxytocin stimulates contraction of uterine smooth muscle by increasing intracellular calcium concentrations; mimicking contractions of normal, spontaneous labor; and transiently impeding uterine blood flow. The uterus has receptors for oxytocin which peak at term in the pregnant woman. Controversy dealing with dosing and delivery of oxytocin for PPH has existed for many years, but it is generally accepted that bolus doses of oxytocin can lead to a decreased systemic vascular resistance and hypotension [53]. The short half of 4–10 min is the basis for its use as an infusion [1]. Oxytocin 20–40 units can be diluted in 1-l normal saline or lactated ringers and titrated to uterine contraction and control of atony. It should be initiated at the clamping of the cord in cesarean sections or immediately after removal of the placenta in vaginal deliveries. Side effects include hypotension as mentioned earlier, possibility for uterine spasm or rupture, and free-water retention due to its ADH-like properties [49].

Methylergonovine (Methergine) is another medication used in the treatment of uterine atony. It is from the ergot alkaloid family. The mechanism of this drug is not exactly fully understood, but it is believed to cause uterine contraction secondary to alpha-adrenergic receptor stimulation [54]. The dose is 0.2 mg intramuscularly every 2–4 h up to five doses [1]. *Special care must be taken in those patients with preexisting hypertension, preeclampsia, or coronary artery disease. The vasoconstrictive properties of methylergonovine can lead to severe hypertension and the sequelae involved in the disease process including stroke and myocardial infarction* [55]. Nausea and vomiting are also of concern with this medication.

Carboprost (Hemabate) is of the prostaglandin F family. It is a synthetic prostaglandin which functions to increase intracellular free-calcium concentrations and increases uterine contractility. Carboprost is given intramuscularly or by intrauterine injection at a dose of 0.25 mg. This dose can be repeated every 15 min up to a total of 2 mg given [1]. *Of special note, carboprost must be used very carefully in those with reactive airways disease as it can lead to severe bronchospasm* [56]. Other side effects include diarrhea, shivering, nausea, and vomiting.

Misoprostol (Cytotec) is another member of the prostaglandin family. The mechanism of action of misoprostol is that of an analogue of prostaglandin E1 causing uterine contraction. It is commonly given per rectum at a dose of 800–1,000 mcg but may also be administered sublingually, buccally, or orally [1]. Side effects include diarrhea, shivering, nausea, and vomiting.

Teratogenicity

Of major concern to the pregnant patient is the safety of the procedures and medications we use as anesthesiologists. During pregnancy, surgery for non-obstetric procedures occurs in up to 2 % of women [57]. Numerous studies have been done over the years pertaining to the effect of anesthetic medications and their presumed effects on the unborn fetus in animals. Ethical and scientific challenges make the possibility of testing our anesthetic drugs in humans virtually impossible.

Teratogenicity is defined as the observation of any significant change in the function or form of a child secondary to prenatal treatment [48]. The teratogenicity of a drug depends upon the dose administered, the route of administration, the species the drug is given to, and the timing of fetal exposure [58]. During the first 2 weeks of human gestation, teratogens are believed to have an all-or-none phenomenon; that is, the fetus is lost or is preserved fully intact. The period from the third to the eighth week of gestation represents the most important time for the fetus, as this is the period of organogenesis [59].

Most anesthetic drugs are known teratogens in animal models, but no detrimental effects have ever been validated in humans [60]. According to Chestnut, teratogenesis in humans has not been associated with the use of any of the commonly used induction agents including the barbiturates, ketamine, propofol, and benzodiazepines or muscle relaxants, inhaled agents, or local anesthetics when they were administered in clinical doses during anesthesia [1]. *Benzodiazepine therapy became controversial after several retrospective studies reported an association between maternal diazepam ingestion during the first trimester and infants with cleft palate, with or without cleft lip. These results were later proven to be unfounded* [61]. Concerns involving the use of nitrous oxide and its possible teratogenic effects remain controversial. The presumed negative effects on the fetus due to nitrous oxide appear to be multifactorial, and with the availability of other inhaled agents with no teratogenic potential, the avoidance of nitrous oxide should be considered. Opioids including morphine and methadone used during pregnancy show no detrimental effects and were associated in pregnant women and their fetus.

We must focus on not only the effects of our anesthetic drugs on the pregnant patient but also the physiologic changes that result from the use of these substances. Of great concern should be the prevention of maternal hypoxemia and the maintenance of placental perfusion. Maternal physiology must be monitored closely. It is extremely important to avoid hypoxia, hypercarbia, hypocarbia, hypotension, and uterine hypertonicity. Maternal hypoxemia can cause uteroplacental vasoconstriction and decreased perfusion leading to hypoxia, acidosis, and possible mortality. Maternal hypercarbia limits the gradient for CO_2 diffusion from fetal to maternal blood and leads to fetal acidosis. End tidal carbon dioxide monitoring should be used to guide ventilation, and arterial blood gas analysis should be considered during prolonged or laparoscopic surgery. Hypocarbia is also problematic as it can potentially cause uteroplacental vasoconstriction and fetal acidosis. The mild hypo-capnia of pregnancy (a usual decrease of $PaCO_2$ of ~4 mmHg) should still be main-tained [59].

In conclusion, we must remain aware of the possibility of the deleterious effects of anesthetics medications and their affect on the fetus. Elective surgery should be delayed until after delivery of the fetus. Emergent surgery should be carried out with a meticulous and careful plan to protect not only the mother but also the fetus.

Chemical Structures

Chemical Structure
41.1 Methylergometrine

Chemical Structure
41.2 Carboprost

Chemical Structure
41.3 Chloroprocaine

Chemical Structure
41.4 Terbutaline

Chemical Structure
41.5 Ritodrine – this
drug has been removed
from the US market

Chemical Structure
41.6 Nifedipine

References

1. Chestnut D, Polley L, Lawrence T, Wong C. Chestnut's obstetric anesthesia. Principle and practice. 4th ed. Philadelphia: Elsevier; 2009.
2. Syme M, Paxton J, Keelan J. Drug transfer and metabolism by the human placenta. Clin Pharmacokinet. 2004;43(8):487–514.
3. Kuhnert BR, Kuhnert PM, Philipson EH, et al. The half-life of 2-chloroprocaine. Anesth Analg. 1986;65:273–8.
4. Ginosar Y, Mirikatani E, Drover D, Cohen S, Riley E. ED50 and ED95 of intrathecal hyperbaric bupivacaine coadministered with opioids for cesarean delivery. Anesthesiology. 2004;100(3):676–82.
5. Carvalho B, Durbin M, Drover DR, Cohen SE, Ginosar Y, Riley ET. The ED50 and ED95 of intrathecal isobaric bupivacaine with opioids for cesarean delivery. Anesthesiology. 2005;103(3):606–12.
6. Horlocker T, Wedel D. Neuraxial anesthesia. In: Longnecker D, Brown D, Newman M, Zapol W, editors. Anesthesia. New York: McGraw-Hill; 2007. p. 993.
7. McDonald J, Chen B, Kwan W. Current diagnosis and treatment: obstetric analgesia and anesthesia. 11th ed. New York: McGraw-Hill; 2013.
8. Hughes S, Levinson G, Rosen M, editors. Shnider and Levinson's anesthesia for obstetrics. 4th ed. Philadelphia: Lippincott Williams and Wilkins; 2002.
9. Polley L, Columb M, Naughton N, Wagner D, Van de Ven C. Relative analgesic potencies of ropivacaine and bupivacaine for epidural analgesia in labor: implications for therapeutic indexes. Anesthesiology. 1999;90(4):944–50.
10. Karabelkar D, Ramanathan S. 2-Chloroprocaine antagonism of epidural morphine analgesia. Acta Anaesthesiol Scand. 1997;41(6):774–8.

11. Pertek J, Haberer J. Effects of anesthesia on postoperative micturition and urinary retention. Ann Fr Anesth Reanim. 1995;14(4):340–51.
12. Brownridge P. Shivering related to epidural blockade with bupivacaine in labour, and the influence of epidural pethidine. Anaesth Intensive Care. 1986;14:412–7.
13. Ralston D, Shnider S. The fetal and neonatal effects of regional anesthesia in obstetrics. Anesthesiology. 1978;48:34–64.
14. Zakowski MI, Krishna R, Grant GJ, Turndorf H. Effect of pH on transfer of narcotics in human placenta during in vitro perfusion. Anesthesiology. 1995;85:A890.
15. Polluck JE. Transient neurologic symptoms: etiology risk factors and management. Reg Anesth Pain Med. 2002;27(6):581–6.
16. Tsui MH, Ngan Kee WD, Ng FF, Lau TK. A double blinded randomized placebo-controlled study of intramuscular pethidine for pain relief in the first stage of labour. Br J Obstet Gynaecol. 2004;111:648–55.
17. Cohen S, Ratner E, Kreitzman T, et al. Nalbuphine is better than naloxone for treatment of side effects after epidural morphine. Anesth Analg. 1992;75:747–52.
18. Hunt C, Naulty J, Bader A, et al. Perioperative analgesia with subarachnoid fentanyl bupivacaine for cesarean delivery. Anesthesiology. 1989;71:535–40.
19. Karaman S, Kocabas S, Uyar M, et al. The effects of sufentanil or morphine added to hyperbaric bupivacaine in spinal anaesthesia for caesarean section. Eur J Anaesthesiol. 2006;23:285–91.
20. Carvalho B, Roland LM, Chu LF, Campitelli 3rd VA, Riley ET. Single-dose, extended-release epidural morphine (DepoDur) compared to conventional epidural morphine for post-cesarean pain. Anesth Analg. 2007;105(1):176–83.
21. Jorgensen H, Wetterslev J, Moiniche S, Dahl J. Epidural local anaesthetics versus opioid-based analgesic regimens on postoperative gastrointestinal paralysis. PONV and pain after abdominal surgery. Cochrane Database Syst Rev. 2001;1:CD001893:1.
22. Friedlander JD, Fox HE, Cain CF, et al. Fetal bradycardia and uterine hyperactivity following subarachnoid administration of fentanyl during labor. Reg Anesth. 1997;22:378–81.
23. Clarke VT, Smiley RM, Finster M. Uterine hyperactivity after intrathecal injection of fentanyl for analgesia during labor: a cause of fetal bradycardia. Anesthesiology. 1994;81:1083.
24. Van de Velde M, Teunkens A, Hanssens M, Vanermeersch E, Verhaeghe J. Intrathecal sufentanil and fetal heart rate abnormalities: a double-blind, double placebo-controlled trial comparing two forms of combined spinal epidural analgesia with epidural analgesia in labor. Anesth Analg. 2004;98(4):1153–9.
25. Rosen M. Recent advances in pain relief in childbirth. Inhalation and systemic analgesia. Br J Anaesth. 1971;43:837–48.
26. Hardman J, Aitkenhead A. Awareness during anaesthesia. Contin Educ Anaesth Crit Care Pain. 2005;5(6):183–185.
27. Rasheed M, Palaria U, Bhadani U, Quadir A. Determination of optimal dose of succinylcholine to facilitate endotracheal pregnant females undergoing elective cesarean section. J Obstet Anaesth Crit Care. 2012;2(2):86–91.
28. Soliday F, Conley Y, Henker R. Pseudocholinesterase deficiency: a comprehensive review of genetic, acquired, and drug influences. ANA J. 2010;78(4):316.
29. Lumley J, Walker A, Marum J, Wood C. Time: an important variable at Caesarean section. J Obstet Gynaecol Br Commonw. 1970;77:10–23.
30. American Society of Anesthesiologists Task Force on Preoperative Fasting. Practice guidelines for preoperative fasting and the use of pharmacologic agents to reduce the risk of pulmonary aspiration. Anesthesiology. 1999;90:896–905.
31. Schug SA, Sidebotham DA, McGuinnety M, et al. Acetaminophen as an adjunct to morphine by patient-controlled analgesia in the management of acute postoperative pain. Anesth Analg. 1998;87:368–72.
32. Lowder JL, Shackelford DP, Holbert D, Beste TM. A randomized, controlled trial to compare ketorolac tromethamine versus placebo after cesarean section to reduce pain and narcotic usage. Am J Obstet Gynecol. 2003;189:1559–62.

33. James PR, Nelson-Piercy C. Management of hypertension before, during, and after pregnancy. Heart. 2004;90(12):1499–504.

34. Uzan J, Carbonnel M, Piconne O, Asmar R, Ayoubi JM. Pre-eclampsia: pathophysiology, diagnosis and management. Vasc Health Risk Manag. 2011;7:467–74.

35. Padden M. HELLP syndrome: recognition and perinatal management. Am Fam Physician. 1999;60(3):829–36.

36. Witlin AG, Sibai BM. Magnesium sulfate therapy in preeclampsia and eclampsia. Obstet Gynecol. 1998;92(5):883–9.

37. Podymow T, August P. Update on the use of antihypertensive drugs in pregnancy. Hypertension. 2008;51:960–9.

38. Kwan WF, Lee C, Chen BJ. A noninvasive method in the differential diagnosis of vecuronium-induced and magnesium-induced protracted neuromuscular block in a severely preeclamptic patient. J Clin Anesth. 1996;8:392–7.

39. Waisman GD, Mayorga LM, Camera MI, et al. Magnesium plus nifedipine: potentiation of hypotensive effect in preeclampsia? Am J Obstet Gynecol. 1988;159:308–9.

40. Snyder SW, Cardwell MS. Neuromuscular blockade with magnesium sulfate and nifedipine. Am J Obstet Gynecol. 1989;161:35–6.

41. Schoonen WM, et al. Do selected drugs increase the risk of lupus? A matched case-control study. Br J Clin Pharmacol. 2010;70(4):588–96.

42. Katz VL, Childress CH. Nifedipine and its indications in obstetrics and gynecology. Obstet Gynecol. 1994;83(4):616–24.

43. Ressel G. ACOG issues recommendations on assessment of risk factors for preterm birth. Am Fam Physician. 2002;65(3):509–10.

44. Haas DM, Imperiale TF, Kirkpatrick PR, Klein RW, Zollinger TW, Golichowski AM. Tocolytic therapy: a meta-analysis and decision analysis. Obstet Gynecol. 2009;113(3):585–94.

45. Simhan HN, Caritis SN. Prevention of preterm delivery. N Engl J Med. 2007;357(5):477–87.

46. Berkman ND, Thorp Jr JM, Lohr KN, et al. Tocolytic treatment for the management of preterm labor: a review of the evidence. Am J Obstet Gynecol. 2003;188(6):1648–59.

47. Horlocker T, Wedel D, Rowlingson J. Regional anesthesia in the patient receiving antithrombotic or thrombolytic therapy: American Society of Regional Anesthesia and Pain Medicine evidence-based guidelines (third edition). Reg Anesth Pain Med. 2010;35(1):64–101.

48. Stoelting RK, Miller RD. Basics of anesthesia, 4th ed. Philadelphia: Churchill Livingstone; 2000. p. 359; Miller RD. Anesthesia. 5th ed. Philadelphia: Churchill Livingstone; 2000; pp. 165, 2059–2060.

49. Birnbach DJ, Browne IM. Anesthesia for obstetrics. Miller's anesthesia. 7th ed. Orlando: Churchill Livingstone; 2009.

50. Ford JB, Roberts CL, Bell JC, et al. Postpartum haemorrhage occurrence and recurrence: a population-based study. Med J Aust. 2007;187:391–3.

51. Klufio CA, Amoa AB, Kariwiga G. Primary postpartum haemorrhage: causes, aetiological risk factors, prevention and management. P N G Med J. 1995;38(2):133–49.

52. American College of Obstetricians and Gynecologists. Postpartum hemorrhage. Practice bulletin no. 76. Washington, DC, October 2006. Obstet Gynecol. 2006;108:1039–47.

53. Bhattacharya S, Ghosh S, Ray D, Mallik S, Laha A. Oxytocin administration during cesarean delivery: randomized controlled trial to compare intravenous bolus with intravenous infusion regimen. Anaesthesiol Clin Pharmacol. 2013;29(1):32–5.

54. de Groot AN, van Dongen PW, Vree TB, et al. Ergot alkaloids: current status and review of clinical pharmacology and therapeutic use compared with other oxytocics in obstetrics and gynaecology. Drugs. 1998;56:523–35.

55. Lin YH, Seow KM, Hwang JL, Chen HH. Myocardial infarction and mortality caused by methylergonovine. Acta Obstet Gynecol Scand. 2005;84:1022.

56. O'Leary AM. Severe bronchospasm and hypotension after 15-methyl prostaglandin F(2alpha) in atonic postpartum haemorrhage. Int J Obstet Anesth. 1994;3:42–4.

57. Crowhurst JA. Anaesthesia for non-obstetric surgery during pregnancy. Acta Anaesthesiol Belg. 2002;53:295–7.

58. Shepard TH. Catalog of teratogenic agents. 7th ed. Baltimore: Johns Hopkins University Press; 1992.
59. Heidemann BH, McClure JH. Changes in maternal physiology during pregnancy. Contin Educ Anaesth Crit Care Pain. 2003;3:65–8.
60. Wilson JG. Environment and birth defects. New York: Academic; 1973. p. 1–82.
61. Shiono PH, Mills JL. Oral clefts and diazepam use during pregnancy. N Engl J Med. 1984;311:919–20.

Chapter 42
Pediatrics

Vanessa Ng, Karina Gritsenko, and Rebecca Lintner

Contents

Introduction

There are numerous specific anatomic, physiologic, and psychological issues that should be understood prior to anesthetizing pediatric patients. In this chapter, we will discuss the basic pharmacologic concepts that relate to drugs commonly used in the anesthetic management of this population.

V. Ng, MD (✉) • K. Gritsenko, MD • R. Lintner, MD
Department of Anesthesiology, Montefiore Medical Center,
Albert Einstein College of Medicine, Bronx, NY, USA
e-mail: vng@montefiore.org; karinagritsenko@googlemail.com;
rlintner@montefiore.org

A.D. Kaye et al. (eds.), *Essentials of Pharmacology for Anesthesia,*
Pain Medicine, and Critical Care, DOI 10.1007/978-1-4614-8948-1_42,
© Springer Science+Business Media New York 2015

Pharmacokinetics in Infants and Children

Infants and children have a larger volume of distribution, smaller proportion of muscle and fat stores, altered protein binding, and immature renal and hepatic function.

Therefore, most medications will have altered pharmacokinetic properties as compared to adults. Any clinician caring for patients in this population must be aware of the age-related alterations in drug absorption, distribution, and elimination since these result in an increased risk of drug overdose and toxicity [1].

Factors Influencing Drug Availability

Protein Binding

The amount of a drug that binds to proteins limits the amount of free drug available. Drugs that are highly protein bound have less available free drug to interact with the drugs targeted receptors.

Neonates and children have a reduced protein binding capacity, which results in more free drug to interact with the drugs target. Reduced protein binding capacity is caused by several factors such as reduced plasma proteins, fetal albumin which has a reduced affinity to bind drugs, and increased competition for acidic binding sites due to increased free fatty acids and unconjugated bilirubin [2, 3].

Body Water

Total body water is highest in infants, representing 80 % of their total body weight versus 60 % in the adult [4]. Water-soluble drugs therefore have higher volumes of distribution and decreased serum levels. Medications dependent upon redistribution into muscle and fat for termination of their clinical effect may have a longer sustained concentration as there is less tissue for redistribution [5].

Cardiac Output

Cardiac output of neonates per kilogram is normally twice that of adults. This increased cardiac output reduces the rate of rise of alveolar concentration of anesthetic inhalational agents as, more anesthetic is removed per unit of time. However, the inhalational agents reach equilibrium between the alveoli and the brain more rapidly as much of the cardiac output of neonates and infants directed to the vessel-rich tissues. These tissues are saturated sooner resulting in faster induction (and faster recovery) as compared to adults [6].

Physiologic Differences

Neonates have increased brain permeability due to an immature blood–brain barrier as compared to adolescents and adults making them more sensitive to sedatives, hypnotics, and narcotics. In addition, incomplete myelination in infants may allow for drugs that are insoluble to cross the blood–brain barrier to cross at a greater rate [7].

Blood Flow Distribution

Administration and absorption of various medications may be altered based on mode of delivery. Intravenous is often the best route of delivery. However, the limiting factor is often the ability to place an IV in this population. Intramuscular injection of medication is affected by variations in blood flow to the muscle. Compared to adults, neonates have a lower muscle mass which could lead to decreased absorption [8]. Topical administration is affected by skin thickness, which is similar in both neonates and adults; however, neonates have a much larger body surface area to body weight ratio, which could lead to a much greater amount of drug absorption [9]. Oral delivery is affected by a variety of factors such as gastric pH (initially alkaline, especially in premature infants), gastrointestinal enzyme activity, volume of gastric juices, gastric emptying rate, and intestinal surface area. Given these factors, it is thought that the rate of drug absorption is slower in neonates [4].

Metabolism and Excretion

Metabolism of drugs dependent on the liver will be decreased in the neonate due to decreased activity of phase I and phase II liver enzymes [10, 11]. In addition, drug metabolism is affected by hepatic blood flow which changes with obliteration of umbilical blood supply as well as closure of the ductus arteriosus [12].

Renal function in preterm and term infants is also less efficient than in adults. Glomerular filtration and tubular function rapidly develops during the first few months of life, and is nearly mature by 20 weeks, and fully mature at two years. Drugs excreted through the kidney will have prolonged pharmacologic levels if kidney function contributes to their elimination [7].

Inhalational Anesthetics

The minimum alveolar concentration (MAC) of an inhalation anesthetic in pediatric patients varies with age. One MAC represents the percent or concentration of an inhaled anesthetic at 1 atm that renders 50 % of patients unresponsive to a surgical stimulus.

Studies have found that infants have a higher MAC than that noted in older children or adults for reasons not clearly understood. Sevoflurane is an inhalational anesthetic that offers an advantage for rapid induction and rapid awakening due to its lower blood solubility, particularly useful in the pediatric population, as it has a less pungent smell than other inhalational agents. In children with congenital cardiac disease, fewer hemodynamic changes have been noted when compared with isoflurane, and it has a greater effect on respiratory depression by decreasing minute ventilation and respiratory frequency as compared with halothane.

Isoflurane has a more pungent odor and does not allow its use for mask induction. This inhalational agent is noted to have less myocardial depression, preservation of the heart rate, and a greater reduction in the cerebral metabolic rate for oxygen.

Desflurane, also pungent in nature, has made it difficult to use it for induction of anesthesia. It has been found to cause an incidence of laryngospasm of 50 % during the gaseous induction of anesthesia in children [13].

Nitrous oxide is a colorless, odorless gas that possesses both analgesic and anxiolytic effects. The drug must be delivered with oxygen to avoid a hypoxic gas mixture and is often used to supplement other inhalation agents. It has low blood–gas partition coefficient resulting in rapid induction and awakening. Although its low potency does not allow for it to be used as a sole anesthetic, it is an extremely useful agent. It is not a trigger for malignant hyperthermia. It increases uptake of sevoflurane on induction via the second gas effect and it also allows easier mask induction due to its neutral odor.

The "steal" induction technique allows the patient to breathe the odorless gas allowing for relaxation while the more pungent inhalant – sevoflurane – is titrated up [14].

Relevant to inhalational anesthetics, as well as other IV anesthetic agents, is emergence delirium, a dissociated state of consciousness in which a child is inconsolable, irritable, uncompromising, or uncooperative with psychomotor agitation in the immediate postoperative period. The incidence of emergence delirium is 12–13 % in children. The incidence of emergence delirium following halothane, isoflurane, sevoflurane, or desflurane ranges from 2 to 55 % [15].

Intravenous Anesthetic Agents

Propofol is a sedative-hypnotic anesthetic agent useful in the induction and maintenance of anesthesia. It is a lipid macroemulsion with egg yolk and soybean oil components. This highly lipophilic drug is painful upon IV injection. It is rapidly distributed into vessel-rich organs accounting for its quick onset, while termination is due to rapid redistribution and hepatic and extrahepatic (kidney and lung) clearance. The dose of propofol required for loss of the eyelash reflex generally increases with decreasing age. Propofol induction dose is 3–4 mg/kg for children younger than 2 years to 2.5–3 mg/kg for older children. Maintenance of general anesthesia requires 200–300 µg/kg/min [16, 17].

Propofol is commonly used in continuous infusions or intermittent boluses for the maintenance of anesthesia in children undergoing procedures in MRI, CT, and interventional radiology and for gastroenterology and oncology procedures. Infusion rates of 200–250 µg/kg/min or greater may be required. A decrease systolic blood pressure and compromise of airway patency and respiration in children are noted with propofol as well as decreased postoperative nausea and vomiting upon emergence.

Ketamine is a phencyclidine derivative that blocks the N-methyl-D aspartate (NMDA) receptor, offering both potent hypnosis and analgesia, preservation of airway reflexes and spontaneous respiration, increasing endogenous catecholamine release, and a small amount of bronchodilation.

Oral ketamine may be used as a sedative, 5–6 mg/kg for children 1–6 years of age, with maximal sedation within 20 min. Induction doses of 1 mg/kg IV yields effective analgesia and sedation with rapid onset. Intramuscular ketamine reaches peak blood levels and clinical effect in 5 min after 3–10 mg/kg. Intramuscular administration of ketamine is an excellent means of sedating the "out of control" patient for IV placement or mildly painful procedures. Simultaneous administration of an anticholinergic will minimize oral secretions. Emergence from ketamine sedation/anesthesia can be marked by diplopia, occasional disturbing dreams, and nausea/vomiting. Use of concomitant midazolam may decrease some of these side effects.

Opioids are important elements of sedation and pain management in children. These medications are also well known to cause central respiratory depression and newborns and infants younger than six months are particularly susceptible due to immaturity of blood–brain barrier and increased levels of free drug [18, 19].

Morphine is the most commonly used opioid in postoperative analgesic management in children and the standard against which all other opioids are compared. It is more hydrophilic than lipophilic resulting in slow brain uptake. Due to its hydrophilic nature and a larger volume of body water in the neonate, morphine has a larger volume of distribution. The large volume of distribution in combination with decreased hepatic metabolism greatly decreases morphine clearance in neonatal patient; thus, many prefer fentanyl for this patient population. Initial dose of morphine is 0.05–0.2 mg/kg IV and may also be administered orally, rectally, transtracheally, and in the epidural and subarachnoid spaces.

Fentanyl is the most commonly used opioid during general anesthesia in pediatrics. It is 100 times more potent than morphine and may be administered IV, IM, epidurally, intrathecally, orally, and transdermally. It is highly lipophilic and crosses the blood–brain barrier rapidly resulting in rapid onset and short duration of action. Given the larger volume of distribution in neonates, concentrations are reduced.

Elimination is prolonged likely due to increased volume of distribution and immature p450 enzymes [20]. Administration of fentanyl also results in prolonged and increased respiratory depression in the neonate versus the adult. Kohentop et al. hypothesize this is due both to prolonged elimination as well as possible increased brain solubility [21]. Usual dose is 1–5 µg/kg IV.

Sufentanil is a synthetic narcotic, five to ten times more potent than fentanyl. It is highly protein bound. Distribution in neonates is increased due to increased volume as well as decreased α1-acid glycoprotein. Elimination is decreased due to immature p450 enzymes and can be further influenced by hepatic blood flow [22]. Dosing of sufentanil is 1 µg/kg IV.

Remifentanil, twice as potent as fentanyl, has also been shown to be an effective part of anesthesia and sedation protocols for a variety of procedures at 0.25–1.0 µg/kg/min continuous infusion. It has a very short half-life due to hydrolysis by nonspecific tissue esterase. It is the only drug for which there is a greater rather than a reduced clearance in neonates [23]. Effective postoperative analgesia is not obtained with remifentanil due to this increased clearance.

Hydrocodone is a semisynthetic opioid and is an orally active analgesic and antitussive, often combined with acetaminophen. It is one-tenth as potent as morphine, and maximum recommended dose of hydrocodone in children 2–12 years is 15 mg over 24 h. It is in often used in neonates. It is eliminated by hepatic enzymes so therefore has an increased half-life [24].

Midazolam is the most commonly used sedative premedicant. It is a short acting, water-soluble benzodiazepine devoid of analgesic properties. The drug is particularly popular because of its short duration and predictable onset. Dose of 0.5–0.75 mg/kg orally peaks ~30 min after administration. Unfortunately, the drug has a very bitter taste though difficult to disguise and has flavored oral preparations. In neonates, it is extremely useful at a dose of 0.1 mg/kg to aid in awake intubations. It has a longer elimination half-life due to decreased hepatic enzyme activity in the neonatal patient [25]. Nasal, rectal, and IM preparations are also available. Intravenous midazolam is excellent for sedation and anxiolysis in patients for minor procedures, with dosing 0.05–0.1 mg/kg and peak effect in 2–3 min.

Diazepam is used less frequently in the pediatric population, as it has a longer duration than midazolam, producing lasting effects for an hour or more. This medication is quite useful for treating muscle spasms, such as torticollis or those experienced by patients with cerebral palsy. Dosing of diazepam is 0.1–0.15 mg/kg intravenously, though painful and not well tolerated; diazepam may also be administered orally or rectally.

Muscle Relaxants

Succinylcholine, a depolarizing muscle relaxant, administered 1.5–2.0 mg/kg IV produces excellent intubating conditions in 60 s with recovery in 6–7 min.

Neonates, infants, and children require a higher dose to demonstrate the same level of muscle relaxation as compared to adults [26]. Succinylcholine is absolutely contraindicated in patients with muscular dystrophy, recent burn injury, spinal cord transaction, and/or immobilization, as well as any child with family history of malignant hyperthermia due to the risk of hyperkalemia, rhabdomyolysis, masseter spasm, and malignant hyperthermia. This drug is relatively contraindicated in all children by the FDA due to infrequent, but reported cases of hyperkalemic cardiac arrest, in which succinylcholine had been administered to children with risk factors not clinically apparent. This drug can be recommended in situations in which ultra rapid onset and short duration of action is of imminent importance (laryngospasm) or when muscle relaxation is required when IV access is not available IM dose of 4 mg/kg.

Nondepolarizing muscle relaxants used in adults are effective in pediatric patients, but because they have a larger percentage of total body water neonates and infants have a larger volume of distribution for these hydrophilic drugs. These patients are also slightly more sensitive to these drugs and so the doses of these agents are the same as for adults, but the duration of action tends to be slightly longer.

Rocuronium has the lowest potency and the fastest onset of action of the currently available nondepolarizing relaxants, 60 s for a 1 mg/kg dose, and is therefore the logical choice for rapid-sequence intubation. The use of rocuronium is limited by its duration of action (30–40 min) and elimination, via hepatic reuptake and biliary excretion.

Cisatracurium is useful in children largely because its elimination is by Hofmann elimination, a process dependent only on pH and temperature. Its onset and offset appears faster in neonates than in infants or children.

Vecuronium has onset and duration of action that is dose dependent. An initial response occurs in 2–4 min, with duration of 30–40 min. Thirty percent is metabolized in the liver and the remaining excreted by the renal and biliary system. Dosing of 0.05–0.1 µg/kg IV, is used for neonates, while older infants and children dosing is similar to adults, between 0.08 and 0.1 µg/kg IV.

Reversal of muscle blockade should be carefully considered in each patient, as the risks associated with inadequate ventilation in small children are great. Muscle twitch should be monitored and reversal agents, neostigmine, 0.05 mg/kg, with 0.015 mg/kg of atropine or 0.01 mg/kg of glycopyrrolate, administered if residual weakness is detected.

Local Anesthetics

Most regional anesthetic techniques can be useful for children undergoing anesthesia and surgery. Choice of local anesthetic is based on the desired duration of action and the toxic effects of local anesthetic solution used. The two classes of local anesthetics include the amides, which undergo enzymatic degradation by the liver and the esters, which are hydrolyzed by plasma cholinesterases. These actions may play a very important role particularly in neonates and infants. Toxicity of local anesthetic solution includes cardiac, peripheral vascular, neurologic, and allergic reactions. Bupivacaine, an amide anesthetic, is the most common agent in infants and children. It is highly bound to α-1 glycoprotein and due to low levels of albumin and α-1 glycoprotein in neonates, the free fraction of this drug may be greater, leading to a greater risk of cardiac toxicity [27].

Ropivacaine is a newer amide local anesthetic used more frequently in pediatric surgery. It is a l-enantiomer with less cardiovascular and central nervous system side effects compared with bupivacaine.

Chloroprocaine, an ester local anesthetic, is advantageous due to its rapid metabolism, minimizing risks of toxicity, especially in patients with preexisting problems such as prematurity or hepatic dysfunction [27].

Adjuvants

Clonidine, an α-2 agonists, has been used as an oral preanesthetic in children for years. Doses of 3–5 mcg/kg result in sedative and anxiolytic effects similar to oral midazolam. Disadvantages include slow onset >30 min and prolonged duration >90 min.

Hydromorphone, while not used as frequently as morphine or fentanyl, is often used when long-term analgesia is required. It is similar to morphine though 3.5 more potent than oral morphine to seven times more potent than IV morphine.

In order to deliver optimal anesthesia care to infants and children, one must truly appreciate the unique nature of this population and the impact that anesthesia can have on their developing physiology.

References

1. Holzman RS, Mancuso TJ, Polaner DM. A practical approach to pediatric anesthesia. Philadelphia: Lippincott Williams and Williams; 2008.
2. Mahmood I. Pediatric pharmacology and pharmacokinetics. In: Developmental pharmacology: impact on pharmacokinetics and PD of drugs. Rockville: Pine House Publishers; 2008. p. 68–107.
3. Ehrnebo M, Agurell S, Jalling B, Boreus LO. Age differences in drug binding by plasma proteins: studies on human foetuses, neonates and adults. Eur J Clin Pharmacol. 1971;3:189–93.
4. Kearns GL, Abdel-Rahman SM, Alander SW, et al. Developmental pharmacology: drug disposition, action, and therapy in infants and children. N Engl J Med. 2003;349(12):1157–67.
5. Roberts F, Freshwater-Turner D. Pharmacokinetics and anaesthesia. Contin Educ Anaesth Crit Care Pain. 2007;7:25–9.
6. Morray JP, Geiduschek JM, Ramamoorthy C, et al. Anesthesia-related cardiac arrest in children: initial findings of the Pediatric Perioperative Cardiac Arrest (POCA) registry. Anesthesiology. 2000;93:6–14.
7. Alcorn J, McNamara PJ. Ontogeny of hepatic and renal systemic clearance pathways in infants: part I. Clin Pharmacokinet. 2002;41:959–98.

8. Greenbalt DJ, Koch-Weaser J. Intramuscular injections of drugs. N Engl J Med. 1976;295(10): 542–6.

9. Choonara I. Percutaneous drug absorption and administration. Arch Dis Child. 1994;71(2):73–4.

10. Jacqz-Aigrain E, Cresteil T. Cytochrome P450–dependent metabolism of dextromethorphan: fetal and adult studies. Dev Pharmacol Ther. 1992;18:161–8.

11. Ward RM, Mirkin BL. Perinatal/neonatal pharmacology. In: Brody TM, Larner J, Minneman KP, editors. Human pharmacology: molecular-to-clinical. 3rd ed. St. Louis: Mosby-Year Book; 1998. p. 873–83.

12. Gow PJ, Ghabrial H, Smallwood RA, et al. Neonatal hepatic drug elimination. Pharmacol Toxicol. 2001;88(1):3–15.

13. Zwass MS, Fisher DM, Welborn LG, et al. Induction and maintenance characteristics of anesthesia with desflurane and nitrous oxide in infants and children. Anesthesiology. 1992;76:373–8.

14. Goldman LJ. Anesthetic uptake of sevoflurane and nitrous oxide during an inhaled induction in children. Anesth Analg. 2003;96(2):400–6.

15. Mason LJ. Pitfalls of pediatric anesthesia: emergence delirium. Richmond: Society for Pediatric Anesthesia; 2004. Retrieved 2012-06-21.

16. Murat I, Billard V, Vernois J, et al. Pharmacokinetics of propofol after a single dose in children aged 1–3 years with minor burns. Comparison of three data analysis approaches. Anesthesiology. 1996;84:526–32.

17. Marik PE. Propofol: therapeutic indications and side-effects. Curr Pharm Des. 2004;10:3639–49.

18. Kupferberg HJ, Way HJ. Pharmacologic basis for the increased sensitivity of the newborn to morphine. J Pharmacol Exp Ther. 1963;141:105–9.

19. Lynn AM, Slattery JT. Morphine pharmacokinetics in early infancy. Anesthesiology. 1987;66: 136–9.

20. Gauntlett IS, Fisher DM, Hertzka RE, et al. Pharmacokinetics of fentanyl in neonatal humans and lambs: effects of age. Anesthesiology. 1988;69:683–7.

21. Koehntop DE, Rodman JH, Brundage DM, et al. Pharmacokinetics of fentanyl in neonates. Anesth Analg. 1986;65:227–32.

22. Lundenberg S, Roelofse J. Aspects of pharmacokinetics and pharmacodynamics of sufentanil in pediatric practice. Paediatr Anaesth. 2010;21:274–9.

23. Ross AK, Davis PJ, Dear GGL, et al. Pharmacokinetics of remifentanil in anesthetized pediatric patients undergoing elective surgery or diagnostic procedures. Anesth Analg. 2001;93:1393–401.

24. Quiding H, Olsson GL, Boreus LO, et al. Infants and young children metabolise codeine to morphine. A study after single and repeated rectal administration. Br J Clin Pharmacol. 1992; 33(1):45–9.

25. Wildt SN, Kearns GL, Hop WC, Murry DJ, Abdel-Rahman SM, Van den Anker JN. Pharmacokinetics and metabolism of oral midazolam in preterm infants. Br J Clin Pharmacol. 2002;50:390–2.

26. Meakin GH, MCKiernan EP, Moris P, et al. Dose-response curve for suxamethonium in neonates, infants, and children. Br J Anesth. 1989;65:655–8.

27. Wilder R. Local anesthetics for the pediatric patient. Pediatr Clin N Am. 2000;47(3):545–58.

Chapter 43
Neurologic Surgery

Allison Spinelli and Robyn Landy

Contents

Introduction to Neurophysiology

Approximately 75–80 ml/100 g/min and white matter about 20 ml/100 g/min. Determinants that regulate CBF include $CMRO_2$, PaO_2, $PaCO_2$, temperature, autoregulation/CPP, and anesthetic drugs [5, 7, 8].

$CMRO_2$ – Normal $CMRO_2$ is 50 ml/min or 3–3.5 ml/100 g/min, about 20 % of total body consumption (250 ml/min). CBF and $CMRO_2$ are directly coupled, meaning increases or decreases in $CMRO_2$ result in a proportional increase or decrease in CBF [5, 7, 8].

PaO_2 – CBF increases when PaO_2 falls below 50 mmHg due to the accumulation of lactic acid [5, 7, 8].

$PaCO_2$ – Between a $PaCO_2$ of 20–80 mmHg CBF is proportional to $PaCO_2$. In general, every 1 mmHg increase or decrease in $PaCO_2$ results in a 1 ml.100 g/min

A. Spinelli, MD (✉) • R. Landy, MD
Department of Anesthesiology, Montefiore Medical Center,
Albert Einstein College of Medicine, Bronx, NY, USA
e-mail: aspinell@montefiore.org; rlandy@montefiore.org

A.D. Kaye et al. (eds.), *Essentials of Pharmacology for Anesthesia,*
Pain Medicine, and Critical Care, DOI 10.1007/978-1-4614-8948-1_43,
© Springer Science+Business Media New York 2015

increase or decrease in CBF. Below a PaCO$_2$ of 20 mmHg, cerebral ischemia may result, and above 80 mmHg, the cerebral vasculature is maximally dilated, in which CBF becomes pressure dependent [5, 7, 8].

Temperature – For every 1 °C decrease in body temperature below 37 °C, CBF and CMRO$_2$ decrease about 7 % [5, 7, 8].

Autoregulation – Is the ability of the cerebral arterioles to constrict or relax in response to changes in perfusion pressure. CPP = MAP – ICP or CVP (whichever is greater). With a CPP between 60 and 150 mmHg, CBF is kept constant; however, above or below these values, autoregulation is lost and CPP is blood pressure dependent (some data suggests autoregulation as low as 50 mmHg; numerous factors shift the autoregulation curve to the right, such as hypertension) [5, 7, 8].

Intracranial Pressure

ICP is normally <10 mmHg. It is determined by the pressure contribution of three volume compartments – brain parenchyma 80–90 %, CSF 5–10 %, and blood 5–10 % – and rises from any increase in any one of these compartments (Monro-Kellie doctrine). However, ICP is maintained over a wide range of intracranial volumes due to several compensatory mechanisms, and there are several ways to decrease ICP intraoperatively: elevation of the head to improve cerebral venous outflow, hyperventilation, osmotic diuretics, CSF drainage, cerebral vasoconstricting drugs, and avoidance of cerebral vasodilating drugs [5, 7, 8].

Intravenous Anesthetics

In general, all intravenous drugs, except ketamine, cause a dose-dependent reduction in both CBF and CMRO$_2$ which leads to a reduction in ICP [5, 7, 8].

Induction Agents

Thiopental (Currently Not Available in the USA)

1. *Class* – Barbiturate.
2. *Mechanism of action* – Acts on the GABA$_A$ receptor in the brain and spinal cord enhancing GABA-mediated chloride currents leading to hyperpolarization of neurons and reduced excitability [5, 7, 8].
3. *Thiopental and neuroanesthesia* – Produces dose-dependent CNS depression. Potent cerebral vasoconstrictor. Reduces CMRO$_2$ in a dose-dependent manner up to a maximum dose at which the EEG becomes flat line (isoelectric). Large

doses can cause cardiovascular depression and may decrease systemic blood pressure to also decrease CPP. Autoregulation of CBF is not altered by barbiturates. Have potent anticonvulsant effects. Believed to provide neuroprotection from focal cerebral ischemia but not likely from global ischemia [5, 7, 8].

4. *Dosing – Adult – Anesthesia*: I.V.: Induction: 3–5 mg/kg, Maintenance: 25–100 mg as needed. *Increased intracranial pressure*: I.V.: Children and Adults: 1.5–5 mg/kg/dose; repeat as needed. *Pediatric – Anesthesia*: *I.V.*: Induction: Infants: 5–8 mg/kg, Children 1–12 years: 5–6 mg/kg. Maintenance: Children: 1 mg/kg as needed. *Increased intracranial pressure*: I.V.: Children: 1.5–5 mg/kg/dose; repeat as needed [10, 11].

5. *Drug interactions* – CNS depressants potentiate its sedative effects. Contrast media and sulfonamides occupy the same protein binding sites and may potentiate its effects by increasing the amount of free drug available [10, 11].

6. *Side effects* – Bradycardia, hypotension, hyperactivity (pediatric), nausea, vomiting, somnolence, porphyria exacerbation, rash, urticaria, pain, swelling, thrombophlebitis, necrosis, hepatitis, respiratory depression, erythema multiforme, Stevens-Johnson syndrome, angioedema, anemia, megaloblastic, TTP, and blood dyscrasias [5, 7, 8, 10, 11].

Propofol

1. *Class* – Isopropylphenol.
2. *Mechanism of action* – Causes global CNS depression through the potentiation of the chloride current mediated through the $GABA_A$ receptor complex. May also cause reduced glutamatergic activity through NMDA receptor blockade [5, 7, 8].
3. *Propofol and neuroanesthesia* – Produces a decrease in both $CMRO_2$ and CBF decreasing ICP. Can critically depress CPP due to a decrease in both CBF and MAP as a result of systemic peripheral vasodilation. Does not alter autoregulation of CBF. In large doses, can produce burst suppression on an EEG which is an endpoint that has been used for the administration of I.V. anesthetics for neuroprotection [5, 7, 8].
4. *Dosing – Adult – Anesthesia* – Induction: 2–2.5 mg/kg. Maintenance: I.V. infusion: Initial: 100–200 mcg/kg/min for 10–15 min; usual maintenance infusion rate: 50–100 mcg/kg/min. I.V. intermittent bolus: 25–50 mg increments as needed. *Pediatric*: *Induction*: I.V.: 3–16 years y/o, 2.5–3.5 mg/kg over 20–30 s; *Maintenance*: I.V. infusion: 2 months to 16 years: 125–300 mcg/kg/min [10, 11].
5. *Drug interactions* – Potentiates nondepolarizing neuromuscular blockers. Fentanyl and alfentanil concentrations may be increased with administration of propofol [10, 11].
6. *Side effects* – Pain at injection site, hypotension, bradycardia, asystole, involuntary muscle movements, respiratory acidosis during weaning, hyperlipidemia, rash, pruritus, anaphylaxis/anaphylactoid reaction, propofol infusion syndrome, cardiac arrest, seizures, opisthotonus, pancreatitis, pulmonary edema, phlebitis, thrombosis, and renal tubular toxicity [5, 7, 8, 10, 11].

Etomidate

1. *Class* – Carboxylated imidazole.
2. *Mechanism of action* – Acts through potentiation of $GABA_A$-mediated chloride channels [5, 7, 8].
3. *Etomidate and neuroanesthesia* – Potent cerebral vasoconstrictor and decreases CBF, $CMRO_2$, and ICP. Produces EEG burst suppression at high doses. Myoclonus may occur and might be associated with an increased frequency of excitatory peaks on EEG [5, 7, 8].
4. *Dosing* – Anesthesia I.V. Induction: Children >10 years and Adults: Initial: 0.2–0.6 mg/kg over 30–60 s; Maintenance: 10–20 mcg/kg/min [10, 11].
5. *Drug interactions* – Fentanyl increases its plasma level and prolongs its elimination half-life. Opioids decrease myoclonus during induction [10, 11].
6. *Side effects* – Nausea, vomiting, injection site pain, transient myoclonus, averting movements, apnea, arrhythmias, bradycardia, tachycardia, decreased cortisol synthesis (shock), hypertension/hypotension, and laryngospasm [5, 7, 8, 10, 11].

Ketamine

1. *Class* – Phencyclidine.
2. *Mechanism of action* – Noncompetitive NMDA receptor antagonist that blocks glutamate. Produces a cataleptic-like state by direct action on the cortex and limbic system. Has analgesic properties [5, 7, 8].
3. *Ketamine and neuroanesthesia* – Unlike the other I.V. anesthetics, it is a cerebral vasodilator with resultant increases in CBF, $CMRO_2$, and ICP. It is not administered if patients have known intracranial disease due to the risk in increasing ICP [5, 7, 8].
4. *Dosing – Adult –* Induction: I.M.: 4–10 mg/kg, I.V.: 0.5–2 mg/kg. Maintenance – supplemental doses of one-half to the full induction dose or a continuous infusion of 0.1–0.5 mg/min. *Pediatric*: I.V.: 0.5–1 mg/kg/dose. Continuous I.V. infusion: 5–20 mcg/kg/min [10, 11].
5. *Drug interactions* – Potentiates nondepolarizing neuromuscular blocking drugs. Combination with theophylline may predispose to seizures. Diazepam attenuates its cardiostimulatory effects and prolongs its elimination half-life. Sympathetic antagonists may unmask its direct myocardial depressant effects. Lithium may prolong its actions [10, 11].
6. *Side effects* – Sialorrhea, anorexia, nausea, vomiting, hypertension, tachycardia, arrhythmias, diplopia, nystagmus, fasciculations, depressed reflexes, hallucinations, bradycardia, hypotension, cystitis, respiratory depression, laryngospasm, increased intraocular pressure, emergence delirium, tonic-clonic movements, and anaphylaxis [5, 7, 8, 10, 11].

Dexmedetomidine

1. *Class* – Selective alpha2-adrenergic agonist.
2. *Mechanism of action* – Activates G-proteins by $alpha_{2a}$-adrenoceptors in the brainstem resulting in inhibition of norepinephrine release; peripheral $alpha_{2b}$-adrenoceptors are activated at high doses or with rapid I.V. administration resulting in vasoconstriction [5, 7, 8].
3. *Dexmedetomidine and neuroanesthesia* – Associated with a decrease in CBF without significant changes in $CMRO_2$ or ICP [5, 7, 8].
4. *Dosing* – Anesthesia; I.V. Initial: Loading infusion of 1 mcg/kg over 10 min. Maintenance infusion of 0.7 mcg/kg/h [10, 11].
5. *Drug interactions* – Potentiates the effects of other CNS depressants and potentiates nondepolarizing neuromuscular blocking drugs [10, 11].
6. *Side effects* – Hypotension, hypertension, nausea, vomiting, bradycardia, xerostomia, hypovolemia, respiratory depression, pleural effusion, agitation, tachycardia, anemia, hyperthermia, hyperglycemia, hemorrhage, pain, oliguria, acidosis, sinus arrest, arrhythmias, atrial fibrillation, ARDS, bronchospasm, hyperkalemia, adrenal insufficiency, leukocytosis, acute renal failure, and acute withdrawal syndrome [5, 7, 8, 10, 11].

Midazolam

1. *Class* – Benzodiazepine.
2. *Mechanism of action* – Binds to stereospecific benzodiazepine receptors on the postsynaptic GABA neuron activating the $GABA_A$ receptor complex [5, 7, 8].
3. *Midazolam and neuroanesthesia* – Decreases both $CMRO_2$ and CBF but to a lesser degree than thiopental or propofol. Does not produce an isoelectric EEG which indicates a ceiling effect on drug-induced decreases in $CMRO_2$. Little to no change in ICP and has been shown to produce no neuroprotective effects. Potent anticonvulsant [5, 7, 8].
4. *Dosing* – *Adults* Anesthesia: I.V.: *Induction*: 0.3–0.35 mg/kg over 20–30 s; *Maintenance*: 0.05 mg/kg as needed, continuous infusion 0.015–0.06 mg/kg/h (0.25–1 mcg/kg/min). *Pediatrics*: *Oral, rectal*: 0.5–0.75 mg/kg as a single dose preprocedure (maximum: 20 mg); *I.M.*: 0.1–0.15 mg/kg maximum total dose: 10 mg. *I.V.*: Infants 6 months–5 years: Initial: 0.05–0.1 mg/kg; maximum total dose: 6 mg. Children 6–12 years: Initial: 0.025–0.05 mg/kg; maximum total dose: 10 mg [10, 11].
5. *Drug interactions* – Reduces MAC of volatile anesthetics. CNS depressants potentiate its sedative effects. Erythromycin inhibits its metabolism and causes a two- to threefold prolongation of its effects. Cimetidine binds to cytochrome P450 and reduces its metabolism [10, 11].

6. *Side effects*: Sedation, nausea, vomiting, injection site pain, hiccups, hypotension, agitation, dystonia, amnesia, diplopia, disinhibition, ataxia, weakness, dysarthria, euphoria, rash, respiratory depression, apnea, cardiac arrest, bradycardia, tachycardia, syncope, paradoxical CNS stimulation, bronchospasm, and anaphylaxis/anaphylactoid reaction [5, 7, 8, 10, 11].

Opioids

1. *Class* – Narcotic.
2. *Mechanism of action* – Stereospecific opioid receptor agonists that act in both the CNS and peripheral tissues activating pain-modulating systems. Presynaptic inhibition of AcH, dopamine, norepinephrine, and substance P. Increases potassium conductance leading to hyperpolarization of cellular membranes [5, 7, 8].
3. *Opioids and neuroanesthesia* – Cerebral vasoconstrictors decreasing CBF and ICP. However, must be used with caution with known intracranial disease because depression of ventilation leads to hypercarbia which can result in increased ICP. Do not produce seizure activity on EEG [5, 7, 8].
4. *Dosing of specific opioids* [10, 11]

    (a) Morphine – Sedation/analgesia – 2–10 mg I.V. (Peds: 0.02–0.1 mg/kg I.V.). Analgesic dosing: 2–20 mg q2–q4 h I.V., IM, SC. Infusion: 0.8–10 mg/h (Peds: sickle cell/cancer pain 0.025–2 mg/kg/h; postop: 0.01–0.04 mg/kg/h).
    (b) Fentanyl – Intubation: 1.5–3 mcg/kg (100–200 mcg). Postop: 0.5–1.5 kg (35–105 mcg). Sedation/analgesia: 0.5 mcg/kg (load); 0.01–0.04 mcg/kg/min (maint). GA (sole agent) Induction: 50–150 mcg/kg. Maint: 0.1–5 mcg/kg/h. GA adjunct: Loading dose: 2–50 mcg/kg; Maint: 0.03–0.1 kg/min.
    (c) Remifentanil – Induction 1–3 mcg/kg over 1 min (70–270 mcg). GA adjunct: Loading dose 0.5–2 mcg/kg (35–140 mcg); bolus 0.5–1 mcg/kg; Maint 0.05–2 mcg/kg/min.
    (d) Sufentanil – GA (minor proc) Ind: 1–2 mcg/kg (70–140), bolus: 10–25 mcg. GA (mod proc): Ind: 2–8 mcg/kg (70–560), bolus: 10–50 mcg; Maint: 0.3–1.5 mcg/kg/h. GA (major proc): 8–30 mcg/kg (560–2,100); bolus 10–50 mcg: Maint 0.5–2.5 mcg/kg/h.
    (e) Alfentanil – Intubation: 20–50 mcg/kg (1,400–3,500). Induction 130–245 mcg/kg (9.1–17.1 mg). Infusion Load 50–75 mcg/kg. Maint 0.5–3 mcg/kg/min.
    (f) Meperidine – Sedation/analgesia: 50–150 mg I.V./IM q3–q4 (Peds 0.5–2 mg/kg I.V./IM), Infusion: 0.3–1.5 mg/kg/h. Post-op shivering 12.5–25 mg I.V.

5. *Drug interactions* – CNS depressants may have a synergistic cardiovascular, respiratory, and sedative effects when combined. Combination of opioids (meperidine) with MAOI can result in respiratory arrest, HTN or hypotension, and hyperpyrexia [10, 11].
6. *Side effects* – Sedation, dizziness, nausea, vomiting, constipation, physical dependence, tolerance, respiratory depression, delayed gastric emptying, hyperalgesia, immunologic and hormonal dysfunction, muscle rigidity, and myoclonus [5, 7, 8, 10, 11].

Muscle Relaxants

1. *Class* – Nondepolarizing and depolarizing neuromuscular blocking drugs
2. *Mechanism of action*

    (a) Nondepolarizing NMBD – Reversibly binds to the postsynaptic nicotinic cholinergic receptor at the neuromuscular junction preventing the binding of acetylcholine which inhibits conduction of nerve impulses causing skeletal muscle paralysis. Can be overcome by increasing Ach in the synaptic cleft [5, 7, 8].

    (b) Depolarizing NMBD – Irreversibly binds to the alpha subunit of the nicotinic cholinergic receptor by mimicking Ach causing prolonged depolarization resulting in muscle paralysis [5, 7, 8].

3. *NMBD and neuroanesthesia* – Do not usually increase ICP unless they induce the release of histamine (atracurium) or cause hypotension. Histamine causes cerebral vasodilation resulting in increased ICP. Succinylcholine may increase ICP during induction through stimulation of muscle spindles, which in turn either directly or indirectly result in increased $CMRO_2$. Because CBF is coupled to $CMRO_2$, CBF also increases leading to increased ICP [5, 7, 8].

4. *Dosing of specific drugs* [10, 11]

    (a) Pancuronium – Intubating dose 0.1 mg/kg. Maintenance dose 0.02 mg/kg
    (b) Rocuronium – Intubating 0.6–1.2 mg/kg (1.2 mg/kg RSI). Main 0.1 mg/kg
    (c) Vecuronium – Intubating 0.1 mg/kg (0.3–0.4 mg/kg RSI). Main 0.02 mg/kg
    (d) Atracurium – Intubating 0.5 mg/kg. Main 0.1 mg/kg
    (e) Cisatracurium – Intubating 0.1 mg/kg (o.4 mg/kg RSI). Main 0.02 mg/kg
    (f) Succinylcholine – Intubating 0.5–1.5 mg/kg

5. *Drug interactions* [5, 7, 8, 10, 11]

    (a) Succinylcholine – Cholinesterase inhibitors prolong phase I block, small doses of nondepolarizing relaxants antagonize phase I block, potentiated by several antibiotics (i.e., streptomycin, aminoglycosides, neomycin, tetracycline, clindamycin), calcium channel blockers (CCB), quinidine, inhalational agents, high doses of local anesthetics, lithium carbonate, magnesium (Mg), and anticonvulsants (phenytoin, carbamazepine)

    (b) Nondepolarizing agents – Effects potentiated by several antibiotics (see above), quinidine, CCB, dantrolene, volatile anesthetics, ketamine, local anesthetics, and Mg

6. *Side effects* – all cause allergic reactions, succinylcholine the most common [5, 7, 8, 10, 11]

    (a) Pancuronium – Tachycardia, increased BP, increased cardiac output
    (b) Atracurium – Dose-dependent release of histamine resulting in hypotension
    (c) Rocuronium/vecuronium/cisatracurium – Do not release histamine or have cardiovascular side effects
    (d) Succinylcholine – Increased ICP (no significant increase in ICP if administered with a standard intubating dose of an induction agent, i.e., propofol,

thiopental), sinus bradycardia, junctional rhythm, cardiac arrest, hyperkalemia, myalgias, trismus, increased intraocular pressure, increased ICP, and increased intragastric pressure

Inhalational Agents

1. *Class* – General anesthetic and volatile anesthetic.
2. *Mechanism of action* – Not fully understood but may alter the activity of neuronal ion channels particularly the fast synaptic neurotransmitter receptors (nicotinic acetylcholine, GABA, and glutamate receptors) [5, 7, 8].
3. *Volatile anesthetics and neuroanesthesia* – In general, all inhalational agents administered higher than 0.5 MAC cause uncoupling between CBF and $CMRO_2$ with a dose-dependent decrease in $CMRO_2$ and increased CBF via vasodilatation [1, 5, 7, 8]. However, it should be noted that at carefully controlled $PaCO_2$ with modest hyperventilation, it has been shown that there is no significant increase in ICP up to1.5 MAC as measured in human studies in which cerebral spinal fluid pressures were transduced (Dr. Milde, Mayo Clinic 0.5 MAC iso and des; Dr. Ebrahim, Cleveland Clinic 0.8 MAC iso and des; Dr. Kaye Tulane Medical Center 1 MAC) [2]. At 0.5 MAC or less, the decrease in $CMRO_2$ counteracts vasodilatation and CBF does not change significantly. May impair autoregulation in a dose-dependent manner; however, in doses less than 1 MAC, it is not clinically significant [5, 7–9]. Do not abolish cerebral vascular responsiveness to changes in $PaCO_2$. The largest increase in CBF occurs with halothane, with less of an effect seen with isoflurane, desflurane, and sevoflurane. Nitrous oxide also increases CBF by causing cerebral vasodilation but, unlike the volatile anesthetics, increases $CMRO_2$ modestly [5, 7, 8]. As a result of increased CBF, ICP increases with all the VA at doses higher than 1 MAC. Of note, it has been shown by Hoffman data that inhalational agents actually have potential benefits in brain tissue oxygenation. Hoffman double brain tissue oxygen levels were determined at inhalational agent doses of 1 MAC or greater utilizing a pH probe placed directly in the human cerebral gyrus (Miura Y) [6].
4. *Dosing of specific VA* [5, 7, 8]

    Minimum alveolar concentration (MAC), the concentration that abolishes movement in response to a noxious stimulus (surgical incision) in 50 % of patients.

    (a) Sevoflurane: MAC 2.1 (neonates have the greatest MAC unlike the other VAs in which 3-month-old infants have the greatest MAC).
    (b) Desflurane: MAC 6.0.
    (c) Isoflurane: MAC 1.2.
    (d) Nitrous Oxide: MAC 0.47.

5. *Drug interactions* [5, 7, 8]

    (a) Isoflurane, desflurane, sevoflurane – Potentiates NMBDs.
    (b) Nitrous oxide – Addition decreases the requirements of other agents. Attenuates the respiratory and cardiovascular effects of VA. Potentiates NMBD (less than other VA).

6. *Side effects* – Nausea, vomiting, agitation, cough, hypotension, laryngospasm, breath holding, bradycardia, tachycardia, somnolence, shivering, sialorrhea, dizziness, hypertension, apnea, arrhythmias, seizures, hepatotoxicity, anaphylactoid reaction, bronchospasm, cardiac arrest, malignant hyperthermia, hyperkalemia, and teratogenic effects (nitrous oxide) [5, 7, 8].

Neuromonitoring

1. Electroencephalogram (EEG) – Is the summation of excitatory and inhibitory postsynaptic electric potentials in the cortical gray matter. Measurements include frequency, amplitude, and duration. Most commonly used in the OR to detect cerebral ischemia or in the ICU for prognostic purposes. In general, EEG waveforms become larger in amplitude and slower in frequency with the use of inhalational or I.V. anesthetics. Exception is nitrous oxide which causes an increase in frequency and a decrease in amplitude. Neuromuscular blockers have no effects [4, 5, 7, 8].

2. Evoked potentials – Measured as sensory, motor, visual, or brainstem auditory evoked potentials. Are electrical stimulus delivered over the course of a nerve and are used to detect injury to the CNS which prevents irreversible injury intraoperatively. Measured in terms of latency, which is the time between the stimulus and the peak amplitude of the generated waveform [3].

   (a) SSEP – Detects injury to the somatosensory pathways, which are supplied by the posterior spinal arteries. Electrical stimuli are applied over the posterior tibial or median nerve with the recording of potentials over the nerve, the spine, and contralateral cortical sensory area over the scalp [3].

   (b) MEP – Detects injury to the motor pathways, which are supplied by the anterior spinal artery. Generated by electrical stimulation of the motor cortex over the scalp with recordings across specific motor nerves (spinal and peripheral) and the innervated muscles themselves [3].

   (c) Drug effects on evoked potentials [5, 7, 8]

      (i) Volatile anesthetics (including nitrous oxide) – order of sensitivity VEP>MEP>SSEP>BAEP. In general, VA increase latency times and decrease amplitude of SSEPs. MEPs are extremely sensitive to VA and at >0.5 MAC will be abolished. Subcortical structures (spinal cord and brainstem) are more resistant to changes in evoked potentials with VA as compared to cortical tissue.

      (ii) IV anesthetics – Generally cause a dose-dependent decrease in EP amplitude and increase in latency time. Exceptions are ketamine and etomidate which increase both latency and amplitude. Opioids produce minimal effect on MEPs or SSEP, even in high doses. If MEPs are being measured, propofol is usually used with a narcotic as total intravenous anesthesia. Neuromuscular blockers have no effect on SSEPs and completely abolish MEPs.

What to Avoid During Intracranial Procedures [5, 7, 8]

1. Movement and coughing – Can lead to bleeding, brain bulging (making surgical exposure difficult), and increased ICP.
2. Direct acting vasodilators (i.e., nitroprusside, nitroglycerin, calcium channel blockers, hydralazine) – Increases CBF and ICP.
3. Ketamine – Increases ICP.
4. Succinylcholine – Increases ICP.

Summary

Many agents, including intravenous and inhalational anesthetics, can significantly influence both cerebral blood flow and intracranial pressure. Understanding this interaction is a vital component of neuroanesthesiology because the use of the wrong anesthetic can be detrimental to patients with central nervous system pathology.

Chemical Structures

Chemical Structure
43.1 Etomidate

Chemical Structure
43.2 Atracurium besylate

Chemical Structure
43.3 Isoflurane

References

1. Bungaard H. Acta Anesth Scanden. 1998;42(6):621–7.
2. Kaye AD, Kucera IJ, Heavner J, Gelb A, Anwar M, Duban M, Ariff S, Craen R, Chang C, Trillo R, Hoffman M. The effects of desflurane vs. isoflurane in patients with intracranial masses. Anesth Analg. 2004;98:1127–32.
3. Kumar A, et al. Evoked potential monitoring in anesthesia and analgesia. Anaesthesia. 2000;55:225–41.
4. Mahla M. The electroencephalogram in the operating room. Sem Anesth. 1997;16:3–13.
5. Miller RD. Miller's anesthesia, 6th ed. 2005, Elsevier, Churchill Livingstone, Philadelphia.
6. Miura Y. Outcome from near-complete but not complete cerebral ischemia as measured by % dead neurons depends on anesthetic agent administered during ischemia in rat model 1.4 % isoflurane, ketamine, fentanyl/nitrous oxide. Anesthesiology. 1998;89:391–400.
7. Morgan Jr GE, Mikhail MS, Murray MJ. Clinical anesthesiology, 4th ed. www.epocrates.com.
8. Stoelting RK, Miller RD. Basics of anesthesia, 5th ed. 2006, Churchill Livingstone, Philadelphia.
9. Takahashi, et al. Sevoflurane 05-1.5 MAC in hyperventilated dogs. BJA. 1993;71(4):551–5.
10. www.epocrates.com.
11. Lexicomp via uptodate.com.

Chapter 44
Liver Disease and Liver Transplantation

Gundappa Neelakanta and Victor Xia

Contents

G. Neelakanta, MD (✉) • V. Xia, MD
Department of Anesthesiology, Ronald Reagan UCLA Medical Center, David Geffen School of Medicine at UCLA, 757 Westwood Plaza, Suite 3325, Los Angeles, CA 90095-7403, USA
e-mail: gneelakanta@mednet.ucla.edu; vxia@mednet.ucla.edu

A.D. Kaye et al. (eds.), *Essentials of Pharmacology for Anesthesia, Pain Medicine, and Critical Care*, DOI 10.1007/978-1-4614-8948-1_44, © Springer Science+Business Media New York 2015

Clinical Pearls

Perioperative risks of surgery in patients with chronic liver disease are increased.

There is no change in drug pharmacokinetics in asymptomatic, chronic hepatitis patients with normal liver function. No drug dose adjustments are necessary. Their perioperative risks after surgery are not increased.

In general, type I drug metabolic functions are affected much earlier in the disease and type II metabolic functions are affected late in the disease.

Factors such a low serum albumin, portosystemic shunts, and decreases in liver blood flow also affect drug pharmacokinetics other than the intrinsic hepatic metabolic function.

Patients with liver disease show increased sensitivity to CNS-acting drugs. Caution is advised with drug doses of anxiolytic, sedative, or hypnotic drugs.

Dose adjustments may be required with non-depolarizing neuromuscular blocking drugs. Cisatracurium is the drug of choice in patients with liver disease.

Isoflurane is considered inhalational drug of choice, but sevoflurane and desflurane are also safe.

No single test of liver function accurately predicts pharmacokinetic behavior of any specific drug.

Careful titration of drugs to their clinical effects and continued vigilance and monitoring for their side effects are critical for safe management of patients with liver disease.

Introduction

Chronic liver disease (CLD) affects more than five million people in the United States and is a significant cause of morbidity and mortality in the world. According to the Centers for Disease Control and Prevention, it was the 12th leading cause of death in the United States in 2007, although according to one study it is estimated to be 8th leading cause of death in the United States [1, 2]. The predominant cause of CLD in the United States is hepatitis C, followed by alcohol and nonalcoholic fatty liver disease. Together, they account for nearly 90 % of all patients. Hepatitis B, cholestatic liver disease, autoimmune disease, and other miscellaneous causes account for a small percentage of all patients with CLD. The disease runs a long and chronic course for many years, but once clinical signs of ascites, bleeding, hepatic encephalopathy (HE), hepatorenal syndrome (HRS), or other complications occur, the mortality rises rapidly. The treatment options for patients with CLD are limited although antiviral therapy with peginterferons and protease inhibitor drugs has remarkably improved survival in patients with hepatitis C. In patients with end-stage liver disease, liver transplantation offers nearly 87 % 1-year and 75 % 5-year survival rates [3]. This option is not available to many patients on the waiting list due to a limited number of donors available in the United States. Approximately 5,600 liver transplants were performed in the United States in 2011, but there were over 15,500 patients on the waiting list.

Surgery in patients with acute liver disease except for liver transplantation is generally avoided and contraindicated due to high mortality. Perioperative risks following surgery in patients with asymptomatic chronic hepatitis patients with normal liver function are not increased [4]. However, the perioperative risk in patients with established cirrhosis is increased. These patients may present for many elective or emergency surgical procedures. These include gastrointestinal endoscopy, transjugular intrahepatic portosystemic shunt (TIPS) procedures, cholecystectomy, liver resection, hernia surgery, orthopedic procedures or sometimes cardiac surgery. Their perioperative risks are higher due to complications of infection, bleeding, encephalopathy, and liver and renal failure [5]. Perioperative mortality independently correlates with severity of liver disease especially in the presence of portal hypertension, type of surgery, and emergency vs. elective surgical procedure. Despite its limitations due to some subjective scoring, Child-Turcotte-Pugh (CTP) score is still used for assessment of severity of liver function. Perioperative mortality ranges from about 10 % in Childs class A to 80 % in Childs class C patients. Recent studies also show correlation of higher MELD (Model for End-Stage Liver Disease) scores with poor outcome and mortality after non-transplant surgery [6]. There is some indication that recent advances in anesthesia and perioperative care may have decreased these risks, but they still remain high.

Liver is the primary organ responsible for elimination of most drugs or toxins in the body by their biotransformation and excretion. Therefore, the fate or pharmacokinetics of administered drugs is expected to be affected in patients with liver disease and cirrhosis. The liver function and drug metabolism are not affected in most patients with early hepatitis, metabolic disease, or hepatic tumors unless associated with cirrhosis.

This article reviews many of the important considerations when selecting anesthetic drugs in patients with CLD presenting for both transplant and non-liver transplant surgery. Drug pharmacokinetic and pharmacodynamic changes specific to CLD are discussed. For a detailed review of specific drugs, the reader should consult other chapters in this book or other references.

Overview of Drug Metabolism in Chronic Liver Disease

The liver is the main site of drug metabolism. Drugs undergo biotransformation by phase I enzymatic reaction followed by phase II conjugation reactions that make them more polar or water soluble, so they may be excreted by the bile or the kidneys. In general, phase I reactions involve oxidation, reduction, hydrolysis, or N-dealkylation of many isozymes of cytochrome P-450 (CYP) system in the hepatocytes. Phase II reactions involve conjugation reactions with sulfates, acetate, glycine, methyl, gluta- thione, and glucuronic acid that make them more polar, biologically inactive, and less toxic. In general, phase I CYP enzymatic reactions are more sensitive to changes in early cirrhosis than phase II reactions. Sequential progressive model of hepatic dys- function proposes that certain cytochrome enzyme functions are affected earlier in cirrhosis followed by other cytochrome enzyme functions later in the disease [7].

Orally administered drugs are absorbed by the gastrointestinal tract and are pre- sented to the liver through the portal vein. Similarly, systemically administered drugs enter the liver by the hepatic blood flow. Hepatic clearance of a drug is the volume of blood that is completely cleared of the drug per unit time through its transit in the liver. Hepatic clearance depends on intrinsic clearance of unbound drug, fraction of unbound drug, and hepatic blood flow. Drugs that are completely cleared of blood through their transit in the liver in a unit time and their clearance approaches that of total hepatic blood flow have an extraction ration of 1.0. Drugs with high hepatic extraction have low bioavailability and their metabolism and bio- availability are dependent on liver blood flow. They are also called blood flow-lim- ited drugs. Examples of such drugs are lidocaine, diphenhydramine, metoprolol, and propofol. Metabolism of these drugs is relatively insensitive to drug binding or enzyme activity. Drugs with low hepatic extraction (extraction ratio <0.3) such as diazepam are enzyme limited and not affected by hepatic blood flow, but changes in drug binding are important in intrinsic clearance of drug. Most drugs have an inter- mediate hepatic extraction ratio between 0.3 and 0.7. Their metabolism will be sig- nificantly affected by all of the three factors of blood flow, drug binding, and intrinsic clearance.

Factors other than direct result of impaired drug metabolism or changes in liver blood flow also play an important role in drug effects seen in CLD. They are dis- cussed in greater detail below.

Serum Albumin

Drugs are transported in blood across various tissues in the body by binding to plasma albumin and some $alpha_2$ glycoprotein. The degree of binding to the albu- min varies and a small proportion of drug carried in the blood is unbound to albu- min. It is the free or the unbound fraction of the drug that determines transfer across the membranes in to the cells or the effector cells. In CLD, the serum albumin level is decreased due to many factors such as decreased absorption, decreased synthesis by the liver, and/or increased loss through the gut. In patients with low serum albumin, a higher fraction of free or unbound drug is carried in blood, which results in a higher concentration of drug at the effect sites or receptors and greater drug effects.

Ascites

Ascites is a major complication of CLD and its onset portends a poor prognosis with a 56 % survival at 3 years. Pathophysiology of ascites is complex, but the central dysfunction is salt and water retention due to splanchnic arteriolar vasodilatation secondary to portal hypertension. Decrease in serum albumin also contributes to formation of ascites. Current treatment regimens involve regular large volume paracentesis with albumin infusion. It is important to understand that the ascitic fluid is in active circulation. The volume of distribution at steady state (Vd_{ss}) of a drug is typically increased. A larger initial dose of drug may be required to achieve an effective plasma concentration, leading to a prolonged duration of action.

Hepatorenal Syndrome

HRS is a functional renal failure due to intense renal vasoconstriction in the presence of portal hypertension in liver disease. Type I HRS is characterized by acute decrease in renal function and has poor prognosis, whereas type II HRS is characterized by low glomerular filtration rate (GFR) and increase in serum creatinine in a chronic but stable disease. Serum creatinine level as an estimation of GFR and renal function in patients with CLD is inaccurate due to decreased muscle mass and impaired conversion of creatine to creatinine. Even the measured creatinine clearance may also be inaccurate due to increased secretion of creatinine in the renal tubules. Presence of HRS complicates pharmacokinetics of drugs that are also significantly excreted by the kidneys.

Portal Vein Thrombosis

Portal vein thrombosis or extrahepatic portal vein obstruction (EHPVO) is most commonly associated with cirrhosis. Other causes of EHPVO due to hepatic tumors or nonmalignant non-cirrhotic conditions are rare. These patients may have an underlying prothrombotic state. Blood supply to the liver is maintained by various undescribed periportal or peribiliary collateral venous networks. They may also develop spontaneous portocaval shunts. Hepatic oxygenation is usually not compromised due to high oxygen supply, low oxygen extraction, and favorable oxygen supply/demand ratio. Liver function is likely to be compromised, but studies of pharmacokinetic data specific to EHPVO are sparse.

Portosystemic Shunts

CLD leads to development of portal hypertension that results in portosystemic shunts predominantly in the esophagus and rectum but may also be developed in intrahepatic and retroperitoneal regions. Surgical portosystemic shunts or creation of TIPS results in similar physiological changes. Bioavailability of drugs such as midazolam, carvedilol, and metoprolol that have high first-pass metabolism or high extraction ratio is increased. Consequently, their initial and maintenance drug dose will need to be decreased.

Hepatic Encephalopathy (HE)

HE is a primary complication of liver disease and heralds poor prognosis. It is manifested by often reversible, neuropsychiatric, personality, or mental status changes in its milder form to development of coma in later stage. The pathophysiology of HE is complex. Ammonia, inflammatory cytokines, manganese, and benzodiazepine-like substances are all implicated in its development. Patients with HE are more sensitive to sedative and hypnotic drugs that are independent of pharmacokinetic changes. Hepatic coma may be precipitated if not careful with drug doses.

Pharmacodynamic Changes

Patients with CLD may also have an altered response to drugs that are independent of pharmacokinetic changes, i.e., pharmacodynamic effects. They show increased sensitivity to CNS-acting drugs such as anxiolytic, sedative, or hypnotic drugs. Increase in sedation to benzodiazepines [8], enhanced analgesia to oxycodone in pretransplant patients [9], and worsening or precipitation of HE after morphine have been clearly demonstrated [10]. They are at higher risk of CNS symptoms of confusion or other neuropsychiatric symptoms from cimetidine or ranitidine due to increased transfer of drug across the blood-brain barrier. Similarly, they have decreased sensitivity to loop diuretics torsemide, bumetanide, and furosemide. Chronotropic response to infusion of isoproterenol is attenuated in patients with CLD due to the downregulation of beta receptors [11]. They are thus less sensitive to beta blockers and show a reduced vascular sensitivity to vasoconstrictors drugs.

Intravenous Anesthetic Agents

Thiopental

The use of thiopental, a barbiturate, as an intravenous anesthetic induction agent in the United States is now replaced by propofol. Its current use is mostly limited to certain neurosurgical cases. Thiopental is extensively metabolized by liver and has a low extraction ratio of <0.2. A pharmacokinetic study in patients with cirrhosis during surgery after a single dose of thiopental showed an increase in unbound fraction, increase in the volume of distribution at steady state (Vd_{ss}), substantial decrease in hepatic clearance (28.3 vs. 18.2 ml/min/kg), and an increase in elimination half-life (t ½) (714 vs. 529 min) compared to normal patients [12]. This study suggests enhanced clinical effects from an increase in unbound fraction of thiopental from a single dose, but significant prolongation of duration of action is unlikely. Dosing adjustments may be necessary during infusions of thiopental in ICU patients. Thiopental induces hepatic CYP enzymes suggesting an increase in dose requirement for induction of anesthesia in patients with alcoholic dependence without liver dysfunction. However, studies in this area are conflicting.

Propofol

Propofol (2,6 diisopropylphenol) is a nonbarbiturate intravenous anesthetic agent that is highly bound to plasma proteins (97–98 %), widely distributed in the tissues, and metabolized mainly by the liver. Its hepatic extraction ratio exceeds 1.0 indicating extrahepatic metabolism, but clinical significance of the extrahepatic metabolism is unknown. Its clearance is limited by total hepatic blood flow and hepatocellular disease is not expected to significantly affect its rate of elimination. Studies in patients with moderate cirrhosis show no significant change in Vd_{ss} or plasma clearance or t ½ of propofol after a single dose of propofol [13]. After an infusion for up to 3.5 h, the Vd_{ss} was significantly increased, but the clearance and elimination did not change significantly [14]. These studies suggest that no change in propofol drug dosing is necessary even after prolonged infusion. Recent studies suggest increasing sensitivity to propofol in severe liver disease. A study in rat with graded cirrhosis model showed increased sensitivity to propofol according to severity of liver disease [15]. A clinical study also showed reduced requirement for propofol in patients with increasing severity of liver dysfunction when monitored by BIS [16]. In this study, plasma levels of propofol at which patients opened their eyes in normal and cirrhotic patients were similar suggesting decrease in drug requirement was unlikely to be due to pharmacodynamic changes of liver disease. Liver disease does not appear to be a risk factor in the development of rare propofol-related infusion syndrome.

Etomidate

Etomidate is a nonbarbiturate, imidazole group, intravenous anesthetic induction agent. In normal patients, it has a large Vd_{ss} (3.7 L/kg) and is rapidly metabolized in the liver with a hepatic extraction ratio of 0.5. In patients with cirrhosis, limited data suggests that Vd_{ss} is doubled and consequently its t ½ is also doubled [17]. Infusions of etomidate up to an hour in patients with cirrhosis did not significantly prolong time to awakening although there was considerable variation between patients.

Etomidate is commonly used for induction of anesthesia in patients with CLD due to its stable hemodynamic properties. A single induction dose of etomidate, however, can cause adrenal suppression for up to 8 h unresponsive to ACTH. The clinical significance of this is unknown. Some suggest that cortisol should be replenished even after single dose of etomidate. But its use for induction of anesthesia during OLT appears to be safe since large doses of steroids are given for immunosuppression in these patients. Use of etomidate in ICU for sedation is contraindicated due to studies suggesting increase in mortality with its use.

Ketamine

Ketamine is a synthetic phenylpiperidine (phencyclidine)-derived anesthetic drug developed in the 1960s. It causes intense analgesia and anesthesia with mostly preserved upper airway reflexes and stable cardiovascular hemodynamics. The anesthetic effect is termed dissociative anesthesia as patients appear dissociated from the environment and yet intensely analgesic. The central effects are mediated via a noncompetitive inhibition of NMDA receptors. In healthy patients, following an IV injection, its onset time is rapid within 2 min and effects lasting for 1–2 h. The Vd_{ss} is 4.6 L/kg with a high plasma clearance of 1.32 L/min and t ½ of 186 min [18]. It is metabolized in the liver, but there is paucity of data regarding its pharmacokinetics in patients with CLD. Continuous infusion of ketamine for the treatment of noncancer complex pain syndrome has been reported to cause hepatotoxicity [19]. However, it is not contraindicated for use during anesthesia in patients with liver disease.

Use of ketamine in anesthesia had waned due to significant side effects of vivid dreams, hallucinations or other psychogenic effects, and nausea or vomiting. But, in recent years, significant resurgence in its use has occurred in view of its beneficial effects in acute and chronic pain.

Midazolam

Midazolam is a short-acting intravenous benzodiazepine used for its hypnotic, anxiolytic, and amnestic effects. As dispensed at a pH of 3.0 at room temperature, it has an open ring structure that makes it water soluble. Following administration, the ring closes at plasma pH increasing its lipid solubility and making it clinically active. It has a fast onset of action and a short half-life of 1.5–3 h. It is highly (96 %) protein bound, is metabolized in the liver via the CYP system, and has hepatic extraction ratio of 0.3–0.5.

Clinical pharmacokinetic studies suggest clearance and elimination of midazolam is dependent on the degree of liver dysfunction. In patients with moderate liver dysfunction, its Vd_{ss} was unchanged, plasma clearance was decreased by about 30 %, and t ½ was prolonged by 25 %, whereas in patients with severe liver disease, its clearance was decreased by half (0.32 vs. 0.62 l/kg/h) and t ½ doubled (3.9 vs. 1.6 h) [8, 20]. Further, increase in central nervous system sensitivity to benzodiazepines has also been demonstrated. Therefore, midazolam needs to be carefully titrated to effect, dose reduced by half, and patients monitored for prolonged drug effects.

Narcotics

Fentanyl

Fentanyl is a semisynthetic narcotic analgesic most familiar to the anesthesiologists. It is 80–100 times more potent than morphine and is highly protein bound (85 %). It is metabolized in the liver by CYP enzymes and has high hepatic extraction. In healthy patients, following an IV dose, it has a rapid onset of action, a very large Vd_{ss} (about 4 L/kg), and t ½ longer than 240 min. Its short duration of action is due to its rapid redistribution. Following repeated doses or infusion of fentanyl, its duration of action is determined by its elimination resulting in prolonged duration of action. Studies in patients with cirrhosis show that the pharmacokinetics of fentanyl is largely unaffected after a single dose. After repeated or continuous or prolonged infusion, accumulation of fentanyl is likely resulting in prolonged duration of action.

Alfentanil

Alfentanil is a short-acting semisynthetic narcotic analgesic ten times more potent than fentanyl. It has a very rapid onset of action, low Vd_{ss} (30 L), and very short elimination. It is highly protein bound and almost exclusively metabolized in the liver by oxidative dealkylation. After a bolus dose of 50 mcg/kg in patients with cirrhosis, the free fraction of drug was higher, Vd_{ss} unchanged, plasma clearance lower (1.6 vs. 3.1 ml/kg/min), and t ½ prolonged (219 vs. 90 min) compared to controls [21]. Thus, alfentanil will exert a prolonged duration of effect in patients with cirrhosis.

Remifentanil

Remifentanil, another semisynthetic narcotic analgesic, is 20 times more potent than alfentanil. Its Vd_{ss} is similar to alfentanil (about 30 L) but very small compared to fentanyl (340 L). Due to its lower pKa of 7.26, remifentanil is rapidly distributed to the tissues. It is metabolized rapidly in the plasma by plasma and tissue cholinesterase but is not affected by pseudocholinesterase deficiency. Its context-sensitive half-time, i.e., time for 50 % decrease in plasma level after a steady-state plasma level following a continuous infusion, is very short. It is about 3.2 min after a 3-h infusion compared to 47 min with alfentanil and 180 min following fentanyl. Its pharmacokinetics is unchanged in patients with liver disease or renal insufficiency [22]. However, patients with liver disease may be more sensitive to ventilatory depressant effect of remifentanil.

Morphine

Morphine is a naturally occurring opioid that has been used as an analgesic for many centuries. Its Vd_{ss} is 3–4 L/kg, about 35 % protein bound, and has a half-life of 1.5–3 h. It is primarily metabolized in the liver by conjugation to morphine 3-glucuronide and morphine 6-glucuronide that is excreted by the kidneys. Extrahepatic metabolism has been described, but its significance is unknown. Its hepatic extraction ratio is 0.7 and plasma concentration is significantly affected by liver blood flow. In patients with cirrhosis, its clearance is reduced by two to threefold, t ½ is approximately doubled to 3–4 h, and central nervous system effects are enhanced [23]. In the presence of HRS, the metabolic conjugates of morphine may accumulate causing toxic CNS side effects. Morphine should be used with caution in patients with cirrhosis and the dosing interval should be increased by 1.5–2 times.

Meperidine

Meperidine is a synthetic opioid and about ten times less potent than morphine. It is metabolized in the liver with formation also of an active metabolite normeperidine. Normeperidine is excreted by the kidneys, but accumulation causes neuroexcitatory effects. In patients with cirrhosis, meperidine bioavailability is increased, clearance is reduced by half, and t ½ is doubled. Formation of normeperidine is also reduced, but its elimination is prolonged. Repeated doses of meperidine should be avoided in patients with cirrhosis.

Neuromuscular Blocking Drugs

Succinylcholine

Succinylcholine is a depolarizing neuromuscular blocking agent (NMB) with a fast onset of action used during rapid sequence intubation. Its onset time to maximum blockade is about 60 s and duration of action about 10 min. It is rapidly metabolized in the plasma by an enzymatic degradation using nonspecific plasma cholinesterase called butyrylcholinesterase (BchE) which is also called pseudocholinesterase or plasma cholinesterase [24]. Almost 90 % of the administered succinylcholine is metabolized in the plasma within the first minute of administration. Only a small fraction of administered drug reaches the site of action.

BchE is synthesized in the liver and has a half-life of about 2 weeks. Due to its long half-life, plasma level of BchE may be normal in patients with acute liver disease but decreased in CLD. The duration of apnea is unlikely to be longer than 20–30 min in patients with CLD as even a 30 % decrease in the level of BchE causes only a modest decrease in the duration of action of succinylcholine.

Pancuronium

Pancuronium is a biquaternary aminosteroid NMB that has a slower onset but long duration of action (1.5–2 h after a dose of 0.15 mg/kg) that is infrequently used during anesthesia in the United States today. It is metabolized by deacetylation that is primarily eliminated by the liver. In patients with cirrhosis, its onset of action is delayed, clearance is decreased by 22 %, and t ½ life is prolonged (208 vs. 114 min) due to 50 % increase in Vd_{ss} [25]. Therefore, a larger initial dose of pancuronium is required resulting in prolonged duration of action.

Vecuronium

Vecuronium is a monoquaternary aminosteroid NMB with an intermediate duration of action. It is about 30 % protein bound, metabolized by deacetylation to partly active metabolites, that is excreted in the bile by the liver. In patients with cirrhosis, at a single dose of 0.1 mg/kg, its pharmacokinetic parameters are largely unaffected with a slightly slower onset of action (2.8 vs. 1.9 min to loss of 100 % twitch height) and time to recovery of twitch heights unaffected [26]. At a dose of 0.2 mg/kg, compared to patients without liver disease, Vd_{ss} was unchanged, clearance was decreased (4.26 vs. 2.73 ml/min/kg), t ½ was prolonged (58 vs. 48 min), and time to recovery of twitch heights was prolonged (130 vs. 62 min) [27]. Similar results have also been shown in patients with liver disease secondary to cholestasis [28]. Therefore, it is likely that its duration of action is prolonged following a higher initial dose or repeated doses.

Rocuronium

Rocuronium is a non-depolarizing NMB with a rapid onset and an intermediate duration of action. Unlike vecuronium, 65–70 % of drug is taken up by the liver and excreted in the bile. Studies of pharmacokinetic data in patients with liver disease are conflicting. A study in patients with moderate cirrhosis showed Vd_{ss} to be unchanged, plasma clearance decreased, and t ½ prolonged. Onset of NMB was not delayed, but recovery of train of four twitches was prolonged [29]. Another study in patients with Childs C disease with ascites showed the Vd_{ss} was increased, t ½ was prolonged, but the clearance was unchanged. Time to initial twitch recovery was not prolonged, but repeated doses resulted in prolonged duration of action [30]. Khalil et al. studied Childs class B patients with mild ascites or encephalopathy and found that Vd_{ss} was increased and t ½ was prolonged. Recovery of twitch heights to 75 and 90 % of control heights was prolonged [31]. It seems clear that in patients with CLD, onset of NMB is slightly delayed due to increase in the volume of distribution. Initial recovery of NMB may not be affected since initial twitch height recovery is due to redistribution of rocuronium. But, the duration of action especially after repeated administration is longer due to increase in t ½ of rocuronium.

Cisatracurium

Cisatracurium is an isomer of atracurium and is three to four times potent than atracurium. It is metabolized in the plasma by a non-liver-dependent, plasma pH, and temperature-dependent spontaneous degradation reaction called Hofmann elimination. Studies in patients undergoing OLT show that its Vd_{ss} is slightly increased, clearance is slightly prolonged, but t ½ is similar. Time to onset of neuromuscular block was 2.4 min vs. 3.3 min probably related hyperdynamic circulation in transplant patients, but time to recovery of twitch to 25 % and twitch recovery index was same. Plasma clearance of laudanosine, a metabolite with neurotoxic side effects, appears to be unchanged in patients with liver disease [32].

Neuromuscular Reversal Drugs

Neostigmine

Neostigmine is a cholinesterase inhibitor used for reversal of neuromuscular blockade. It is water soluble and an ionized compound and therefore excreted by kidneys. Its duration of action is not affected by liver disease [33].

Inhalational Anesthetic Agents

Inhalational anesthetic agents historically have been associated with liver toxicity. Older anesthetic agents chloroform, trichloroethylene, divinyl ether, tribromoethanol, and methoxyflurane all caused direct hepatotoxicity that resulted in centrilobular liver necrosis. The introduction of halothane in 1956 marked a milestone in inhalational anesthesia, but it soon became apparent that it also caused hepatotoxicity. Mild increase in transaminase was observed in up to 30 % of patients. But severe form of hepatotoxicity was rare with an estimated incidence of 1 in 3,000 or less. Obese patients under conditions of hypoxia after repeat exposure to halothane were identified as at risk of halothane hepatitis. There were two pathways identified in the pathophysiology of halothane hepatitis. It was either due to production of cellular cytotoxic reactive metabolites that are produced under hypoxic conditions in certain patients or due to an immune response to halothane metabolite-modified hepatic protein cellular antigen in certain individuals following repeat exposure to halothane [34]. Halothane is no longer used in the United States today.

Subsequently, introduced agents enflurane and isoflurane are metabolized in the liver to a much lower extent. Halothane is metabolized up to 20 %, enflurane 2–4 %, and isoflurane 0.2 %. In the United States at present, sevoflurane and desflurane and to a smaller extent isoflurane are the only inhalational agents used during anesthesia. Sevoflurane is extensively metabolized in vitro, but in vivo, its metabolism is limited to about 5 %, due to its low blood gas solubility. Sevoflurane has not been shown to produce any reactive metabolite that mediates liver injury. Only a very minute fraction, 0.01 % of administered dose of desflurane is metabolized in the liver. The modern anesthetic agents have been in use for over two decades and reports of hepatitis following exposure to isoflurane, sevoflurane, or desflurane are extremely rare [35–37]. Although clearly associated with their use, determination of causality is difficult in the absence of specific immunological or other tests.

Other considerations for use of inhaled anesthetic agent in liver disease include its effect on liver blood flow and hepatic oxygen supply demand ratio. All inhaled anesthetics decrease liver blood flow, but isoflurane causes the least decrease in liver blood flow. Effects of sevoflurane on hepatic blood flow appear to be similar to isoflurane. Given the potential for worsening of existing liver function due to decrease in liver blood flow, isoflurane is considered the drug of choice for patients with CLD and during liver transplantation. However, sevoflurane or desflurane is also considered safe in these patients. Recently, xenon has been studied in patients with liver disease and may be considered as an ideal anesthetic. It is not degraded in the body and has minimal effects on cardiovascular hemodynamics or liver blood flow, but high cost prohibits its use at the current time.

Antifibrinolytic Drugs

Epsilon aminocaproic acid (ECA) and tranexamic acid are used as antifibrinolytic drugs during liver transplantation. They are both competitive inhibitors of plasminogen activator and noncompetitive inhibitor of plasmin. In normal patients, following an initial dose of 10 g of ECA, its half-life was estimated at 77 min and 65–78 % of administered drug is excreted unchanged in the urine.

Tranexamic acid is six to ten times more potent than ECA. Following an IV dose of 1 g, its Vd_{ss} was estimated to be 8–10 l, t ½ of about 2 h, and over 95 % of drug excreted unchanged in the urine within 24 h [38]. The half-life may be prolonged to 24–48 h in patients with renal failure.

No dosage adjustments of ECA or tranexamic acid are necessary in patients with CLD unless HRS is also present.

Miscellaneous Drugs

Lidocaine

Lidocaine is metabolized rapidly in the liver by oxidative N-dealkylation to produce monoethylglycinexylidide (MEG-X) and glycinexylidide. Less than 10 % is excreted in kidney unchanged. Lidocaine has a high extraction ratio and its metabolism is therefore dependent on hepatic blood flow. Plasma level in patients with liver disease is two to three times higher, clearance is decreased by 30 %, and t ½ is prolonged two to three times compared to 1.5–2 h observed in healthy patients. Its dose should be decreased by a factor of 2 or 3 in severe liver disease.

Metoclopramide

Metoclopramide is biotransformed in the liver and has an extraction ratio of 0.2. Its clearance is decreased by half and t ½ prolonged to 15 h vs. 5 h in healthy volunteers [39]. The dose should be reduced by half especially if the patient also has concomitant renal failure.

Ondansetron

Ondansetron, a 5-HT_3 antagonist is an antiemetic and is extensively metabolized by the liver. Following a single intravenous dose of 8 mg of ondansetron in patients with liver disease, its bioavailability was increased, clearance reduced, and elimination prolonged compared to healthy volunteers. The t ½ increased from 5.65 h in healthy volunteers to 10–19.7 h in patients with liver disease depending upon the severity of disease [40]. No change in single dose is necessary, but repeated doses should be limited to 8 mg/day.

A summary of pharmacokinetic changes in liver disease of drugs discussed above is summarized in Table 44.1.

Table 44.1 Summary of pharmacokinetic changes in liver disease of common anesthetic drugs

Drug	Protein binding and hepatic extraction ratio	Volume of distribution at steady state	Clearance	Elimination half-life	Clinical significance in patients with liver disease
Thiopental	85 %, 0.2	Increased	Decreased	Prolonged	Probable enhanced clinical effects, but no change in single dose, decrease dose for infusion
Propofol	97–98 %, 1.0	No change, increased after infusion	No change	No change	No change in single dose, decrease dose after prolonged infusion
Etomidate Ketamine	75 %, 0.5	Increased × 2		Decreased by ½	No change in single dose Safe to use as single dose or for short infusions
Midazolam	96 %, 0.3–0.5	No change	Decreased by 30–50 %	Prolonged	Decrease dose especially after repeat doses, increased CNS sensitivity
Fentanyl	85 %, high				Recovery from single dose unaffected due to distribution
Alfentanil Remifentanil	92 %	No change	Decreased	Prolonged	Prolonged duration of effect Not metabolized in the liver, probable increase in cerebral sensitivity
Morphine	35 %, 0.7		Decreased by 2–3 times	Increased by 2–3 times	Decrease dose by 1–5 to 2 times, increase in cerebral sensitivity
Meperidine Succinylcholine	63 %		Decreased by half	Increased by 2	Avoid repeat doses Slight increase in duration of apnea in chronic liver disease but not in acute liver disease
Pancuronium	11–29 %	Increased by 50 %	Decreased	Prolonged	Onset delayed, increase initial dose, prolongation of effect
Vecuronium	30 %	No change with 0.1 mg/kg	No change (0.1 mg/kg), decreased with 0.2 mg/kg	No change or prolonged	No change with 0.1 mg/kg, prolonged duration after 0.2 mg/kg

(continued)

Table 44.1 (continued)

Drug	Protein binding and hepatic extraction ratio	Volume of distribution at steady state	Clearance	Elimination half-life	Clinical significance in patients with liver disease
Rocuronium	30 %	No change or increased	Decreased	Prolonged	Duration of action prolonged after repeat doses
Cisatracurium		Slight increase	Slight prolongation	No change	Not metabolized in the liver, no change in drug doses
Lidocaine	60–80 %, high		Decreased by 30 %	Increased by 2–3 time	Decrease dose by 2–3 times
Metoclopramide	40 %, 0.2		Decreased 50 %	Prolonged 2–3 times	Decrease dose by half
Ondansetron	78 %		Decreased	Prolonged	No change in single dose, decrease frequency for repeat dose

Conclusion

Liver, a major metabolic organ in the body, is unique and has many functions other than biotransformation of drugs. Commonly performed liver function tests do not accurately quantitate the degree of metabolic dysfunction of the liver. Even specific tests such as lidocaine MEG-X test and antipyrine or indocyanine green clearance tests of drug metabolism do not accurately assess or predict the pharmacokinetic changes of drugs in patients with liver disease. Some drugs undergo phase I reactions that may be significantly affected by hepatocellular disease but not by cholestatic disease. Factors other than intrinsic metabolic insufficiency due to liver disease such as changes in liver blood flow, serum albumin, portosystemic shunts, or pharmacodynamic sensitivity also play a significant part in drug metabolism and their effect. Further, considerable interindividual variability exists in response to many drugs in patients with liver disease. Ultimately, it is difficult to consistently predict clinical effects of any given drug in patients with liver disease. Therefore, careful titration of drug to its clinical effects and continued vigilance and monitoring for its side effects are critical in any patient with liver disease.

Chemical Structures

Chemical Structure 44.1   Cisatracurium besylate

**Chemical Structure
44.2** Aminocaproic acid

**Chemical Structure
44.3** Tranexamic acid

References

1. Xu JQ, Kochanek KD, Murphy SL, Tejada-Vera B. Deaths: final data for 2007. National vital statistics reports, vol. 58, no 19. Hyattsville: National Center for Health Statistics; 2010.
2. Asrani S, Kamath P, Pedersen R, et al. Liver related mortality in the US is underestimated. Hepatology. 2010;52:408. A169.
3. Organ Procurement and Transplantation Network. http://optn.transplant.hrsa.gov/data/. Accessed 10 Jun 2014.
4. Runyon BA. Surgical procedures are well tolerated by patients with asymptomatic chronic hepatitis. J Clin Gastroenterol. 1986;8(5):542-4.
5. Friedman LS. The risk of surgery in patients with liver disease. Hepatology. 1999;29(6): 1617-23.
6. Teh SH, Nagorney DM, Stevens SR, Offord KP, Therneau TM, Plevak DJ, Talwalkar JA, Kim WR, Kamath PS. Risk factors for mortality after surgery in patients with cirrhosis. Gastroenterology. 2007;132(4):1261-9.
7. Verbeeck RK. Pharmacokinetics and dosage adjustment in patients with hepatic dysfunction. Eur J Clin Pharmacol. 2008;64(12):1147-61.
8. MacGilchrist AJ, Birnie GG, Cook A, Scobie G, Murray T, Watkinson G, Brodie MJ. Pharmacokinetics and pharmacodynamics of intravenous midazolam in patients with severe alcoholic cirrhosis. Gut. 1986;27(2):190-5.
9. Tallgren M, Olkkola KT, Seppälä T, Höckerstedt K, Lindgren L. Pharmacokinetics and ventilatory effects of oxycodone before and after liver transplantation. Clin Pharmacol Ther. 1997;61(6):655-61.
10. Laidlaw J, Read AE, Sherlock S. Morphine tolerance in hepatic cirrhosis. Gastroenterology. 1961;40:389-96.
11. Ramond MJ, Comoy E, Lebrec D. Alterations in isoprenaline sensitivity in patients with cirrhosis: evidence of abnormality of the sympathetic nervous activity. Br J Clin Pharmacol. 1986;21(2):191-6.
12. Pandele G, Chaux F, Salvadori C, Farinotti M, Duvaldestin P. Thiopental pharmacokinetics in patients with cirrhosis. Anesthesiology. 1983;59(2):123-6.
13. Servin F, Desmonts JM, Haberer JP, Cockshott ID, Plummer GF, Farinotti R. Pharmacokinetics and protein binding of propofol in patients with cirrhosis. Anesthesiology. 1988;69(6): 887-91.
14. Servin F, Cockshott ID, Farinotti R, Haberer JP, Winckler C, Desmonts JM. Pharmacokinetics of propofol infusions in patients with cirrhosis. Br J Anaesth. 1990;65(2):177-83.
15. Li Z, Chen X, Meng J, Deng L, Ma H, Csete M, Xiong L. ED50 and recovery times after propofol in rats with graded cirrhosis. Anesth Analg. 2012;114(1):117-21.
16. Wu J, Huang SQ, Chen QL, Zheng SS. The influence of the severity of chronic virus-related liver disease on propofol requirements during propofol-remifentanil anesthesia. Yonsei Med J. 2013;54(1):231-7.
17. van Beem H, Manger FW, van Boxtel C, van Bentem N. Etomidate anaesthesia in patients with cirrhosis of the liver: pharmacokinetic data. Anaesthesia. 1983;38(Suppl):61-2.
18. Clements JA, Nimmo WS, Grant IS. Bioavailability, pharmacokinetics, and analgesic activity of ketamine in humans. J Pharm Sci. 1982;71(5):539-42.
19. Noppers IM, Nietsers M, Aarts LPHJ, Bauer MCR, Drewes AM, Dahan A, Sarton EY. Drug-induced liver injury following a repeated course of ketamine treatment for chronic pain in CRPS type 1 patients: a report of 3 cases. Pain. 2011;152:2173-8.
20. Trouvin JH, Farinotti R, Haberer JP, Servin F, Chauvin M, Duvaldestin P. Pharmacokinetics of midazolam in anaesthetized cirrhotic patients. Br J Anaesth. 1988;60(7):762-7.
21. Ferrier C, Marty J, Bouffard Y, Haberer JP, Levron JC, Duvaldestin P. Alfentanil pharmacokinetics in patients with cirrhosis. Anesthesiology. 1985;62(4):480-4.

22. Dershwitz M, Hoke JF, Rosow CE, Michałowski P, Connors PM, Muir KT, Dienstag JL. Pharmacokinetics and pharmacodynamics of remifentanil in volunteer subjects with severe liver disease. Anesthesiology. 1996;84(4):812–20.

23. Hasselström J, Eriksson S, Persson A, Rane A, Svensson JO, Säwe J. The metabolism and bioavailability of morphine in patients with severe liver cirrhosis. Br J Clin Pharmacol. 1990;29(3):289–97.

24. Davis L, Britten JJ, Morgan M. Cholinesterase. Its significance in anaesthetic practice. Anaesthesia. 1997;52(3):244–60.

25. Duvaldestin P, Agoston S, Henzel D, Kersten UW, Desmonts JM. Pancuronium pharmacokinetics in patients with liver cirrhosis. Br J Anaesth. 1978;50(11):1131–6.

26. Arden JR, Lynam DP, Castagnoli KP, Canfell PC, Cannon JC, Miller RD. Vecuronium in alcoholic liver disease: a pharmacokinetic and pharmacodynamic analysis. Anesthesiology. 1988;68(5):771–6.

27. Lebrault C, Berger JL, D'Hollander AA, Gomeni R, Henzel D, Duvaldestin P. Pharmacokinetics and pharmacodynamics of vecuronium (ORG NC 45) in patients with cirrhosis. Anesthesiology. 1985;62(5):601–5.

28. Lebrault C, Duvaldestin P, Henzel D, Chauvin M, Guesnon P. Pharmacokinetics and pharmacodynamics of vecuronium in patients with cholestasis. Br J Anaesth. 1986;58(9):983–7.

29. van Miert MM, Eastwood NB, Boyd AH, Parker CJ, Hunter JM. The pharmacokinetics and pharmacodynamics of rocuronium in patients with hepatic cirrhosis. Br J Clin Pharmacol. 1997;44(2):139–44.

30. Magorian T, Wood P, Caldwell J, Fisher D, Segredo V, Szenohradszky J, Sharma M, Gruenke L, Miller R. The pharmacokinetics and neuromuscular effects of rocuronium bromide in patients with liver disease. Anesth Analg. 1995;80(4):754–9.

31. Khalil M, D'Honneur G, Duvaldestin P, Slavov V, De Hys C, Gomeni R. Pharmacokinetics and pharmacodynamics of rocuronium in patients with cirrhosis. Anesthesiology. 1994;80(6):1241–7.

32. De Wolf AM, Freeman JA, Scott VL, Tullock W, Smith DA, Kisor DF, Kerls S, Cook DR. Pharmacokinetics and pharmacodynamics of cisatracurium in patients with end-stage liver disease undergoing liver transplantation. Br J Anaesth. 1996;76(5):624–8.

33. Bevan DR, Donati F, Kopman AF. Reversal of neuromuscular blockade. Anesthesiology. 1992;77(4):785–805.

34. Kenna JG, Jones RM. The organ toxicity of inhaled anesthetics. Anesth Analg. 1995;81(6 Suppl):S51–66.

35. Singhal S, et al. Sevoflurane hepatotoxicity: a case report of sevoflurane hepatic necrosis and review of the literature. Am J Ther. 2010;17(2):219–22.

36. Martin JL, et al. Hepatotoxicity after desflurane anesthesia. Anesthesiology. 1995;83(5):1125–9.

37. Nicoll A, et al. Repeated exposure to modern volatile anaesthetics may cause chronic hepatitis as well as acute liver injury. BMJ Case Rep. 2012. doi:10.1136/bcr-2012-006543.

38. Nilsson IM. Clinical pharmacology of aminocaproic and tranexamic acids. J Clin Pathol Suppl (R Coll Pathol). 1980;14:41–7.

39. Magueur E, Hagege H, Attali P, Singlas E, Etienne JP, Taburet AM. Pharmacokinetics of metoclopramide in patients with liver cirrhosis. Br J Clin Pharmacol. 1991;31(2):185–7.

40. Figg WD, Dukes GE, Pritchard JF, Hermann DJ, Lesesne HR, Carson SW, Songer SS, Powell JR, Hak LJ. Pharmacokinetics of ondansetron in patients with hepatic insufficiency. J Clin Pharmacol. 1996;36(3):206–15.

Part IV
Special Topics

Chapter 45
Black Box FDA Warnings and Legal Implications

Meghan Lane-Fall

Contents

The US Food and Drug Administration (FDA) is broadly charged with ensuring food, drug, device, and cosmetic safety for products marketed and sold in the United States [1]. The FDA is part of the Department of Health and Human Services (HHS), which is comprised of 11 divisions including the National Institutes of Health and Centers for Medicare and Medicaid Services. The HHS Secretary is a member of the President's Cabinet; as such, HHS and its divisions fall into the executive branch of the US government.

Food and drug regulation in the United States can be traced back to the nineteenth century, with the formation of the Division of Chemistry [2]. The FDA (then known as the Bureau of Chemistry) began to take its current form in 1906, with the passage of the Pure Food and Drug Act. The Act was passed in part as a response to the patent medicine industry and the proliferation of adulterated food. The Bureau of Chemistry eventually became the Food, Drug, and Insecticide Administration. The shortened FDA name was adopted in 1930 [2].

M. Lane-Fall, MD, MSHP
Department of Anesthesiology and Critical Care,
University of Pennsylvania, Philadelphia, PA, USA
e-mail: meghan.lane-fall@uphs.upenn.edu

A.D. Kaye et al. (eds.), *Essentials of Pharmacology for Anesthesia,*
Pain Medicine, and Critical Care, DOI 10.1007/978-1-4614-8948-1_45,
© Springer Science+Business Media New York 2015

The FDA's current jurisdiction (Box 45.1) includes most products meant for human or animal consumption, application, or implantation [1]. The FDA is tasked with ensuring that products under its purview are safe. For those products purporting to have therapeutic benefits, effectiveness must also be demonstrated. To address issues of safety and effectiveness, the FDA requires that drugs undergo pre-market approval and that they be labeled with safe use directions. This requirement dates back to 1938, with the passage of the Food, Drug, and Cosmetic Act during Franklin D. Roosevelt's administration [2].

Box 45.1: Products Under FDA Jurisdiction as of 2013 [1]
Blood and blood products
Cosmetics
Drugs (including supplements)
Food (human and animal)
Medical devices (including mobile medical apps)
Radiation-emitting products
Tobacco
Vaccines

As part of its continuous evaluation of drug safety, the FDA issues periodic notifications about ongoing safety reviews, guidance to health-care professionals who utilize or prescribe certain drugs, and public health advisories. In 2010, the FDA consolidated all of these communications into Drug Safety Communications to simplify the transmission of drug safety information [3]. One important type of Drug Safety Communication is the "boxed warning," also known as a "black box warning." The boxed warning is the highest level of warning issued by the FDA.

FDA boxed warnings are issued when there are important safety issues that must be considered in prescribing of a drug [4]. These warnings must be placed in a prominent boxed section in the prescribing information for the drug of concern. Boxed warnings may be required at the time of a new drug's approval, as occurred with prasugrel (Effient®) [5], but are more commonly added after the FDA becomes aware of drug-related adverse effects. Boxed warnings are usually based on clinical data but may also be informed by preclinical or laboratory studies [4, 5]. Numerous drugs commonly used in anesthesia practice carry an FDA boxed warning (Table 45.1). Additionally, there are other drugs with boxed warnings that the anesthesia practitioner may encounter (Table 45.2). Finally, there are a number of drugs of interest to the anesthesia practitioner about which the FDA has issued safety warnings but not boxed warnings (Table 45.3). The FDA hosts a website listing drugs that have had any type of drug safety communication [3]. However, there is no FDA-maintained list of drugs with boxed warnings [4]. Rather, individual drugs can be interrogated on the websites of the FDA [6] or individual drug manufacturers. Other compendia of drug information such as the

Table 45.1 Drugs with boxed warnings that are commonly used in anesthetic or critical care practice [6]

Drug (date of most recent available labeling)	Indication	Reason for boxed warning	Alternatives
Antiemetics			
Droperidol (Inapsine®) 12/2001	Nausea and vomiting; neuroleptic anesthesia	Prolonged QT interval, torsades de pointes	Ondansetron[b], metoclopramide prochlorperazine, promethazine, propofol[c]
Metoclopramide (Reglan®) 9/2011	Nausea and vomiting; gastroparesis	Tardive dyskinesia	Ondansetron[b], droperidol, prochlorperazine, promethazine, propofol[c]
Prochlorperazine (Compazine®) 12/2010	Nausea and vomiting	Increased risk of mortality (cardiovascular, infectious) in elderly patients with dementia-related psychosis	Ondansetron[b], droperidol, metoclopramide, promethazine, propofol[c]
Promethazine (Phenergan®) 9/2009	Nausea and vomiting	Tissue damage on extravasation or intra-arterial injection, potentially fatal respiratory depression in pediatric patients <2 years, worsening of Parkinsonian symptoms in older patients	Ondansetron[b], droperidol, prochlorperazine, promethazine, propofol[c]
Antimicrobials			
Fluoroquinolones: ciprofloxacin (Cipro®), levofloxacin (Levaquin ®), moxifloxacin (Avelox®), norfloxacin (Noroxin®), ofloxacin 4/2012 (levofloxacin)	Prophylaxis and treatment of bacterial infections	Tendinitis, tendon rupture, exacerbation of muscle weakness in myasthenic patients	Depends on targeted pathogen
Analgesics and anxiolytics			
Acetaminophen (Tylenol®) – mandates boxed warning when added to other drugs	Acute and chronic pain	Hepatotoxicity in doses exceeding 4,000 mg daily (adults)	NSAIDs, opioids, regional/ neuraxial analgesia
Buprenorphine (Buprenex®, Butrans®) 7/2012	Opioid withdrawal, chronic pain	Respiratory depression, diversion/misuse, overdose if patch exposed to heat, overdose with accidental ingestion by children	Other opioids, NSAIDs, acetaminophen

(continued)

Table 45.1 (continued)

Drug (date of most recent available labeling)	Indication	Reason for boxed warning	Alternatives
Fentanyl patch (Duragesic® patch) 7/9/2012	Acute and chronic pain	Respiratory depression, diversion/misuse, overdose with CYP3A4 inhibitors, overdose if patch exposed to heat, overdose with accidental exposure in children	Other opioids, NSAIDs, acetaminophen, regional/neuraxial analgesia
Hydromorphone (Dilaudid®, Dilaudid-HP®, Exalgo®) 3/2013	Acute and chronic pain	Respiratory depression, diversion/misuse, overdose with high potency version, overdose with crushing/chewing extended release version, overdose with accidental ingestion by children	Other opioids, NSAIDs, acetaminophen, regional/neuraxial analgesia
Ketorolac (Toradol®) 3/2013	Acute pain	Cardiovascular events, myocardial infarction and stroke; GI events, bleeding, ulcer, perforation; renal impairment; bleeding risk; hypersensitivity including anaphylaxis; contraindicated in pregnant women or nursing mothers; should be used for <5 days	Acetaminophen, ibuprofen, opioids
Methadone (Dolophine®) 7/2012	Opioid withdrawal, chronic pain	Respiratory depression, QT prolongation, torsades de pointes, overdose with accidental ingestion by children, should be prescribed by professionals knowledgeable in using opioids for chronic pain	Shorter-acting opioids, NSAIDs, acetaminophen, regional/neuraxial analgesia
Midazolam (Versed®) 6/2010	Anxiety, procedural sedation	Respiratory depression; in older patients, risk of impaired psychomotor function, syncope, falls; seizures in neonates; use only in hospitals or ambulatory care settings	Anxiety, low doses; procedural sedation, fentanyl, propofol
Nonselective NSAIDs: ibuprofen (Advil®, Motrin®) 9/2007	Acute and chronic pain	Cardiovascular events, myocardial infarction and stroke; GI events, bleeding, ulcer, perforation	Short-term use of nonselective NSAIDs; acetaminophen, opioids, regional/neuraxial analgesia

Oxymorphone (Opana®) 7/2012	Acute and chronic pain	Respiratory depression, diversion/misuse, overdose if mixed with alcohol, overdose with accidental ingestion by children	Other opioids, NSAIDs, acetaminophen, regional/neuraxial analgesia
Local anesthetics			
Bupivacaine[d] (Marcaine®) 1/2012	Local, regional, neuraxial anesthesia	Cardiac arrest when 0.75 % solution used for obstetrical epidural anesthesia, chondrolysis when used for continuous intra-articular infusion	Lower concentration of bupivacaine for obstetrical anesthesia, avoidance of intra-articular infusion (e.g., single-shot or continuous nerve blockade, neuraxial anesthesia)
Other drugs			
Amiodarone[d] (Cordarone®) 11/2011	Atrial fibrillation	Hypersensitivity pneumonitis, hepatotoxicity, heart block	Metoprolol, diltiazem
Bumetanide (Bumex®) 1/2010	Fluid overload	Profound diuresis with water and electrolyte depletion	Lower doses, furosemide, hydrochlorothiazide
Dantrolene (Dantrium®) – oral formulation only 7/2012	Treatment of malignant hyperthermia, neuroleptic malignant syndrome, spasticity	Hepatic injury/hepatitis (potentially fatal)	Malignant hyperthermia, none; spasticity, baclofen, diazepam
Low-molecular-weight heparins: dalteparin (Fragmin®), enoxaparin (Lovenox®) 4/2011 (enoxaparin)	Prophylactic or therapeutic anticoagulation	Spinal/epidural hematoma risk with neuraxial anesthesia	Unfractionated heparin
Nimodipine (Nimotop®) 1/2006	Hypertension in subarachnoid hemorrhage	Hypotension when contents of oral capsules extracted and injected intravenously	Nicardipine, oral dosing of nimodipine
Protamine 1/2008	Reversal of heparin anticoagulation	Severe hypotension, catastrophic pulmonary vasoconstriction, cardiovascular collapse, noncardiogenic pulmonary edema; not to be used in bleeding not associated with heparin exposure	(None)

(continued)

Table 45.1 (continued)

Drug (date of most recent available labeling)	Indication	Reason for boxed warning	Alternatives
Quetiapine (Seroquel®) 11/2011	Psychosis	Increased risk of mortality (cardiovascular, infectious) in elderly patients with dementia-related psychosis, suicidality in children and young adults with concomitant psychiatric disease	Haloperidol
Sodium nitroprusside (Nipride®) 8/2007	Hypertension	Cyanide intoxication, hypotension	Nitroglycerin, nicardipine
Succinylcholine (Anectine®) 9/2010	Neuromuscular blockade	Rhabdomyolysis with hyperkalemia	Non-depolarizing neuromuscular blockers
Warfarin (Coumadin®) 10/2011	Therapeutic anticoagulation	Major or fatal bleeding	Unfractionated or low-molecular-weight heparins, dabigatran, rivaroxaban

SSRI selective serotonin reuptake inhibitor, *SNRI* serotonin-norepinephrine reuptake inhibitor

[a]List may not be comprehensive, as the FDA does not maintain a repository of boxed warnings

[b]Ondansetron carries FDA warnings about QT prolongation but does not have a boxed warning on its labeling as of 11/2012

[c]Propofol may be used off-label in subhypnotic doses (e.g., 10–20 mg IV bolus) for treatment of nausea or vomiting

[d]Does not contain a boxed warning at the beginning of its package labeling as many boxed warning drugs do but does contain a boxed warning in the body of the labeling

Table 45.2 Drugs with boxed warnings that may be of interest to anesthesiologists [6]

Drug (date of most recent available labeling)	Indication	Reason for boxed warning	Alternatives
Analgesics			
Codeine 2/2013	Acute and chronic pain	Respiratory depression after tonsillectomy/ adenoidectomy in pediatric patients with ultrarapid metabolism or with sleep apnea	Acetaminophen
COX-2 inhibitors – celecoxib (Celebrex®), rofecoxib (Vioxx®) 11/2012 (celecoxib)	Acute and chronic pain	Cardiovascular events (myocardial infarction, stroke)	Nonselective NSAIDs, acetaminophen, opioid analgesics
Anticoagulants and antiplatelet agents			
Clopidogrel (Plavix ®) 12/2011	Antiplatelet therapy in acute coronary syndrome, after coronary stent implantation	Subtherapeutic drug levels leading to thrombotic events in slow metabolizers (CYP2C19 variants) or with co-administration of drugs inhibiting CYP2C19 (esomeprazole, omeprazole, azole antifungals, cimetidine)	Higher dose clopidogrel (e.g., 600 mg daily), triple antiplatelet therapy (e.g., clopidogrel, aspirin, and cilostazol)
Rivaroxaban (Xarelto®) 3/2013	Anticoagulant therapy in non-valvular atrial fibrillation or after surgery	Risk of thrombosis with abrupt discontinuation, risk of spinal/epidural hematoma with neuraxial procedures	Warfarin
Ticlopidine (Ticlid®)	Antiplatelet therapy	Neutropenia, agranulocytosis, thrombotic thrombocytopenic purpura, aplastic anemia	Clopidogrel
Other drugs			
Levothyroxine[a] (Synthroid®) 9/2012	Hypothyroidism	Should not be used for weight loss in euthyroid patients	None
Perflutren microbubble contrast agents (Definity®, Optison®) 10/2011	Suboptimal echocardiographic images	"Serious cardiopulmonary reactions, including fatalities" – should not be given intra-arterially or to patients with intracardiac shunts	None
Metformin[a] (Glucophage®) 1/2009	Diabetes mellitus type 2	Lactic acidosis	Sulfonylureas, insulin
Terbutaline (Brethine®)	Premature labor	>48–72 h use: maternal arrhythmia or death	Ritodrine, nifedipine, magnesium sulfate
Naltrexone (Vivitrol®) 10/2010	Alcohol dependence, opioid dependence	Hepatocellular injury; contraindicated in acute hepatitis or liver failure	Alcohol dependence, disulfiram; opioid dependence, methadone; buprenorphine
Propylthiouracil 7/2011	Hyperthyroidism	Liver injury, liver failure	Methimazole

[a]Does not contain a boxed warning at the beginning of its package labeling as many boxed warning drugs do but does contain a boxed warning in the body of the labeling

Table 45.3 FDA safety warnings from 2008 to 2013 potentially of interest to anesthesiologists [3]

Drug (date of safety warning)	Indication	Reason for safety warning	Alternatives
Antimicrobials			
Cefepime (Maxipime®) 6/2012	Prophylaxis and treatment of bacterial infections	Nonconvulsive status epilepticus in patients with creatinine clearance <60 mL/min	Depends on targeted pathogen
Ceftriaxone (Rocephin®) 4/2009	Prophylaxis and treatment of bacterial infections	Particulate formation occurs when mixed with calcium-containing fluids (including Ringer's lactate)	Depends on targeted pathogen
Linezolid (Zyvox®) 10/2011	Prophylaxis and treatment of bacterial infections	Serotonin syndrome when co-administered with serotonergic medications (clomipramine, SSRIs, SNRIs)	Depends on targeted pathogen
Other drugs			
Benzocaine 4/2011	Topical anesthesia	Methemoglobinemia	Lidocaine
Bupivacaine (Marcaine®), chloroprocaine (Nesacaine®), lidocaine (Xylocaine®), mepivacaine (Carbocaine), ropivacaine (Naropin®) 12/2010	Local, regional, neuraxial anesthesia	Chondrolysis when used for continuous intra-articular infusion	Avoidance of intra-articular infusion (e.g., single-shot or continuous nerve blockade, neuraxial anesthesia)
Adenosine (Adenocard®), amiodarone (Cordarone®) 5/2011	Supraventricular tachycardia	Prefilled glass syringes can break off in IV administration sets	Alternate formulation
Heparin 12/2012	Prophylaxis and treatment of thrombosis, stroke prophylaxis in atrial fibrillation	Old and new formulations have different potency	(Check drug strength prior to administration)
Methylene blue 10/2011	Vasoplegia, body fluid labeling	Serotonin syndrome when co-administered with serotonergic medications (clomipramine, SSRIs, SNRIs)	Vasoplegia, direct or indirect vasoconstrictors (e.g., phenylephrine, ephedrine, epinephrine, etc.); fluid labeling, isosulfan blue
Proton pump inhibitors: esomeprazole (Nexium®), lansoprazole (Prevacid®), omeprazole (Prilosec®), pantoprazole (Protonix®) 2/2012	Prophylaxis and treatment of gastric ulcers	*Clostridium difficile* diarrhea	Histamine (H2) receptor blockers, sucralfate
Sildenafil (Revatio®) 8/2012	Pulmonary hypertension, erectile dysfunction	Pulmonary hypertension and heart failure leading to death in children ages 1–7	Nifedipine, nitric oxide, inhaled epoprostenol

Physicians' Desk Reference have boxed warning information, but the accuracy of this data is dependent on the publisher [4].

This chapter highlights one class of drugs, antiemetics, which carry boxed warnings. The medicolegal implications of boxed warnings are also addressed.

Antiemetic Drugs

There are multiple classes of drugs used primarily for the prevention and treatment of postoperative nausea and vomiting (PONV), most of which have either an FDA boxed warning (Table 45.1) or other safety warning (Table 45.3). In this section, we consider three commonly used antiemetic agents: droperidol, ondansetron, and promethazine.

Droperidol

Droperidol (Inapsine®), primarily a dopamine receptor antagonist, is used for both neuroleptic anesthesia (higher doses) and for prophylaxis and treatment of nausea and vomiting (low doses). Droperidol is chemically related to the typical antipsychotic haloperidol, which also possesses antiemetic properties.

Droperidol causes a dose-dependent prolongation of the QT interval in susceptible individuals. This side effect prompted the FDA to issue a boxed warning for droperidol in 2001 [7]. The boxed warning for droperidol is somewhat unusual in that it severely limits the practitioner's ability to use the drug: "Because of potential for serious proarrhythmic effects and death, use only when response to other treatment is unacceptable (due to lack of efficacy or intolerable adverse effects." The warning goes on to say that a 12-lead ECG should be obtained prior to droperidol administration and that the use of droperidol is contraindicated in patients with known or suspected QT prolongation.

The droperidol boxed warning decision was controversial for at least three reasons. First, the FDA based its decision on review of 65 unique cases (273 reports) of arrhythmia associated with droperidol use, along with 2 European studies using droperidol doses in excess of 50 times the dose used for PONV in the United States. Second, droperidol appears to be more efficacious in the treatment of PONV than ondansetron. Third, droperidol had a large (roughly 30 %) market share at the time the warning was issued. The use of droperidol dropped by 90 % after the warning's issuance [7, 8].

In 2005, the FDA reconsidered droperidol's boxed warning, holding an advisory panel consisting of anesthesiologists, pharmacologists, cardiologists, and patient representatives [8]. The FDA acknowledged the controversial decision but ultimately decided that there was insufficient clinical evidence to retract the warning.

Despite the boxed warning, anesthesiologists continue to use droperidol for the treatment of PONV, albeit less frequently than alternative drugs such as the serotonin receptor antagonists. It should be noted that the doses of droperidol used for PONV, 0.625–1.25 mg, are below the FDA's "minimum approved dose" of 2.5 mg. As such, using these smaller doses is considered an "off-label" use of the drug not covered by the product labeling [8]. Despite the apparent low risk of QT prolongation with antiemetic doses of droperidol, it should be used cautiously when co-administered with other drugs known to prolong the QT interval (e.g., inhaled anesthetics, propofol, succinylcholine, metoclopramide).

Ondansetron

Ondansetron (Zofran®) and related drugs granisetron and dolasetron are serotonin receptor (5HT-3) antagonists used for prophylaxis and treatment of nausea and vomiting, especially in postoperative settings or with administration of chemotherapy. Ondansetron, similar to droperidol, prolongs the QT interval in a dose-dependent fashion. Unlike droperidol, however, ondansetron does not have a boxed warning. The risk of QT prolongation and torsades de pointes prompted the FDA to remove the highest dose of ondansetron, 32 mg, from the market [3]. Ondansetron is a less efficacious antiemetic than droperidol and more readily prolongs the QT interval, but it remains popular in clinical practice.

Promethazine

Promethazine (Phenergan®) is a phenothiazine derivative that inhibits dopamine and muscarinic cholinergic receptors. It is in the same drug class as prochlorperazine. The FDA issued a black box warning for promethazine that has three components [3]. First, there is a risk of severe tissue damage, including gangrene, if promethazine extravasates into tissues or if it is injected intra-arterially. Second, there is an increased risk of mortality for patients with dementia-related psychosis when promethazine or atypical antipsychotics are used. Third, promethazine can cause respiratory depression in patients younger than 2 years of age.

Implications for Using Drugs with Boxed Warnings

The prescriber's responsibility with respect to the FDA is twofold. First, providers serve as an important source of post-market information for the FDA. If providers suspect an adverse drug reaction, they should consider submitting a report to the FDA via its MedWatch system so that safety information can be updated, if appropriate [9]. Second, the FDA expects providers to be aware of drug safety warnings, which are published on the FDA website, on drug manufacturers' websites, and in drug packaging inserts. The FDA hosts a Twitter feed, an RSS (really simple syndication) feed, and an audio podcast about drug safety that facilitate dissemination of drug information to providers [5].

The FDA does not place restrictions on providers' ability to use drugs with boxed warnings [10]. Rather, the warnings are intended to offer guidance to providers so that they can decide whether to use alternate agents or adjust dosage in high-risk patients. Nevertheless, assignment of a boxed or other safety warning does sometimes prompt providers to drastically curtail their use of a drug or drug class [4], as occurred with antidepressant medications in the early twenty-first century [11] and with droperidol as previously discussed.

The use of drugs with FDA boxed warnings can be justified in the appropriate clinical scenario but may still pose some medicolegal risk. As an example, more than 40 legal opinions related to metoclopramide have been filed since its black box warning was issued [12]. It is unclear how many, if any, of the related lawsuits were settled or decided in favor of plaintiffs, but it seems prudent for providers to clearly document their reasoning for using drugs with boxed warnings if they opt to do so.

References

1. Food and Drug Administration. FDA Fundamentals. 2013. http://www.fda.gov/AboutFDA/Transparency/Basics/ucm192695.htm. Accessed 27 Jul 2013.
2. Food and Drug Administration. Research tools on FDA history. 2013. http://www.fda.gov/AboutFDA/WhatWeDo/History/ResearchTools/default.htm. Accessed 25 Jul 2013.
3. Food and Drug Administration. Drug safety communications. 2013. http://www.fda.gov/Drugs/DrugSafety/ucm199082.htm. Accessed 25 Jul 2013.
4. Cheng CM, Guglielmo BJ, Judy M, Auerbach AD. Coverage of FDA medication boxed warnings in commonly used drug information resources. Arch Intern Med. 2010;170(9):831–3.
5. Marks NS, Weiss K. Boxed warnings and other FDA communication tools. Am Fam Physician. 2010;81(3):259–260.
6. Food and Drug Administration. FDA approved drug products. 2013. http://www.accessdata.fda.gov/scripts/cder/drugsatfda/index.cfm. Accessed 27 Jul 2013.
7. Matlock A, Allan N, Wills B, Kang C, Leikin JB. A continuing black hole? The FDA boxed warning: an appeal to improve its clinical utility. Clin Toxicol. 2011;49(6):443–7.
8. Gan TJ. "Black box" warning on droperidol: a report of the FDA convened expert panel [1]. Anesth Analg. 2004;98(6):1809.
9. Food and Drug Administration. MedWatch: the FDA safety information and adverse event reporting program. 2013. http://www.fda.gov/Safety/MedWatch/default.htm. Accessed 27 Jul 2013.
10. O'Connor NR. FDA boxed warnings: how to prescribe drugs safely. Am Fam Physician. 2010;81(3):298–303.
11. Libby AM, Orton HD, Valuck RJ. Persisting decline in depression treatment after FDA warnings. Arch Gen Psychiatry. 2009;66(6):633–9.
12. Ehrenpreis ED, Deepak P, Sifuentes H, Devi R, Du H, Leikin JB. The metoclopramide black box warning for tardive dyskinesia: effect on clinical practice, adverse event reporting, and prescription drug lawsuits. Am J Gastroenterol. 2013;108(6):866–72.

Chapter 46
Drug-Induced QT Prolongation

Elizabeth A. Valentine, Alan David Kaye, Jackie V. Abadie, and Adam M. Kaye

Contents

E.A. Valentine, MD (✉)
Department of Anesthesiology and Critical Care, Perelman School of Medicine at the
University of Pennsylvania, Philadelphia, PA 19104, USA
e-mail: elizabeth.valentine@uphs.upenn.edu

A.D. Kaye, MD, PhD
Department of Anesthesiology, Tulane Medical Center, New Orleans, LA, USA

Department of Anesthesiology, Louisiana State University Health Sciences Center,
New Orleans, LA, USA
e-mail: alankaye44@hotmail.com

J.V. Abadie, MD
Department of Anesthesiology, Alton Ochsner Clinic, New Orleans, LA, USA
e-mail: jakqs25@yahoo.com

A.M. Kaye, PharmD
Thomas J. Long School of Pharmacy and Health Sciences, University of the Pacific,
3601 Pacific Avenue, Stockton, CA, USA
e-mail: akaye@pacific.edu

A.D. Kaye et al. (eds.), *Essentials of Pharmacology for Anesthesia,*
Pain Medicine, and Critical Care, DOI 10.1007/978-1-4614-8948-1_46,
© Springer Science+Business Media New York 2015

Introduction

The QT interval is the electrocardiographic (ECG) representation of ventricular depolarization and repolarization as measured from the beginning of the QRS complex to the end of the T wave. The normal QT interval varies inversely with heart rate and is frequently reported as a QT corrected (QTc). The most common correction is Bazett's formula, which divides the measured QT interval by the square root of the RR interval [1]. The American Heart Association and American College of Cardiology Foundation (AHA/ACCF) expert writing group recommends that a QTc value greater than the 99th percentile should be considered abnormally prolonged; this corresponds to a QTc >470mx for otherwise healthy males and >480 ms for otherwise healthy females [2]. Drug-induced increases in QTc >60 ms above baseline are also potentially arrhythmogenic [2]. Symptoms of long QT include palpitations, syncope, seizure-like activity, arrhythmias, and sudden cardiac death.

QT prolongation can be congenital or acquired. Most cases of acquired QT prolongation are drug induced, and QTc prolongation is one of the most common causes of restriction or withdrawal of a drug after initial marketing [3]. Many drugs administered in the perioperative period have the potential to prolong the QT interval and ventricular repolarization. It has been suggested the hospitalized patients may be at higher risk for potentially fatal arrhythmias as compared to the outpatient population due to age, underlying comorbidities, and the potential for drug-induced QTc prolongation via polypharmacy and rapid intravenous administration [2].

Abnormal ventricular repolarization may precipitate malignant ventricular dysrhythmias such as torsades de pointes (TdP), a polymorphic ventricular tachycardia first described by Dessertenne in which the ventricular QRS axis appears to "twist" around an isoelectric axis (Fig. 46.1) [4]. While generally self-limited, TdP may degenerate into ventricular fibrillation and result in sudden cardiac death.

[Drug Class and] Mechanism of Action

The action potential of a ventricular myocyte consists of five phases (Fig. 46.2) [5]. Phase 0 consists of rapid depolarization, resulting from rapid sodium influx through fast sodium (Na^+) channels and a decreased permeability to potassium (K^+) efflux. Phase 1 is a phase of early repolarization caused by the opening of an outward K^+ channel. Phase 2 is the plateau phase, caused by the activation of slow inward calcium (Ca^{2+}) channels. Repolarization occurs during phase 3, during which Ca^{2+} channels are inactivated and K^+ efflux occurs via both rapid (I_{kr}) and slow (I_{ks}) potassium rectifier currents. It is this phase that is most important in the pathophysiology of QT prolongation and ventricular arrhythmias. Phase 4 is the resting membrane potential, maintained by a membrane-bound Na^+–K^+ ATPase at approximately −90 mV.

I_{kr} blockade results in a delay of rapid repolarization (Phase 3) and prolongation of duration of the action potential, reflected clinically by QT prolongation on the

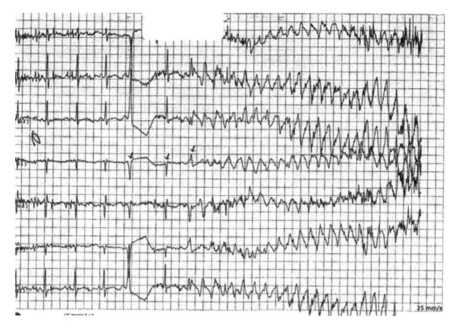

Fig. 46.1 Characteristic short-long-short on ECG rhythm strip preceding episode of torsades de pointes (With kind permission from Springer Science + Business Media: Benson et al. [66], Figure 3, and any original (first) copyright notice displayed with material)

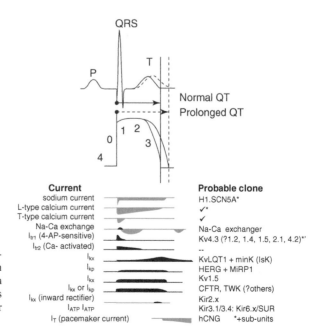

Fig. 46.2 Typical myocardial action potential (With kind permission from Springer Science + Business Media: Rowan and Darbar [67], Figure 1)

Table 46.1 Patient risk factors for QT prolongation and torsades de pointes [2, 12, 16, 17, 64]

Female
Advanced age
Family history or occult history of congenital long QT syndrome
Previous history of drug-induced torsades de pointes
Prolonged baseline QT
Multiple QT-prolonging agents
Treatment with drugs that interfere with metabolism of QT-prolonging agents
Structural heart disease
Hypokalemia
Hypomagnesemia
Hypocalcemia
Hepatic impairment
Bradycardia

ECG. Nearly all drugs that cause QT prolongation block I_{kr} [6, 7]. A strong correlation has been demonstrated between a drug's ability to block I_{kr} and its potential to cause ventricular arrhythmias and sudden cardiac death [8]. Prolonged repolarization may result in early afterdepolarizations (EADs). When EADs reach a threshold voltage, extrasystolic ventricular beats may occur. His-Purkinje and mid-myocardial (M cells) have been shown to be particularly susceptible to EADs when exposed to QT-prolonging drugs [9–11]. Heterogeneity in ventricular repolarization, also known as dispersion of refractoriness, may lead to zones of unidirectional block, which in turn may lead to a myocardium vulnerable to reentrant tachycardias and TdP [12–15].

Drug-induced TdP is frequently preceded by a characteristic "short-long-short" sequence on ECG (Fig. 46.1) [12, 16]. This typically begins with a premature ectopic beat followed by a compensatory pause. A subsequent sinus beat may have a prolonged QT with a deformed TU complex. A second premature beat following this "long QT" beat, typically occurring near the peak of the distorted TU wave complex known as the vulnerable period, may then precipitate a ventricular arrhythmia such as TdP.

Indications and Clinical Pearls

Though most patients receiving QT-prolonging medications have no detrimental sequelae, several risk factors exist that may predispose patients to TdP. In one study, nearly all patients with episodes of TdP attributed to noncardiac medication had one or more risk factors [17]. Risk factors associated with TdP may be found in Table 46.1. Additional studies have demonstrated subclinical mutations in genes causing congenital long QT syndrome (LQTS) in patients with drug-induced QT prolongation and TdP [18, 19]. Hospitalized patients may be at a higher risk of developing TdP with QT-prolonging drugs than outpatients, due to multiple risk factors, multiple QT-prolonging agents, and rapid intravenous administration [2].

While antiarrhythmic agents are perhaps the most commonly recognized contributor to QT prolongation, many other drugs and drug classes have been associated with QT prolongation (Table 46.2). Many of these agents are used in the perioperative

Table 46.2 Drugs that may cause QT prolongation and torsades de pointes [65]

Generic name	Brand name
Albuterol	Proventil, Ventolin
Alfuzosin	Uroxatral
Amantadine	Symmetrel
Amiodarone	Cordarone, Pacerone
Amisulpride	Solian
Amitriptyline	Elavil
Amphetamine	Dexedrine, Adderall
Arsenic trioxide	Trisenox
Artenimol-piperaquine	Eurartesim
Astemizole	Hismanal
Atazanavir	Reyataz
Atomoxetine	Strattera
Azithromycin	Zithromax
Bedaquiline	Sirturo
Bepridil	Vascor
Chloral hydrate	Noctec
Chloroquine	Aralen
Chlorpromazine	Thorazine
Ciprofloxacin	Cipro
Cisapride	Propulsid
Citalopram	Celexa
Clarithromycin	Biaxin
Clomipramine	Anafranil
Clozapine	Clozaril
Cocaine	Cocaine
Desipramine	Pertofrane
Dexmethylphenidate	Focalin
Diphenhydramine	Benadryl, Nytol
Disopyramide	Norpace
Dobutamine	Dobutrex
Dofetilide	Tikosyn
Dolasetron	Anzemet
Domperidone	Motilium
Dopamine	Intropin
Doxepin	Sinequan
Dronedarone	Multaq
Droperidol	Inapsine
Ephedrine	Broncholate, Rynatuss
Epinephrine	Primatene, Bronkaid

(continued)

Table 46.2 (continued)

Generic name	Brand name
Eribulin	Halaven
Erythromycin	Erythrocin, E.E.S.
Escitalopram	Lexapro, Cipralex
Famotidine	Pepcid
Felbamate	Felbatol
Fenfluramine	Pondimin
Fingolimod	Gilenya
Flecainide	Tambocor
Fluconazole	Diflucan
Fluoxetine	Prozac, Sarafem
Foscarnet	Foscavir
Fosphenytoin	Cerebyx
Galantamine	Reminyl
Gatifloxacin	Tequin
Gemifloxacin	Factive
Granisetron	Kytril
Halofantrine	Halfan
Haloperidol	Haldol
Ibutilide	Corvert
Iloperidone	Fanapt
Imipramine	Tofranil
Indapamide	Lozol
Isoproterenol	Isuprel, Medihaler-Iso
Isradipine	Dynacirc
Itraconazole	Sporanox
Ketoconazole	Nizoral
Lapatinib	Tyverb
Levalbuterol	Xopenex
Levofloxacin	Levaquin
Levomethadyl	Orlaam
Lisdexamfetamine	Vyvanse
Lithium	Lithobid, Eskalith
Mesoridazine	Serentil
Metaproterenol	Alupent
Methadone	Methadose, Dolophine
Methylphenidate	Concerta, Ritalin
Midodrine	ProAmatine
Mirtazapine	Remeron
Moexipril/HCTZ	Uniretic
Moxifloxacin	Avelox
Nicardipine	Cardene
Nilotinib	Tasigna
Norepinephrine	Levophed
Nortriptyline	Pamelor
Octreotide	Sandostatin
Ofloxacin	Floxin
Olanzapine	Zyprexa

Table 46.2 (continued)

Generic name	Brand name
Ondansetron	Zofran
Oxytocin	Pitocin
Paliperidone	Invega
Paroxetine	Paxil
Pentamidine	Nebupent, Pentam
Perflutren lipid microspheres	Definity
Phentermine	Adipex, Fastin
Phenylephrine	Neosynephrine
Phenylpropanolamine	Accutrim, Dexatrim
Pimozide	Orap
Probucol	Lorelco
Procainamide	Procan, Pronestyl
Protriptyline	Vivactil
Pseudoephedrine	Pediacare, Sudafed
Quetiapine	Seroquel
Quinidine	Cardioquin, Quinaglute
Ranolazine	Ranexa
Risperidone	Risperdal
Ritodrine	Yutopar
Ritonavir	Norvir
Roxithromycin	Rulide
Salmeterol	Serevent
Sertindole	Serlect
Sertraline	Zoloft
Sevoflurane	Ultane
Sibutramine	Meridia
Solifenacin	VESIcare
Sotalol	Betapace
Sparfloxacin	Zagam
Sunitinib	Sutent
Tacrolimus	Prograf
Tamoxifen	Nolvadex
Telithromycin	Ketek
Terbutaline	Brethine
Terfenadine	Seldane
Thioridazine	Mellaril
Tizanidine	Zanaflex
Tolterodine	Detrol
Trazodone	Desyrel
Trimethoprim-sulfa	Bactrim, Septra
Trimipramine	Surmontil
Vandetanib	Caprelsa
Vardenafil	Levitra
Venlafaxine	Effexor
Voriconazole	Vfend
Ziprasidone	Geodon

setting. As many as 80 % of patients may demonstrate significant QT prolongation in the perioperative setting, although the occurrence of TdP is rare [20]. Exposure to multiple agents makes identifying the causative drug difficult when it occurs. Other concomitant risk factors during the surgical period such as electrolyte derangements, decreased temperatures, and surgical stress may also contribute to arrhythmias.

Many agents specific to the perioperative period are known to affect the QT interval. The volatile agents have been shown to prolong the QT interval via inhibition of the I_{kr} current [21–32]. Each volatile agent may affect potassium currents differently, causing varying degrees of prolongation [22, 25, 26]. Several studies suggest that volatile agents have no significant effect on QT prolongation [23, 27]. Evidence is conflicting as to whether propofol leads to QT prolongation or TdP [28, 33–35]. Several studies have demonstrated that both depolarizing and non-depolarizing muscle relaxants can cause significant QT prolongation [33, 36–38].

While many opioids affect potassium channels, not all cause QT prolongation or TdP [39–44]. Fentanyl, codeine, and buprenorphine have been shown to block potassium channels, but do not seem to have a noticeable effect on QT interval [44]. Distribution of levomethadyl was discontinued in 2003 due to the risk of adverse cardiac events such as QT prolongation, TdP, and cardiac death [45]. Propoxyphene was withdrawn from the US market in 2010 due to its propensity to cause QT prolongation [46]. In 2006, the Food and Drug Administration (FDA) issued a public health advisory and black box warning regarding the risk of QT prolongation and TdP in patients receiving methadone [47]. It has been recommended that patients undergoing methadone therapy should obtain a baseline ECG prior to initiating therapy as well as periodic ECGs throughout therapy to monitor for QT prolongation [42].

Several antiemetics used during the perioperative period have been associated with QT prolongation and TdP. In 2001, the FDA issued a black box warning for droperidol regarding the potential for drug-induced QT prolongation and TdP [48]. Despite the black box warning, some suggest that droperidol used at lower doses is a safe and effective antiemetic [49–51]. Though the serotonin 5-hydroxytryptamine (5-HT$_3$) receptor antagonists have increased in popularity for antiemetic prophylaxis, these agents have also been found to prolong the QT interval [37, 52–54]. The FDA has issued safety alerts regarding the potential QT prolongation with dolasetron, ondansetron, and granisetron [55–57]. In one study, 5-HT$_3$ blockers were found to have similar effects on QT prolongation as droperidol at clinically significant doses [58]. When used together, ondansetron and droperidol have not been found to prolong QT interval more than either drug alone [59].

Most episodes of TdP are self-limited. The American College of Cardiology/American Heart Association and the European Society of Cardiology guidelines recommend magnesium sulfate 2 g intravenously as a first-line agent to terminate TdP, irrespective of serum magnesium level [60]. This therapy may be repeated. The underlying protective mechanism of magnesium is unknown. Repletion of potassium to levels >4.5 mmol/L may also be considered [60]. Temporary transvenous overdrive pacing or isoproterenol infusion may be used in an attempt to abolish pauses that may trigger TdP. Immediate nonsynchronized DC cardioversion should be initiated for patients with unstable TdP or TdP that degenerates into ventricular fibrillation [61].

Dosing Options

It is important for clinicians to be cognizant of which drugs commonly cause QT prolongation, as well as the fact that multiple QT-prolonging drugs can have an additive effect. Patients with congenital long QT syndrome should not receive QT-prolonging agents. While QT prolongation is not strictly related to drug dosing, it may be prudent to decrease or limit the dosing of QT-prolonging drugs to patients with ECG evidence of or risk factors for QT prolongation. When possible, alternative drugs should be utilized.

Drug Interactions

Nearly all QT-prolonging drugs block the rapid component of ventricular repolarization. In most cases, risk increases as the plasma drug concentration increases, although some drugs can prolong the QT interval and induce TdP at any dose. Notably, class IA antiarrhythmics have been shown to cause QT prolongation at lower or even subtherapeutic doses [62]. Polypharmacy with multiple QT-prolonging medications can have an additive effect.

It is also important to recognize that any drug that inhibits the metabolism of QT-prolonging agents can result in drug accumulation. This accumulation may worsen the proarrhythmic effects. While there is individual variability in drug metabolism, the majority of QT-prolonging drugs are metabolized via the CYP450 enzymes, most notably CYP3A4 and CYP2D6. Clinicians should familiarize themselves with drugs not only that induce QT prolongation but also that may inhibit these enzymes [63].

Side Effects/Black Box Warnings

A black box warning is the strongest warning required by the Food and Drug Administration (FDA) for a prescription medication. It is reserved for medications for which medical studies have demonstrated a significant risk of serious or potentially life-threatening adverse effects. Several drugs used in the perioperative period – including methadone, droperidol, and thioridazine – have received a black box warning for their ability to cause QT prolongation. Others – such as ondansetron and haloperidol – have had additional warnings added to the labeling because of their ability to prolong the QT intervals. Still others – including astemizole, cisapride, grepafloxacin, levacetylmethadol, mesoridazine, sertindole, terfenadine, and terodiline – have been withdrawn from the market due to QT-prolonging effects [64]. Drugs with a known potential to cause QT prolongation may be found in Table 46.2.

Summary

TdP is an uncommon but potentially life-threatening ventricular arrhythmia. QT prolongation, either congenital or acquired, is a risk factor for this occurrence. Many drugs have the ability to prolong the QT interval, and these drugs may have an additive effect. Hospitalized patients may be especially at risk for QT prolongation.

For patients receiving QT-prolonging medication, particularly multiple QT-prolonging medications, consideration should be given to periodic ECG monitoring as outpatients or for continuous telemetry while in the hospital setting. QT-prolonging drugs should be avoided in patients with predisposing factors for long QT syndrome when at all possible. Other risk factors, such as electrolyte abnormalities, should be considered and promptly treated.

TdP may be responsive to magnesium therapy or chemical or electrical overdrive pacing in addition to standard ACLS protocols. If TdP degenerates into ventricular fibrillation, standard ACLS maneuvers should be utilized.

Clinical Structures

Clinical Structure
46.1 Droperidol

References

1. Bazett HC. An analysis of the time-relations of electrocardiograms. Heart. 1920;7:353.
2. Drew BJ, Ackerman AJ, Funk M, Gibler WB, Kligfield P, Menon V, et al. Prevention of torsade de pointes in hospital settings: a scientific statement from the American Heart Association and the American College of Cardiology Foundation. JACC. 2010;55:934–47.
3. Lasser KE, Allen PD, Woolhandler SJ, Himmelstein DU, Wolfe SM, Bor DH. Timing of new black box warnings and withdrawals for prescription medications. JAMA. 2002;287:2215–20.

4. Dessertenne F. La tachycardia ventriculaire à deux foyers opposes variables. Arch Mal Coeur. 1966;59:263–72.
5. Barrett KE, Barman SM, Boitano S, Brooks HL, editors. Ganong's review of medical physiology. 24th ed. New York: McGraw-Hill; 2012.
6. Mitcheson JS, Chen J, Lin M. A structural basis for drug-induced long QT syndrome. Proc Natl Acad Sci U S A. 2000;97:12329–33.
7. Sanguinetti MC, Jiang C, Curran ME, Keating MT. A mechanistic link between an inherited and an acquired cardiac arrhythmia: HERG encodes the I_{kr} potassium channel. Cell. 1995;81: 299–307.
8. Debruin ML, Pettersson M, Meyboom RH, Hoes AW, Leufkens HGM. Anti-HERG activity and the risk of drug-induced arrhythmias and sudden death. Eur Heart J. 2005;26:590–7.
9. Antzelevitch C. Role of transmural dispersion of repolarization in the genesis of drug-induced torsades de pointes. Heart Rhythm. 2005;2:S9–15.
10. Roden DM, Hoffman BF. Action potential prolongation and induction of abnormal automaticity by low quinidine concentrations in canine Purkinje fibers: relationship to potassium and cycle length. Circ Res. 1985;56:857–67.
11. Sicouri S, Antzelevitch C. Drug-induced afterdepolarizations and triggered activity occur in a discrete subpopulation of ventricular muscle cells (M cells) in the canine heart: quinidine and digitalis. J Cardiovasc Electrophysiol. 1993;4:48–58.
12. Gupta A, Lawrence AT, Krishnan K, Kavinsky CJ, Trohman RG. Current concepts in the mechanisms and management of drug-induced QT prolongation and torsade de pointes. Am Heart J. 2007;153:891–9.
13. Roden DM, Lazarra R, Rosen M, Schwartz PJ, Towbin J, Vincent GM. Multiple mechanisms in the long-QT syndrome. Current knowledge, gaps, and future directions. The SADS Foundation Task Force on LQTS. Circulation. 1996;94:1996–2012.
14. El-Sharif N, Caref EB, Yin H, Restivo M. The electrophysiological mechanism of ventricular arrhythmias in the long QT syndrome: tridimensional mapping of activation and recovery patterns. Circ Res. 1996;79:474–92.
15. El-Sharif N, Caref EB, Chinushi M, Restivo M. Mechanism of arrhythmogenicity of the short-long cardiac sequence that precedes ventricular tachycardias in the long QT syndrome. J Am Coll Cardiol. 1999;33:1415–23.
16. Yap YJ, Camm AJ. Drug induced QT prolongation and torsades de pointes. Heart. 2003;89: 1363–72.
17. Zelster D, Justo D, Halkin A, Prokhorov V, Heller K, Viskin S. Torsade de pointes due to noncardiac drugs: most patients have easily identifiable risk factors. Medicine. 2003;82:282–90.
18. Makita N, Horie M, Nakamura T, Tomohiko A, Sasaki K, Yokoi H, et al. Drug-induced long-QT syndrome associated with a subclinical SCN5A mutation. Circulation. 2002;106:1269–74.
19. Yang P, Kanki H, Drolet B, Yang T, Wei J, Viswanathan PC, et al. Allelic variants in long-QT disease genes in patients with drug-associated torsades de pointes. Circulation. 2002;105: 1943–8.
20. Nagele P, Pal S, Brown F, Blood J, Miller JP, Johnston J. Postoperative QT interval prolongation in patients undergoing noncardiac surgery under general anesthesia. Anesthesiology. 2012;117:321–8.
21. Aypar E, Karagoz AH, Ozer S, Celiker A, Ocal T. The effects of sevoflurane and desflurane anesthesia on QTc interval and cardiac rhythm in children. Paediatr Anaesth. 2007;17: 563–7.
22. Karagoz AH, Basgul E, Celiker V, Aypar U. The effect of inhalational anaesthetics on QTc interval. Eur J Anaesthesiol. 2005;22:171–4.
23. Scuderi PE. Sevoflurane and QTc prolongation: an interesting observation, or a clinically significant finding? Anesthesiology. 2010;113:772–5.
24. Han DW, Park K, Jang SB, Kern SE. Modeling the effect of sevoflurane on corrected QT prolongation: a pharmacodynamic analysis. Anesthesiology. 2010;113:806–11.
25. Riley DC, Schmeling WT, Al-Wathiqui MH, Kampine JP, Wartlier DC. Prolongation of the QT interval by volatile anesthetics in chronically instrumented dogs. Anesth Analg. 1988;67:741–9.

26. Schmeling WT, Warltier DC, McDonald DJ, Madsen KE, Atlee JL, Kampine JP. Prolongation of the QT interval by enflurane, isoflurane, and halothane in humans. Anesth Analg. 1991;72: 137–44.
27. Silay E, Kati I, Tekin M, Guler N, Huseyinoglu UA, Coskuner I, et al. Comparison of the effects of desflurane and sevoflurane on the QTc interval and QT dispersion. Acta Cardiol. 2005;60:459–64.
28. Kazanci D, Unver S, Karadeniz U, Iyican D, Koruk S, Yilmaz MB, et al. A comparison of the effects of desflurane, sevoflurane, and propofol on QT, QTc, and P dispersion on ECG. Ann Card Anaesth. 2009;12:107–12.
29. Yildrim H, Adanir T, Atay A, Katircioglu K, Savaci S. The effects of sevoflurane, isoflurane and desflurane on QT interval of the ECG. Eur J Anaesthesiol. 2004;21:566–70.
30. Whyte SD, Booker PD, Buckley DG. The effects of propofol and sevoflurane on the QT interval and transmural dispersion of repolarization in children. Anesth Anal. 2005;100:71–7.
31. Saussine M, Massad I, Raczka F, Davy JM, Frapier JM. Torsades de pointes during sevoflurane in a child with congenital long QT syndrome. Paediatr Anaesth. 2006;16:63–5.
32. Tacken MC, Bracke FA, Van Zundert AA. Torsades de pointes during sevoflurane anesthesia and fluconazole infusion in a patient with long QT syndrome. Acta Anaesthesiol Belg. 2011;62:105–8.
33. Michaloudis DG, Kanakoudis FS, Petrou AM, Konstantinidou AS, Pollard BJ. The effects of midazolam or propofol followed by suxamethonium on the QT interval in humans. Eur J Anaesthesiol. 1996;13:364–8.
34. Saarnivaar L, Hiller A, Oikkonen M. QT interval, heart rate and arterial pressures using propofol, thiopentone, or methohexitone for induction of anaesthesia in children. Acta Anaesthesiol Scand. 1993;37:419–23.
35. Irie T, Kaneko Y, Nakajima T, Saito A, Kurabayashi M. QT interval prolongation and torsades de pointes induced by propofol and hypoalbuminemia. Int Heart J. 2010;51:365–6.
36. Saarnivaara L, Lindgren L. Prolongation of QT interval during induction of anaesthesia. Acta Anaesthesiol Scand. 1983;27:126–30.
37. Keller GA, Ponte ML, Di Girolamo G. Other drugs acting on nervous system associated with QT-interval prolongation. Curr Drug Saf. 2010;5:105–11.
38. Saarnivaara L, Klemola UM, Lindgren L. QT interval of the ECG, heart rate and arterial pressure using five non-depolarizing muscle relaxants for intubation. Acta Anaesthesiol Scand. 1988;32:623–8.
39. Adler A, Viskin S, Bhulyan ZA, Eisenberg E, Rosso R. Propoxyphene-induced torsades de pointes. Heart Rhythm. 2011;8:1952–4.
40. Krantz MJ, Kutinsky IB, Robertson AD, Mehler PS. Dose-related effects of methadone on QT prolongation in a series of patients with torsade de pointes. Pharmacotherapy. 2003;23:802–5.
41. Krantz MJ, Garcia JA, Mehler PS. Effects of buprenorphine on cardiac repolarization in a patient with methadone-related torsades de pointes. Pharmacotherapy. 2005;25:611–4.
42. Stringer J, Welsh C, Tommaselio A. Methadone-associated QT interval prolongation and torsades de pointes. Am J Health Syst Pharm. 2009;66:825–33.
43. Wieneke H, Conrads H, Wolstein J, Breuckmann F, Gastpar M, Erbel R, et al. Levo-alpha-acetylmethadol (LAAM) induced QTc-prolongation-results from a controlled clinical trial. Eur J Med Res. 2009;14:7–12.
44. Katchman AN, McGroary KA, Kilborn MJ, Kornick CA, Manfredi PL, Woosley RL, et al. Influence of opioid agonists on cardiac human ether-a-go-go-related gene K(+) currents. J Pharmacol Exp Ther. 2002;303:688–94.
45. Food and Drug Administration [Internet]. [Updated 2003 Sept; cited 2013 Feb 27]. FDA safety alert: Orlaam (levomethadyl acetate hydrochloride). Available from: http://www.fda.gov/Safety/MedWatch/SafetyInformation/SafetyAlertsforHumanMedicalProducts/ucm153332.htm.
46. Food and Drug Administration [Internet]. [Updated 2010 Nov; cited 2013 Feb 27]. FDA drug safety communication: propoxyphene: withdrawal – risk of cardiac toxicity. Available from: www.fda.gov/safety/medwatch/safetyinformation/safetyalertsforhumanmedicalproducts/ucm234389.htm.

47. Food and Drug Administration [Internet]. [Updated 2006 Nov; cited 2013 Feb 27]. FDA public health advisory: methadone use for pain control may result in death and life-threatening changes in breathing and heart beat. Available from: http://www.fda.gov/Drugs/DrugSafety/PostmarketDrugSafetyInformationforPatientsandProviders/DrugSafetyInformationfor HeathcareProfessionals/PublicHealthAdvisories/ucm124346.htm.

48. Food and Drug Administration [Internet]. [Updated 2001 Feb; cited 2013 Feb 27]. FDA safety alert: Inapsine (droperidol). Available from: http://www.fda.gov/Safety/MedWatch/SafetyInformation/SafetyAlertsforHumanMedicalProducts/ucm172364.htm.

49. Halloran K, Barash PG. Inside the black box: current policies and concerns with the United States Food and Drug Administration's highest drug safety warning system. Curr Opin Anaesthesiol. 2010;23:423–7.

50. White PF. Droperidol: a cost-effective antiemetic for over thirty years. Anesth Anal. 2002; 95:789–90.

51. Nutall GA, Eckerman KM, Jacob KA, Pawlaski EM, Wigersma SK, Marienau MES, et al. Does low-dose droperidol administration increase the risk of drug-induced QT prolongation and torsade de pointes in the general surgical population? Anesthesiology. 2007;107:531–6.

52. Turner S, Matthews L, Pandharipande P, Thompson R. Dolasetron-induced torsades de pointes. J Clin Anesth. 2007;19:622–5.

53. Boike SC, Ilson B, Zariffa N, Jorkasky DK. Cardiovascular effects of i.v. granisetron at two administration rates and of ondansetron in healthy adults. Am J Health Syst Pharm. 1997;54: 1172–6.

54. Benedict CR, Arbogast R, Martin L, Patton L, Morrill B, Hahne W. Single-blind study of the effects of intravenous dolasetron mesylate versus ondansetron on electrocardiographic parameters in normal volunteers. J Cardiovasc Pharmacol. 1996;28:53–9.

55. Food and Drug Administration [Internet]. [Updated 2001 Sept; cited 2013 Feb 27]. FDA alert: Anzemet (dolasetron mesylate) tablet and injection detailed view: safety labeling changes approved by FDA center for drug evaluation and research (CDER). Available from: http://www.fda.gov/Safety/MedWatch/SafetyInformation/ucm187424.htm.

56. Food and Drug Administration [Internet]. [Updated 2012 Jun; cited 2013 Feb 27]. FDA drug safety communication: new information regarding QT prolongation with ondansetron (Zofran). Available from: http://www.fda.gov/Drugs/DrugSafety/ucm310190.htm.

57. Food and Drug Administration [Internet]. [Updated 2011 Apr; cited 2013 Feb 27]. FDA alert: Kytril (granisetron hydrochloride) intravenous injection: safety labeling changes approved by FDA center for drug evaluation and research (CDER). Available from: http://www.fda.gov/Safety/MedWatch/SafetyInformation/ucm254261.htm.

58. Charbit B, Albaladejo P, Funck-Brentano C, Legrand M, Samain E, Marty J. Prolongation of QTc interval after postoperative nausea and vomiting treatment by droperidol or ondansetron. Anesthesiology. 2005;6:1094–100.

59. Charbit B, Alvarez JC, Dasque E, Abe E, Démolis JL, Funck-Brentano C. Droperidol and ondansetron-induced QT interval prolongation: a clinical drug interaction study. Anesthesiology. 2008;109:206–12.

60. Zipes DP, Camm AJ, Borggrefe M, Buxton AE, Chaitman B, Fromer M, et al. ACC/AHA/ESC 2006 guidelines for management of patients with ventricular arrhythmias and the prevention of sudden cardiac death: a report of the American College of Cardiology/American Heart Association Task Force and the European Society of Cardiology Committee for Practice Guidelines (Writing Committee to Develop Guidelines for management of patients with ventricular arrhythmias and the prevention of sudden cardiac death). J Am Coll Cardiol. 2006;48: e247–346.

61. Berg RA, Hemphill R, Abella BS, Aufderheide TP, Cave DM, Hazinski MF, et al. Part 8.2: management of cardiac arrest: 2010 American Heart Association Guidelines for cardiopulmonary resuscitation and emergency cardiovascular care. Circulation. 2010;122:S685–705.

62. Lazzara R. Antiarrhythmic drugs and torsades de pointes. Eur Heart J. 1994;14:H88–92.

63. Michalets EL. Update: clinically significant cytochrome P-450 drug interactions. Pharmacotherapy. 1998;18:84–112.

64. Roden DM. Drug-induced prolongation of the QT interval. N Engl J Med. 2004;350:1013–22.
65. AZ CERT [Internet]. [Updated 2013 Jan 2; cited 2013 Feb 27]. QT drugs to avoid. Available from: http://www.azcert.org/drugs_to_avoid.pdf.
66. Benson MR, Kotagal V, Oral H. A 26-year-old woman with recurrent loss of consciousness. J Gen Intern Med. 2011;26(12):1509.
67. Rowan SB, Darbar D. Genetic and molecular basis of arrhythmias. In: Yan G, Kowey PR, eds. Management of cardiac arrhythmias. 2nd ed. New York: Humana Press; 2011:65–86.

Chapter 47
Drugs and Cancer Propagation

Amit Prabhakar, Alan David Kaye, and Richard D. Urman

Contents

A. Prabhakar, MD, MS
Department of Anesthesiology, Louisiana State University
Health Sciences Center, New Orleans, LA, USA
e-mail: aprab1@lsuhsc.edu

A.D. Kaye, MD, PhD (✉)
Department of Anesthesiology, Tulane Medical Center, New Orleans, LA, USA

Department of Anesthesiology, Louisiana State University Health Sciences Center,
New Orleans, LA, USA
e-mail: alankaye44@hotmail.com

R.D. Urman, MD, MBA
Department of Anesthesiology, Perioperative and Pain Medicine, Brigham and Women's
Hospital, Harvard Medical School, Boston, MA, USA

Center for Perioperative Management and Medical Informatics, Brigham and Women's
Hospital, Boston, MA, USA
e-mail: urmanr@gmail.com

A.D. Kaye et al. (eds.), *Essentials of Pharmacology for Anesthesia,*
Pain Medicine, and Critical Care, DOI 10.1007/978-1-4614-8948-1_47,
© Springer Science+Business Media New York 2015

Introduction

Cancer is one of the most significant healthcare issues in both the developed and undeveloped world. The American Cancer Society projects that over 1,638,910 new cancer cases and over 577,190 cancer-related deaths will occur in the United States alone this year. The most prevalent cancers in the United States are breast, prostate, lung, and gastrointestinal, respectively [1].

Tireless research has greatly enhanced our knowledge base on cancer in recent years. Despite this, much is still needed to be learned about both cancer physiology and treatment. Current treatment modalities range from surgical excision, radiation, chemotherapy, to immunotherapy. The advent of more sensitive and specific screening tests has allowed for some cancers to be detected much earlier. This has given physicians the advantage of providing the patient with quicker treatment and better surgical options.

Opioid pharmacotherapy, in particular, has served as the mainstay in the treatment of acute and chronic cancer pain. However, both animal and human models have shown that opioid use can cause suppression of both the innate and acquired immune responses. This suppression may not only predispose patients to opportunistic infections but may also expedite the progression of cancer via metastasis [2, 3].

This chapter will examine the common modalities used to treat cancer pain, including opioid pharmacotherapy, surgery, and regional anesthesia, and explain how these may actually alter the tumor microenvironment and promote disease progression, metastasis, and recurrence.

Opioid Overview

Opioids are derived from opium poppy (Papaver somniferum) and are some of the most commonly prescribed medications to treat severe pain. Opium was first described as having medicinal use in the 1700s. Opioids used in the clinical setting today can be classified as either natural (codeine, morphine), semisynthetic (oxycodone, hydrocodone), fully synthetic (fentanyl, methadone, tramadol), or endogenous (endorphin, enkephalins, dynorphin) [4]. These ligands bind to four different opioid receptors; mu, delta, kappa, and nociceptin. It is important to note that the mu-opioid receptor mediates the analgesic activity of morphine and its congeners. Molecular analysis has found that these receptors are classic seven-transmembrane domain G protein-coupled receptors [5]. Once these receptors are ligand bound, their subunits go on to interact with several different downstream effector systems [5]. Opioid receptor expression is dictated by individual cell microenvironments that are influenced by both proinflammatory cytokines and growth factors [6]. Molecular and modern imaging techniques have confirmed an increase in the presence of opioid receptors in human cancers compared to normal tissue [4].

Opiates and the Immune System

Various forms of anesthesia and analgesia have all been found to exert an effect on both cellular and humoral immunity. These effects have been quantified by measuring fluctuations of key substances involved in normal immune response such as cytokines IL-2, IL-10, IL-12, and IFN-gamma [7]. While research remains limited, morphine and its congeners have been found to exert effects on almost all cells in the immune system including macrophages, neutrophils, T cells, and natural killer cells [8]. NK cells are vital to the rejection of tumor cells and viruses. Morphine can directly exert effects on immune cells expressing opioid receptors. Morphine has also been found to have indirect effects via the central nervous system and hypothalamic-pituitary axis activation [8].

It should be noted that the degree of opiate-induced immunosuppression is dependent on the specific opioid being used. Franchi et al. conducted an in vivo study of rats and examined their immune responses to different opioids [9]. They found that both morphine and fentanyl decreased NK cell function and increased metastasis. However, buprenorphine, a partial mu-receptor agonist, was actually found to have a more favorable immune profile devoid of intrinsic immunosuppressive activity [10]. Li et al. found that patients given high-dose fentanyl after esophageal cancer surgery showed a reduction in NK cell number assessed in peripheral blood when compared to presurgery [11].

Other Factors Alter Effectiveness of the Immune System

Intravenous Anesthetic Agents

Melamed et al. investigated the effect of various intravenous anesthetic agents on rodents injected with tumor cells [12]. There work revealed that ketamine, thiopental, and propofol all lead to decreased levels and effectiveness of NK cells [12]. Rats treated with ketamine were found to have 5.5 times the number of tumor cells compared to control rats. Rats treated with thiopental were found to have twice the number of tumor cells compared to the control rats [12]. Further studies revealed that conjugate products from propofol-DHA and propofol-EPA inhibited cellular adhesion, migration, and apoptosis of MDA-MB-31 breast cancer cells [13].

Inhalational Agents

Inhalational agents have also been shown to modulate the immune response by suppressing NK cell function [14, 15]. Mice models have shown that both isoflurane and halothane attenuate the interferon stimulation of NK cytotoxicity. Sevoflurane has also been found to alter cytokine release by NK and NK-like cells. General anesthesia leads to reduced circulation of NK cells in patients undergoing elective orthopedic surgeries [16]. The many variables associated with inhalational agents have made quantifying the magnitude of the immunosuppression difficult and further research is required.

Surgery and the Immune System

Further analysis in order to isolate the effects of opiates has proven difficult due to the suppressive effect major surgery itself has on cellular immunity. The surgical stress response results in the release of numerous proinflammatory cytokines that have been shown to either directly or indirectly promote tumor progression [17]. In rodents, surgical stress itself has been found to result in decreased NK cell activity and enhanced tumor cell metastasis. The neuro-sympatho-endocrine system also plays a key role in perioperative immunosuppression by the release of catecholamines and glucocorticoids [17]. Both catecholamines and glucocorticoids have been found to suppress cell-mediated immunity and affect cell migration and cell invasiveness [17]. Buprenorphine was found to actually reverse the surgical stress-induced increase in tumor metastasis in rodents [9]. The inflammatory response to surgery results in a cascade of chain reactions leading to cytokine release. In particular, IL-6 and IL-1beta have been shown to upregulate the expression of vascular endothelial growth factor, a key component to angiogenesis [17].

Factors That Contribute to Angiogenesis and Metastasis

Angiogenesis is defined as the growth of new vessels from preexisting blood vessels. During the early stages of tumor growth, immune cells are capable of recognizing stressed tumor cells and promote an effective immune response resulting in tumor death. However, in solid tumors that grow beyond $1–2 \text{ mm}^3$, hypoxia-induced tumor cell growth factor secretion can lead to angiogenesis [8]. This is compounded by the ability of some cancer cells to continually change their antigenic makeup and allow the evasion of the immune system. Morphine has been found to influence several key aspects of angiogenesis related to tumor growth and vascular permeability.

Molecular Factors

Ecimovic et al. studied the expression of NET1 in the presence of morphine. MDA-MB-231 (estrogen-positive) and MCF7 (estrogen-negative) breast cancer cells were incubated with morphine and an increase in cell proliferation over the control was observed. NET1 gene product plays an essential role in actin reorganization which can contribute to increased cellular migration and invasion [18].

Dysregulated expression of cyclin D1 is another key feature of angiogenesis and tumor growth. Cyclin D1 results in increased cell cycle progression and survival. Gupta et al. have found that clinically relevant doses of morphine stimulate endothelial cyclin D1 and subsequent cell cycle progression and survival by stimulating protein kinase B phosphorylation [5].

Morphine has also been implicated in the release of nitric oxide from endothelial cells [19]. Nitric oxide-dependent mitogen-activated protein kinase and protein kinase B phosphorylation can then act downstream to result in VEGF release [20, 21]. Therefore, while morphine stimulates nitric oxide and MAPK phosphorylation, it also indirectly results in VEGF receptor activation. Nitric oxide also stimulates the production of cyclooxygenase (COX) and subsequent production of prostaglandin E2 (PGE2). PGE2 is known to enhance angiogenesis. It has also been shown that selective COX-2 inhibitors are capable of inhibiting tumor progression [22–24]. Chronic morphine administration was also found to result in upregulation of COX-2 gene and PGE2 in breast tumors in A/J mice [25].

Vascular Integrity

Alteration in vascular permeability is another key component for angiogenesis. Endothelial cell integrity is maintained by several different junctions including adherens, gap, and tight. cAMP is a key regulator of endothelial barrier permeability [26]. Opioid receptor coupling and signaling by G (alpha i) inhibitory subunits lead to inhibition of adenylate cyclase, decreased cAMP, and an increase in barrier permeability in vitro [27, 28]. Interestingly, this increase in permeability can be blocked by pretreatment with methylnaltrexone, a mu-opioid receptor antagonist. Chronic exposure to opioids is actually associated with an increase in cAMP production [27]. This switch from G (alpha i) signaling to G (beta-gamma) signaling is postulated to be related to opioid tolerance [29].

Despite these findings, morphine has also been found to inhibit angiogenesis in certain animal models. Morphine inhibited tumor growth and prevented angiogenesis in a study using Lewis lung carcinoma cells [30].

Morphine's Promigratory Effect

Shanahan et al. performed a bioresponse assay in which they injected mice with morphine every 12 h for 3 days and then collected their serum. The serum was then used to test cell migration in a modified Boyden chamber assay towards control medium or medium added with 2 % serum prepared from morphine- and saline-treated mice (book pg 86). Researchers found that serum from morphine-injected mice was a much more potent chemoattractant than serum from the saline-injected mice. The addition of naloxone did not attenuate the migration induced by morphine-treated serum thus proving that the pro-migratory effect observed was not due to the presence of residual morphine in the serum. However, the pro-migratory effect was voided after the morphine-treated serum was heated. This has led investigators to postulate that an indirect effect of morphine treatment on cell migration was observed and contribute the effect to heat sensitive factors that are present in serum after pharmacologically active concentrations of morphine have been eliminated from circulation [31].

The Roles of Pain and Anxiety

Pain has been known to influence both the sympathetic and immune systems. There is evidence that uncontrolled pain by itself can stimulate cancer proliferation and spread and that the control of pain, by any method, is paramount for prevention. A prospective study followed patients who complained of both widespread and regional pain over an 8-year span [32]. This study found an association between reporting of widespread pain and death from cancer in both the medium and long term [32]. Smith et al. found that the use of intrathecal pumps in patients with refractory pain leads to better quality of life and improved survival [33]. Sassamura et al. found that pain control by either morphine or sciatic nerve neurectomy resulted in reduced tumor growth and lung metastasis in mice inoculated with painful tumors in the hind paw [34].

Anxiety has also been shown to create an environment that supports cancer growth and suppresses the immune system [7]. Stefanki et al. examined the effects of stress and immune function in rats [35]. Rats were injected with tumor cells and placed in situations that involved hostile interactions. Investigators found that rats that showed submissive behavior also had increases in lung tumor retention [35]. Human studies have examined the effect of chronic stress in patients during the periods of breast cancer diagnosis and surgery [36]. It was found that stress served as a significant predictor of lowered NK cell lysis [36]. Stress was also found to serve as a significant predictor of the proliferative response of peripheral blood lymphocytes to different proteins [36].

Is One Method of Cancer Analgesia Better than Others for Surgery?

Regional Anesthesia

Regional anesthesia has been postulated to influence the long-term outcome of cancer surgery in three ways [7, 37]. Firstly, regional anesthesia may attenuate the intrinsic immunosuppression induced from surgery [38]. Secondly, patients who receive regional anesthesia often do not require as much opioid therapy postoperatively, thus avoiding the immunosuppressive effects that accompany opioid use [39]. Lastly, use of regional anesthesia lessens the amount of general anesthesia needed [7]. Studies have shown that patients who undergo regional anesthesia have lower plasma levels of cortisol and epinephrine and better T-cell function postoperatively compared to patients who did not [40, 41]. Another small study of 32 patients found that regional anesthesia resulted in decreased levels of VEGF and TNF-B postoperatively, both key markers for inflammation and metastatic potential [42].

Local Anesthetics

Local anesthetics have been shown to have beneficial effects in the setting of cancer surgery and tumor suppression. Both lidocaine and ropivacaine have been found to provide direct inhibition of cancer cell proliferation [43, 44]. Lidocaine was found to inhibit the epidermal growth factor receptor (EGFR) in tongue cancer cells [43]. This inhibition of EGF also subsequently led to a reduction in the tyrosine kinase activity that stimulates EGFR [43]. Ropivacaine has been found to inhibit the proliferation of human colon adenocarcinoma cancer cells in a dose-dependent manner [44]. Research remains limited and further studies are needed to confirm the clinical significance of these findings.

Epidural Anesthesia and Analgesia

The use of epidural anesthesia has been well known to reduce the amount of anesthetic and analgesic agents used in the perioperative and postoperative period. It has been postulated that epidural anesthesia results in attenuation of the surgical stress response, thus limiting the extent of immunosuppression [45].

Prostate Cancer

Biki et al. performed a retrospective analysis to determine if the utilization of epidural anesthesia provided any benefit over conventional anesthetic methods in relation to cancer recurrence and metastasis [46]. They analyzed 225 patients undergoing radical prostatectomy and divided patients into two groups. One group underwent conventional general anesthesia with opioids. The other group was treated with a combination of epidural and general anesthesia. The study defined biochemical recurrence as an increase in prostate-specific antigen (PSA) compared with its immediate postoperative nadir. The follow-up interval was 2.8–12.8 years. After adjusting for tumor size, Gleason score, and preoperative PSA, Biki et al. found a 57 % decrease in the recurrence of cancer in patients who received the combination of epidural and general anesthesia compared to patients receiving general anesthesia and opiates [46]. However, limitations to this study must be mentioned. First, because this is a retrospective study, there is a potential for unidentified confounding factors. Questions were also raised due to lack of specific documentation of the medications and duration of treatment in the epidural patients.

Tsui et al. conducted a similar retrospective analysis of 99 patients looking also at the rate of disease recurrence [47]. Median follow-up time was 4.5 years and biochemical recurrence was defined as $PSA > 0.2$ ng/ml. Their analysis found no difference between patients who received epidural anesthesia compared to those in the general anesthesia group. Limitations to this study include small sample size subsequently leading to possible type 2 error.

More recently, retrospective studies from both Wuethrich et al. and Forget et al. found that epidural anesthesia was associated with a decrease in cancer progression and recurrence [48, 49]. Further evidence is needed in order to clearly identify the potential benefits epidural analgesia plays in the role of prostate cancer surgery [46, 47].

Ovarian Cancer

De Oliveira et al. published a retrospective analysis of 182 patients with ovarian cancer who underwent cytoreductive ovarian debulking [45]. Each patient in this study underwent general anesthesia and there were no patients who only received epidural anesthesia. Induction was performed with fentanyl 2–3 mcg/kg, midazolam 0.02–0.04 mg/kg, and propofol 1.5–2.5 mg/kg. Sevoflurane was used as the maintenance agent. Researchers identified the primary end point as time to recurrence, defined as $CA\text{-}125 > 21$ u/ml. The secondary end point was time to death.

Patient health records were analyzed for 3–9 years and stratified into three groups. The first group consisted of 127 patients who did not receive either epidural anesthesia or analgesia. The second group consisted of 26 patients who received epidural anesthesia both intraoperatively and postoperatively. The third group consisted of 29 patients who received epidural anesthesia and analgesia for postoperative pain control only. Thus, out of 182 patients, 127 received only intravenous opioids for intraoperative and postoperative control, while 55 patients received epidural anesthesia [45].

Kaplan-Meier survival curves were obtained and a log-rank test was used in order to compare median survival and time to recurrence between groups. Patients who received preoperative epidurals had an increased time to recurrence of ovarian cancer at 73 months compared to patients who either did not receive any epidurals or those who received epidurals for postoperative pain control only. Patients who did not receive epidurals had an average of 38 months ($p < 0.001$) time to recurrence. Patients who received epidurals for postoperative pain control only had an average of 33 months time to recurrence [45]. It must be noted that this study did have a confounding variable bias. Neither operative care nor postoperative care was standardized.

Colon Cancer

Gottaschalk et al. retrospectively examined 699 patients with colon cancer for 7 years [50]. Investigators separated the patients into two groups and compared the time to recurrence between them. The first group of patients underwent colorectal surgery with epidural anesthesia. The second group underwent colorectal surgery under general anesthesia. Median follow-up time for the study was 1.8 years. Cancer recurrence was detected in 16 % of patients who did not receive epidurals compared to 13 % of patients who did receive epidurals [50].

It must be noted that patients who received epidural therapy shared certain characteristics. More males than females received epidural therapy. These patients also had lower American Society of Anesthesiologists classification scores, worse tumor grades, and received lower FiO_2 intraoperatively. Also these patients underwent different surgical procedures, received greater crystalloid volume, had higher estimated blood loss, and were more likely to receive radiation and chemotherapy [50].

Multivariable analysis of this study showed no association between the use of epidurals and the time to recurrence of cancer ($p = 0.043$). Post hoc analysis of nine pairwise interactions indicated that only age expressed a linear effect. Stratification between patients <64 years old and those >64 years old revealed that patients >64 years old experienced better outcomes with the use of epidurals.

Christopherson et al. performed a prospective multicenter analysis of colon cancer patients called Cooperative Study Number 345 (CSN345) [51]. Investigators randomized 1,021 patients into two groups who either only received general anesthesia or those treated with epidural anesthesia supplemented with general anesthesia. Patients were followed for 30 days to an end point of death.

During the 30-day postoperative period, the two groups did not have significant differences in either death or major complications. Christopherson et al. further expanded on the trial by employing multivariable analysis to construct log regression survival models. These models were used to analyze pathological stage, type of anesthesia used, and other variables. The models showed that patients without metastases who had epidural anesthesia had improved survival within 1.46 years ($p = 0.012$). However, after 1.46 years, the type of anesthesia used did not affect survival. Epidural anesthesia had no effect on survival in patients with metastasis. Christopherson et al. stated that their investigation was preliminary and further co-variables, such as cause of death, need to be further examined [51].

Other Significant Studies

The effects of regional anesthesia on long-term cancer survival in patients were also studied in a randomized prospective trial that involved 446 patients at 23 clinical sites [52]. This study focused on abdominal procedures with the goal of complete surgical excision of cancers. Surgical procedures included esophagectomy, gastrectomy, nephrectomy, cystectomy, radical hysterectomy, and open prostatectomy.

Patient populations were divided into two groups. One group received epidural anesthesia both intraoperatively and postoperatively while the other group opioid-based postoperative analgesia. The primary end point was identified as cancer-free survival. The secondary end point was all causes of mortality. These end points were measured at 5-year increments for up to 15 years. Both cancer recurrence and survival from the date of surgery were recorded. Investigators that collected follow-up data were blinding to exposure status in an attempt to minimize bias. Both groups of patients received standardized premedication, intraoperative monitoring, and induction and maintenance anesthesia. Epidural catheters were inserted in the thoracic region with continuous infusions of ropivacaine supplemented with either fentanyl or meperidine. The epidurals were kept in for approximately 3 days post-operatively [52].

Extrapolated data found the median time to recurrence of cancer or death in patients who received epidural anesthesia was 2.6 years. The median time to recurrence of cancer or death in the non-epidural group was 2.8 years ($p=0.61$, hazard ratio 0.95, CI 0.76–1.17). Further analysis of the data identified significant predictors of early death or cancer recurrence. These include patient age ($p<0.001$), sex, and risk from red blood cell transfusion. Of note, the epidural group did not show any negative predictors. Strengths of this study include large sample size, randomization, and adequate follow-up time. However, weaknesses of study include exclusion criteria for smaller effects that may still be of considerable clinical importance, particularly for individual cancer types. The study also lacked power ($n=446$).

Approximately 29 other prospective clinical trials are underway currently with more clinical trials anticipated [52]. These will help to further elucidate the role of epidural anesthesia in the context of oncology care.

Paravertebral Block

Paravertebral blocks are a commonly used alternative to epidural anesthesia. These blocks have been found to be maximally beneficial for unilateral thoracic surgery such as breast cancer excision and are also associated with a reduced adverse event profile when compared to epidural anesthesia [53, 54].

The most significant findings related to paravertebral blocks were published by Exadaktylos et al. [55]. They conducted a retrospective analysis of 129 patients with breast cancer who underwent simple mastectomy with axillary clearance over a 1-year span. The patients were divided into two main groups. One group was given general anesthesia with postoperative intravenous morphine. The other group was given a paravertebral block with general anesthesia. Patients who underwent wide local excision and sentinel axillary lymph node procedures were excluded because these operations did not require paravertebral blocks and were seen as less extensive [55].

The paravertebral block was standardized among patients with a 0.2 ml/kg bolus of 0.25 % levobupivacaine before induction of general anesthesia. The infusion for each patient was scheduled for 48 h postoperatively. It is important to note that the same anesthetist placed all of the paravertebral catheters, the same surgeon performed all operations, the same oncologist cared for each patient, and the same general anesthesia protocol was used for each patient.

Cancer recurrence or metastasis was documented in 6 % of patients who received the paravertebral block. However, patients who received only general anesthesia and morphine were documented to have a 24 % rate of cancer recurrence or metastasis. Multivariable analysis also indicated that the risk of recurrence was less after the adjustment for both tumor histological grade and degree of axillary involvement. The study is limited because it is both retrospective and nonrandomized. The authors also mention that other confounding variables such as tumor size, margin size, chemotherapy regimes, and the amount of postoperative analgesia used further limited the study [55].

Investigators at the Cleveland Clinic are currently conducting a prospective, multicenter clinical trial with an enrollment of approximately 1,100 patients over a 5-year span [56]. This trial will test the hypothesis that local or metastatic recurrence after breast cancer surgery is lower with the utilization of paravertebral block and light sedation compared to recurrence from general anesthesia and opiate use. Until further studies are performed, the potentially protective effects of paravertebral blocks in regard to metastasis and recurrence must be considered with caution.

Conclusion

The financial cost of the care and treatment of cancer patients places a huge financial burden on the already taxed American healthcare system. While the medical community has made great strides to better understand cancer physiology, much is still needed to be done. Research shows that both cell-mediated and humoral-mediated immunities are suppressed by anesthetics and analgesics. Regional anesthesia has been associated with a reduction of metastasis and surgical site infections and improved long-term survival rates. However, further research is needed in order to fully understand its role in oncologic treatment plans. While the use of morphine and other opiates during the perioperative period may solely contribute to cancer metastasis and recurrence, it is more probable that this effect is multifactorial. The clinical anesthesiologist needs to be cognizant of these factors when preparing for both cancer pain management and cancer surgery.

Chemical Structures

Chemical Structure
47.1 Morphine

Chemical Structure
47.2 Ropivacaine

Chemical Structure
47.3 Levobupivacaine

References

1. American Cancer Society. Cancer facts & figures 2012. Atlanta: American Cancer Society; 2012.
2. Vallejo R, de Leon-Casasola O, Benyamin R. Opioid therapy and immunosuppression: a review. Am J Ther. 2004;11(5):354–65. Epub 2004/09/10.
3. McCarthy L, Wetzel M, Sliker JK, Eisenstein TK, Rogers TJ. Opioids, opioid receptors, and the immune response. Drug Alcohol Depend. 2001;62(2):111–23. Epub 2001/03/14.
4. Gupta K. Iatrogenic angiogenesis. In: Parat MO, editor. Morphine and metastasis. Dordrecht: Springer; 2013: chap 5.

5. Gupta M, Yunfang L, Gupta K. Opioids as promoters and regulators of angiogenesis. In: Maragoudakis ME, Papadimitriou E, editors. Angiogenesis: basic science and clinical applications. Kerala: Transworld Research Network. 2007; p. 303–17.

6. Borner C, Kraus J, Schroder H, Ammer H, Hollt V. Transcriptional regulation of the human mu-opioid receptor gene by interleukin-6. Mol Pharmacol. 2004;66:1719–26.

7. Snyder, Greenberg. Effect of anaesthetic technique and other perioperative factors on cancer recurrence. Br J Anaesth. 2010;105(2):106–15.

8. Koodie L, Roy S. Morphine and immunosuppression in the context of tumor growth and metastasis. In: Parat MO, editor. Morphine and metastasis. Dordrecht: Springer; 2013: chap 3.

9. Franchi S, Panerai AE, Sacerdote P. Buprenorphine ameliorates the effect of surgery on hypothalamus-pituitary-adrenal axis, natural killer cell activity and metastatic colonization in rats in comparison with morphine and fentanyl treatment. Brain Behav Immun. 2007;21(6): 767–74.

10. Sacerdote P. Opioid-induced immunosuppression. Curr Opin Support Palliat Care. 2008;2(1):14–8.

11. Li W, Tang HZ, Jiang YB, Xu MX. Influence of different doses of fentanyl on T-lymphocyte and subpopulations and natural killer cells of patients with esophageal tumor during preoperation and postoperation. Ai Zheng. 2003;22(6):634–6.

12. Melamed R, Bar-Yosef S, Shakhar G, Shakhar K, Ben-Eliyahu S. Suppression of natural killer cell activity and promotion of tumor metastasis by ketamine, thiopental, and halothane, but not by propofol: mediating mechanisms and prophylactic measures. Anesth Analg. 2003;97:1331–9.

13. Siddiqui RA, Zerouga M, Wu M, Castillo A, Harvey K, Zaloga GP, Stillwell W. Anticancer properties of propofol-docosahexaenoate and propofol-eicosapentaenoate on breast cancer cells. Breast Cancer Res. 2005;7:R645–54.

14. Markovic SN, Knight PR, Murasko DM. Inhibition of interferon stimulation of natural killer cell activity in mice anesthetized with halothane or isoflurane. Anesthesiology. 1993;78(4):700–6. Epub 1993/04/01.

15. Hole A, Unsgaard G. The effect of epidural and general anaesthesia on lymphocyte functions during and after major orthopaedic surgery. Acta Anaesthesiol Scand. 1983;27(2):135–41. Epub 1983/04/01.

16. Brand JM, Kirchner H, Poppe C, Schmucker P. The effects of general anesthesia on human peripheral immune cell distribution and cytokine production. Clin Immunol Immunopathol. 1997;83:190–4.

17. Shilling AM, Mohamed T. Perioperative morphine and cancer recurrence. In: Parat MO, editor. Morphine and metastasis. Dordrecht: Springer; 2013: chap 9.

18. Ecimovic P, Murray D, Doran P, McDonald J, Lambert DG, Buggy DJ. Direct effect of morphine on breast cancer cell function in vitro: role of the NET1 gene. Br J Anaesth. 2011;107:916–23.

19. Stefano GB, Hartman A, Bilfinger TV, Magazine HI, Liu Y, Casares F, Goligorsky MS. Presence of the mu3 opiate receptor in endothelial cells: coupling to nitric oxide production and vasodilation. J Biol Chem. 1995;270:30290–3.

20. Gupta K, Kshirsagar S, Chang L, Schwartz R, Law PY, Yee D, Hebbel RP. Morphine stimulates angiogenesis by activating proangiogenic and survival promoting signaling and promotes breast tumor growth. Cancer Res. 2002;62:4491–8.

21. Poonawala T, Levay-Young BK, Hebbel RP, Gupta K. Opioids heal ischemic wounds in the rat. Wound Repair Regen. 2005;13:165–74.

22. Chang SH, Liu CH, Conway R, Han DK, Nithipatikom K, Trifan OC, Lane TF, Hla T. Role of prostaglandin e2-dependent angiogenic switch in cyclooxygenase 2-induced breast cancer progression. Proc Natl Acad Sci. 2004;101:591–6.

23. Griffin RJ, Williams BW, Wild R, Cherrington JM, Park H, Song CW. Simultaneous inhibition of the receptor tyrosine kinase activity of vascular endothelial, fibroblast, and platelet-derived growth factors suppresses tumor growth and enhances tumor radiation response. Cancer Res. 2002;62:4491–8.

24. Leahy KM, Ornberg RL, Wang Y, Zweifel BS, Koki AT, Masferrer JL. COX-2 inhibition by celecoxib reduces proliferation and induces apoptosis in angiogenic endothelial cells in vivo. Cancer Res. 2002;62:625–31.

25. Farooqui M, Li Y, Rogers T, Poonawala T, Griffin RJ, Song CW, Gupta K. COX-2 inhibitor celecoxib prevents chronic morphine-induced promotion of angiogenesis, tumour growth, metastasis and mortality, without compromising analgesia. Br J Cancer. 2007;97:1523–31.

26. Moore TM, Chetham PM, Kelly JJ, Stevens T. Signal transduction and regulation of lung endothelial cell permeability: interaction between calcium and cAMP. Am J Physiol. 1998;275:L203–22.

27. Al-Hasani R, Bruchas MR. Molecular mechanisms of opioid receptor-dependent signaling and behavior. Anesthesiology. 2011;115:1363–81.

28. Sharma SK, Nirenberg M, Klee WA. Morphine receptors as regulators of adenylate cyclase activity. Proc Natl Acad Sci. 1975;72:590–4.

29. Gintzler AR, Chakrabarti S. Post opioid receptor adaptations to chronic morphine; altered functionality and associations of signaling molecules. Life Sci. 2006;79:717–22.

30. Koodie L, Ramakrishnan S, Roy S. Morphine suppresses tumor angiogenesis through a HIF-1alpha/p38MAPK pathway. Am J Pathol. 2010;177:984–97.

31. Shanahan H, Parat MO, Buggy D. Could opioids affect cancer recurrence or metastases? Current experimental and translational evidence. In: Parat MO, editor. Morphine and metastasis. Dordrecht: Springer; 2013: chap 6.

32. Macfarlane GJ, McBeth J, Silman AJ. Widespread body pain and mortality: prospective population based study. BMJ. 2001;323:662–5.

33. Smith TJ, Staats PS, Deer T, Stearns LJ, Rauck RL, Boortz-Marx RL, Buchser E, Catala E, Bryce DA, Coyne PJ, Pool GE. Randomized clinical trial of an implantable drug delivery system compared with comprehensive medical management for refractory cancer pain: impact on pain, drug-related toxicity, and survival. J Clin Oncol. 2002;20:4040–9.

34. Sasamura T, Nakamura S, Lida Y, Fujii H, Murata J, Saiki I, Nojima H, Kuraishi Y. Morphine analgesia suppresses tumor growth and metastasis in a mouse model of cancer pain produced by orthotopic tumor inoculation. Eur J Pharmacol. 2002;441:185–91.

35. Stefanski V, Ben-Eliyahu S. Social confrontation and tumor metastasis in rats: defeat and beta-adrenergic mechanisms. Physiol Behav. 1996;60:277–82.

36. Andersen BL, Farrar WB, Golden-Kreutz D, Kutz LA, MacCallum R, Courtney ME, Glaser R. Stress and immune responses after surgical treatment for regional breast cancer. J Natl Cancer Inst. 1998;90:30–6.

37. Sessler DI. Does regional analgesia reduce the risk of cancer recurrence? A hypothesis. Eur J Cancer Prev. 2008;17:269–72.

38. O'Riain SC, Buggy DJ, Kerin MJ, Watson RW, Moriarty DC. Inhibition of the stress response to breast cancer surgery by regional anesthesia and analgesia does not affect vascular endothelial growth factor and prostaglandin E2. Anesth Analg. 2005;100:244–9.

39. Moller JF, Nikolajsen L, Rodt SA, Ronning H, Carlsson PS. Thoracic paravertebral block for breast cancer surgery: a randomized double-blind study. Anesth Analg. 2007;105:1848–51.

40. Murphy GS, Szokol JW, Marymont JH, Avram MJ, Vender JS. The effects of morphine and fentanyl on the inflammatory response to cardiopulmonary bypass in patients undergoing elective coronary artery bypass graft surgery. Anesth Analg. 2007;104(6):1334–42, table of contents. Epub 2007/05/22.

41. Ahlers O, Nachtigall I, Lenze J, Goldmann A, Schulte E, Hohne C, Fritz G, Keh D. Intraoperative thoracic epidural anaesthesia attenuates stress-induced immunosuppression in patients undergoing major abdominal surgery. Br J Anaesth. 2008;101(6):781–7. Epub 2008/10/17.

42. Looney M, Doran P, Buggy DJ. Effect of anesthetic technique on serum vascular endothelial growth factor C and transforming growth factor beta in women undergoing anesthesia and surgery for breast cancer. Anesthesiology. 2010;113(5):1118–25.

43. Sakaguchi M, Kuroda Y, Hirose M. The antiproliferative effect of lidocaine on human tongue cancer cells with inhibition of the activity of epidermal growth factor receptor. Anesth Analg. 2006;102:1103–7.

44. Martinsson T. Ropivacaine inhibits serum-induced proliferation of colon adenocarcinoma cells in vitro. J Pharmacol Exp Ther. 1999;288:660–4.
45. de Oliveira Jr GS, Ahmad S, Schink JC, Singh DK, Fitzgerald PC, McCarthy RJ. Intraoperative neuraxial anesthesia but not postoperative neuraxial analgesia is associated with increased relapse-free survival in ovarian cancer patients after primary cytoreductive surgery. Reg Anesth Pain Med. 2011;36(3):271–7.
46. Biki B, Mascha E, Moriarty DC, Fitzpatrick JM, Sessler DI, Buggy DJ. Anesthetic technique for radical prostatectomy surgery affects cancer recurrence: a retrospective analysis. Anesthesiology. 2008;109(2):180–7.
47. Tsui BC, Rashiq S, Schopflocher D, Murtha A, Broemling S, Pillay J, Finucane BT. Epidural anesthesia and cancer recurrence rates after radical prostatectomy. J Can Anaesth. 2010;57(2):107–12.
48. Wuethrich PY, Hsu Schmitz SF, Kessler TM, Thalmann GN, Studer UE, Stueber F, Burkhard FC. Potential influence of the anesthetic technique used during open radical prostatectomy on prostate cancer-related outcome: a retrospective study. Anesthesiology. 2010;113(3):570–6.
49. Forget P, Tombal B, Scholtes JL, Nzimbala J, Meulders C, Legrand C, Van Cangh P, Cosyns JP, De Kock M. Do intraoperative analgesics influence oncological outcomes after radical prostatectomy for prostate cancer? Eur J Anaesthesiol. 2011;28:830–5.
50. Gottschalk A, Ford JG, Regelin CC, You J, Mascha EJ, Sessler DI, Durieux ME, Nemergut EC. Association between epidural analgesia and cancer recurrence after colorectal cancer surgery. Anesthesiology. 2010;113(1):27–34.
51. Christopherson R, James KE, Tableman M, Marshall P, Johnson FE. Long-term survival after colon cancer surgery: a variation associated with choice of anesthesia. Anesth Analg. 2008;107(1):325–32.
52. Myles PS, Peyton P, Silbert B, Hunt J, Rigg JR, Sessler DI. Perioperative epidural analgesia for major abdominal surgery for cancer and recurrence-free survival: randomised trial. BMJ. 2011;342:d1491.
53. Schnabel A, Reichl SU, Kranke P, Pogatzki-Zahn EM, Zahn PK. Efficacy and safety of paravertebral blocks in breast surgery: a meta analysis of randomized controlled trials. Br J Anaesth. 2010;105:842–52.
54. Wenk M, Schug SA. Perioperative pain management after thoracotomy. Curr Opin Anaesthesiol. 2011;24:8–12.
55. Exadaktylos AK, Buggy DJ, Moriarty DC, Mascha E, Sessler DI. Can anesthetic technique for primary breast cancer surgery affect recurrence or metastasis? Anesthesiology. 2006;105(4):660–4.
56. Sessler DI, Ben-Eliyahu S, Mascha EJ, Parat MO, Buggy DJ. Can regional analgesia reduce the risk of recurrence after breast cancer? Methodology of a multicenter randomized trial. Contemp Clin Trials. 2008;29(4):517–26.

Chapter 48
Lipid-Lowering Agents

Scott D. Friedman and Brian McClure

Contents

Introduction

One of the most important jobs as an anesthesiologist is to reduce the incidence of adverse perioperative outcome and reduce the incidence of morbidity and mortality associated with various surgeries. Historically, this has been done through applying various medical therapies perioperatively and even postoperatively. Searching for the best therapies is a constant, ongoing pursuit to better the field of anesthesiology. Two huge examples of this ongoing pursuit to find medical therapies to reduce morbidity and mortality in the perioperative period include the use of pre-incision prophylactic antibiotics and perioperative beta-blockade. Another huge modality that is

S.D. Friedman, MD • B. McClure (✉)
Department of Anesthesiology, Tulane University School of Medicine,
New Orleans, LA, USA
e-mail: sdf4444@gmail.com; brian.mcclure@hcahealthcare.com

A.D. Kaye et al. (eds.), *Essentials of Pharmacology for Anesthesia,*
Pain Medicine, and Critical Care, DOI 10.1007/978-1-4614-8948-1_48,
© Springer Science+Business Media New York 2015

gaining interest is the use of 3-hydroxy-3-methylglutaryl-coenzyme A (HMG-CoA) reductase inhibitors, also known as statins, as well as other lipid-lowering drugs.

Statins are the prototypical lipid-lowering drugs that have shown promise in improving perioperative outcomes in reducing morbidity and mortality. Although statins are the prototypical medications for lowering lipids, other drugs with lipid-lowering affects have also shown promise. This review chapter will give an overview of the pharmacology of statins, summarize the mechanisms of the beneficial effects of statins, provide an overview of the evidence in the use of statins in the perioperative period, and also provide information on newer and less researched lipid-lowering drugs and their effect on morbidity and mortality if given perioperatively (Fig. 48.1).

Drug Classes

Statins

Statins are the gold standard for lowering cholesterol. This class of medications was originally created through extraction from a genus of fungal class Ascomycetes, *Penicillium citrinum*. In vivo, the initial and prototypical statin applicable to humans was mevastatin. Mevastatin ultimately was converted into lovastatin, the first FDA-approved statin used for therapeutic cholesterol-lowering capabilities. Lovastatin was isolated from the fungus *Aspergillus terreus* [1]. Over time, numerous statins with lipid-lowering effects have been studied, researched, and created and have now become one of the most convincing therapies in the treatment of coronary artery disease and other atherosclerotic and embolic disease states [4, 32].

There are six major derivatives of statins: lovastatin, pravastatin, simvastatin, atorvastatin, fluvastatin, and rosuvastatin (Fig. 48.2). All of these variations have a structure similar to HMG-CoA, which is what gives statins their reversible and competitive inhibitory effects on HMG-CoA [1].

Pharmacology

As mentioned before, statins are competitive inhibitors of HMG-CoA reductase, which converts HMG-CoA to mevalonate (Fig. 48.3). This initial step is the rate-limiting step in the synthesis of cholesterol. Statins decrease low-density lipoprotein (LDL) through a multistep process that occurs initially in the liver hepatocytes. Statins interfere with hepatic cholesterol synthesis, which leads to an enhanced expression of the LDL receptor gene. The increase in triggered transcription factors then signals an increase in the synthesis of LDL receptors, which also limits degradation of LDL receptors. Finally, this increased number of LDL receptors augments the removal of LDL from the blood [1, 2]. Another theory as to how statins ultimately lower LDL levels is through the removal of LDL precursors. These precursors,

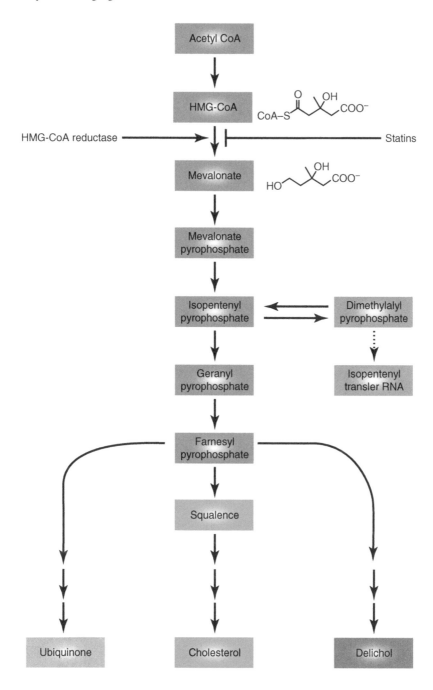

Fig. 48.1 Acetyl-CoA pathway to its end points

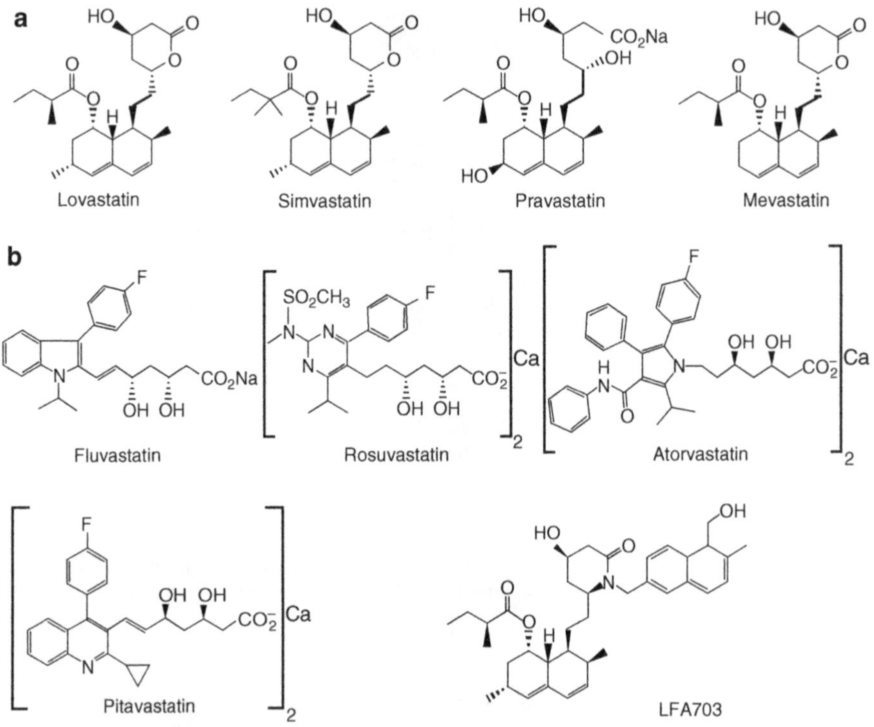

Fig. 48.2 Examples of different statins

Fig. 48.3 Rate-limiting step in the pathway of cholesterol

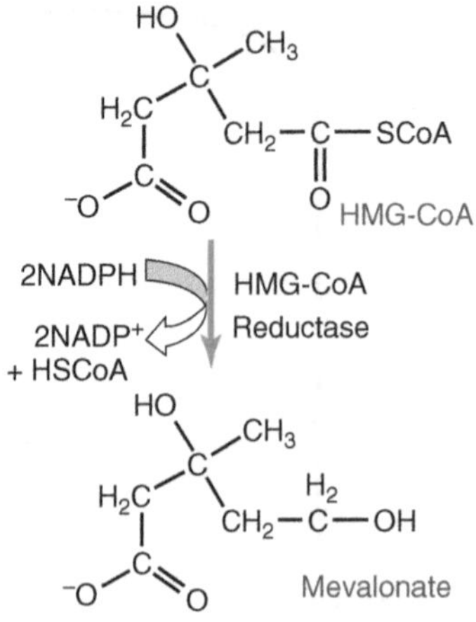

very-low-density lipoprotein and intermediate-density lipoprotein (VLDL and IDL), are made up of apoB-100. The increased numbers of LDL receptors function to eliminate apoB-100 and ultimately decrease further LDL production [1, 3].

Pharmacokinetics

Statins are primarily metabolized via hepatic enzymes and the cytochrome P450 3A4 hydroxylation pathway. Intestinal absorption of statins can reach up to 85 % after oral intake. The main form of drug elimination is via hepatic biliary excretion with less than 2 % recovered in the urine [22]. All statins are either administered in their active, B-hydroxy acid, form or as inactive lactones, which require transformation into active B-hydroxy acid forms. The already active statins, atorvastatin, pravastatin, fluvastatin, and rosuvastatin, are capable of inhibiting HMG-CoA reductase prior to undergoing transformation. However, the inactive statins, simvastatin and lovastatin, must first be transformed in the liver to their respective B-hydroxy acids prior to having downstream effects. Due to the transformation process required for activation, these statins undergo high intestinal clearance and first-pass metabolism and have a low systemic availability (5–30 %). Food has been shown to reduce the rate of statin absorption as well. Most statins reach a maximum plasma concentration in about 1–4 h. However, rosuvastatin and atorvastatin, two of the long-acting statins, have half-lives of 15–20 h with a maximum plasma concentration of 2–4 h. The longer half-lives yield greater efficacy of cholesterol-lowering capability [15].

Mechanism of Lipid-Dependent Effects of Statins

Multiple studies have demonstrated the effects of statin use on reducing coronary events in multiple patient populations, including men, women, African American, diabetics, smokers, and hypertensive patients [9–14]. It has been proven that reduction in LDL cholesterol concentration can potentially prevent cardiovascular disease, such as myocardial infarction (MI). There is a 25–30 % reduction in mortality when statin derivatives are used for primary and secondary prevention of cardiovascular disease in patients 60–80 years of age [5, 33, 34] (Fig. 48.4).

Mechanism of Lipid-Independent Effects of Statins

Studies have proven that statins have multiple cholesterol-related cardiovascular benefits. These studies have also proven that statins also provide other cholesterol-independent effects on protecting the cardiovascular system. The main studied cholesterol-independent benefits include the anti-inflammatory response, antithrombosis, enhanced fibrinolysis, vasodilation, and decreased platelet reactivity. These are described below and are outlined in Fig. 48.5 [6].

Anti-inflammatory

The figure below (Fig. 48.6) graphically helps demonstrate the anti-inflammatory effects of statins. One of the many by-products of the cholesterol synthesis pathway is isoprenoids. The entire cholesterol synthesis pathway is disrupted by statins

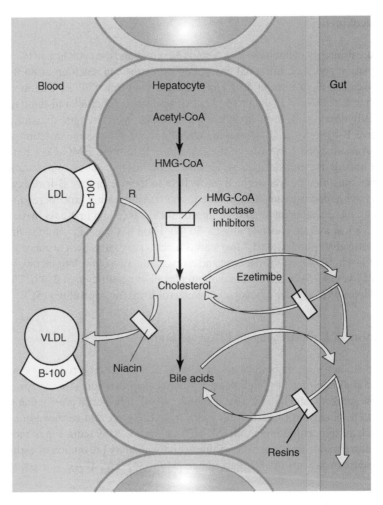

Fig. 48.4 Mechanism of Lipid-Dependent Effects of Statins. *Source*: Katzung et al. [3], http://www.accessmedicine.com/

influence on inhibiting HMG-CoA reductase. Therefore, the inhibition of HMG-CoA in turn downregulates and inhibits the formation of isoprenoids. The inhibition of isoprenoids in turn prevents downstream inflammatory signaling via the obstruction of Rho and Ras. Rho and Ras are two inflammatory signals in the human body. Rho eventually activates nuclear factor, NF-κB, which signals inflammatory responses and reduces endothelial nitric oxide synthase. Therefore, through a multistep inhibition pathway, statins inhibit Rho and Ras and help to inhibit the inflammatory pathway [7].

Another important anti-inflammatory effect of statins is through their effect on the cytokine pathway and inhibiting plaque rupture [8]. Many studies have shown that fatal postoperative MIs are a result of plaque rupture and that this

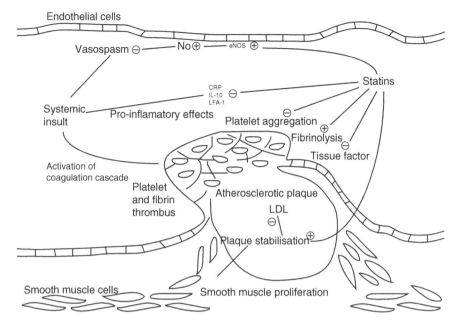

Fig. 48.5 Summary of relevant pleiotropic effects of statins. *NO* nitric oxide, *eNOS* endothelial nitric oxide synthase, *CRP*, C-reactive protein, *IL-10* interleukin-10, *LFA-1* leukocyte function antigen-1, *LDL* low-density lipoprotein (Modified from Gajendragadkar et al. [6])

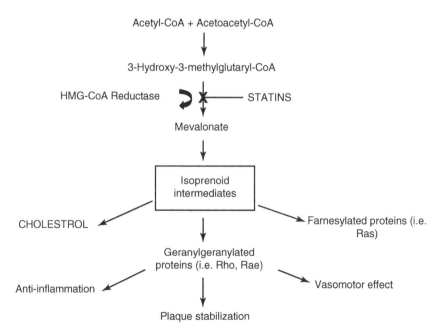

Fig. 48.6 Pharmacology of statins. The mevalonate pathway is demonstrated with the corresponding G proteins affected by reduced flux through isoprenoid intermediates to formation of cholesterol (Modified from Williams and Harken [7])

adverse event occurs secondary to rupture just as often as perioperative oxygen/ supply mismatch. Statins have been shown to be effective at inhibiting the pro-inflammatory cytokines (IL-1, IL-6, and IL-8) and increasing the anti-inflammatory cytokine (IL-10). Figure 48.5 graphically demonstrates these effects [6]. All of these combined effects have an overall capability of reducing the possibility of plaque rupture by stabilizing the lipid core and decreasing the inflammation of the cells in the fibrous cap [8, 9]. Reducing the incidence of plaque rupture has helped to reduce the incidence of adverse cardiovascular outcomes in medical patients [9–14].

Lastly, the idea of continuing statins postoperatively has gained a lot of attention over the years. Surgery on the human body causes a massive amount of inflammatory markers to be released into circulation. Studies have shown that the discontinuation of statins postoperatively has led to an increase in cardiovascular events. These adverse events are secondary to an increase in CRP and other proinflammatory markers, which were being inhibited while on statin therapy [11].

Vasodilation

There are multiple pathways in which statins ultimately have an effect on vasodilation. Probably the most important pathway affected involves the nitric oxide pathway. Nitric oxide is a powerful vasodilator in the human body, as well as an important cellular signaling molecule. Nitric oxide bioavailability is rapidly increased with the use of statins [12, 13]. Statins, as stated before, inhibit HMG-CoA reductase, which then upregulates endothelial nitric oxide synthase (Fig. 48.5) [6]. Other lipid-independent vasodilatory effects of statins include reduced expression of intercellular adhesion molecule, such as E-selectin; upregulation of heme oxygenase 1 by monocytes; inhibition of angiotensin II-induced reactive oxygen species (ROS) production through downregulation of angiotensin 1 receptors; and inhibition of activation of Rac, a small G protein that contributes to nicotinamide adenine dinucleotide phosphate [NAD(P)H].

Antithrombosis and Anticoagulation

Antithrombotic effects of statins can be endothelium dependent and endothelium independent. Statins cause thrombolysis by increasing endothelial thrombotic expression and altering the balance between plasminogen activator inhibitor and tissue plasminogen activator [14]. Moreover, statins can manipulate effects on coagulation factors V, VII, and XII. It is postulated that statins reduce the inflammatory atherosclerotic processes that lead to plaque instability [8, 10]. This reduction can therefore help reduce morbidity and mortality associated with perioperative cardiovascular disease.

Adverse Effects and Drug-Drug Interactions of Statins

Myopathy

Rhabdomyolysis is an idiosyncratic destruction of muscle tissue leading to renal failure. This devastating disease state is the most serious adverse effect of statin medications. Although this may occur secondary to statin use only, this adverse effect is most commonly associated with drug-drug interactions. These drug-drug interactions include but are not limited to gemfibrozil, 38 %; cyclosporine, 4 %; digoxin, 5 %; warfarin, 4 %; macrolide antibiotics, 3 %; mibefradil, 2 %, which has been voluntarily withdrawn from the US market; and azole antifungals, 1 % [16, 17]. Cerivastatin was notorious for causing myopathic complications, which is why this agent is no longer available commercially in the United States. Although rhabdomyolysis is a serious complication, cases of fatalities secondary to statin use are extremely rare. The rate of deaths due to rhabdomyolysis is 0.15 deaths per one million prescriptions [18]. Despite this rare complication, statins are considered among the safest class of medications available on today's market [16, 19].

Hepatotoxicity

The beneficial aspect of statins in the clinical prevention of coronary heart disease greatly outweighs the adverse effects that statins can have on other areas of the body. Statins have been associated with a low incidence of hepatotoxicity. The most common adverse effect associated with statins is transaminitis, in which hepatic enzyme levels are elevated in the absence of proven hepatotoxicity. Transaminitis, however, is usually asymptomatic, reversible, and dose related [16]. However, there is increasing incidence of chronic liver diseases, including nonalcoholic fatty liver disease and hepatitis C, when using statins in patients with high cardiovascular risk [17]. Due to the increasing numbers of hepatotoxicity associated with these lipid-lowering drugs, monitoring alanine aminotransferase (ALT) is a basic recommended lab test for patients while taking statins. The ALT has normal values of 10–40 U/L in male and 7–35 U/L in female [1, 17].

Diabetes Mellitus

Diabetes is quickly becoming one of the most common noncommunicable disease processes in the world. It has unquestionably become the most challenging health concern of the twenty-first century. In a relatively recent development, statins have been associated with a potential increased risk of developing diabetes [20]. The risk increases with age and appears greatest in patients over 60 years of age [21].

Niacin

Niacin (nicotinic acid) is a member of the B vitamin family. Natural niacin is found in many fruits, vegetables, meats, and grains and is one of the oldest known cholesterol-lowering drugs. Although niacin is often given as a vitamin supplement (35 mg/day), it must be given at doses well above the vitamin requirement to have lipid-lowering effects (1–3 g/day).

Niacin has multiple mechanisms of action. They reduce LDL by reducing the production and release of LDL from the liver. They have an effect on triglycerides by reducing the release of free fatty acids stored in fat cells. The overall effect is a 10–20 % reduction in LDL, a 20–50 % reduction in triglycerides, and a 15–35 % increase in HDL.

There are two main types of nicotinic acid preparations and both have fairly significant side effects and drug-drug interactions. The immediate release form of niacin is inexpensive and available OTC. It is highly recommended that the use of immediate-release niacin not be used for cholesterol lowering without monitoring by a physician. The extended release, although better tolerated, does have a higher potential to cause liver damage. Both forms of niacin have a common drug-drug interaction with blood pressure medications, and a strict record of blood pressures should be kept while taking this group of lipid-lowering drugs.

The most common side effect associated with niacin is flushing, which is a result of vasodilation. Other side effects include liver enzyme abnormalities, an elevated blood glucose and hemoglobin A1C, gout, gastrointestinal symptoms (nausea, vomiting, diarrhea, and ulcers), and muscle toxicity if combining this class with statins or fibrates. The recommendation for nicotinic acid is to refrain from taking this class of medications if you have diabetes, liver disease, an active peptic ulcer, arterial bleeding, or unexplained liver enzyme elevations.

Bile Acid Resins

The most common bile acid sequestrants are cholestyramine and colestipol, with a typical dose of around 10 g/day. This class of lipid-lowering medication acts like superglue in the intestine. The normal bile acid-cholesterol complex is reabsorbed into the bloodstream and carried back to the liver which recycles the cholesterol component. Bile acid resins bind bile acids from the liver and prevent it from being reabsorbed into the circulatory system and are then eliminated in the stool. The overall effect of this pathway disruption is a 15–30 % reduction of LDL, while raising HDL up to 5 %. Welchol (colesevelam hydrochloride) is a newer agent that also binds bile acids and is approved as both a lipid-lowering and glucose-lowering agent. The exact mechanism by which it improves glycemic control is unknown.

One "good" drug-drug interaction is the use of bile acid sequestrants in conjunction with statins. This combination has been proven to reduce LDL more than 40 %. The main side effect of these medications is bloating and other gastrointestinal symptoms (heartburn, constipation, and abdominal pain). Therefore, it is recommended that these medications be taken with large amounts of fluids to avoid stomach and intestinal effects. They have also been shown to increase triglycerides in patients who already have an elevated triglyceride level and have also been shown to reduce the body's ability to absorb oral medications and vitamins.

Fibric Acid Derivatives

The main effect of fibrates (1,200 mg/day) is in lowering triglycerides and, to a lesser extent, in increasing HDL levels (5–20 %). They work by affecting the actions of key enzymes in the liver, enabling the liver to absorb more fatty acids and therefore reducing the production of triglycerides. Fibrates do have a minor affect on lowering LDL (10–15 %), but are not considered first-line therapy. There is an increased risk of myopathy and rhabdomyolysis when combined with statins and therefore should never be prescribed with statins. Other known drug-drug interactions occur with warfarin and oral diabetic drugs. Close monitoring of bleeding time and blood sugar is required in patients who combine these drugs. Fibrates have few side effects, with the most common being gastrointestinal complaints (nausea, vomiting, diarrhea, and gas). Few studies have shown an increase in gallstones and gallbladder surgery in people taking fibrates for lowering cholesterol.

Cholesterol Absorption Inhibitors

The most commonly prescribed cholesterol absorption inhibitor is ezetimibe, better known as Zetia (10 mg/day). This new class of drug, which first became available in 2002, lowers cholesterol by preventing it from being absorbed in the intestine. By itself, ezetimibe can reduce cholesterol by about 18 %, but when paired with other statins, LDL levels can be reduced by as much as 25 % more than with statins alone. The side effects of cholesterol absorption inhibitors are minor in comparison with other lipid-lowering drugs and include back, stomach, and joint pain and should not be used in conjunction with fibrates. When used with bile acid sequestrants, the absorption of ezetimibe can be reduced by around 50 %. However, the benefits of ezetimibe come with a cost of around $60 for a 1-month supply.

Summary

Prior to 2002, there were no recommendations for the perioperative use of statins. In 2002, the American College of Cardiology/American Heart Association/National Heart, Lung, and Blood Institute organized the *Clinical Advisory on the Use and Safety of Statins* to investigate the increased incidence of rhabdomyolysis noted with cervistatin and make recommendations for the use of statins. This newly formed group and their investigators sparked a huge wave of journals and studies looking to prove the beneficial effects of statins. The risk factors linked with an increased incidence of rhabdomyolysis included advanced age, renal or hepatic dysfunction, diabetes, hypothyroidism, patients in the perioperative period, and medications that interfere with statin metabolism (antifungals, calcium channel blockers, cyclosporines, and amiodarone). Because of this finding, the Advisory Committee originally suggested discontinuing the use of statins in the perioperative period [24]. However, more and more studies later began to prove that the few reported cases of rhabdomyolysis in patients not on cerivastatin might have been related to medications other than statins. Finally, in 2005, Schouten et al. found no increased risk of myopathy and no rhabdomyolysis in patients on statins in the perioperative period. It is now recognized that the rare incidence of rhabdomyolysis is heavily outweighed by the observed reduction in perioperative risk and postoperative death in patients undergoing noncardiac as well as cardiac surgery [25].

Also in 2002, the National Cholesterol Education Program Expert Panel on Detection, Evaluation, and Treatment of High Blood Cholesterol in Adults issued their recommendations for patients with known coronary artery disease, vascular disease, stroke, or diabetes. They suggested that low-density lipoprotein cholesterol (LDL-C) levels be kept below 100 mg/dl [26]. By 2004, recommendations again suggested statin use to achieve LDL-C levels below 100 mg/dl in patients with known coronary artery disease, with even more benefit if suggested to be optimally kept below 70 mg/dl in patients with known coronary artery disease who also possess additional risk factors such as diabetes, hypertension, obesity, smoking, and acute coronary syndromes [27].

Further, in 2007, studies by LeManach et al. and Schouten et al. looked at the effects of discontinuing statin therapy in the perioperative period for patients who were long-term statin users and undergoing major vascular surgery. The lipid-lowering effects from statins take days to weeks to reverse, so the effects from short-term withdrawal could be linked to the lipid-independent or pleiotropic effects that are connected with their use as discussed previously. The pleiotropic effects (antioxidant, anti-inflammatory decreases in C-reactive protein production; plaque-stabilizing actions; decreased endothelin-1 production; increases in nitric oxide synthase production; and reduction in platelet aggregation) linked with statin use may be lost acutely and may be the main reason for the observed cardiovascular benefits found in patients who continue their use in the perioperative period [23].

Patients presenting for coronary artery bypass grafting or vascular surgery should have statin therapy initiated before surgery. The ACC/AHA 2007 perioperative guidelines state, "In patients undergoing vascular surgery with or without clinical risk factors, statin use is reasonable [28]." The perioperative timing of statin initiation in these patients is not certain however. The ACC/AHA 2007 guidelines strongly recommend continuation of statin therapy in patients already on therapy undergoing noncardiac or cardiac surgery and deem it reasonable to consider statin therapy in patients with risk factors who are undergoing intermediate-risk procedures [28]. Statins should also be initiated immediately in patients who experience an acute coronary syndrome postoperatively [29], and it is logical to assume that patients who qualify for chronic statin therapy and who are presenting for elective vascular surgery should be initiated on therapy prior to having surgery.

Overall, there have been countless studies involving statins and other lipid-lowering drugs and their use in the preoperative, perioperative, and postoperative phases of anesthesia. It has been shown in depth that statins are beneficial for preventing and reducing morbidity and mortality when given for cardiac, vascular, and noncardiac surgical patients. It is the general consensus and the basic guidelines of the ACC/AHA to maintain these benefits and continue to promote the use of statins and other lipid-lowering drugs as described throughout this entire chapter.

Acknowledgements The editors and publisher would like to thank Drs. Alan Kaye and Phillip Kalarickal for contributing to the chapter on this topic in the prior edition. It has served as the foundation for the chapter.

References

1. Mahley RW, Bersot TP. Chapter 35: Drug therapy for hypercholesterolemia and dyslipidemia. In: Brunton LL, Lazo JS, Parker KL, editors. Goodman & Gilman's The pharmacological basis of therapeutics, 11th ed. New York: McGraw-Hill; 2006.
2. Aguila-Salinas CA, Barrett H, Schonfeld G. Metabolic modes of action of the statins in the hyperlipoproteinemias. Atherosclerosis. 1998;141:203–7.
3. Katzung BG, Masters SB, Trevor AJ. Basic and clinical pharmacology. 11th ed. New York: McGraw-Hill companies; 2009.
4. Biccard BM. A peri-operative statin update for non-cardiac surgery. Part I: the effects of statin therapy on atherosclerotic disease and lessons learnt from statin therapy in medical (non-surgical) patients. Anaesthesia. 2008;63:52–64.
5. Williams D, Feely J. Pharmacokinetic-pharmacodynamic drug interactions with HMG-CoA reductase inhibitors. Clin Pharmacokinet. 2002;41(5):343–70.
6. Gajendragadkar PR, Cooper DG, Walsh SR, et al. Novel uses for statins in surgical patients. Intl J Surg. 2009;7:285–90.
7. Williams TM, Harken AH. Statins for surgical patients. Ann Surg. 2008;247:30–7.
8. Rosenson RS, Tagney CC. Antiatherothrombotic properties of statins: implications for cardiovascular event reduction. JAMA. 1998;279:1643–50.
9. Cohen MC, Artz TH. Histological analysis of coronary artery lesions in fatal postoperative myocardial infarction. Cardiovasc Pathol. 1999;8:133–9.
10. Dawood MM, Gupta DK, Southern J, et al. Pathology of fatal perioperative myocardial infarction; implications regarding pathophysiology and prevention. Intl J Cardiol. 1996;57:37–44.
11. Li JJ, Li YS, Chen J, et al. Rebound phenomenon of inflammatory response may be a major mechanism responsible for increased cardiovascular events after abrupt cessation of statin therapy. Med Hypotheses. 2006;66:1199–204.
12. Werner N, Nickenig G, Laufs U. Pleiotropic effects of HMG-CoA reductase inhibitors. Basic Res Cardiol. 2002;97:105–16.
13. Wolfrum S, Jensen KS, Liao JK. Endothelium-dependent effects of statins. Arterioscler ThrombVasc Biol. 2003;23:729–36.
14. Manach YL, et al. Statin therapy within the perioperative period. Anesthesiology. 2008;108:1141–6.
15. Rossi S, editor. Australian medicines handbook 2006. Adelaide: Australian Medicines Handbook; 2006.

16. Armitage J. The safety of statins in clinical practice. Lancet. 2007;370:1781–90.
17. Calderon RM, et al. Statins in the treatment of dyslipidemia in the presence of elevated liver aminotransferase levels: a therapeutic dilemma. Mayo Clin Proc. 2010;85:349–56.
18. Ballantyne CM, Corsini A, Davidson MH, et al. Risk for myopathy with statin therapy in high-risk patients. Arch Intern Med. 2003;163:553–64.
19. Black DM. A general assessment of the safety of HMG CoA reductase inhibitors (statins). Curr Artheroscler Rep. 2002;4:34–41.
20. Ridker PM, Danielson E, Fonseca FA, JUPITER Study Group, et al. Rosuvastatin to prevent vascular events in men and women with elevated C-reactive protein. N Engl J Med. 2008; 359:2195–207.
21. Sattar N, Preiss D, Murray HM, et al. Statins and risk of incident diabetes: a collaborative meta-analysis of randomized statin trials. Lancet. 2010;375:735–42.
22. Corsini A, Bellosta S, Baetta R, et al. New insights into the pharmacodynamic and pharmaco-kinetic properties of statins. Pharmacol. Ther. 1999;84:413–28.
23. Schouten O, Hoeks SE, Welten G, et al. Effect of statin withdrawal on frequency of cardiac events after vascular surgery. Am J Cardiol 2007;100:316–20.
24. American College of Cardiology/American Heart Association/National Heart Lung Blood Institute. Clinical advisory on the use and safety of Statins. J Am Coll Cardiol. 2002;40:567–72.
25. Schouten O, Kertai MD, Bax JJ, et al. Safety of perioperative statin use in high-risk patients undergoing vascular surgery. Am J Cardiol. 2005;95:658–60.
26. Third Report of the National Cholesterol Education Program (NCEP). Expert panel on detection evaluation and treatment of high blood cholesterol in adults (Adult Treatment Panel III) final report. Circulation. 2002;106:3143–421.
27. Grundy SM, Cleeman JL, Merz CN, et al. Implications of recent trials for the national cholesterol education program adult treatment Panel III guidelines. Circulation. 2004;110:227–39.
28. Fleisher LA, Beckman JA, Brown KA, et al. ACC/AHA 2007 guidelines on perioperative cardiovascular evaluation and care for noncardiac surgery. A report of the American college of cardiology/American heart association task force on practice guidelines. Circulation. 2007;116:e418–99.
29. Fonarow GC, Wright RS, Spencer FA, Fredrick PD, Dong W, Every N, French WJ. Effect of stain use within the first 24 hours of administration for acute myocardial infarction on early morbidity and mortality. Am J Cardiol. 2005;96:611–6.
30. National Confidential Enquiry into Patient Outcome and Death. Report-abdominal aortic aneurysm: a service in need of surgery? London: NCEPOD; 2005. http://www.ncepod.org.uk/2005report2/Downloads/AAA_report.doc2005.
31. Conte MS, Bandyk DF, Clowes AW, et al. Risk factors, medical therapies and perioperative events in limb salvage surgery: observations from the PREVENT III multicenter trial. J Vasc Surg. 2005;42:829–36; discussion 836–7.
32. Bicard BM. A peri-operative statin update for non-cardiac surgery. Part II: statin therapy for vascular surgery and peri-operative statin trial design. Anaesthesia. 2008;63:162–71.
33. American Heart Association. Cardiovascular disease statistics. 2006. Available at: http://www.americanheart.org/presenter.jhtml?identifier=4478.
34. British Heart Foundation statistics website. CVD mortality in Europe. 2005. Available at: http://www.heartstats.org/topic.asp?id=753.

Chapter 49
Serotonin Syndrome

Julie A. Gayle, Jacqueline Volpi Abadie, Adam M. Kaye, and Alan David Kaye

Contents

J.A. Gayle, MD (✉)
Department of Anesthesiology, Louisiana State University Health Sciences Center,
New Orleans, LA 70112, USA
e-mail: jgayle@lsuhsc.edu

J.V. Abadie, MD
Department of Anesthesiology, Alton Ochsner Clinic, New Orleans, LA 70112, USA
e-mail: jakqs25@yahoo.com

A.M. Kaye, PharmD
Thomas J. Long School of Pharmacy and Health Sciences, University of the Pacific,
3601 Pacific Avenue, Stockton, CA 95211, USA
e-mail: akaye@pacific.edu

A.D. Kaye, MD, PhD
Department of Anesthesiology, Louisiana State University Health Sciences Center,
New Orleans, LA 70112, USA

Department of Anesthesiology, Tulane Medical Center, New Orleans, LA USA
e-mail: alankaye44@hotmail.com

A.D. Kaye et al. (eds.), *Essentials of Pharmacology for Anesthesia,*
Pain Medicine, and Critical Care, DOI 10.1007/978-1-4614-8948-1_49,
© Springer Science+Business Media New York 2015

Introduction

Serotonin syndrome or "serotonin toxicity" is a potentially life-threatening condition caused by excessive serotonergic activity in the nervous system. The majority of cases of serotonin syndrome are iatrogenic resulting from a synergistic combination of two or more serotonergic drugs or medications. As the number of available serotonergic drugs increases, so does their use in clinical practice. An increase in the incidence of serotonin syndrome or at least the reporting of these incidents has been noted. The content below describes the mechanism of action of serotonergic drugs and medications and how they contribute to the development of serotonin syndrome. Clinical features and diagnostic criteria as well as treatment of serotonin syndrome are discussed. Important drug interactions, side effects, and Food and Drug Administration (FDA) warnings are highlighted. Special emphasis is placed on drugs and medications commonly used by anesthesia and critical care providers that may precipitate serotonin syndrome.

Drug Class and Mechanism of Action

Serotonin syndrome and its spectrum of symptoms are a product of the overactivation of both the central and peripheral serotonin receptors due to high levels of serotonin. Serotonin (5-hydroxytryptamine [5-HT]) is formed from the decarboxylation and hydroxylation of tryptophan, which is then stored in vesicles and released into the synaptic cleft when stimulated. 5-HT is metabolized by monoamine oxidase A (MAOA) into 5-hydroxindoleacetic acid. There are at least seven families of 5-HT receptors to which serotonin can bind [1–3]. There is no single receptor that is responsible for serotonin syndrome; however, several studies provide evidence that the 5-HT2A receptors are the most important receptors involved in the development of serotonin syndrome [1, 3, 4].

Serotonin can act both peripherally and centrally. Peripheral serotonin is produced primarily in the enterochromaffin cells of the gastrointestinal (GI) tract. It functions to stimulate vasoconstriction, uterine contraction, bronchoconstriction, GI motility, and platelet aggregation. Central serotonin is present in the midline raphe nuclei of the brainstem from the midbrain to the medulla. It functions to inhibit excitatory neurotransmission and to modulate wakefulness, attention, affective behavior (anxiety and depression), sexual behavior, appetite, thermoregulation, motor tone, migraine, emesis, nociception, and aggression [1, 3, 5].

Several animal studies show that high levels of noradrenaline are seen during the course of serotonin syndrome, which may also contribute to the symptoms [4, 6]. N-Methyl-D-aspartate (NMDA) receptor antagonists, gamma-aminobutyric acid (GABA), and dopamine have also been proposed to play a role in serotonin syndrome, but their impact is still unclear [3, 6].

Table 49.1 Drugs commonly implicated in inducing serotonin syndrome by mechanism

Inhibitors of serotonin reuptake

Selective serotonin reuptake inhibitors (SSRIs): fluoxetine, paroxetine, sertraline, citalopram, fluvoxamine

Serotonin-norepinephrine reuptake inhibitors (SNRIs): venlafaxine, desvenlafaxine, duloxetine, milnacipran

Tricyclic antidepressants (TCAs): amitriptyline, nortriptyline, protriptyline clomipramine, imipramine, desipramine, trimipramine, amoxapine, doxepin, maprotiline

Dopamine-norepinephrine reuptake inhibitors: bupropion

Serotonin modulators: trazodone, nefazodone

Phenylpiperidine opioids: fentanyl, dextromethorphan

5-HT3 receptor antagonists: ondansetron, granisetron

Local anesthetics: cocaine

Herbal supplements: St. John's wort (*Hypericum perforatum*)

Tramadol

Meperidine

Methadone

MDMA (ecstasy)

Inhibitors of serotonin metabolism

Monoamine oxidase inhibitors (MAOIs): St. John's wort, linezolid, methylene blue, tranylcypromine, selegiline, phenelzine, isocarboxazid, furazolidone, Syrian rue

Increase serotonin synthesis

L-tryptophan

Increase serotonin release

Amphetamines and amphetamine derivatives: methamphetamine, fenfluramine, phentermine

Dopamine agonists: L-dopa and bromocriptine

MDMA (ecstasy)

Ethanol

Cocaine

Lithium

Serotonin receptor agonism

Antidepressants: buspirone, trazodone, mirtazapine

Antimigraines: triptans, valproic acid, carbamazepine

Ergot alkaloid derivatives: methylergonovine, ergotamine

Fentanyl

Metoclopramide

Buspirone

Lysergic acid diethylamide (LSD)

Increases sensitivity of postsynaptic receptor

Lithium

Adapted from reference [3]

There are multiple mechanisms by which drugs can cause serotonin syndrome (Table 49.1). The mechanisms are as follows: inhibition of serotonin reuptake, inhibition of serotonin metabolism, increased serotonin synthesis, increased serotonin release, serotonergic receptor agonism, and increased sensitivity of postsynaptic receptors. Another mechanism involves the inhibition of certain cytochrome P450 (CYP450) enzymes by the SSRIs themselves, including CYP2D6 and CYP3A4 [7]. Inhibition results in the accumulation of certain serotonergic drugs (venlafaxine, methadone, tramadol, oxycodone, risperidone, dextromethorphan, and phentermine), which are usually metabolized by these enzymes. This creates an exacerbation loop, where the SSRI inhibits the metabolism of a certain drug, which in turn increases serotonergic activity. Several studies discuss this mechanism to be important in the development of serotonin syndrome with the concomitant use of an SSRI with tramadol [3, 8–10]. Many drugs, in addition to SSRIs, can inhibit these enzymes, resulting in accumulation of serotonergic drugs that are being used simultaneously. Ciprofloxacin has been reported to cause serotonin syndrome via its CYP3A4 inhibition [11]. A second example is a case report of serotonin syndrome caused by the concomitant use of citalopram and fluconazole, which suggested that the inhibition of CYP2C19 by fluconazole resulted in the accumulation of its substrate, citalopram [3, 12].

Clinical Features and Diagnosis

The diagnosis of serotonin syndrome is purely clinical. Therefore, clinical suspicions should rise when a patient displays signs and symptoms of the syndrome following administration or dose increase of drugs known to act on the serotonergic system. Clinical manifestations of serotonin syndrome are described in terms of changes in mental status, autonomic function, and neuromuscular status (Table 49.2). The clinician should have high index of suspicion of this diagnosis should a patient who has been exposed to drugs with serotonergic activity develop a fever and altered mental status, autonomic instability, and increased (lower) limb rigidity [14].

Several diagnostic criteria have been proposed for serotonin syndrome. The most recent diagnostic criteria are the Hunter Serotonin Toxicity Criteria (HSTC). When compared to the gold standard of diagnosis by a medical toxicologist, the HSTC are sensitive (84 %) and specific (97 %). The Hunter Criteria include the use of a serotonergic agent plus one out of five of the following: spontaneous clonus, inducible clonus plus agitation or diaphoresis, ocular clonus plus agitation or diaphoresis, tremor and hyperreflexia, hypertonia, and a temperature above 38 °C plus ocular or inducible clonus [3, 10, 11]. The presence of clonus and hyperreflexia is most important for the diagnosis; however, severe muscle rigidity may mask these symptoms. Prominent features of life-threatening cases include hyperthermia (>38.5 °C), peripheral hypertonicity, and truncal rigidity. These symptoms have shown a high risk of progression to respiratory failure [11]. There are some nonspecific laboratory abnormalities that may be seen in serotonin syndrome which include leukocytosis, low bicarbonate, and elevated creatinine and transaminases. Serum serotonin concentrations do not correlate with the severity of this syndrome [3, 15].

The differential diagnoses for serotonin syndrome are extensive. It includes neuroleptic malignant syndrome (NMS), malignant hyperthermia, anticholinergic

Table 49.2 Clinical manifestations associated with serotonin syndrome

Changes in mental status[b]
Agitation[a]
Delirium
Anxiety
Disorientation
Restlessness
Lethargy
Hallucinations
Autonomic dysfunction[b]
Hypertension
Tachycardia
Tachypnea
Hyperthermia[a] (temperature above 38 °C)
Arrhythmias
Flushed skin
Diaphoresis[a]
Dilated pupils
Vomiting
Shivering
Neuromuscular changes[b]
Clonus[a] (spontaneous or inducible, ocular)
Tremor[a]
Muscle rigidity
Hyperreflexia[a]
Hypertonia

Adapted from reference [13]

[a]Italics are *signs/symptoms* fulfilling Hunter Criteria for serotonin syndrome (see text for details of specific combination of symptoms)

[b]Clinical pearl for remembering signs and symptoms of serotonin syndrome: acronym *CAN* (Changes in mental status, Autonomic dysfunction, Neuromuscular changes)

toxicity, serotonergic discontinuation syndrome, sympathomimetic drug intoxication, meningitis, encephalitis, heat stroke, and central hyperthermia [3]. The main differential diagnosis is NMS which often has a slower onset, is associated with hyperthermia (>38 °C), and has a much higher mortality [16]. Table 49.3 summarizes some of the clinical features and diagnostic aids that differentiate NMS, malignant hyperthermia, and serotonin syndrome.

During the preoperative evaluation, emphasis should be placed on the history of ingested substances including prescription drug use, over-the-counter medication and dietary supplement use, illicit substance use, and any recent changes in dosing or addition of new drugs to a drug regimen. The onset and description of symptoms and the presence of any comorbidity are of utmost importance. Certain comorbidities, such as depression and chronic pain, may clue the clinician into the use of drugs that can precipitate serotonin syndrome [3]. Hypertension, atherosclerosis,

Table 49.3 Differentiating serotonin syndrome among common presentations

	Serotonin syndrome	Neuroleptic malignant syndrome	Malignant hyperthermia
Onset and resolution	Develops within 24 h	Develops over days to weeks	Develops in minutes or within 24 h
	Resolves within 24 h of treatment	Resolves within days to weeks with treatment	
Causative agents	Serotonin agonists	Dopamine antagonists	Halogenated inhalational anesthetics or depolarizing muscle relaxants
Neuromuscular changes	Hyperreactivity	Muscular rigidity and bradyreflexia	Rigidity and hyporeflexia
Treatment agents	Discontinue serotonergic agents; benzodiazepines[a]; cyproheptadine[b]	Bromocriptine	Dantrolene

Adapted from references [3, 13, 15]

[a]Benzodiazepines for sedation (i.e., lorazepam 1–2 mg IV per dose in adults)

[b]Cyproheptadine if agitation and abnormal vital signs persist with benzodiazepines and supportive care (initial adult dose 12 mg PO or OGT)

and hyperlipidemia are all associated with reduced endothelial MAO activity which affects serotonin metabolism [17]. Also, a higher incidence of serotonin syndrome has been reported in patients with end-stage renal disease who are on selective serotonin reuptake inhibitors (SSRIs) and hemodialysis. These patients are prone to developing serotonin toxicity, suggesting that this increased toxicity could be related to a decrease in renal function [3, 4]. Furthermore, predisposing factors such as inherited or acquired deficits in peripheral serotonin metabolism may contribute to the development of serotonin syndrome. The preexisting conditions illustrated above coupled with the use of serotonergic drugs increase the chances of serotonin syndrome [17].

Treatment

The keys to management are discontinuing all serotonergic agents, supportive care via stabilizing vital signs, giving oxygen in order to keep oxygen saturation greater than 94 %, administering intravenous fluids, continuous cardiac monitoring, sedation with benzodiazepines, and possible administration of serotonin antagonists. With treatment, serotonin syndrome usually resolves within 24 h. Treatment for mild cases includes discontinuing the serotonergic agent, supportive care with oxygen and intravenous fluids, sedation with benzodiazepines, and observation for at least six hours [3]. Benzodiazepines provide anxiolysis and control of seizures

Table 49.4 Management of serotonin syndrome

Principles of management	Specific treatments
Discontinue serotonergic agents	See Table 49.3 for drugs associated with serotonin syndrome
Supportive care	Supplemental oxygen
	Intravenous fluids
	Continuous cardiac monitoring
Treat mild symptoms	Continue supportive care
Hypertension	Stabilize vital signs
Tachycardia	Cooling measures
Agitation	Benzodiazepines
Tremor, clonus	Observation for at least 6 h
Treat moderate symptoms	Supportive care, benzodiazepines
Hypertension, tachycardia, agitation, tremor	Cyproheptadine (5HT antagonist) for severe agitation and abnormal vital signs not responsive to benzodiazepines
Ocular clonus	Admit for cardiac monitoring and observation
Hyperthermia (temperature 40 °C)	
Treat severe symptoms	Immediate sedation, intubation, and ventilation with paralysis (use non-depolarizing agent)
Autonomic instability (extreme swings in blood pressure and heart rate)	Esmolol or nitroprusside for severe hypertension and/or tachycardia
Hyperthermia (temperature >41.1 °C)	Cooling measures
Muscle rigidity	Admit to intensive care unit
Delirium	

or muscle hyperreactivity [16]. Moderate cases can be treated as above plus the addition of a serotonin antagonist and admission to the hospital for cardiac monitoring and observation. In severe life-threatening cases, the patient should be treated as above plus sedation, intubation, ventilation, and paralysis in the intensive care unit [1, 3, 15]. Refer to Table 49.4 for an overview of management based on symptom severity.

The management of mild hypertension and tachycardia includes benzodiazepines. Diazepam, a GABA mimetic, has been studied the most and has shown to blunt the hyperadrenergic symptoms of serotonin syndrome [1, 5, 6]. Therefore, diazepam not only works to sedate the patient but can also correct mild hypertension and tachycardia and reduce fever [3, 6]. If a patient exhibits severe hypertension and tachycardia, short-acting esmolol or nitroprusside should be used. It is recommended to avoid long-acting agents like propranolol because these agents can cause hypotension and can mask tachycardia. Masking tachycardia is undesirable because tachycardia can be used to follow treatment response and patient improvement [1, 18]. If a patient presents with hypotension, which can commonly occur with the concomitant use of propranolol and MAOIs, the preferred treatment is a low dose of direct-acting sympathomimetics, including norepinephrine, epinephrine, and phenylephrine [1, 3].

If a patient still remains agitated after the use of benzodiazepines and stabilization of vital signs, serotonin antagonists can be administered. More specifically, 5-HT2A receptor antagonists seem to be the most effective. Animal studies have shown that due to their 5-HT2A receptor antagonism, both cyproheptadine and chlorpromazine in high doses can be used to prevent hyperthermia and lethality in serotonin syndrome. Cyproheptadine is a more potent 5-HT2A receptor antagonist and therefore may be more effective [3, 4]. However, cyproheptadine does not shorten the time course of serotonin syndrome [19, 20].

Minimizing excess muscle activity and cooling measures can be used to treat hyperthermia. Antipyretics are not useful for the treatment of hyperthermia in serotonin syndrome because the high temperature is secondary to increased muscle activity and not due to a change in the hypothalamic temperature set point [1, 5]. For temperatures greater than 41.1 °C, the patient should be sedated; paralyzed with non-depolarizing agents, such as vecuronium; and intubated. Succinylcholine should not be used due to the risk of hyperkalemia and possible worsening of rhabdomyolysis [3, 15].

Dantrolene, used as treatment for malignant hyperthermia, has not proven to be efficacious in the treatment of serotonin syndrome in animal models [4]. Bromocriptine, a dopamine agonist used to treat neuroleptic malignant syndrome, may exacerbate serotonin syndrome by increasing serotonin levels [1, 3]. Neither of these agents plays a role in the treatment of serotonin syndrome.

Drug Interactions

The reported drug interactions that have caused serotonin syndrome are continuing to increase and include many different combinations of serotonergic drugs. Some of the reported drug combinations are listed in Table 49.5. The most well-known combination is an SSRI with a MAOI. However, the combination of any two serotonergic drugs can precipitate this syndrome and therefore should be used sparingly or with great caution [3]. The lesser known MAOIs, such as linezolid and some opioid analgesics, have serotonergic activity. When combined with serotonergic medications, drugs like linezolid may precipitate serotonin syndrome. The phenylpiperidine opioids (meperidine, tramadol, methadone, and propoxyphene) exhibit weak serotonin reuptake inhibitor qualities. All have been involved in serotonin toxicity reactions with MAOIs, some fatal [21]. Life-threatening cases tend to occur with the use of an irreversible MAOI or with combinations of serotonergic drugs rather than with just the use of an SSRI alone [1, 3, 22].

Although serotonin syndrome is uncommon, it has potential to complicate the administration of drugs frequently used in anesthetic practice. For example, combining meperidine or tramadol with an SSRI or a MAOI is known to increase the risk of serotonin syndrome. Methylene blue, a phenothiazine derivative with a structure similar to antipsychotic drugs, is a dye used intraoperatively to facilitate surgical progress. In the presence of serotonergic medications, methylene blue can lead to a surge in plasma serotonin levels and precipitate serotonin syndrome [23].

Table 49.5 Reported drug combinations causing serotonin syndrome	**MAOIs**
	MAOIs with SSRIs or SNRIs or TCAs or opiates
	Methylene blue with paroxetine or clomipramine
	Phenelzine with meperidine
	SSRIs
	SSRIs with MAOIs or SNRIs or TCAs or opiates or triptans
	Fluoxetine with carbamazepine or phentermine or fentanyl
	SNRIs (venlafaxine)
	SNRIs with MAOIs or TCAs or opiates or triptans
	Venlafaxine with mirtazapine and tramadol
	Venlafaxine with amitriptyline and meperidine
	Venlafaxine with methadone and fluoxetine
	Venlafaxine with methadone and sertraline
	Venlafaxine with tramadol and trazodone and quetiapine
	Opiates: (tramadol)
	Opiates with MAOIs or SSRIs or SNRIs or triptans
	Tramadol alone
	Tramadol with mirtazapine and olanzapine
	Antibiotics
	Ciprofloxacin with venlafaxine and methadone
	Fluconazole with citalopram
	Linezolid with SSRIs or tapentadol
	Adapted from reference [3]

Case reports of serotonin syndrome implicate drugs commonly given in the perioperative period such as fentanyl and ondansetron. Fentanyl, a phenylpiperidine opioid, administered to patients who received the preoperative SSRIs citalopram or sertraline precipitated serotonin syndrome. Ondansetron, a 5-HT3 receptor blocker commonly used for postoperative nausea prophylaxis, administered with mirtazapine triggered serotonin syndrome [23]. Given the lack of evidence regarding individual susceptibility and dose-responsive activation of serotonin syndrome, anesthesia providers should avoid using combinations of drugs known to precipitate the syndrome [16].

Side Effects/Black Box Warnings

> The Food and Drug Administration (FDA) has issued warnings alerting healthcare professionals and the public to life-threatening serotonin syndrome resulting from the combined use of 5-hydroxytryptamine receptor agonists (triptans) with certain antidepressants. Triptans are a commonly prescribed migraine drug and when combined with an SSRI or SNRI may precipitate serotonin syndrome.

Methylene blue, a heterocyclic aromatic chemical compound, is used to treat methemoglobinemia, vasoplegic syndrome, ifosfamide-induced encephalopathy, and cyanide poisoning. Methylene blue is also used as a dye in certain diagnostic and therapeutic applications. Because it is a potent monoamine oxidase inhibitor, methylene blue increases serotonin levels by decreasing levels of monoamine oxidase A, an enzyme responsible for breaking down serotonin in the brain. In July 2011, the FDA issued a Drug Safety Communication warning regarding the potential drug interaction between methylene blue and serotonergic psychiatric medications. At that time, the FDA recommended that methylene blue should not be given to patients taking serotonergic drugs except under emergent conditions. In October 2011, the FDA issued an update stating that most of the cases of serotonin syndrome as reported to their Adverse Event Reporting System (AERS) resulted from the intravenous administration of methylene blue (1–8 mg/kg) to patients taking specific serotonergic medications (SSRIs, SNRIs, and clomipramine) in the setting of parathyroid surgery. A similar FDA Safety Communication was issued about linezolid (Zyvox) in July 2011. The FDA received reports of serotonin syndrome in patients on serotonergic psychiatric medications following administration of linezolid, even after discontinuation of the serotonergic psychiatric medications [24].

Summary

The possibility of serotonin syndrome presenting in the perioperative setting directly correlates with the increasing use of psychiatric medications in all types of patient populations. Interactions with antibiotics and other drugs outside of the operative arena make serotonin syndrome a real possibility in the critical care settings as well. Because serotonin syndrome is strictly a clinical diagnosis, healthcare professionals providing anesthesia and pain management as well as critical care should be knowledgeable of the clinical features of serotonin syndrome and drugs that may precipitate it. Early diagnosis and appropriate treatment are crucial to halting the progression of this potentially life-threatening condition.

References

1. Boyer EW, Shannon M. The serotonin syndrome. N Engl J Med. 2005;352:1112–20.
2. Morgan GE, Mikhail MS, Murray MJ. Lange – clinical anesthesiology. 4th ed. New York: McGraw-Hill; 2006.
3. Volpi-Abadie J, Kaye AM, Kaye AD. Serotonin syndrome. Ochsner J. 2013;13(4):533–40.

4. Koichi N, Yoshino T, Yui K, Katoh S. Potent serotonin (5-HT) 2A receptor antagonists completely prevent the development of hyperthermia in an animal model of the 5-HT syndrome. Brain Res. 2001;890:23–31.

5. Dvir Y, Smallwood P. Serotonin syndrome: a complex but easily avoidable condition. Gen Hosp Psychiatry. 2008;30:284–7.

6. Nisijima K, Shioda K, Yoshino T, Takano K, Kate S. Diazepam and chlormethiazole attenuate the development of hyperthermia in an animal model of serotonin syndrome. Neurochem Int. 2003;43:155–64.

7. Mitchell PB. Drug interaction of clinical significance with selective serotonin reuptake inhibitors. Drug Saf. 1997;17:390–406.

8. Lange-Asschenfeldt C, Weigmann H, Hiemke C, Mann K. Serotonin syndrome as a result of fluoxetine in a patient with tramadol abuse: plasma level-correlated symptomatology. J Clin Psychopharmacol. 2002;22:440–1.

9. Mason BJ, Blackburn KH. Possible serotonin syndrome associated with tramadol and sertraline coadministration. Ann Pharmacother. 1997;31:175–7.

10. Ables AZ, Nagubilli R. Prevention, diagnosis, and management of serotonin syndrome. Am Fam Physician. 2010;81(9):1139–42.

11. Lee J, Franz L, Goforth HW. Serotonin syndrome in a chronic-pain patient receiving concurrent methadone, ciprofloxacin and venlafaxine. Psychosomatics. 2009;50:638–9.

12. Levin TT, Cortes-Ladino A, Weiss M, Palomba ML. Life-threatening serotonin toxicity due to a citalopram-fluconazole drug interaction: case reports and discussion. Gen Hosp Psychiatry. 2008;30:372–7.

13. Walsh J. Serotonin syndrome. Anaesthesia tutorial of the week 166. 18 Jan 2010 from www.totw.anaesthesiologists.org.

14. Peck T, Wong A, Norman E. Anaesthetic implications of psychoactive drugs. Contin Educ Anaesth Crit Care Pain. 2010;10(6):177–81.

15. Boyer EW, Traub SJ, Grayzel J. Serotonin syndrome. UpToDate. 2010. Retrieved 28 Sep 2011, from UpToDate.com.

16. Chinniah S, French JLH, Levy DM. Serotonin and anaesthesia. Contin Educ Anaesth Crit Care Pain. 2008;8(2):43–5.

17. Guo SL, Wu TJ, Liu CC, Ng CC, Chien CC, Sun HL. Meperidine-induced serotonin syndrome in a susceptible patient. Br J Anaesth. 2009;103(3):369–70.

18. Dunkley EJC, Isbister GK, Sibbritt D, Dawson AH, Whyte IM. The hunter serotonin toxicity criteria: simple and accurate diagnostic decision rules for serotonin toxicity. QJM. 2003;96:635–62.

19. Graudins A, Stearman A, Chan B. Treatment of serotonin syndrome with cyproheptadine. J Emerg Med. 1998;16:615–9.

20. McDaniel WW. Serotonin syndrome: early management with cyproheptadine. Ann Pharmacother. 2001;35:870–3.

21. Gillman PK. Monoamine oxidase inhibitors, opioid analgesics and serotonin toxicity. Br J Anaesth. 2005;95(4):434–41.

22. Isbister GK, Bowe SJ, Dawson A, Whyte IM. Relative toxicity of selective serotonin reuptake inhibitors (SSRIs) in overdose. J Toxicol Clin Toxicol. 2004;42:277–85.

23. Altman CS, Jahangiri MF. Serotonin syndrome in the perioperative period. Anesth Analg. 2010;110(2):526–8.

24. Jones D, Story DA. Serotonin syndrome and the anaesthetist. Anaesth Intensive Care. 2005;33:181–7.

Part V
New Vistas in Pharmacology

Chapter 50
Novel Psychoactive Substances: Synthetic Cathinones and Cannabinoid Receptor Agonists

Ethan O. Bryson

Contents

Introduction

The synthesis of "designer drugs" intended to mimic the effects of chemically similar controlled substances while circumventing existing drug laws has grown exponentially since the turn of the century. These novel psychoactive substances (NPSs) have been introduced into the market with some regularity over the previous century in response to regulations which outlaw the use of existing agents, but more recently the Internet has allowed for worldwide distribution and encouraged NPS production on a global scale. These synthetic compounds contain modified molecular structures similar enough to controlled or illegal substances so as to produce a similar effect in the user but different enough so as to not fall under the same restrictions placed on the production, distribution, possession, and use of the parent compound.

E.O. Bryson, MD
Departments of Anesthesiology and Psychiatry,
The Mount Sinai School of Medicine, New York, NY, USA
e-mail: ethan.bryson@mountsinai.org

A.D. Kaye et al. (eds.), *Essentials of Pharmacology for Anesthesia,*
Pain Medicine, and Critical Care, DOI 10.1007/978-1-4614-8948-1_50,
© Springer Science+Business Media New York 2015

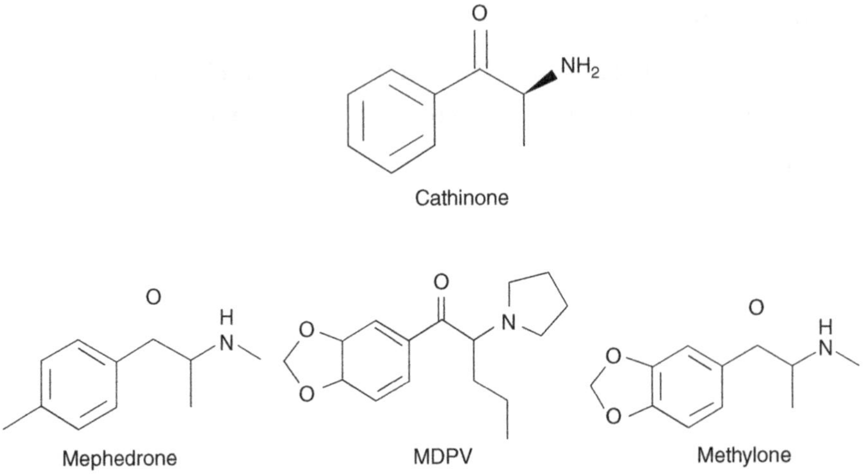

Fig. 50.1 Chemical structure of the naturally occurring compound cathinone and the three most common synthetic cathinones found in commercial "bath salt" preparations

These drugs are often produced clandestinely with little or no quality control processes, and there is a wide variation in chemical content among commercial preparations purported to be the same product. Typically the existence of a new NPS comes to the attention of law enforcement or the medical community only after users begin to die in large numbers or present to hospitals for treatment with heretofore unseen symptoms.

Synthetic Cathinones

Known as "bath salts" or "plant food" and sold in packaging clearly labeled "not for human consumption," this NPS often contains a variety of psychoactive and inert compounds. Most prominent among the ingredients is a group of chemically similar sympathomimetic compounds known as cathinones. First isolated from *Catha edulis* (khat) over 100 years ago, cathinone has long been recognized as a stimulant and has been consumed for these and its antidepressant properties. Cathinone was recognized as a drug with high potential for abuse and classified by the DEA as a schedule I drug in the 1970s [1]. Current bath salt formulations typically contain any combination of three major synthetic cathinones: the semisynthetic beta-keto derivative of phenethylamine, mephedrone (1-(4-methylphenyl)-2-methylaminopropan-1-one), MDPV (3,4-methylenedioxypyrovalerone), or methylone (3,4-methylenedioxymethcathinone) (Fig. 50.1). Until recently, mephedrone (also known as "drone," "MCAT," "meow," or "meow, meow") was considered by many to be one of the "legal highs," compounds which provide the user with a subjective experience similar to that provided by illegal drugs such as cocaine, though it has been illegal in

Table 50.1 Relative effect of the synthetic cathinones on catecholamine receptors

Receptor type	Mephedrone	MDPV	Methylone
Dopamine	+++	+++	+++
Norepinephrine	++	+++	+++
Serotonin	+++	+	++

the United States since 2011. Mephedrone is structurally related to cathinone and chemically similar to ephedrine, cathine, and other amphetamines [2]. Cathinone was ubiquitous in several NPS products until it was banned in 2010 and subsequently replaced with synthetic derivatives. Because it is an analog of a compound classified as an illegal drug, attempts to curb mephedrone use were first made under the Federal Analog Act, though its distribution and use has been illegal under the DEA Schedule I since from October 2011.

First synthesized in 1929, mephedrone was not widely abused until it became available commercially in 2003. Following several deaths attributed to its recreational use, mephedrone was first made illegal in the country where most of the drug had been previously synthesized (Israel) in 2008. Prompted by increased use observed by law enforcement, Sweden outlawed mephedrone use later that year. Currently, the drug is illegal in most countries but is still widely available in large quantities over the Internet [3]. Experience suggests that future generations of NPS products will contain both illegal substances and compounds that have yet to be identified and scheduled.

Users of bath salts typically insufflate the dry powder nasally, though it has also been taken orally or rectally, injected, or smoked [4]. These drugs produce subjective effects of euphoria and psychomotor agitation similar to that produced by 3,4-methylenedioxymethamphetamine (MDMA) and cocaine [5] and auditory or visual hallucinations such as those produced by the more classic serotonergic hallucinogens *N,N*-dimethyltryptamine (DMT), lysergic acid diethylamide (LSD), psilocybin, and mescaline [6].

Mechanism of Action

The clinical and subjective effects of the synthetic cathinones are similar to the effects of MDMA, cocaine, and methamphetamine, though not identical, and the mechanism of action of these drugs is somewhat different (Table 50.1). While commercial preparations may include any combination of active compounds, it is helpful to look at the more commonly isolated substances.

Mephedrone and methylone both stimulate the release of dopamine from central nervous system dopaminergic nerve terminals and simultaneously prevent dopamine reuptake, producing effects similar to those of cocaine [7]. Mephedrone is relatively nonselective catecholamine releaser which produces hypertension via stimulation of peripheral alpha-adrenergic receptors and tachycardia through activation of beta-adrenergic receptors, similar to that of methamphetamine [8].

Though it is not known through exactly what mechanism mephedrone produces this cardiovascular response, given its structural similarity to methamphetamine, it is likely that this is caused by the release of norepinephrine from peripheral sympathetic nerves. Both mephedrone and methylone are transporter substrates and not blockers. Like cocaine, both of these agents appear to be nonselective for particular transporters. A decrease in serotonin reuptake in the central nervous system is the likely mechanism for these drugs' reported antidepressant properties.

Methylenedioxypyrovalerone (MDPV) is the main compound isolated from patients admitted to hospital emergency departments with "bath salt" overdose in the United States [9] and likely is the primary active ingredient in current preparations [10]. It is a potent catecholamine-selective transporter blocker that is not a transporter substrate and inhibits dopamine reuptake with weaker effect on serotonin in the same way the structurally similar cathinone pyrovalerone does [11]. When compared to cocaine and amphetamine, MDPV was found to be 50 times more potent in blocking dopamine reuptake and 10 times more potent in blocking norepinephrine and displays a high selectivity for catecholamine reuptake blocking. Given these findings, it is likely that bath salt preparations containing MDPV have a high potential for abuse, and it is likely that clinicians will see an increasing number of patients admitted with symptoms related to cardiovascular stimulation as the use of these NPSs becomes more widespread.

Adverse Effects

The synthetic stimulants found in commercial bath salt preparations have been implicated in a number of acute and chronic untoward events. Presumably these drugs are sought out for their purported effects of intense stimulation, alertness, and euphoria. Some users have reported mild sexual stimulation and feelings of empathy similar to those reported by users of the entactogen ecstasy (MDMA). Adverse or unwanted effects reported by some users include distressing feelings of anxiety and agitation with some developing paranoid delusions and hallucinations. These hallucinations are typically of a violent nature with threatening intruders and a feeling of intense fearfulness and have resulted in high-profile violent episodes involving law enforcement. Insomnia, inability to concentrate, difficulty with memory, and headaches are common, and some users have developed tremors, muscle twitching, chest pain, and seizures. Encephalopathy due to hyponatremia has been reported [12], resulting from an excessive thirst, similar to what was reported with MDMA use in the early 1990s [13].

Synthetic Cannabinoid Receptor Agonists

Marketed with names such as "Spice Gold," "herbal incense," or "K2" and labeled clearly as "not for human consumption," these products are little more than dried vegetable matter sprayed with synthetic cannabinoids [14]. The active ingredient in

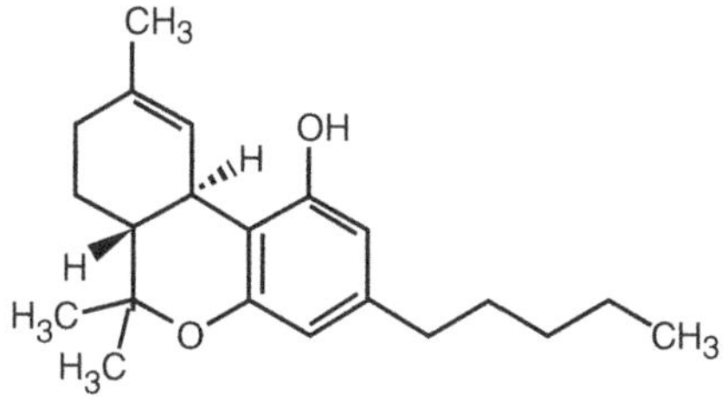

Fig. 50.2 Chemical structure of the naturally occurring compound THC and synthetic cannabinoid receptor agonists from the JWH and CP class. Note that all three compounds have markedly different structures

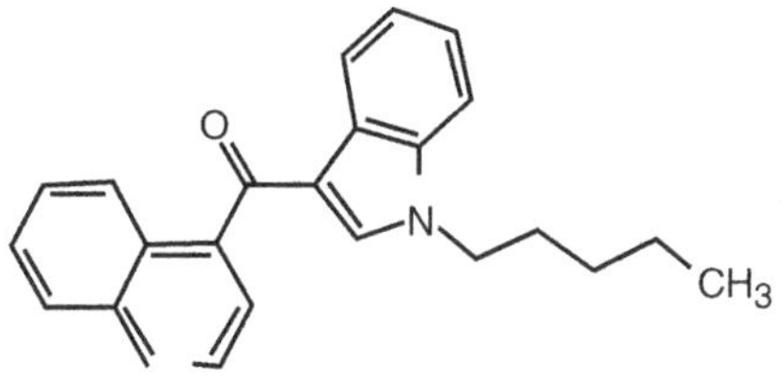

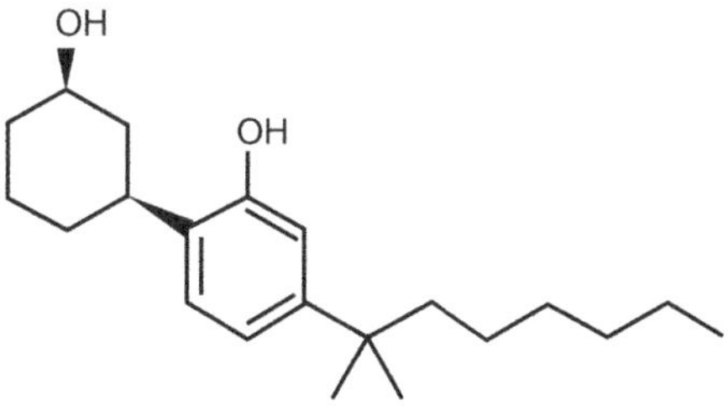

these synthetic cannabinoid products was designed to stimulate the cannabinoid receptors, particularly the CB1 cannabinoid receptors concentrated in the brain, much in the same way delta-9 tetrahydrocannabinol (THC) does. Though their effects are similar to the effects of THC, these synthetic cannabinoids are structurally different, bind to receptors with different affinities, and have not yet been tested in humans. The two most common synthetic cannabinoids found in these over-the-counter preparations are JWH 018, first synthesized in 1995 by Clemson University researcher John W. Huffman, PhD, and a synthetic cannabinoid created by Pfizer called CP 47,497 (Fig. 50.2).

Synthetic cannabinoids are smoked or eaten in the same manner as marijuana. They are rapidly absorbed through the lungs and produce a wide range of psychological and central nervous system (CNS) effects that peak in 15 min but unlike THC may persist for 12–24 h depending on the dose [15]. Users report feelings of euphoria, heightened sensory perception, and a distortion of space and time similar to marijuana [16]. In some patients these sensations are distressing, and some users have reported feelings of anxiety, dysphoria, as well as nausea and vomiting [17]. In patients with underlying psychiatric disorders, aggravation of psychotic states has been reported [18]. Generalized CNS depression leading to drowsiness and sleep typically follows the initial psychomotor agitation. When synthetic cannabinoids are ingested via the oral route, the bioavailability is variable but considerably lower due to issues with adsorption and first-pass metabolism by the liver. The onset of effects is slower and may persist longer [19].

Mechanism of Action

There are two main classes of synthetic cannabinoid molecules, those related to the JWH compounds developed by John W. Huffman at Clemson University and those related to the CP compounds developed by Pfizer. Both classes are structurally different from THC but were designed to bind to the same CB1 and CB2 cannabinoid receptors. The CB1 receptor is expressed primarily in the hippocampus, basal ganglia, neocortex, amygdala, and cerebellum of the mammalian brain but is found throughout the body in lesser numbers. Though also expressed in the brain, the CB2 receptor is much less dense. Most research has focused on the CB1 receptor.

Synthetic cannabinoid receptor agonists belonging to the JWH class make up the majority of agents isolated from commercial preparations. Their affinity for the cannabinoid receptors is much greater and their effects are significantly more pronounced. JWH 018 has an affinity for the CB1 receptor that is four times that of THC and an affinity for the CB2 receptor that is ten times that of THC [20]. Unlike THC, however, these synthetic agents are full agonists and bind more tightly to their target receptors [21].

Synthetic cannabinoid receptor agonists belonging to the CP class also differ considerably from the classic cannabinoid structure of THC. CP-47,497 has a greater affinity for the CB1 receptor than THC [22] and is also 28 times more potent [23].

Other less common synthetic cannabinoid receptor agonists found in commercial preparations include members of the HU class developed at Hebrew University and the benzoylindoles. Unlike members of the JWH and CP class, the HU agonists are structurally very similar to THC. HU-210, for example, binds tightly to both the CB1 and CB2 receptors but is over 100 times more potent than naturally occurring THC [24]. Little is known about synthetic cannabinoid receptor agonists belonging to the benzoylindole class. Both AM-694 and RCS-4 have been isolated from commercial preparations, and both compounds have been shown to bind tightly to the CB1 and CB2 receptors [25].

Adverse Effects

Because these synthetic agents bind more tightly to the endogenous cannabinoid receptors, the effects of acute intoxication mirror those of cannabis intoxication but are more pronounced and prolonged. Hypertension, tachycardia, agitation, insomnia, and other psychiatric effects can persist for days. Prolonged use has been associated with physical dependence and discontinuation with a withdrawal syndrome [26]. Synthetic cannabinoid receptor agonists have been associated with learning and memory difficulty in animals [27], but these tests have not been carried out on humans. There likely exists a much greater risk for the development of acute psychosis in users of these synthetic products, perhaps because commercial preparations do not contain cannabidiol, a compound with antipsychotic properties that is found in naturally occurring cannabis [28]. At this point, nothing is known about the long-term effects these agents have on the human body, but their similar structure to known carcinogens has prompted some to suspect they may turn out to be considerably more toxic than is currently thought.

Summary

NPS drugs are attractive to users for a number of reasons. As novel compounds they are not detected in standard toxicology screens and may frequently used by persons who are subject to random drug tests [29]. While some tests are available for specific compounds that are commonly seen in most commercially available preparations, their use is not currently widespread. As many of these agents are not (yet) scheduled, they remain inexpensive and readily available. One can purchase an NPS drug in a retail store (they are available in so-called "head" shops and even gas stations in many parts of the country) or via the Internet. The typical NPS is marketed as a "natural" substance and users may believe that as such it is somehow safer than the currently illegal drugs many are more familiar with. Unfortunately little is known about the long-term effects these drugs have on the human body and psyche, and we are just beginning to understand the pharmacology of some of the newer agents.

References

1. Advisory Council on the Misuse of Drugs. Consideration of cathinones. 2012. http://www.namsdl.org/documents/ACMDCathinonesReport.pdf. Accessed 18 Nov 2012.
2. Schifano F, Albanese A, Fergus S, Stair JL, Deluca P, Corazza O, Davey Z, Corkery J, Siemann H, Scherbaum N, Farre' M, Torrens M, Demetrovics Z, Ghodse AH. Mephedrone (4-methyl-methycathinone; 'meow meow'): chemical and pharmacological and clinical issues. Psychopharmacology. 2011;214:593–602.
3. Ayres TC, Bond JW. A chemical analysis examining the pharmacology of novel psychoactive substances freely available over the internet and their impact on public (ill) health. Legal highs or illegal highs? BMJ Open. 2012;2:e977.
4. Motbey CP, Hunt GE, Bowen MT, Artiss S, McGregor IS. Mephedrone (4-methyl-methycathinone, 'meow'): acute behavioural effects and distribution of Fos expression in adolescent rats. Addict Biol. 2012;17:409–22.
5. Hadlock GC, Webb KM, McFadden LM, Chu PW, Ellis JD, Allen SC, Andrenyak DM, Vieira-Brock PL, German CL, Hanson GR, Flecknstein AE. 4-methyl-methycathinone (mephedrone): neuropharmacological effects of a designer stimulant of abuse. J Pharmacol Exp Ther. 2011;339:530–6.
6. Winstock A, Mitcheson L, Ramsey J, Davies S, Puchnarewicz M, Marsden J. Mephedrone: use, subjective effects and health risks. Addiction. 2011;106:1991–6.
7. Kehr J, Ichinose F, Yoshitake S, Goiny M, Sievertsson T, Nyberg F, Yoshitake T. Mephedrone, compared with MDMA (ecstasy) and amphetamine, rapidly increases both dopamine and 5-HT levels in nucleus accumbens of awake rats. Br J Pharmacol. 2011;164:1949–58.

8. Baumann MH, Ayestas Jr MA, Partilla JS. The designer methcathinon analogs, mephedrone and methylone, are substrates for monoamine transporters in brain tissue. Neuropsychopharmacology. 2012;37:1192–203.

9. Borek HA, Holstege CP. Hyperthermia and multiorgan failure after abuse of 'bath salts' containing 3,4-methylenedioxypyrovalerone. Ann Emerg Med. 2012;60:103–5.

10. Spiller HA, Ryan ML, Weston RG, Jansen J. Clinical experience with and analytical confirmation of 'bath salts' and 'legal highs' (synthetic cathinones) in the United States. Clin Toxicol. 2011;49:499–505.

11. Baumann MH, Partilla JS, Thorndike EB, Hoffman AF, Holy M, Rothman RB, Goldberg SR, Lupica CR, Sitte HH, Brandt SD, Tella SR, Cozzi NV, Schindler CW. Powerful cocaine-like actions of 3,4-methylenedioxypyrovalerone (MDPV), a principal constituent of psychoactive 'bath salts' products. Neuropharmacology. 2013;38(4):552–62.

12. Sammler EM, Foley PL, Lauder GD, Wilson SJ, Goudie AR, O'Riordan JI. A harmless high? Lancet. 2010;376:742.

13. DeMaria Jr S, Bryson EO, Frost EA. Anesthetic implications of acute methylenedioxymethamphetamine intoxication in a patient with traumatic intracerebral hemorrhage. Middle East J Anesthesiol. 2009;20(2):281–4.

14. Bryson EO, Frost EAM. Marijuana, nitrous oxide and other inhaled drugs: spotlight on chemically altered cannabis. In: Bryson EO, Frost EAM, editors. Perioperative addiction. New York: Springer Science and Business Media; 2011.

15. Simmons JR, Skinner CG, Williams J, Kang CS, Schwartz MD, Willis BK. Intoxication from smoking "spice". Ann Emerg Med. 2011;57:187–8.

16. Schifano F, Corazza O, Deluca P. Psychoactive drug or mystical incense? Overview of the online available information on spice products. J Cult Ment Health. 2009;2:137–44.

17. Canning J, Ruha A, Pierce R, Torrey M, Reinhart S. Severe GI distress after smoking JWH-018. Clin Toxicol. 2010;48:618.

18. Hurst D, Loeffler G, McLay R. Psychosis associated with synthetic cannabinoid agonists: a case series. Am J Psychiatr. 2011;168:1119.

19. British Medical Association. Therapeutic uses of cannabis. London: Harwood Academic Publishers; 1997.

20. Hauffman J. Cannabimimetic indoles, pyrroles and indenes: structure activity relationships and receptor interactions. In: Reggio PH, editor. The cannabinoid receptors. New York: Humana Press; 2009. p. 49–94.

21. ElSohly MA, Gul W, Elsohly KM, Murphy TP, Madgula VL, Khan SI. Liquid chromatography-tandem mass spectrometry analysis of urine specimens for K2 (JWH-018) metabolites. J Anal Toxicol. 2011;35:487–95.

22. Auwarter V, Dressen S, Weinmann W, Muller M, Putz M, Ferreiros N. "Spice" and other herbal blends: harmless incense or cannabinoid designer drugs? J Mass Spectrom. 2009;44:832–7.

23. Weissman A, Milne GM, Melvin Jr LS. Cannabimimetic activity from CP-47,497, a derivative of 3-phenylcyclohexanol. J Pharmacol Exp Ther. 1982;223:516–23.

24. Felder CC, Joyce KE, Briley EM, Mansouri J, Mackie K, Blond O, Lai Y, Ma AL, Mitchell RL. Comparison of the pharmacology and signal transduction of the human cannabinoid CB1 and CB2 receptors. Mol Pharmacol. 1995;48(3):443–50.

25. HUtter M, Broecker S, Kneisel S, Auwarter V. Identification of the major urinary metabolites in man of seven synthetic cannabinoids of the aminoalkylindole type present as adulterants in 'herbal mixtures' using LC-MS/MS techniques. J Mass Spectrom. 2012;47:54–65.

26. Zimmermann US, Winkelmann PR, Pilhatsch M, Nees JA, Spanagel R, Schulz K. Withdrawal phenomena and dependence syndrome after the consumption of "spice gold". Dtsch Arztebl Int. 2009;106(27):464–7.

27. Ferrari F, Ottani A, Vivoli R, Giuliani D. Learning impairment produced in rats by the cannabinoid agonist HU 210 in a water-maze task. Pharmacol Biochem Behav. 1999;64:555–61.

28. Zuardi AW, Crippa JA, Hallak JE, Moreira FA, Guimaraes FS. Cannabidiol, a cannabis sativa constituent, as an antipsychotic drug. Braz J Med Biol Res. 2006;39:421–9.

29. Loeffler G, Hurst D, Penn A, Yung K. Spice, bath salts, and the U.S. Military: the emergence of synthetic cannabinoid receptor agonists and cathinones in the U.S. Armed Forces. Mil Med. 2012;177(9):1041–8.

Chapter 51
New Vistas in Anesthetics, IV Induction Agents

John Pawlowski

Contents

Introduction

Since the advent of thiopental in the 1930s, there has been a proliferation of intravenous induction agents used in anesthesia practices. While all of these induction agents share the common features of rapid sedation and hypnosis, they all have side effects that are both common to all and unique to the specific class of pharmacologic drug [1]. This chapter will focus on the most popular anesthetic classes currently and will introduce several new and, perhaps, improved induction agents that may provide more reliable sedation with more predictable recovery and more limited side effects.

J. Pawlowski
Division of Thoracic Anesthesia, Beth Israel Deaconess Medical Center, Boston, MA, USA
e-mail: jpawlows@bidmc.harvard.edu

A.D. Kaye et al. (eds.), *Essentials of Pharmacology for Anesthesia, Pain Medicine, and Critical Care*, DOI 10.1007/978-1-4614-8948-1_51,
© Springer Science+Business Media New York 2015

Table 51.1 General classes of anesthetic agents, sedative actions, and purported mechanisms of action

	Group 1	Group 2	Group 3
Agents	Etomidate, propofol	Ketamine, nitrous oxide, xenon, cyclopropane	Barbiturates, halo alkyls
Actions	*Potent hypnotics*	*Potent analgesics*	*Potent hypnotics*
	Weak immobilizers	Weak hypnotics	*Potent immobilizers*
		Weak immobilizers	
Mechanisms	GABA-A receptors ($\alpha1$ and $\beta3$ subunits)	NMDA, AMPA, nACh, HCN1 receptors	GABA-A, TREK, NMDA, AMPA, nACh

Abbreviations: *GABA* gamma aminobutyric acid, *NMDA* N-methyl-D-aspartate (glutamate), *AMPA* alpha-amino-3-hydroxy-5-methyl-4-isoxazole propionic acid, *nACh* nicotinic acetyl choline, *HCN1* hyperpolarization-activated cyclic nucleotide-gated channel 1, *TREK* TWIK-related K+

Any discussion of induction agents should start with a general review of the features of an anesthetic and the groups of anesthetics and their described mechanisms of action (see Table 51.1). Anesthetic agents cause varying degrees of hypnosis, analgesia, immobilization, and amnesia [2]. The last property of amnesia will be addressed separately with the mention of the benzodiazepine class of medications. The first three properties of hypnosis, analgesia, and immobility have predictable distribution of actions among the groups listed in Table 51.1. These constellations of features are probably due to the different mechanisms of actions.

The anesthetic agents that qualify as intravenous induction agents must be able to produce a rapid state of unconsciousness in the patient. Since the intravenous (IV) route of administration results in almost immediate therapeutic drug concentrations, the IV induction agent remains the preferred type of induction agent to practicing anesthesiologists. This chapter will focus on the current and the new intravenous induction agents. Many of these agents have been extensively used and studied in human populations. Several of the newer and more promising induction agents, however, are described with animal studies alone.

Many of the newer compounds will have limited human clinical data, however, such that the pharmacologic mechanisms of action represent the results of animal studies, cellular experiments, and limited human experiences [3]. Unless specifically mentioned, all pharmacokinetic and pharmacodynamics data presented in the text and in the figures will be human data. All human data that deals with dosage schedules and clinical effects must be read with a degree of suspicion, due to the small number of healthy volunteers who often comprise the cohort in human investigational drug protocols. Conclusions as to the effectiveness of any new drug on whole populations are merely the speculation of the author.

This chapter will compare newer agents with those in current clinical use. Specific comparisons will be made regarding speed of onset, duration of action, rate of metabolism, and route of elimination. Where evidence exists, specific populations and pathologic conditions that may alter the predicted performance of the induction agent will be mentioned.

In general, most of the IV induction agents have effects on the gamma-amino butyric acid (GABA)-A type receptor in neural tissues. Where more detailed mechanisms are known or suggested, this chapter will mention the different mechanisms and will postulate on the potential clinical implications. The reader should realize that most of the clinical experiences are early, preliminary, and often confined to a healthy segment of the human adult population.

The specific types and examples of new IV induction agents that will be mentioned in this chapter are the *benzodiazepine* agents (*remimazolam* and *JM-1232*), the *etomidate* derivatives (*MOC-etomidate*, *carboetomidate*, *DMMM*, and *CMMM*), the *propofol* derivatives (*fos-propofol* and *PF0713*), and the *propanidid* derivative (*THRX-918661*). In addition, the opioid *remifentanil* will also be discussed, even though its mechanism of action is very different from the other IV induction agents. In certain specific clinical situations, however, remifentanil is very useful as an induction agent to provide short-term surgical anesthetic conditions.

Drug Class and Mechanism of Action

While the most popular and current intravenous agents represent a half dozen distinct classes of compounds, many of these agents share common mechanisms of action (Table 51.2). *Dexmedetomidine* is an alpha-2 agonist. *Etomidate* is an imidazole that increases the activity of the gamma aminobutyric acid (GABA) receptor as does *methohexital*, a barbiturate; *midazolam*, a benzodiazepine; and *propofol*, an isopropylphenol compound. *Ketamine*, a phencyclidine, acts as an NMDA receptor antagonist. Therefore, for most of the IV induction agents, the mechanism by which they produce sedation and hypnosis is through the activation of GABA-A. The GABA-A receptor is a pentameric formation that encircles a chloride channel (see Fig. 51.1). Usually this pentameric rosette consists of 2 alphas, 2 betas, and 1 gamma subunit. Activation of the central chloride channel results in the enhancement of inhibitory activity in the central nervous system, which can result in sedation, in anxiolysis, and decreases in abnormal neural activity seizures and spastic muscular activity. In fact, as many as 18 different subunits of the GABA-A receptor have been identified to date, and it is the arrangement of these subtypes into pentamers that may confer the unique properties of GABA activation [4]. The potential usefulness of a nonsedating anxiolytic or an antiepileptic that does not disturb the memory process should be clear to most readers.

Table 51.2 Current induction agents, general classes, and purported mechanisms of action

Drug	Class	Mechanism of action
Dexmedetomidine	Alpha-2	Alpha-2
Etomidate	Imidazole	GABA-A
Ketamine	Phencyclidine	NMDA
Methohexital	Barbiturate	GABA-A
Midazolam	Benzodiazepine	GABA-A
Propofol	Isopropyl phenol	GABA-A

Fig. 51.1 Pentameric
structure of the GABA
receptor

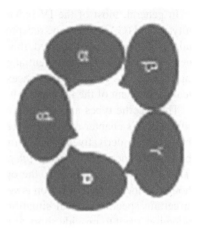

Indications/Clinical Pearls

Among the *benzodiazepine* class of medications, *remimazolam* [5] and *JM-1232* [6] offer potential utility as IV induction agents. Remimazolam provides a rapid onset of unconsciousness within 1–2 min, which is faster than midazolam. In addition, the volume of distribution is small and the metabolism is both rapid and predictable – making remimazolam a drug with fast onset and fast offset. Hydrolyzed by esterases, remimazolam is converted to an inactive metabolite. Remimazolam enjoys a nearly constant context-sensitive halftime, even when given as an infusion for up to 6 h [7]. The ester hydrolysis represents the "soft drug" technology, which can produce reliable metabolism of the drug, even in patients with significant liver and kidney disease [8].

The compound JM-1232 is a distinct isoindoline derivative that is chemically different from the other benzodiazepines but that does act as a full agonist at the benzodiazepine site on the GABA-A receptor and that is fully reversed by the antagonist flumazenil. The speed of onset of sedation for JM-1232 is faster than that of midazolam and is almost as rapid as propofol. Results in animals suggest some analgesic properties of JM-1232, but this has not been verified in humans.

Among the *etomidate* derivatives, *methoxycarbonyl-etomidate* (*MOC-etomidate*) shares the hemodynamic stability with that of etomidate [9]. MOC-etomidate acts as an ultrashort-acting induction agent with little adrenal suppression [10], which is a side effect of etomidate. Unfortunately, the active metabolite of MOC-etomidate has anesthetic properties and can result in a slow awakening, especially after a prolonged infusion. This exaggerated context-sensitive halftime of MOC-etomidate has prompted the development of other etomidate derivatives. Two such derivatives, *dimethyl MOC-metomidate* (*DMMM*) and *cyclopropyl MOC-metomidate* (*CPMM*), may exhibit better pharmacokinetic properties than MOC-etomidate. DMMM and CPMM both show slower metabolism via esterases and, therefore, represent more promising anesthetic agents for repeated doses or prolonged infusions. CPMM in particular demonstrates a more rapid recovery from anesthesia and more rapid resolution from adrenal suppression than does MOC-etomidate. Human trials of CPMM are scheduled to start soon in the United States.

To reduce the pain of injection from propofol, several *propofol* derivatives have been developed. *Fos-propofol* contains a phosphate moiety that renders the molecule more polar and allows the drug to be injected in an aqueous solution with minimal local site pain on injection. As a prodrug, fos-propofol is converted via alkaline phosphatase to propofol in the blood stream. This prodrug conversion delays the onset of action as well as lowers the peak concentrations, when compared to an equipotent bolus injection of propofol. There is less apnea seen with a bolus of fos-propofol [11] than with a bolus of propofol. Unfortunately, fos-propofol injection is associated with a severe burning sensation in the genital and anal regions. This type of burning sensation is seen with the injection of other phosphate medications, and this symptom may eventually preclude the use of fos-propofol as an induction agent.

Another propofol derivative, *PF0713*, is a diastereomer with a larger side group than propofol that produces rapid induction of unconsciousness and little to no pain on injection. The reduction in pain may be due to a diminished aqueous phase concentration of PF0713 compared with propofol. The increased potency of PF0713 versus propofol suggests the possibility that a single enantiomer may show improved clinical actions when compared to a racemic mixture.

A newer sedative hypnotic, *THRX-918661*, is a *propanidid* derivative that exhibits esterase hydrolysis. In animals, THRX-918661 produces a rapid onset of unconsciousness with a similar recovery profile to that of propofol. Less potent than propofol, doses of THRX-918661 need to be 3 times larger to accomplish similar levels of sedation. The metabolism by esterases presents the possibility that THRX-918661 can represent another "soft drug," with predictable metabolism.

Finally, the synthetic opioid *remifentanil* is in current use and can be used as an induction agent of sorts in specific clinical applications. Remifentanil provides profound analgesia and a rapid onset and offset. Painful procedures of a short duration can be performed painlessly with the use of a remifentanil bolus, such as manipulation of a shoulder dislocation or a retrobulbar block of the eye. While awareness can occur, the memory is seldom painful or distressing. Remifentanil is a "soft drug" with a rapid half-life and a near-constant context-sensitive halftime, making it useful in patients with liver or kidney dysfunction and good in both repeated boluses and as an infusion.

Dosing Options

Most of the newer agents have defined dosage schedules for the induction of surgical anesthesia. Many of these agents also have infusion dosage schedules, due to their relatively constant context-sensitive halftimes. Table 51.3 lists the published and probable dosing for human adults for both bolus induction and infusion of these agents.

Table 51.3 Intravenous induction agents

Drug	Dose	Onset (minutes)	Duration (hours)
Propofol	1–2 mg/kg	1	1
Midazolam	0.5 mg/kg	3	2
Fentanyl	10 mcg/kg	3	1
Methohexital	1–2 mg/kg	1	2
Remimazolam	0.3 mg/kg	1.5	0.2
Dexmedetomidine	0.8 mcg/kg	10	2
Remifentanil	0.3 mcg/kg	1.5	0.2
Etomidate	0.2 mg/kg	1	3
MOC-etomidate	20 mg/kg	2	1
Fos-propofol	6.5 mg/kg	3	1
Ketamine	1 mg/kg	1	3

Please note that these schedules represent an estimate by the author, based on human or animal data and from preliminary experimental or limited clinical experiences. All medications should be titrated to clinical effect. All patients should be monitored for vital signs and for unwanted side effects. Appropriate resuscitation equipment should be available whenever an anesthetic induction agent is administered.

Drug Interactions

The combination of sedatives can result in additive or even potentiated clinical effects. Certain GABA agonists can have lethal consequences. For example, ethanol, barbiturates, chloral hydrate, or chlormethiazole can produce fatal respiratory arrests either alone or in combination, due to a common mechanism of direct opening of the chloride channel associated with the GABA receptor. In contrast, benzodiazepines only facilitate the opening of the chloride channel through an indirect effect on the efficiency of GABA binding to the receptor. Thus, benzodiazepines seldom produce respiratory arrests.

Side Effects/Black Box Warnings

The administration of benzodiazepines to patients who are on antiretroviral therapy has been associated with prolonged sedation and respiratory arrest. The mechanism for this interaction seems to be the common route of metabolism through the cytochrome P450 pathway. Therefore, medications that share the mode of metabolism can lead to extended effects. Benzodiazepines also have synergistic effects on opioid- and propofol-induced respiratory depression. The newer benzodiazepine, remimazolam, would be expected to have similar synergistic actions.

Summary

A number of current and newer intravenous induction agents allow for the continued practice of safe and rapid administration of medications to induce a loss of consciousness with possible additional effects of analgesia, amnesia, and immobility [12]. The mechanism for most induction agents is an effect on GABA receptors, although several important distinctions between GABA agonists and other mechanisms were made. Several promising new drugs and several alternative mechanisms were also suggested. The general concept of "soft drugs" was advanced and several clinical examples were given.

Chemical Structures

**Chemical Structure
51.1** Remimazolam

**Chemical Structure
51.2** Dexmedetomidine

**Chemical Structure
51.3** Methohexital

Chemical Structure
51.4 Fospropofol

References

1. Brunton LL, Chabner BA, Knollmann BC, editors. Goodman and Gilman's the pharmacological basis of therapeutics. 12th ed. USA: McGraw-Hill Companies, Inc; 2011.
2. Miller RD, Eriksson LI, Fleisher LA, Weiner-Kronish JP, Young WL, editors. Miller's anesthesia. 7th ed. Philadelphia: Churchill Livingstone; 2010.
3. Sneyd JR, Rigby-Jones AE. New drugs and technologies, intravenous anaesthesia is on the move (again). Br J Anaesth. 2010;105(3):246–54.
4. Nutt DJ, Malizia AL. New insights into the role of the GABA-A- benzodiazepine receptor in psychiatric disorder. Br J Psychiatry. 2001;179:390–6.
5. Sneyd JR. Remimazolam. Anesth Analg. 2012;115:217–9.
6. Nishiyama T, Chiba S, Yamada Y. Antinociceptive property of intrathecal and intraperitoneal administration of a novel water-soluble isoindolin-1 derivative, JM-1232 in rats. Eur J Pharmacol. 2008;596:56–61.
7. Wiltshire HR, Kilpatrick GJ, Tilbrook GS, Borkett KM. A placebo- and midazolam-controlled phase I single ascending dose study evaluating the safety, pharmacokinetics and pharmacodynamics of remimazolam (CNS-7056): Part II. Population pharmacokinetic and pharmacodynamics modeling and simulation. Anesth Analg. 2012;115:284–96.
8. Egan TD. Is anesthesiology going soft? Trends in fragile pharmacology. Anesthesiology. 2009;111:229–30.
9. Forman SA. Clinical and molecular pharmacology of etomidate. Anesthesiology. 2011; 114(3):695–707.
10. Ge RL, Pejo E, Haburcak M, Husain SS, Forman SA, Raines DE. Pharmacological studies of methoxycarbonyl etomidate's carboxylic acid metabolite. Anesth Analg. 2012;115:305–8.
11. Candiotti KA, Gan TJ, Young C, Bekker A, Sum-Ping ST, Kahn R, Lebowitz P, Littman JJ. A randomized, open-label study of the safety and tolerability of fospropofol for patients requiring intubation and mechanical ventilation in the intensive care unit. Anesth Analg. 2011;113(3):550–6.
12. Pawlowski J. Moderate and deep sedation techniques. In: Ernst A, Herth FJF, editors. Principles and practice of interventional pulmonology. New York: Springer; 2013.

Chapter 52
New Vistas in Neuromuscular Blockers

Matthew T. Murrell and John J. Savarese

Contents

What Is the Need for New Neuromuscular-Blocking Drugs?

The medication drawer of a modern anesthesiology workstation may contain up to five neuromuscular-blocking drugs (NMBs): succinylcholine, vecuronium, rocuronium, and possibly pancuronium and cisatracurium. With such an extensive armamentarium for providing muscle relaxation, why would an anesthesiologist require additional compounds? Although the depolarizing neuromuscular-blocking compound succinylcholine has been at anesthesiologists' disposal since 1952 [1] and remains the sole short-acting neuromuscular-blocking agent capable of providing adequate conditions for rapid tracheal intubation, succinylcholine nevertheless possesses an adverse effect profile well known to all practicing anesthesiologists: muscle fasciculations, hyperkalemia, cardiac arrest, and increased intraocular and intracranial pressures. Vecuronium, rocuronium, and pancuronium all possess a much more favorable adverse effect profile, but all three exhibit altered pharmacokinetics in the setting of end-organ perturbations. Cisatracurium is currently the only clinically available nondepolarizing neuromuscular-blocking compound with

M.T. Murrell, MD, PhD (✉) • J.J. Savarese, MD
Department of Anesthesiology, Weill Cornell Medical College, New York, NY, USA
e-mail: mtm9006@med.cornell.edu

A.D. Kaye et al. (eds.), *Essentials of Pharmacology for Anesthesia,*
Pain Medicine, and Critical Care, DOI 10.1007/978-1-4614-8948-1_52,
© Springer Science+Business Media New York 2015

organ-independent metabolism and thus a lack of cumulative effects [2, 3]; however, this compound has an intermediate duration of action, a high potency, and therefore a relatively slow onset of action insufficient for rapidly securing a patient's airway. Clearly, additions to the current armamentarium of neuromuscular-blocking compounds would prove useful in clinical practice, and the search for new molecules to fill the clinical voids has been ongoing since the 1970s.

Another force driving the search for novel neuromuscular-blocking compounds arises from the elucidation and general recognition of the adverse effects of perioperative residual neuromuscular blockade. What were once thought to be clinically insignificant amounts of residual blockade [4] are now recognized as significant causes of perioperative adverse events including visual disturbances, hypoxemia, aspiration, and tracheal reintubation [5–9]. Although there remains disagreement about the ideal manner in which to monitor intraoperative and perioperative neuromuscular blockade, practitioners surveyed in both the United States and Europe generally recognize that a train-of-four (TOF) ratio greater than or equal to 90 % is considered the standard of care prior to tracheal extubation [10]. An initial step toward addressing these issues and ensuring safe care of patient in the perioperative period has been achieved with sugammadex, a gamma cyclodextrin, and possibly also with the newer compound calabadion, an acyclic member of the cucurbit(n) urils family. Better and more consistent use of neuromuscular monitoring in the perioperative setting will also reduce the morbidity resultant from residual neuromuscular blockade. However, the full resolution of the problem lies in the development of neuromuscular-blocking molecules with improved pharmacokinetics over and distinct reversal mechanisms from those drugs currently employed in clinical practice.

The Ideal Neuromuscular-Blocking Drug and Novel Drug Development

As early as 1975, the need for several NMBs with distinct characteristics to fill specific clinical roles was recognized: a rapidly acting NMB with short duration and minimal cardiovascular (both autonomic and hemodynamic) side effects to supplant succinylcholine, an intermediate-acting NMB without cumulative effect, and a long-acting NMB lacking significant hemodynamic effects [11]. Around the same time, anesthesiologists recognized the characteristics of the desired ideal NMB: a rapid onset of action, a lack of cumulative effect (organ-independent activity neutralization), a favorable cardiovascular side effect profile, and complete reversibility at any time point of blockade [12–15]. Although several of the subsequently developed neuromuscular-blocking compounds have fulfilled some of these criteria, none to date possess all these characteristics.

Identifying molecules that can satisfy all these ideal requirements is a difficult task. Our increased knowledge of the structure-activity relationships for neuromuscular-blocking compounds has begun to elucidate how different sites on a given molecule can confer changes in potency, duration of action, and cardiovascular side effects (including alterations in autonomic activity and histamine release). Nevertheless, the process of identifying candidate molecules, assessing their potency, pharmacokinetics, and adverse effect profiles in animal models, and subsequently engineering structural changes in attempt to confer the desired activity profile in promising candidate molecules is a time-consuming and expensive process. The pitfalls of novel drug development can be highlighted by the clinical course of rapacuronium, the most recent neuromuscular-blocking compound to be released in the United States. After extensive preclinical development and testing, which revealed a rapid onset of action similar to that of succinylcholine and a duration shorter than that of mivacurium [16], the drug was withdrawn from the market in 2001 due primarily to bronchoconstriction events [17, 18].

In order to have clinical relevance, any novel neuromuscular-blocking compound must possess adequate potency to permit a reasonable dosing range; however, a rapid onset of action is another desired characteristic of candidate compounds, and as potency increases, the rapidity of onset typically decreases [19–21]. Moreover, a rapid onset of action can be aided by a rapid clearance or metabolism of the drug [22]. Both of these factors, in addition to a stable hemodynamic profile, must be identified in a single candidate molecule in order to proceed with further preclinical and clinical testing. Identifying a compound with the desired potency and onset of action is a process of trial and error involving structure-activity relationship testing in vivo. One means of ensuring rapid clearance and shortened duration of effect is identifying and developing a novel class of molecules with a predictable, organ-independent inactivation mechanism.

The Newest Emerging Class of Neuromuscular-Blocking Molecules: Fumarates

The olefinic isoquinolinium diester fumarates are the most recent class of neuromuscular-blocking molecules possessing significant clinical potential. Gantacurium (Fig. 52.1a) and CW002 (Fig. 52.1b), both enantiomeric fumarates, are the first two molecules in this class of neuromuscular-blocking drugs to be tested. The inactivation mechanism, L-cysteine adduction at the central fumarate double bond, is unique to this class of neuromuscular-blocking molecules and represents a novel reversal paradigm as well as organ-independent kinetics.

Gantacurium is an ultrashort-acting nondepolarizing neuromuscular-blocking drug whose inactivation is mediated via two principal mechanisms: cysteine adduction [23] and pH-sensitive hydrolysis at the ester linkage of the molecule [24] (Fig. 52.2). In humans, gantacurium has an ED_{95} of 0.19 mg/kg, representing a relatively modest potency [25] but likely contributing, along with rapid clearance, to its rapid onset of action. Maximum neuromuscular blockade occurred within 90 s following the administration of $1.5xED_{95}$ gantacurium and within 60 s following higher doses.

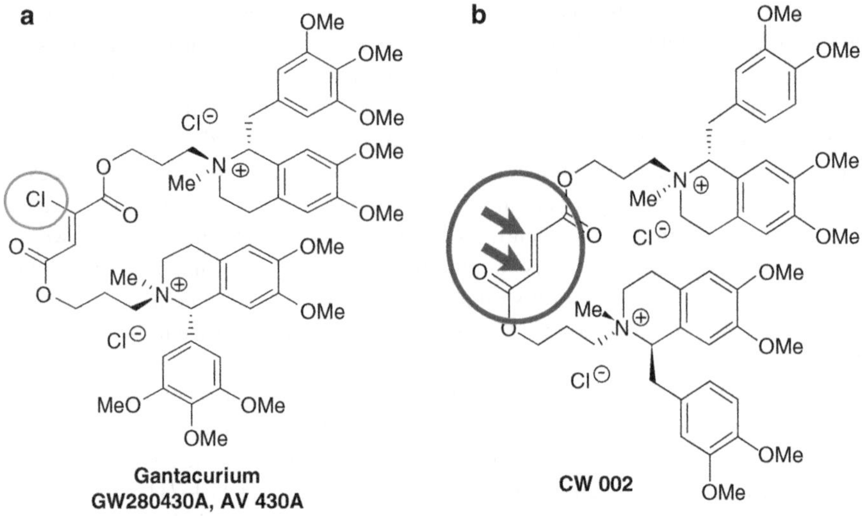

Fig. 52.1 The chemical structures of gantacurium (**a**) and CW002 (**b**). The chlorine (**a**, *red circle*) substituted at the olefinic double bond of gantacurium was designed to accelerate the inactivation of the molecule in the presence of L-cysteine. CW002 (**b**) lacks a halogen substitution at the fumarate component (*blue circle*) and undergoes L-cysteine adduction and inactivation at a slower rate (Reproduced with permission from Savarese et al. [27])

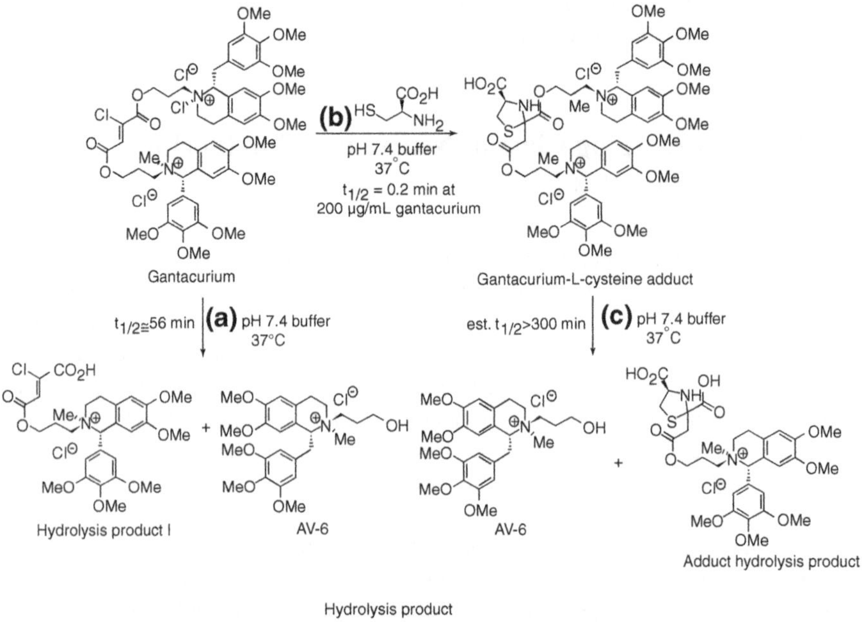

Fig. 52.2 Degradation of gantacurium. At pH 7.4 and 37 °C (**a**), the molecule undergoes slow alkaline hydrolysis. In the presence of L-cysteine (**b**), rapid formation of an adduct intermediate occurs; this adduction product then undergoes slow alkaline hydrolysis (**c**) (Reproduced with permission from Savarese et al. [27])

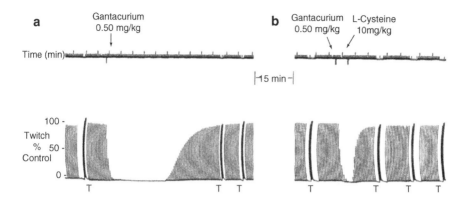

Fig. 52.3 Representative mechanomyographic measurements of gantacurium-induced neuromuscular blockade and its antagonism using L-cysteine in an anesthetized rhesus monkey. Panel (**a**) depicts the neuromuscular blockade produced by 0.5 mg/kg gantacurium (representing approximately 5xED$_{95}$). Panel (**b**) One minute after injection of a second dose of 0.5 mg/kg, the administration of 10 mg/kg L-cysteine restored twitch and train-of-four (*T*) to baseline within 2 min (Reproduced with permission from Savarese et al. [27])

Thus, gantacurium possesses kinetics very similar to those of succinylcholine, the molecule gantacurium was designed to replace. Although transient cardiovascular effects emerged at doses of 3xED$_{95}$ and histamine release occurred in humans at doses of 4xED$_{95}$ [25], the propensity of gantacurium to provoke these types of adverse effects was less than that observed with mivacurium [26], another short-duration nondepolarizing drug that has been removed from the clinical market for economic reasons. The inactivation of gantacurium, as mentioned, occurs via both slow pH-sensitive hydrolysis ($t_{1/2}$ 56 min) and rapid L-cysteine adduction ($t_{1/2}$ 0.2 min), the latter resulting in an adduct product of extremely low potency that itself undergoes alkaline hydrolysis to form inactive products (Fig. 52.2).

The antagonism of gantacurium by the addition of exogenous L-cysteine is extremely rapid, with reduction of total duration of neuromuscular block from approximately 10 min with spontaneous recovery to 3 min with 10 mg/kg L-cysteine administered 1 min after a gantacurium dose that completely abolished twitch response [27]. Figure 52.3 depicts the rapidity of blockade antagonism produced by the administration of L-cysteine as measured with mechanomyography.

Although gantacurium possessed a rapid speed of onset, an ultrashort duration, and an acceptable side effect profile that was highly attractive to clinical application, problems with production and marketing prevented this molecule from entering the pharmacopeia. Efforts are ongoing to develop other ultrashort-acting fumarate neuromuscular-blocking molecules possessing rapidity of onset and cysteine reversibility with superior side effect profiles to that of gantacurium. This type of molecule would be well positioned to replace the use of succinylcholine in many clinical situations.

The most recent isoquinolinium diester neuromuscular-blocking drug to undergo both nonhuman primate and human testing is CW002 (Fig. 52.1b), which is

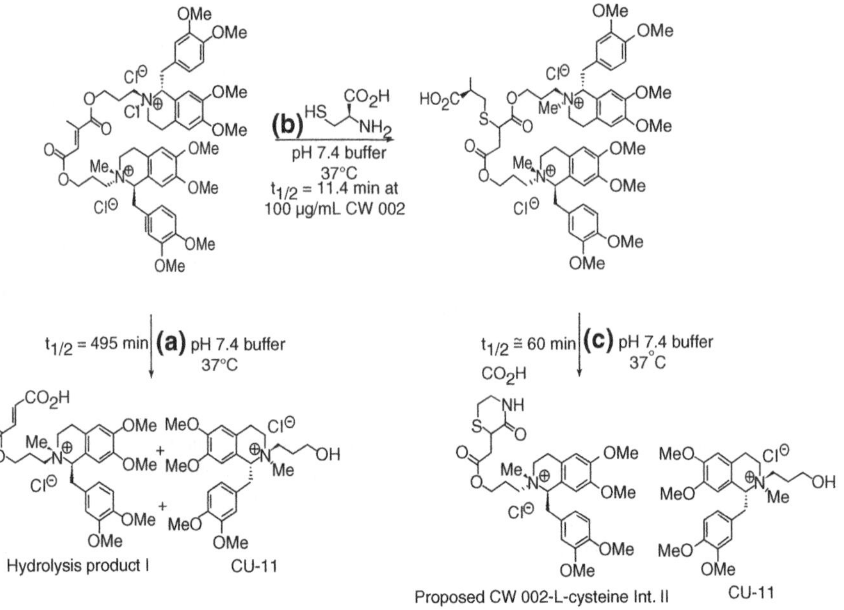

Fig. 52.4 Degradation of CW002. CW002 undergoes slow alkaline hydrolysis at pH 7.4 and 37 °C (**a**). In the presence of L-cysteine (**b**), an adduction intermediate is formed which is approximately 70-fold less potent than CW002. This adduction intermediate itself undergoes alkaline hydrolysis (**c**) (Reproduced with permission from Savarese et al. [27])

currently in a phase I human trial. CW002 differs in structure from gantacurium in that its fumarate is symmetrical and lacks halogen substitution. This results in less activation of the olefinic carbon atoms and therefore a slower L-cysteine adduction reaction and inactivation of the molecule.

CW002, as with gantacurium, undergoes both alkaline hydrolysis ($t_{1/2}$ 495 min) and a more rapid L-cysteine adduction reaction ($t_{1/2}$ 11.4 min), although both of these processes are slower than those for gantacurium (Fig. 52.4). The CW002 L-cysteine adduction product (Fig. 52.4) is approximately 70-fold less potent than CW002.

CW002 thus has an approximately threefold longer duration of action than gantacurium (approximately 28 min versus 10 min, respectively) in nonhuman primates and can be classified as an intermediate duration of action neuromuscular blocker [27]. The comparable recovery time for cisatracurium under identical conditions is approximately 58 min [27].

Although longer in duration than gantacurium, CW002 is a more potent molecule, with an ED_{95} of 0.05 mg/kg in nonhuman primates [28]. This increased potency could be expected to make the onset of action slower than that of gantacurium; however, CW002 at doses of $3 \times ED_{95}$ produces complete neuromuscular blockade within 1 min. Thus, CW002 is a potential intermediate duration nondepolarizing drug which might produce conditions for tracheal intubation in humans within approximately 90 s or possibly less. This quality, combined with the ability to

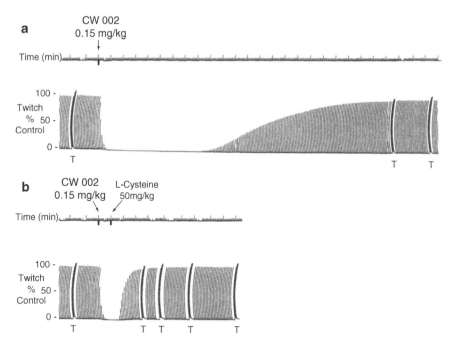

Fig. 52.5 Representative mechanomyographic measurements of CW002-induced neuromuscular blockade and its antagonism using L-cysteine in an anesthetized rhesus monkey. Panel (**a**) depicts the neuromuscular blockade produced by injection of 0.15 mg/kg CW002 (approximately 4xED$_{95}$). One hour following this first dose, injection of 50 mg/kg L-cysteine 1 min after the administration of 0.15 mg/kg CW002 restored twitch and train-of-four (*T*) to baseline within 2 and 3 min, respectively (Reproduced with permission from Savarese et al. [27])

rapidly inactivate the molecule at any point during neuromuscular blockade with the administration of L-cysteine, makes CW002 an attractive clinical candidate.

L-cysteine inactivation of CW002 occurs via the same reaction as that for gantacurium, although more slowly due to the lack of an "activating" halogen substitution at the fumarate of CW002. Nevertheless, the administration of L-cysteine 60 s after a 4xED$_{95}$ dose of CW002 restores neuromuscular function to normal within 3 min (Fig. 52.5) [27]. Thus, as with the ultrashort-acting molecule gantacurium, the duration of action of even an intermediate duration isoquinolinium fumarate like CW002 can be tailored to the clinical duration required via the administration of L-cysteine.

Unlike rapacuronium, neither CW002 nor gantacurium interacts with M2 or M3 airway receptors [29] and is unlikely therefore to result in bronchoconstriction by this mechanism. Although gantacurium at doses several times ED$_{95}$ resulted in moderate cardiovascular changes and histamine release in humans, studies to date with CW002 reveal a more promising safety profile. In animals, doses of 20–80xED$_{95}$ resulted in only modest hemodynamic effects with no bronchoconstriction or significant histamine release [30]. The CW002 safety profile evident in dogs and non-human primates is currently being assessed in a human phase I trial.

In summary, the isoquinolinium diester fumarate compounds and L-cysteine reversal represent an important potential change to the current clinical armamentarium of neuromuscular-blocking drugs. Ideally, clinical anesthesiologists would have at their disposal an intermediate duration compound like CW002 for use in cases of moderate length, where the neuromuscular-blocking activity could be terminated easily at any point with L-cysteine. Moreover, there is still a definite clinical need for an ultrashort-acting compound with an excellent adverse effect safety profile superior to that of gantacurium that would serve as a replacement for succinylcholine and an improvement over the previously available mivacurium. Such an ultrashort-acting compound would provide a tool for a wide array of clinical scenarios including rapid tracheal intubation, short surgical procedures requiring limited periods of paralysis, and as an accompaniment to agents like propofol and remifentanil during total intravenous anesthesia. The fumarates and related compounds could have considerable impact on future clinical practice.

References

1. Foldes FF, McNall PG, Borrego-Hinojosa JM. Succinylcholine: a new approach to muscular relaxation in anesthesiology. N Engl J Med. 1952;247:596–600.
2. Belmont MR, Lien CA, Quessy S, Abou-Donia MM, Abalos A, Eppich L, Savarese JJ. The clinical neuromuscular pharmacology of 51W89 in patients receiving nitrous oxide/opioid/barbiturate anesthesia. Anesthesiology. 1995;82(5):1139–45.
3. Lepage JY, Malinovsky JM, Malinge M, Lechevalier T, Dupuch C, Cozian A, Pinaud M, Souron R. Pharmacodynamic dose-response and safety study of cisatracurium (51W89) in adult surgical patients during N2O-O2-opioid anesthesia. Anesth Analg. 1996;83(4):823–9.
4. Ali HH, Wilson RS, Savarese JJ, Kitz RJ. The effect of tubocurarine on indirectly elicited train-of-four muscle response and respiratory measurements in humans. Br J Anaesth. 1975;47:570–4.
5. Eriksson LI, Sato M, Severinghaus JW. Effect of a vecuronium-induced partial neuromuscular block on hypoxic ventilatory response. Anesthesiology. 1993;78:693–9.
6. Kopman AF, Yee PS, Neuman GG. Relationship of the train-of-four fade ratio to clinical signs and symptoms of residual paralysis in awake volunteers. Anesthesiology. 1997;86:765–71.
7. Berg H, Viby-Mogensen J, Mortensen CR, Engbaek J, Skovgaard LT, Krintel JJ. Residual neuromuscular block is a risk factor for postoperative pulmonary complications after atracurium, vecuronium and pancuronium. Acta Anaesthesiol Scand. 1997;41:1095–103.
8. Murphy GS, Szokol JW, Marymount JH, Greenberg SB, Avram MJ, Vender JS. Residual neuromuscular blockade and critical respiratory events in the postanesthesia care unit. Anesth Analg. 2008;107:130–7.
9. Murphy GS, Szokol MD, Avram MJ, Greenberg SB, Marymount JH, Vender JS, Gray J, Landry E, Gupta DK. Intraoperative acceleromyography monitoring reduces symptoms of muscle weakness and improves quality of recovery in the early postoperative period. Anesthesiology. 2011;115:946–54.
10. Naguib M, Kopman AF, Lien CA, Hunter JM, Lopez A, Brull SJ. A survey of current management of neuromuscular block in the United States and Europe. Anesth Analg. 2010;111:110–9.
11. Savarese JJ, Kitz RJ. Does clinical anesthesia need new neuromuscular blocking agents? Anesthesiology. 1975;42:236–9.
12. Busfield D, Child KJ, Clarke AJ, Davis B, Dodds MG. Br J Pharmacol. 1968;33:609–29.

13. Kitz RJ, Karis JH, Ginsburg S. A study *in vitro* of new short acting nondepolarizing neuromuscular blocking agents. Biochem Pharmacol. 1969;18:871–81.
14. Ginsburg S, Kitz RJ, Savfarese JJ. Neuromuscular blocking activity of a new series of quaternary N-substituted choline esters. Br J Pharmacol. 1971;43:107–26.
15. Savarese JJ, Kitz RJ. The quest for a short-acting nondepolarizing neuromuscular blocking agent. Acta Anaesthesiol Scand. 1973;53(suppl):43–58.
16. Wierda JM, Beaufort AM, Kleef UW, et al. Preliminary investigations of the clinical pharmacology of three short-acting nondepolarizing neuromuscular blocking agents, Org 9453, Org 9489 and Org 9487. Can J Anaesth. 1984;41:213–20.
17. Jooste E, Klafter F, Hirshman CA, et al. A mechanism for rapacuronium-induced bronchospasm: M2 muscarinic receptor antagonism. Anesthesiology. 2003;98:906–11.
18. Jooste EH, Sharma A, Zhang Y, et al. Rapacuronium augmentsacetylcholine-induced bronchospasm via positive allosteric interactions at the M3 muscarinic receptor. Anesthesiology. 2005;103:1195–203.
19. Bowman WC, Rodger IW, Houston J, et al. Structure: action relationships among some desacetoxy analogues of pancuronium and vecuronium in the anesthetized cat. Anesthesiology. 1988;69:57–62.
20. Wastila WB, Maehr RB, Turner GL, et al. Comparative pharmacology of cisatracurium (51W89), atracurium, and five isomers in cats. Anesthesiology. 1996;85:169–77.
21. Kopman AF. Pancuronium, gallamine, and d-tubocurarine compared: is speed of onset inversely related to drug potency? Anesthesiology. 1989;70:915–20.
22. Bevan DR. Neuromuscular blocking drugs: onset and intubation. J Clin Anesth. 1997; 9:36S–9.
23. Boros EE, Samano V, Ray JA, Thompson JB, Jung DK, Kaldor I, et al. Neuromuscular blocking activity and therapeutic potential of mixed-tetrahydroisoquinolinium halofumarates and halosuccinates in rhesus monkeys. J Med Chem. 2003;46:2502–15.
24. Savarese JJ, Belmont MR, Hashim MA, Mook RA, Boros EE, Samano V, et al. Preclinical pharmacology of GW280430A (AV430A) in the rhesus monkey and in the cat. Anesthesiology. 2004;100:835–45.
25. Belmont MR, Lien CA, Tjan J, Bradley E, Stein B, Patel SS, Savafrese JJ. Clinical pharmacology of GW280430A in humans. Anesthesiology. 2004;100:768–73.
26. Lien CA, Belmont MR, Heerdt PM. GW280430A: pharmacodynamics and potential adverse effects. Anesthesiology. 2005;102:862–3.
27. Savarese JJ, McGilvra JD, Sunaga H, Belmont MR, Van Ornum SG, Savard PM, Heerdt PM. Rapid chemical antagonism of neuromuscular blockade by L-cysteine adduction to and inactivation of the olefinic (double-bonded) isoquinolinium diester compounds gantacurium (AV430A), CW002 and CW001. Anesthesiology. 2010;113:58–73.
28. Belmont MR, Savard P, Vasquez A, et al. A promising cysteine-reversible intermediate duration neuromuscular blocker in rhesus monkeys. Anesthesiology. 2007;107:A986.
29. Sunaga H, Zhang Y, Savarese JJ, et al. Gantacurium and CW002 do not potentiate muscarinic receptor-mediated airway smooth muscle constriction in guinea pigs. Anesthesiology. 2010;112:892–9.
30. Heerdt PM, Malhotra JK, Pan BY, Sunaga H, Savarese JJ. Pharmacodynamics and cardiopulmonary side effects of CW002, a cysteine-reversible neuromuscular blocking drug in dogs. Anesthesiology. 2010;112:910–6.

Chapter 53
Patient-Controlled Analgesia: The Importance of Effector Site Pharmacokinetics

Pamela P. Palmer and Mike A. Royal

Contents

Introduction

Opioid transit across the blood-brain barrier (BBB) and into the central nervous system (CNS) is complex and is dependent on a drug's specific physiochemical properties, such as lipophilicity, molecular size, degree of protein binding and ionization, as well as physiological factors, such as metabolism and drug clearance. More recently, drug equilibration from the systemic circulation to the CNS has been determined to be significantly governed by a dynamic interplay between influx and efflux membrane transporter pumps and synergy between transporters and metabolizing enzymes. In combination with physicochemical and physiological factors, these transporter systems regulate CNS opioid receptor exposure and effectively

P.P. Palmer, MD, PhD (✉) • M.A. Royal, MD, MBA, JD
AcelRx Pharmaceuticals, Inc, Redwood City, CA, USA
e-mail: ppalmer@acelrx.com

A.D. Kaye et al. (eds.), *Essentials of Pharmacology for Anesthesia,*
Pain Medicine, and Critical Care, DOI 10.1007/978-1-4614-8948-1_53,
© Springer Science+Business Media New York 2015

determine analgesic onset, as well as the magnitude and duration of pharmacodynamic (PD) effects, including side effects. The infamous and colorful bank robber "Slick Willie" Sutton suggested that the reason he robbed banks was "because that's where they keep the money" [1]. Following Sutton's lead, we should look to the CNS, not traditional venous pharmacokinetic (PK) parameters, to better understand and more appropriately select opioids and routes of administration for various clinical use scenarios.

Variables Regulating Opioid Pharmacokinetics

When administered as an IV bolus, opioid venous plasma concentrations typically reflect two phases: the alpha phase primarily due to rapid distribution from systemic circulation to body tissues and the beta phase due to metabolism and clearance mechanisms. The initial distribution phase relates to physicochemical properties, such as lipophilicity and ionization, of the opioid. Route of administration can dramatically affect this initial PK phase, especially with lipophilic drugs, with more extended absorption routes (e.g., oral, transmucosal) counteracting the rapid distribution phase, resulting in more consistent drug concentrations over time compared to IV bolus administration.

During the elimination phase, opioids primarily undergo hepatic metabolism through oxidation, dealkylation, hydrolysis, and conjugation. Each of these metabolic pathways is designed to produce metabolites that are more hydrophilic than the parent compound and thereby easier to excrete via urine. Phase I enzymatic reactions (oxidation and hydrolysis) are performed by various cytochrome P450 (CYP) enzyme systems, e.g., CYP3A4 or CYP2D6, which modify the structure of the drug. Several opioids are metabolized by CYP2D6 to compounds with greater potency than the parent (i.e., codeine to morphine, hydrocodone to hydromorphone, and tramadol to its M1 metabolite, (+)R-O-desmethyl-tramadol) [2]. Additionally, CYP2D6 and to a lesser extent CYP3A4 are subject to frequent polymorphisms that may result in patient-to-patient variability in primary metabolism to inactive or active metabolites resulting in highly variable outcomes, including toxicity on the one hand or inadequate analgesia on the other. Phase II reactions involve conjugation with glucuronic acid (via uridine 5'-diphospho-glucuronosyl-transferases [UGT], primarily UGT2B7), sulfate, glutathione, or amino acids to create less lipophilic conjugates eventually excreted in the urine or bile.

Variability in metabolic pathways can be critically important for opioids that have active metabolites, as biotransformation can result in an active metabolite with equal or greater potency. Table 53.1 presents the major metabolic pathways and metabolite activity for the commonly used parenteral opioids in postoperative pain management.

Table 53.1 Major metabolites of commonly used parenteral opioids for postoperative pain management

Opioid	Metabolic pathway	Major metabolites	Analgesic activity	Adverse effect
Morphine	UGTB27	M3G	N	Nausea, neuroexcitatory effects
		M6G	Y	Prolonged duration especially with renal insufficiency
Fentanyl	CYP3A4	Norfentanyl	N	n/a
Hydromorphone	UGTB27	H3G	N	Nausea, neuroexcitatory effects
	UGT1A3	H6G	Y	Prolonged duration especially with renal insufficiency
Meperidine	CYP3A4, CYP2B6	Normeperidine	N	Seizures
Sufentanil	CYP3A4	Norsufentanil	N	n/a

Source: Modified from Smith [2]

CYP cytochrome P450, *H3G* hydromorphone-3-glucuronide, *H6G* hydromorphone-6-glucuronide, *M3G* morphine-3-glucuronide, *M6G* morphine-6-glucuronide, *UGT* UDP-glucuronosyl-transferase

The Blood-Brain Barrier

Aside from the classic distribution and elimination mechanisms that regulate opioid PK, it is now clear that CNS drug levels are governed by more than just these well-known processes. The BBB is much more than a physical barrier as, along with the gut mucosa, these membranes contain various influx and efflux transporters that modulate opioid entry through a dynamic energy-dependent gating process [3, 4]. Membrane transporters, such as P-glycoprotein (P-gp), are multispecific transport proteins that not only mediate the BBB (and gut) passage of numerous endogenous compounds but are important in determining the onset, magnitude, and duration of the (PD) effects of opioids and other centrally acting drugs. P-gp appears to have developed as a primary mechanism to protect the body from exogenous toxins and transports substances/drugs, against a concentration gradient, from the brain, gonads, or other organs into the gut, urine, or bile [5]. For oral analgesics, P-gp has an important "gatekeeper" function (eliminating drug into the gut lumen) and should be considered as part of the "first-pass effect," especially when administered with a P-gp inducer.

In summary, opioids can have widely disparate PK/PD based on route of administration, physicochemical properties, variability of metabolic pathways, production of active metabolites, and whether the parent drug is a substrate for membrane transporters, such as P-gp [6]. Opioids with active metabolites that are also P-gp substrates, e.g., morphine glucuronides, will have far greater variability in analgesic effect and potential for unanticipated adverse events, particularly late-onset sedation and respiratory depression [7]. Therefore, the anticipated onset, magnitude, and duration of opioid analgesic effects can become quite complex.

Effector Site Pharmacokinetics

The true correlation to opioid PD is clearly the local CNS effector site drug concentration and not the venous drug concentration that is classically used to determine PK parameters, such as C_{max} (peak venous plasma concentration), T_{max} (time to C_{max}), and $t_{1/2}$ (elimination half-life). Furthermore, simply changing the route of delivery of an opioid from IV to transmucosal, for example, can dramatically affect even these classic PK parameters. The previous discussion of opioid distribution, elimination, and membrane transporters suggests that there is a need for a better understanding of effector site PK as opposed to venous plasma PK. As systemic opioids must enter the CNS to be effective, plasma concentration plotted against effect generates a reverse or counterclockwise hysteresis relationship due to the time delay in crossing in and out of the BBB (Fig. 53.1) [8]. Initially as the plasma concentration rises, the analgesic response magnitude is low as the drug moves from systemic circulation to the effector site. As the CNS concentration rises (even as plasma concentration begins to fall), analgesia (or the likelihood of a side effect) increases. CNS levels (and pain relief) eventually decline with the elimination of drug from the body by metabolism and clearance mechanisms.

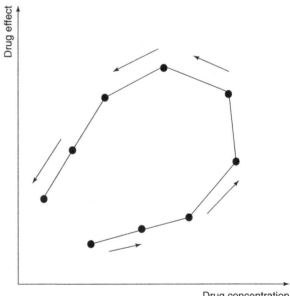

Fig. 53.1 Reverse hysteresis loop for opioid analgesic effect (Source: Lorenzini et al. [8])

Table 53.2 Plasma-CNS equilibration half-life ($t_{1/2ke0}$) values

Opioid	$t_{1/2ke0}$ (min)
Morphine-6-glucuronide [9]	384
Morphine [9]	168
Hydromorphone [10]	46
Meperidine [10]	10
Fentanyl [11]	6.6
Sufentanil [11]	6.2

Source: Lotsch [9]; Shafer and Flood [10]; Scott et al. [11]

The Importance of $t_{1/2ke0}$ and CST$_{1/2}$

When discussing effector site PK, the plasma/effector site equilibration half-life ($t_{1/2ke0}$) and the context sensitive halftime (CST$_{1/2}$) are two parameters that are more reflective of the PD of a specific opioid and route of administration than traditional PK parameters.

The $t_{1/2ke0}$ is experimentally determined by measuring an objective sign of opioid CNS effect (EEG or pupillometry are two popular methods) and comparing the kinetics of this effect with the measured drug concentration in the venous plasma, thereby determining the time required for "equilibration" between the effector site and the plasma concentration. For opioids that are highly lipophilic and are not efflux transporter substrates, such as fentanyl and sufentanil, this equilibration occurs rapidly as these drugs rapidly escape out of the aqueous plasma environment into the lipid bilayers of the CNS [9]. For hydrophilic drugs that have limited ability to transit into lipophilic environments and, in addition, are substrates for efflux transporters, such as morphine, this equilibration can take hours, and the equilibration of active metabolites, such as morphine-6-glucuronide (M6G), can take even longer (Table 53.2). So it is easy to see that while the venous C_{max} of IV bolus morphine may be reached in a minute after administration, this classic PK parameter is of little benefit when determining the timing of onset of action of the drug or its peak effect.

The CST$_{1/2}$ of a drug is defined as the time from C_{max} to 50 % of C_{max} following discontinuation of drug administration. Route of delivery (e.g., IV vs. transmucosal) and duration of the delivery (bolus vs. infusion) are key determining variables for CST$_{1/2}$. Similar to $t_{1/2ke0}$ being a more accurate measure of onset of opioid effect, the CST$_{1/2}$ is a more accurate measure of offset of the opioid effect rather than the traditional elimination half-life or $t_{1/2}$. While total body drug stores may take hours to be eliminated following IV delivery of an opioid, reflecting a long $t_{1/2}$, the plasma concentration of the drug, which reflects the concentration presented to the CNS, may be dramatically reduced in less than an hour after administration. Therefore, by measuring the time to 50 % reduction of circulating drug levels instead of total body stores, the CST$_{1/2}$ is a more accurate reflection of the offset of effect of the drug. This, of course, can be complicated by extremely delayed $t_{1/2ke0}$ drugs such as morphine.

New Insights into Opioids Used for IV PCA

Historically, IV morphine has commonly been considered the "gold standard" for PCA use. In light of effector site PK analysis, one might reach the conclusion that morphine's PK/PD characteristics are not optimal for PCA use [12]. Additionally, morphine has been associated with a relatively high adverse event (AE) rate in the literature [13]. The $t_{1/2ke0}$ concept may be helpful in understanding why this might be so. While IV morphine has about the same alpha distribution and beta elimination $t_{1/2}$ as IV fentanyl or sufentanil (1.7 min vs. 1.7 or 1.4 min, and 177 min vs. 219 or 164 min, respectively), these latter drugs have $t_{1/2ke0}$ values of 6.6 and 6.2 min, respectively, whereas the $t_{1/2ke0}$ for morphine is 168 min (25 times longer) and its M6G metabolite is more than twice longer still at 384 min [14]. The consequence of prolonged $t_{1/2ke0}$ values is that, while the venous plasma PK are not significantly different for these drugs, morphine will have a much slower onset compared to fentanyl or sufentanil when given at equianalgesic doses. Add to this the even slower BBB penetration of M6G, and the potential consequences of the erratic and delayed onset of peak drug effect is apparent. While one can use a loading dose of morphine in hopes of overcoming its longer $t_{1/2ke0}$ and, thereby, speeding its onset of action, the consequence can be prolonged residence time in the CNS with the potential for adverse events continuing long after drug administration has stopped. The typical short PCA lockout time of 6–10 minute for this slow $t_{1/2ke0}$ opioid increases the risk of dose stacking and delayed adverse events.

On the other hand, duration of effect is often seen as the limiting factor making fentanyl and sufentanil less viable for optimal IV PCA use. For these rapid CNS-equilibrating opioids, the short $t_{1/2ke0}$ means that the venous PK is more truly reflective of the effector site PK, and, therefore, if the chosen route of delivery results in rapid distribution of drug away from the circulation, the $CST_{1/2}$ will be short, resulting in a rapid exit from the CNS and short duration of action overall. This is why using these opioids for IV PCA often results in patients having to frequently redose to maintain sufficient analgesia. Alternate routes of administration, which prolong the $CST_{1/2}$, may help to optimize the use of these lipophilic opioids for PCA use.

Novel Opioid Formulation to Optimize $t_{1/2ke0}$ and $CST_{1/2}$

One product in development is the Sufentanil NanoTab® PCA System (Zalviso™ AcelRx Pharmaceuticals, Redwood City, CA) which allows patients to self-administer very small 15 mcg sublingual sufentanil microtablets as often as every 20 minute via a preprogrammed handheld device. Compared to IV administration of sufentanil, the slower absorption of sufentanil across the sublingual mucosa offsets the rapid distribution phase and "flattens" the plasma concentration time curve resulting in a median $CST_{1/2}$ that is 18-fold longer (2.5 hr versus 0.14 hr for IV sufentanil) [15]. The physicochemical properties of sufentanil allow the sublingual route to be an attractive option for drug delivery, and the route, in turn, optimizes the effector site PK for this drug for PCA delivery.

An analysis of a recently conducted Phase 3 open-label, randomized, active comparator study in 359 patients at 26 US sites after open abdominal surgery or total knee or hip arthroplasty who received either sublingual sufentanil administered via a handheld PCA device with a 20 minute lockout interval ($n=177$) or IV PCA morphine 1 mg with a 6 minute lockout interval ($n=180$) may be instructive in understanding how $CST_{1/2}$ and $t_{1/2ke0}$ can be used to benefit patient outcome [16]. Patients had their pain controlled using IV opioids in the operating room and recovery room. When ready for discharge from the recovery room, opioids were stopped until the patient had at least a 5/10 or greater on a 0–10 numerical rating scale, at which point study drug was initiated. The primary efficacy measure was the Patient Global Assessment of Method of Pain Control over the 48 hour study period (PGA-48), with success defined as the percentage of patients reporting "good" or "excellent" ratings on a 4-point scale of poor, fair, good, or excellent. Overall, 78.5 % versus 65.6 % achieved good or excellent ratings ("success") for the NanoTab System versus IV PCA morphine groups, respectively, demonstrating that the NanoTab System was noninferior to IV PCA morphine based on the prespecified 95 % confidence interval (CI) around the difference in success rates ($p<0.001$ using the one-side Z-test against the preset -15 % noninferiority margin) as well as statistically superior in favor of the NanoTab System ($p=0.007$) based on the lower limit of the 95 % CI ($+3.69$ %) not crossing zero.

That the Sufentanil NanoTab System was equally efficacious is perhaps not as impressive as the fact that the noninvasive NanoTab System demonstrated better pain intensity differences (PID; Fig. 53.2) and pain relief (PR) scores (data not shown) in the first 4 hr after initial dosing than IV PCA morphine. In a demonstration of the benefit of a shorter $t_{1/2ke0}$, PID and PR scores for the NanoTab PCA System showed a numerical improvement compared to IV PCA morphine as early as 45 minute and significantly superior PID and PR scores at 1, 2, and 4 hour after initiation of treatment ($p<0.01$). The effect of a longer $CST_{1/2}$ due to the sublingual route (2.5 hr) can be seen in the fact that over the duration of the 48 hour study, the least squares mean interdosing interval for sublingual sufentanil tablets was 1.35 hour, much longer than the $CST_{1/2}$ of IV sufentanil (0.14 hr = 8 min). As previously discussed, the shorter $t_{1/2ke0}$ also may reduce the potential for AEs by avoiding dose stacking. Possibly reflecting this advantage, the NanoTab System had statistically fewer patients with oxygen desaturations below 95 % with oxygen supplementation compared to IV PCA morphine ($p=0.028$; Fig. 53.3). This data may also reflect the higher therapeutic index of sufentanil (26,000) compared to morphine (70) in preclinical studies [17].

Summary

A third or more of patients report inadequate treatment for moderate-to-severe postoperative pain after inpatient surgery [18, 19] or ambulatory surgery [20, 21] despite the use of IV PCA and other modalities [22]. Undertreatment of pain is associated

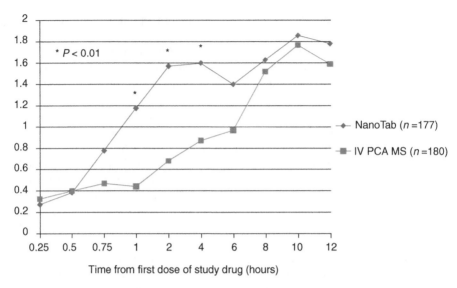

Fig. 53.2 Mean pain intensity difference (PID) per evaluation time point

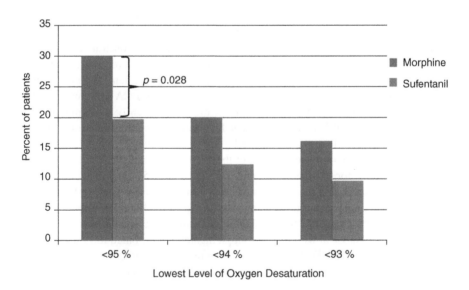

Fig. 53.3 Oxygen desaturation events

with well-characterized and potentially dangerous consequences [23]. These untoward events increase healthcare utilization and cost and reduce patient satisfaction which impacts reimbursement under the Hospital Consumer Assessment of Healthcare Providers and Systems (HCAHPS) [24].

Commonly utilized opioids for postoperative IV PCA are limited by relatively slow penetration into the CNS, active metabolites that complicate both analgesia and adverse events, and highly variable efflux transporter effects which can substantially affect the analgesic response and potential for significant adverse events. Potent lipophilic opioids (e.g., fentanyl, sufentanil) with a short $t_{1/2ke0}$ might be better suited for PCA approaches if the shortcomings of IV administration (short $CST_{1/2}$) could be overcome. Novel routes of administration may soon offer an approach to avoid these limitations and offer postoperative pain relief that is noninvasive and free of the errors associated with IV PCA use, while maintaining the desired patient-controlled feature that has been documented to result in higher patient satisfaction [25, 26].

Chemical Structures

Chemical Structure
53.1 Sufentanil

Chemical Structure
53.2 Fentanyl

References

1. Willie Sutton. the source for all the notorious details. http://williesutton.com/index.html. Accessed 16 Aug 2012.
2. Smith H. The metabolism of opioid agents and the clinical impact of their active metabolites. Clin J Pain. 2011;27:824–38.
3. Girardun F. Molecular biology of the blood-brain and the blood-cerebrospinal fluid barriers: similarities and differences. Dialogues Clin Neurosci. 2006;8:311–21.
4. Redzic Z. Molecular biology of the blood-brain and the blood-cerebrospinal fluid barriers: similarities and differences. Fluids Barriers CNS. 2011;8(3):1–23. Available at http://www.fluidsbarrierscns.com/content/8/1/3.
5. Sharom FJ, DiDiodado G, Yu X, Ashbourne JD. Interaction of the P-glycoprotein multidrug transporter with peptides and ionophores. J Biol Chem. 1995;270:10334–41.
6. Wandel C, Kim R, Wood M, Wood A. Interaction of morphine, fentanyl, sufentanil, alfentanil, and loperamide with the efflux drug transporter P-glycoprotein. Anesthesiology. 2002;96:913–20.
7. Huwyler J, Drewe J, Klusemann C, Fricker G. Evidence for P-glycoprotein-modulated penetration of morphine and morphine-6-glucuronide into brain capillary endothelium. Brit J Pharmacol. 1996;118:1879–85.

8. Lorenzini KI, Daali Y, Dayer P, Desmeules J. Pharmacokinetic-pharmacodynamic modelling of opioids in healthy human volunteers. A minireview. Basic Clin Pharmacol Toxicol. 2012; 110:219–26.

9. Lötsch J. Pharmacokinetic-pharmacodynamic modeling of opioids. J Pain Symptom Manag. 2005;29(5 Suppl):S90–103.

10. Shafer SL, Flood PD. The pharmacology of opioids in geriatric patients. In: Silverstein JH, Rooke GE, Reves JG, McLeskey CH, editors. Geriatric anesthesiology. New York: Springer Science; 2007. p. 209.

11. Scott JC, Cooke JE, Stanski DR. Electroencephalographic quantitation of opioid effect: comparative pharmacodynamics of fentanyl and sufentanil. Anesthesiology. 1991;74:34–42.

12. Barietta JF. Clinical and economic burden of opioid use for postsurgical pain: focus on ventilatory impairment and ileus. Pharmacotherapy. 2012;32(9 Pt 2):12S–8.

13. Oderda GM, Evans RS, Lloyd J, et al. Cost of opioid-related adverse drug events in surgical patients. J Pain Symptom Manag. 2003;25:276–83.

14. Scholz J, Steinfath M, Schultz M. Clinical pharmacokinetics of alfentanil, fentanyl, and sufentanil. Clin Pharmacother. 1996;31:275–92.

15. Gan TJ, Palmer PP, Royal M. Optimizing a drug for PCA delivery: the clinical importance of $CST_{1/2}$ and $t_{1/2ke0}$. Poster A1298 presented at the Annual Meeting of the American Society of Anesthesiologists, October 12, 2013, San Francisco, CA. http://www.asaabstracts.com. Accessed 04 Jun 2014.

16. Melson T, Boyer DL, Minkowitz H, Palmer PP, Royal M. Sufentanil NanoTab PCA System versus IV PCA morphine for postoperative pain: a randomized, open-label, active-comparator trial. Poster A3087 presented at the Annual Meeting of the American Society of Anesthesiologists, October 14, 2013, San Francisco, CA. http://www.asaabstracts.com. Accessed 04 Jun 2014.

17. Mather LE. Opioids: a pharmacologist's delight! Clin Exp Pharmacol Physiol. 1995;22:833–6.

18. Warfield CA, Kahn CH. Acute pain management: programs in US hospitals and experiences and attitudes among US adults. Anesthesiology. 1995;83:1090–4.

19. Apfelbaum JL, Chen C, Mehta SS, Gan TJ. Postoperative pain experience: results from a national survey suggest postoperative pain continues to be undermanaged. Anesth Analg. 2003;97:534–40.

20. McGrath B, Elgendy H, Chung F, et al. Thirty percent of patients have moderate to severe pain 24 h after ambulatory surgery: a survey of 5,703 patients. Can J Anesth. 2004;51:886–91.

21. Rawal N, Hylander J, Nydahl PA, et al. Survey of postoperative analgesia following ambulatory surgery. Acta Anaesth Scand. 1997;41:1017–22.

22. Constantini R, Affaitati G, Fabrizio A, Giamberardino MA. Controlling pain in the postoperative setting.et al. Int J Clin Pharmacol Ther. 2011;49:116–27.

23. Sinatra R. Causes and consequences of inadequate management of acute pain. Pain Med. 2010;11:1859–71.

24. US Department of Health and Human Services, Centers for Medicare and Medicaid. HCAHPS: Patients' perspectives of care survey. http://www.cms.gov/HospitalQualityInits/30_HospitalHCAHPS.asp. Accessed 13 Aug 2012.

25. Ballantyne JC, Carr DB, Chalmers TC, et al. Postoperative patient-controlled analgesia: meta-analyses of initial randomized controlled trials. J Clin Anesth. 1993;5:182–93.

26. Hudcova J, McNicol ED, Quah CS, et al. Patient controlled opioid analgesia versus conventional opioid analgesia for postoperative pain, Cochrane Database Syst Rev. 2006;(4):CD003348. doi:10.1002/14651858. CD003348.pub2.

Chapter 54
Understanding Anesthesia-Induced Memory Loss

Agnieszka A. Zurek and Beverley A. Orser

Contents

This chapter is based, in part, on a lecture presented at the meeting of the Association of American Anesthesiologists in April 2013.

A.A. Zurek
Department of Physiology, University of Toronto,
Medical Sciences Building, 1 King's College Circle,
Room 3318, Toronto, ON M5S 1A8, Canada

B.A. Orser (✉)
Department of Physiology, University of Toronto,
Medical Sciences Building, 1 King's College Circle,
Room 3318, Toronto, ON M5S 1A8, Canada

Department of Anesthesia, University of Toronto,
123 Edward Street, Room 1204,
Toronto, Ontario M5G 1E2, Canada

Department of Anesthesia, Sunnybrook Health Sciences Centre,
2075 Bayview Avenue, Toronto, ON M4N 3M5, Canada
e-mail: beverley.orser@utoronto.ca

A.D. Kaye et al. (eds.), *Essentials of Pharmacology for Anesthesia,*
Pain Medicine, and Critical Care, DOI 10.1007/978-1-4614-8948-1_54,
© Springer Science+Business Media New York 2015

Introduction

Despite the widespread use of general anesthetics in operating rooms and intensive care units, the understanding of the mechanisms of action of these drugs remains limited. Increasing knowledge of the molecular mechanisms underlying general anesthesia is important both to advance drug development and to ensure appropriate use of currently available drugs. Anesthetics are also effective probes for exploring the biological basis of cognition and cognitive disorders.

The prevailing concept of the anesthetic state is that it does not result from global neurodepression but rather represents a constellation different of behavioral end points that together allow patients to tolerate surgical trauma. The four key therapeutic end points of anesthesia are memory loss (amnesia), immobility, unconsciousness, and analgesia. These desired effects are accompanied by a multitude of adverse effects, including cardiovascular instability, hypothermia, emesis, respiratory depression, and postoperative cognitive dysfunction [1] (Fig. 54.1). One major goal of anesthesia research is to identify the specific receptors and neuronal networks underlying the various therapeutic and undesirable effects. The ultimate aim is to develop new compounds that are capable of selectively modulating these receptors and that can be used in combination to create a "safer" anesthetic state.

This chapter focuses on our laboratory efforts to identify the mechanisms underlying the memory-blocking properties of anesthetics. We first outline the rationale for studying memory loss as it relates to disorders such as intraoperative awareness and postoperative cognitive dysfunction. We then describe studies identifying receptors that are highly and preferentially expressed in regions of the brain that play a critical role in anesthesia-induced memory loss. Finally, we present results suggesting that activation of these memory-blocking receptors contributes to memory deficits in the postoperative period.

Why Study Anesthesia-Induced Memory Loss?

Understanding how anesthetics cause memory loss is of considerable interest, as some patients experience insufficient amnesia and unexpected recall of adverse surgical events. The incidence of explicit recollection of surgical events that occur during general anesthesia, a disorder referred to as "intraoperative awareness," is approximately 1.3 per 1,000 patients [2, 3]. The incidence of possible awareness, whereby patients recall events during anesthesia and surgery that cannot be substantiated by operating room personnel, may be as high as 2.4 per 1,000 patients [2]. Given that over 40 million patients undergo anesthesia in North America each year (American Society of Anesthesiologists), thousands of patients may be at risk for serious psychological harm.

At the opposite end of the spectrum of memory disorders associated with anesthesia are the persistent memory deficits that some patients experience. A decline in cognitive performance after general anesthesia is commonly referred to as postoperative cognitive dysfunction (POCD) [4–6]. In the International Study on POCD, approximately

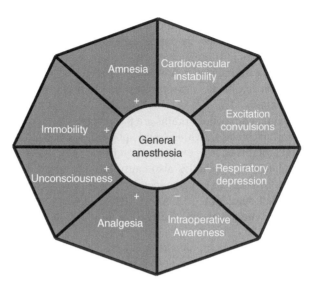

Fig. 54.1 Anesthesia has both desirable and undesirable end points. General anesthetics cause the therapeutic end points of amnesia, immobility, unconsciousness, and analgesia (shown in *blue*). Cardiovascular instability, convulsions, respiratory depression, and intraoperative awareness are potential negative consequences of anesthesia (shown in *red*) (Modified from Urban et al. [1])

37 % of young adults and 41 % of older patients exhibited cognitive deficits in the days immediately following surgery, with the deficits persisting for up to 3 months in 6 to 13% of patients [4]. Loss of explicit memory and impairment of executive function (which involves skills such as decision-making or planning follow-up appointments) are common features of POCD [7, 8].

The duration of general anesthesia is an independent predictor of cognitive dysfunction, and anesthetics are thereby implicated as a potential causative factor in POCD [6]. However, POCD also occurs in patients undergoing regional anesthesia and conscious sedation, which suggests that inflammation and sedative drugs are contributing factors [8, 9]. Other factors that may contribute to poor performance on psychometric tests include the patient's underlying illness, disrupted sleep during the hospital stay, the stress and novelty of the hospital environment, and postoperative pain [4, 7].

Cognitive deficits after surgery represent a serious concern as they are associated with poor long-term outcome, premature retirement, loss of independence, and increased long-term mortality [7]. Unfortunately, no treatments or preventive measures are available for POCD. Thus, studies of laboratory animals are required to disentangle the role of anesthesia from the myriad of other potential contributing factors. As described below, research to elucidate the molecular basis of POCD and to identify potential therapeutic strategies is in progress.

Animal Studies to Elucidate Mechanisms of Postoperative Memory Deficits

Studies using rodent models have shown that a clinically relevant dose of the inhaled anesthetic isoflurane or sevoflurane can impair anterograde spatial memory, as well as retrograde spatial and recognition memory, and that such deficits persist for days to weeks after exposure [10–13]. Neuronal damage and cognitive deficits in rodents are positively correlated with the duration of anesthesia and the number of exposures [14]. Readers interested in a more detailed summary of recent studies of anesthesia-induced neurotoxicity are referred to a commentary [15] and a special issue on anesthetic neurotoxicity and neuroplasticity of the British Journal of Anaesthesia [16].

Fetal and newborn brains are particularly vulnerable to the neurotoxic properties of anesthetics, which cause apoptotic neuronal death by increasing proapoptotic proteins such as caspase-3, cyclin D1, and Bcl-2-interacting protein [17–20]. Inhalational anesthetics also cause mitochondrial dysfunction and increase the levels of reactive oxygen species in neurons, which further contribute to apoptotic cell death [21–23]. At peak periods of brain development, anesthetics can reduce synaptogenesis, thereby causing a sustained reduction in the number of synapses [24].

In the adult brain, inhaled and intravenous anesthetics have been shown to promote the development of Alzheimer's disease-related cytopathology [25–31]. Transgenic mouse models of Alzheimer's disease are more susceptible to anesthetic-induced increases in cytokine levels and cognitive deficits than wild-type mice [32]. Exposure to anesthetics increases amyloid-beta aggregation and tau hyperphosphorylation [28–31, 33]. However, the mechanisms underlying anesthetic-induced memory loss in adult brains without any preexisting neuropathology are unknown.

Molecular Basis of Memory Loss During Anesthesia

Our recent laboratory studies have focused on the mechanisms underlying anesthesia-induced memory loss. Most general anesthetics cause their primary end points by acting on specific ion channels in the brain and spinal cord [34]. In particular, γ-aminobutyric acid type A (GABA$_A$) receptors are inhibitory receptors in the brain that are targets for most general anesthetics and intravenous sedative drugs [34, 35], including the volatile anesthetics sevoflurane, desflurane, and isoflurane and the intravenous anesthetics etomidate, propofol, barbiturates, and benzodiazepines (Fig. 54.2).

GABA$_A$ receptors are chloride-permeable ion channels that assemble from 5 subunits encoded by 19 different genes. The particular subunit composition of the receptors influences their pharmacological, physiological, and biophysical properties, as well their regional and cellular patterns of expression. GABA$_A$ receptors are categorized into two main groups, synaptic and extrasynaptic, according to their proximity to the synapse [36]. Synaptic receptors are transiently stimulated by high concentrations of GABA to generate fast inhibitory postsynaptic currents [36]. Extrasynaptic receptors are composed of $\alpha5$, $\beta3$, and $\gamma2$ subunits or, alternatively, $\alpha4/\alpha6$, $\beta2/\beta3$, and δ subunits. These receptors are activated by low, ambient

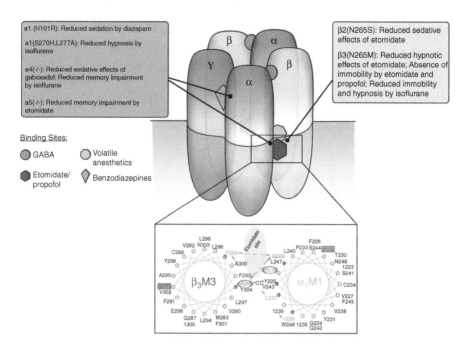

Fig. 54.2 GABA$_A$ receptors are targets for anesthetics. GABA$_A$ receptors are targets for many neurodepressive drugs, including etomidate, propofol, most inhaled anesthetics, benzodiazepines, and barbiturates. The approximate locations of binding sites for some of these compounds are indicated in the diagram. Binding of anesthetics to different isoforms of the GABA$_A$ receptors causes various behavioral end points of anesthesia, and specific genetic mutations in GABA$_A$ receptor isoforms cause insensitivity to specific end points of anesthesia. Specific mutations that have been associated with reduced sensitivity to anesthetics are outlined in the *yellow* and *green boxes* (Modified from Wang and Orser [69])

concentrations of GABA to generate a tonic current [36–39] that reduces neuronal excitability [40, 41].

Our recent studies have focused on extrasynaptic α5-subunit-containing GABA$_A$ (α5GABA$_A$) receptors, which are abundantly expressed in the hippocampus, a brain structure that is essential for learning and memory recall [42]. These receptors are highly sensitive to many classes of neurodepressive drugs, including the general anesthetics isoflurane, midazolam, and propofol [43–45]. These drugs bind directly to the receptors or interact with water-filled binding cavities and act as positive allosteric modulators that markedly increase opening of the integral ion channel [34, 46]. Anesthetics such as propofol also reduce receptor desensitization (closure of the ion channel while the agonist remains bound to the receptor) [47]. Together, the increase in receptor activation and the reduction in desensitization allow channels to remain in the open conducting state for prolonged periods [45].

Anesthetic-Induced Amnesia and α5GABA_A Receptors

Behavioral studies of humans and laboratory animals have shown that the expression and function of α5GABA_A receptors regulate memory behaviors. Reducing α5GABA_A receptor activity through pharmacological inhibition (by the selective inverse agonist L-655,708) or through genetic knockdown of the gene encoding the α5 subunit (to generate *Gabra5–/–* mice) improves performance for certain memory tasks. L-655,708 also enhances long-term potentiation of excitatory synaptic plasticity in the hippocampus, a molecular substrate of memory [48]. Conversely, drugs that increase the activity of α5GABA_A receptors, such as the intravenous anesthetic etomidate, cause memory deficits and prevent the induction of long-term synaptic plasticity [49, 50].

Studies with genetically modified mice have further implicated α5GABA_A receptors in drug-induced memory loss. Wild-type mice treated with a low dose of etomidate were unable to learn a fear-conditioning task during treatment [49]. In contrast, *Gabra5–/–* mice treated with etomidate and wild-type mice co-treated with etomidate and L-655,708 formed new memories during training on the fear-conditioning task [49]. Collectively, these results show that α5GABA_ARs are required for the acute memory blockade induced by etomidate (Fig. 54.3).

In recent studies, we have examined whether α5GABA_A receptors also contribute to long-term memory deficits that persist after elimination of the anesthetic. In a preclinical mouse model, we showed that a single, 1-h treatment with isoflurane or sevoflurane caused learning and memory deficits for contextual fear memory and object recognition memory for at least 48 h [51, 52]. Such memory loss occurred at a time when concentrations of anesthetic in the brain were undetectable or at the limits of detection [51].

More importantly, pharmacological or genetic inhibition of α5GABA_A receptors prevented these memory deficits [51, 52]. This result suggests that α5GABA_A receptors are required for triggering postanesthetic memory deficits and contribute to the memory deficits observed after anesthesia. Ongoing studies are evaluating the effectiveness of α5GABA_A receptor inhibitors for treating memory deficits after intravenous anesthesia in rodents and nonhuman primates.

Inflammation-Induced Memory Loss and α5GABA_A Receptors

Systemic inflammation after major surgery may also contribute to postoperative memory loss. The levels of many proinflammatory cytokines, including tumor necrosis factor-α, interleukin 1β (IL-1β), and interleukin 6, are markedly increased in the circulation and brain after surgery [53–55]. These cytokines, which are released from macrophages at the site of injury, stimulate innate immune responses in the brain and activate resident microglia to release additional cytokines.

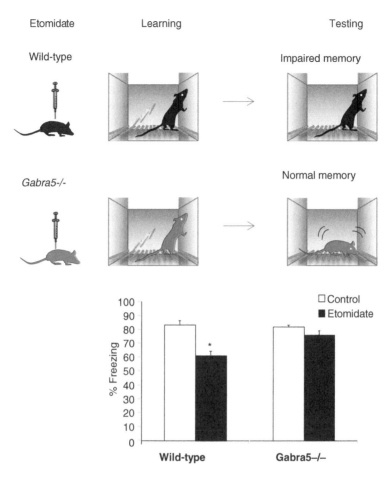

Fig. 54.3 α5GABA$_A$ receptors contribute to memory blockade by etomidate. Wild-type mice and mice lacking the α5GABA$_A$ receptor (*Gabra5−/−*) were injected with a low dose of etomidate (4 mg/kg) and were immediately trained on the fear-conditioning memory task. During training, an aversive foot shock was presented in a novel context, and the mice learned to associate the foot shock with the context. During the testing phase, mice were reintroduced into the context. Mice that remembered the aversive context remained immobile or "froze" during testing, as evidenced by a higher percentage of time spent freezing. Wild-type mice treated with etomidate had impairment of memory performance, as indicated by reduced freezing. In contrast, *Gabra5−/−* mice treated with etomidate showed normal memory performance. These results indicate that α5GABA$_A$ receptors are necessary for the amnestic action of etomidate under these experimental conditions (Modified from Cheng et al. [49])

Rodent models of various types of surgery, including hepatectomy, splenectomy, and orthopedic tibial osteotomy, have confirmed that inflammation is associated with postoperative memory deficits [53, 56–58]. In particular, increased levels of cytokines were associated with memory loss for certain hippocampus-dependent tasks, such as contextual fear-conditioning and spatial navigational memory [53, 56].

Innovative strategies aimed at reducing memory deficits after surgery and anesthesia have included treatment with anti-inflammatory drugs or selective antagonists for certain proinflammatory cytokine receptors [53, 59]. For example, the anti-inflammatory antibiotic minocycline [53] and the COX-2 inhibitor parecoxib [60] reduce cognitive deficits associated with postoperative inflammation in a mouse model. A major limitation of this approach is that reductions in the immune response could delay wound healing or increase the risk of postoperative infection. Therefore, we have studied an alternative approach to identify and target specific receptors in the hippocampus that mediate the memory-blocking effects of proinflammatory cytokines.

We recently investigated whether systemic inflammation increases the expression of $\alpha5GABA_A$ receptors in hippocampal neurons. We found that IL-1β enhances the activity and surface expression of $\alpha5GABA_A$ receptors, an effect that contributes to memory deficits [61]. The increased expression of $\alpha5GABA_A$ receptors depended on binding of IL-1β to the interleukin-1 receptor and involved activation of p38 mitogen-activated protein kinase-dependent signaling pathways [61]. Importantly, memory performance was impaired in wild-type mice in which systemic inflammation was induced by injection of the bacterial endotoxin lipopolysaccharide or IL-1β, but *Gabra5−/−* mice did not exhibit such memory deficits. Pharmacological inhibition of $\alpha5GABA_A$ receptors also reduced memory deficits induced by systemic inflammation (Fig. 54.4). Collectively, these results suggest that proinflammatory cytokines contribute to memory deficits by enhancing the number of functional inhibitory $\alpha5GABA_A$ receptors in the brain. Animal models have shown that anesthetics further stimulate the release of proinflammatory cytokines [62], which may exacerbate memory deficits.

Anesthetic-Induced Memory Loss: Where Do We Go from Here?

The results summarized above raise many questions. For example, does a reduction in the expression levels of $\alpha5GABA_A$ receptors contribute to intraoperative awareness? Polymorphisms exist in the human gene that encodes the $\alpha5$ subunit [63], but whether such polymorphisms increase the risk of awareness in patients is unknown. Additionally, it will be of great interest to determine whether inverse agonists that preferentially inhibit $\alpha5GABA_A$ receptors can either prevent or treat memory loss associated with anesthesia in patients.

It will also be important to determine whether different classes of anesthetics differ in their ability to cause postoperative cognitive deficits. For example, preliminary studies in rodent models have shown that sevoflurane but not desflurane causes an increase in reactive oxygen species and subsequent cell death in the young brain [64, 65]. The sedative dexmedetomidine may also be neuroprotective rather than neurotoxic [66–68]. Lastly, studies in both animals and humans should help in

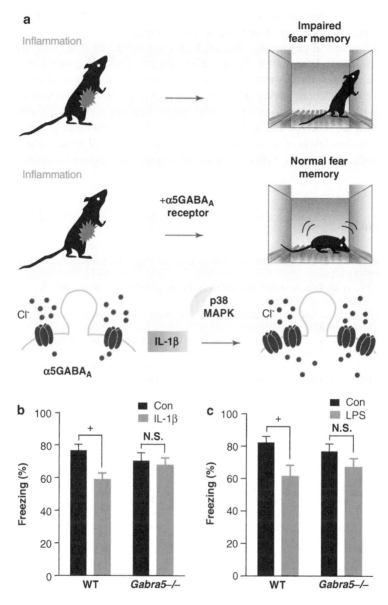

Fig. 54.4 Systemic inflammation triggers memory deficits and increased surface expression of α5GABA_A receptors. (**a**) The impairment of fear memory by systemic inflammation could be prevented by pharmacological or genetic inhibition of α5GABA_A receptors in mice. These memory deficits may be triggered by the binding of interleukin-1β (IL-1β) to the interleukin-1 receptor and the triggering of increased α5GABA_A receptor expression through p38 MAPK-dependent signaling pathways. Wild-type (WT) but not *Gabra5−/−* mice showed impairment of fear memory, as indicated by a reduction in time spent freezing, after systemic injection of (**b**) interleukin-1β or (**c**) an endotoxin (Modified from Wang et al. [61])

determining whether the cognitive deficits associated with inflammation can be reduced without impairing or delaying wound healing.

From a practical perspective, high-risk patients should be informed about the risks of cognitive deficits after anesthesia and surgery, and appropriate precautions should be taken, such as writing down critical information about drugs and treatment recommendations during the postoperative period. Family members or other care providers may wish to accompany patients to ensure that postoperative care instructions are received and recorded correctly. Also, the exposure of health care personnel to low levels of anesthetics should be minimized until we develop a better understanding of the long-term consequences of anesthetic-induced neurotoxicity.

References

1. Urban BW, et al. Concepts and correlations relevant to general anaesthesia. Br J Anaesth. 2002;89(1):3–16.
2. Sebel PS, et al. The incidence of awareness during anesthesia: a multicenter United States study. Anesth Analg. 2004;99(3):833–9.
3. Mashour GA, et al. Intraoperative awareness: from neurobiology to clinical practice. Anesthesiology. 2011;114:1218–33.
4. Monk TG, et al. Predictors of cognitive dysfunction after major noncardiac surgery. Anesthesiology. 2008;108(1):18–30.
5. Moller JT. Postoperative cognitive decline: the extent of the problem. Eur J Anaesth. 1998;15(6):765–7.
6. Moller JT, et al. Long-term postoperative cognitive dysfunction in the elderly ISPOCD1 study. ISPOCD investigators. International Study of Post-Operative Cognitive Dysfunction. Lancet. 1998;351(9106):857–61.
7. Price CC, et al. Type and severity of cognitive decline in older adults after noncardiac surgery. Anesthesiology. 2008;108(1):8–17.
8. Newman S, et al. Postoperative cognitive dysfunction after noncardiac surgery – a systematic review. Anesthesiology. 2007;106(3):572–90.
9. Heyer EJ, et al. A study of cognitive dysfunction in patients having carotid endarterectomy performed with regional anesthesia. Anesth Analg. 2008;107(2):636–42.
10. Culley DJ, et al. Long-term impairment of acquisition of a spatial memory task following isoflurane-nitrous oxide anesthesia in rats. Anesthesiology. 2004;100(2):309–14.
11. Culley DJ, et al. The memory effects of general anesthesia persist for weeks in young and aged rats. Anesth Analg. 2003;96(4):1004–9.
12. Crosby C, et al. Spatial memory performance 2 weeks after general anesthesia in adult rats. Anesth Analg. 2005;101(5):1389–92.
13. Palanisamy A, et al. Rats exposed to isoflurane in utero during early gestation are behaviorally abnormal as adults. Anesthesiology. 2011;114(3):521–8.
14. Yu D, et al. Repeated exposure to propofol potentiates neuroapoptosis and long-term behavioral deficits in neonatal rats. Neurosci Lett 2013;534:41–6.
15. Jevtovic-Todorovic V, et al.. Anaesthetic neurotoxicity and neuroplasticity: an expert group report and statement based on the BJA Salzburg Seminar. Br J Anaesth. 2013;111(2):143–51.
16. Hemmings Jr HC, et al. Special issue on anaesthetic neurotoxicity and neuroplasticity. Br J Anaesth. 2013;110(Supplement 1):i1–2.
17. Soriano SG, et al. Ketamine activates cell cycle signaling and apoptosis in the neonatal rat brain. Anesthesiology. 2010;112(5):1155–63.

18. Liang G, et al. Isoflurane causes greater neurodegeneration than an equivalent exposure of sevoflurane in the developing brain of neonatal mice. Anesthesiology. 2010;112(6):1325–34.
19. Bercker S, et al. Neurodegeneration in newborn rats following propofol and sevoflurane anesthesia. Neurotox Res. 2009;16(2):140–7.
20. Walker SM, et al. Effects of intrathecal ketamine in the neonatal rat evaluation of apoptosis and long-term functional outcome. Anesthesiology. 2010;113(1):147–59.
21. Zhu CL, et al. Isoflurane anesthesia induced persistent, progressive memory impairment, caused a loss of neural stem cells, and reduced neurogenesis in young, but not adult, rodents. J Cereb Blood Flow Metab. 2010;30(5):1017–30.
22. Sanchez V, et al. General anesthesia causes long-term impairment of mitochondrial morphogenesis and synaptic transmission in developing rat brain. Anesthesiology. 2011; 115(5):992–1002.
23. Boscolo A, et al. The abolishment of anesthesia-induced cognitive impairment by timely protection of mitochondria in the developing rat brain: the importance of free oxygen radicals and mitochondrial integrity. Neurobiol Dis. 2012;45(3):1031–41.
24. Lunardi N, et al. General anesthesia causes long-lasting disturbances in the ultrastructural properties of developing synapses in young rats. Neurotox Res. 2010;17(2):179–88.
25. Xie ZC, et al. The common inhalation anesthetic isoflurane induces caspase activation and increases amyloid beta-protein level in vivo. Ann Neurol. 2008;64(6):618–27.
26. Zhen Y, et al. Nitrous oxide plus isoflurane induces apoptosis and increases beta-amyloid protein levels. Anesthesiology. 2009;111(4):741–52.
27. Perucho J, et al. Anesthesia with isoflurane increases amyloid pathology in mice models of Alzheimer's disease. J Alzheimers Dis. 2010;19(4):1245–57.
28. Planel E, et al. Anesthesia leads to tau hyperphosphorylation through inhibition of phosphatase activity by hypothermia. J Neurosci. 2007;27(12):3090–7.
29. Planel E, et al. Anesthesia-induced hyperphosphorylation detaches 3-repeat tau from microtubules without affecting their stability in vivo. J Neurosci. 2008;28(48):12798–807.
30. Run XQ, et al. Anesthesia induces phosphorylation of Tau. J Alzheimers Dis. 2009;16(3): 619–26.
31. Planel E, et al. Acceleration and persistence of neurofibrillary pathology in a mouse model of tauopathy following anesthesia. FASEB J. 2009;23(8):2595–604.
32. Lu Y, et al. Anesthetic sevoflurane causes neurotoxicity differently in neonatal naive and Alzheimer disease transgenic mice. Anesthesiology. 2010;112(6):1404–16.
33. Tan WF, et al. Tau hyperphosphorylation is associated with memory impairment after exposure to 1.5% isoflurane without temperature maintenance in rats. Eur J Anaesthesiol. 2010;27(9): 835–41.
34. Hemmings HC Jr, et al. Emerging molecular mechanisms of general anesthetic action. Trends Pharmacol Sci. 2005;26(10):503–10.
35. Franks NP, et al. Molecular and cellular mechanisms of general anaesthesia. Nature. 1994;367(6464):607–14.
36. Farrant M, et al. Variations on an inhibitory theme: phasic and tonic activation of $GABA_A$ receptors. Nat Rev Neurosci. 2005;6(3):215–29.
37. Sur C, et al. Autoradiographic localization of $\alpha 5$ subunit-containing $GABA_A$ receptors in rat brain. Brain Res. 1999;822(1–2):265–70.
38. Scimemi A, et al. Multiple and plastic receptors mediate tonic $GABA_A$ receptor currents in the hippocampus. J Neurosci. 2005;25(43):10016–24.
39. Mody I. Distinguishing between $GABA_A$ receptors responsible for tonic and phasic conductances. Neurochem Res. 2001;26(8–9):907–13.
40. Bonin RP, et al. $\alpha 5 GABA_A$ receptors regulate the intrinsic excitability of mouse hippocampal pyramidal neurons. J Neurophysiol. 2007;98(4):2244–54.
41. Bieda MC, et al. A major role for tonic $GABA_A$ conductances in anesthetic suppression of intrinsic neuronal excitability. J Neurophysiol. 2004;92(3):1658–67.
42. Crestani F, et al. Trace fear conditioning involves hippocampal $\alpha 5 GABA_A$ receptors. Proc Natl Acad Sci. 2002;99(13):8980–5.

43. Caraiscos VB, et al. Selective enhancement of tonic GABAergic inhibition in murine hippo-
    campal neurons by low concentrations of the volatile anesthetic isoflurane. J Neurosci. 2004;
    24(39):8454–8.
44. Bai D, et al. The effect of propofol on baseline current mediated by GABA$_A$ receptors over-
    shadows its effect on IPSCs in cultured hippocampal neurons. Can J Anaesth. 1998;45:A48.
45. Bai D, et al. Distinct functional and pharmacological properties of tonic and quantal inhibitory
    postsynaptic currents mediated by gamma-aminobutyric acid(A) receptors in hippocampal
    neurons. Mol Pharmacol. 2001;59(4):814–24.
46. Akk G, et al. Structural studies of the actions of anesthetic drugs on the gamma-aminobutyric
    acid type A receptor. Anesthesiology. 2010;115(6):1338–48.
47. Bai D, et al. The general anesthetic propofol slows deactivation and desensitization of GABA$_A$
    receptors. J Neurosci. 1999;19(24):10635–46.
48. Martin LJ, et al. α5GABA$_A$ receptor activity sets the threshold for long-term potentiation and
    constrains hippocampus-dependent memory. J Neurosci. 2010;30(15):5269–82.
49. Cheng VY, et al. α5GABA$_A$ receptors mediate the amnestic but not sedative-hypnotic effects
    of the general anesthetic etomidate. J Neurosci. 2006;26(14):3713–20.
50. Martin LJ, et al. Etomidate targets alpha 5 gamma-aminobutyric acid subtype A receptors to
    regulate synaptic plasticity and memory blockade. Anesthesiology. 2009;111(5):1025–35.
51. Saab BJ, et al. Memory impairment after isoflurane can be prevented by pretreatment with the
    α5GABA$_A$ receptor inverse agonist L-655,708. Anesthesiology. 2010;113(5):1061–71.
52. Zurek AA, et al. Inhibition of α5 γ-Aminobutyric acid type A receptors restores recognition
    memory after general anesthesia. Anesth Analg. 2012;114(4):845–55.
53. Cibelli M, et al. Role of interleukin-1β in postoperative cognitive dysfunction. Ann Neurol.
    2010;68(3):360–8.
54. Terrando N, et al. Tumor necrosis factor-α triggers a cytokine cascade yielding postoperative
    cognitive decline. Proc Natl Acad Sci U S A. 2010;107(47):20518–22.
55. Ni Choileain N, et al. Cell response to surgery. Arch Surg. 2006;141(11):1132–40.
56. Cao XZ, et al. Postoperative cognitive deficits and neuroinflammation in the hippocampus
    triggered by surgical trauma are exacerbated in aged rats. Prog Neuro-Psychopharmacol Biol
    Psychiatry. 2010;34(8):1426–32.
57. Wan YJ, et al. Cognitive decline following major surgery is associated with gliosis, beta-amyloid
    accumulation, and tau phosphorylation in old mice. Crit Care Med. 2010;38(11):2190–8.
58. Wan Y, et al. Postoperative impairment of cognitive function in rats: a possible role for
    cytokine-mediated inflammation in the hippocampus. Anesthesiology. 2007;106(3):436–43.
59. Terrando N, et al. The impact of IL-1 modulation on the development of lipopolysaccharide-
    induced cognitive dysfunction. Crit Care. 2010;14(3):R88.
60. Peng M, et al. The cyclooxygenase-2 inhibitor parecoxib inhibits surgery-induced proinflam-
    matory cytokine expression in the hippocampus in aged rats. J Surg Res. 2012;178(1):E1–8.
61. Wang D-S, et al. Memory deficits induced by inflammation are regulated by α5-subunit-
    containing GABA$_A$ receptors. Cell Rep. 2012;2(3):488–96.
62. Wu X, et al. The inhalation anesthetic isoflurane increases levels of proinflammatory TNF-α,
    IL-6, and IL-1 beta. Neurobiol Aging. 2012;33(7):1364–78.
63. Kim Y. et al. Human gamma-aminobutyric acid-type A receptor alpha 5 subunit gene (GABRA5):
    characterization and structural organization of the 5' flanking region. Genomics 1997;42:378–87.
64. Zhang Y, et al. The mitochondrial pathway of anesthetic isoflurane-induced apoptosis. J Biol
    Chem. 2010;285(6):4025–37.
65. Zhang Y, et al. Anesthetics isoflurane and desflurane differently affect mitochondrial function,
    learning, and memory. Ann Neurol. 2012;72(4):630.
66. Ma DQ, et al. Dexmedetomidine produces its neuroprotective effect via the α(2A)-adrenoceptor
    subtype. Eur J Pharmacol. 2004;502(1–2):87–97.
67. Rajakumaraswamy N, et al. Neuroprotective interaction produced by xenon and dexmedetomi-
    dine on in vitro and in vivo neuronal injury models. Neurosci Lett. 2006;409(2):128–33.
68. Sanders RD, et al. Dexmedetomidine attenuates isoflurane-induced neurocognitive impair-
    ment in neonatal rats. Anesthesiology. 2009;110(5):1077–85.
69. Wang DS, et al. Inhibition of learning and memory by general anesthetics. Can J Anaesth.
    2011;58(2):167–77.

Chapter 55
Novel Targets of Current Analgesic Drug Development

Jeffrey A. Katz and Honorio T. Benzon

Contents

Introduction

The development of new pharmaceutical agents for the treatment of pain seems at first like an ideal target for pharmaceutical companies. There is an enormous unmet need with a vast potential market. For many years, opioids and NSAIDs have remained the mainstay treatments in chronic pain [1], and while the advent of anti-epileptic drugs and antidepressant medications into the indication arena for chronic and neuropathic pain has been helpful, it is far from adequate to meet the demands for controlling both acute and chronic pain [2]. Hence, the pursuit of new novel medications for pain seems a rational action, but further insight shows how difficult the task truly is, not to mention the financial risks of such innovation [3].

J.A. Katz, MD (✉) • H.T. Benzon, MD
Department of Anesthesiology, Northwestern University
Feinberg School of Medicine, Chicago, IL, USA
e-mail: paindude@gmail.com; hbenzon@nmff.org

A.D. Kaye et al. (eds.), *Essentials of Pharmacology for Anesthesia,*
Pain Medicine, and Critical Care, DOI 10.1007/978-1-4614-8948-1_55,
© Springer Science+Business Media New York 2015

In 2011 and 2012, 16 new analgesic drugs were approved by the US FDA. None of them targeted new mechanisms or receptors; they were all reformulations of existing drugs such as opioids or old drugs approved for new conditions [4]. This situation of pursuing "safe" drug development persists, with efforts to pursue medications such as other SNRIs like TD-9855 [5], modified formulations of hydrocodone (benzhydrocodone) [6], or topical clonidine (ARC-4558, Arcion Therapeutics) [7]. This situation reflects the difficulty in defining the goal in pain management but also reflects our poor understanding of the mechanisms of pain. The goal in pain treatment is actually difficult to pinpoint. Pain is crucial for our survival as a species, so it is not all pain we want stopped, only the pain that causes suffering or dysfunction. Blocking a physiologic process crucial to our survival as a species is akin to controlling the symptom of thirst, too much control, and the results can be lethal. Pain drug development is thus hampered by a lack of a clear target outcome.

Drug development in pain management is further hampered by limited understanding of pain processes. Receptors, transmitters, agonists, and antagonists are often identified, but when we create ligands to target any of these processes, we have little idea what other effects they may have. Who knew with their initial development that NSAIDs might raise blood pressure and cause MIs, CVAs, and potentially death [8]? Similarly, the anti-nerve growth factor drugs when developed had unpredictable (and unclear) results on arthritis progression that resulted in a temporary delay in development by the FDA, but ultimately trials were allowed to resume with additional precautions [9]. With any physiologic target, if we don't know where else that physiology is relevant, severe consequences may result and may only be seen once millions of people are exposed to it, compared to the mere thousands (at most) that might be exposed during phase I–III drug development [10]. For example, it is entirely possible that targeting a receptor on nociceptive nerve fibers in thousands of patients in trials may seem safe, but once in the general population that same receptor may be critical for maintaining blood flow in atherosclerotic coronary arteries following MI; this wouldn't be seen until many patients post-MI had been exposed. Hence, the common statement seen in so many basic science pain research articles, "this receptor/neurotransmitter/neurokinin/etc. appears to be a potential target for controlling pain," ignores possible other roles of these processes, with medications targeting them having disastrous results in the population at large.

With the above in mind, this chapter will address several areas where medications are in development for pain management (Box 55.1). By the time the book is published, some of these may no longer be in development while other targets are being pursued, but for now it appears that the cannabinoids, TRPA1 antagonists, anti-nerve growth factor agents, and spicamycin derivatives have potential and are in active development. Others will be briefly mentioned as well, but the selection here is in no way meant to suggest one compound has greater potential than another; we just had to start somewhere. It should be noted that none of these classes of drugs are true analgesics, similar to the NSAIDs, antiepileptic drugs, antidepressants, and all other non-opioid medications. While opioids actually blunt both the nociceptive input from peripheral pain fibers as well as affecting the perception of that reduced input, all other drugs seem to only alter the hyperalgesic conditions that appear after injury. So far, nothing is in development that can yet supplant opioids from their position of being the only true analgesics.

Cannabinoids

The development of cannabinoid receptor agonists for analgesia demonstrates the remarkable disconnect that can exist between animal models of pain pharmacology and human response. *Cannabis sativa* has been noted historically for over 4,000 years in its role for hemp and medicinal purposes, including analgesia [11]. The cannabinoid receptors, CB1 and CB2, belong to the G protein-coupled receptor family. While it seems that CB1 is primarily found in the CNS and peripheral neurons (along with many other organs in the body from testis and fat to endothelium), CB2 is mainly found in lymphoid organs and cells of the immune system. However, under certain neuroinflammatory situations, CB2 can be found on microglia in the CNS [11]. Interestingly, the endogenous ligands to these receptors, the endocannabinoids, are reminiscent of prostaglandins in that they are not stored in vesicles but are the result of an "enzymatic cleavage of a phospholipid precursor in the cell membrane by a specific phospholipase D" [11].

Animal data strongly suggests that the primary active substance in cannabis, Δ^9-tetrahydrocannabinol (THC), has profound analgesic properties [12]. Numerous animal models in a variety of induced pain states showed that agonism of both CB1 and CB2 receptors can give marked analgesia [13–17]. However, human data is far less impressive, with oral THC failing to raise pain thresholds or having no effect on postoperative pain in some studies. While higher oral THC doses were more effective for postoperative pain, side effects became notable [18–20]. Studies in neuropathic pain states, such as HIV neuropathy or brachial plexus avulsions, have shown successful reductions in pain; while some view a 30 % reduction in these conditions as only moderate, given the notoriously resistant nature of the pain in these conditions, this degree of relief becomes more impressive [11].

Several cannabinoid medications are currently available: dronabinol (Marinol oral tablets, Δ^9-THC, schedule III), nabilone (Cesamet, a synthetic oral analog of

Δ^9-THC, schedule II), and cannabis extract (Sativex, mostly Δ^9-THC and cannabi-diol as an oromucosal spray). Dronabinol and nabilone are approved in the USA, but not for pain; they are indicated for the treatment of nausea and vomiting associated with cancer chemotherapy and for anorexia with weight loss in AIDS [21]. Sativex, currently not approved in the USA, is indicated for symptomatic relief of cancer pain and for the neuropathic pain and spasticity in adults with multiple sclerosis [22].

One of the major concerns with pursuing the cannabinoid receptors for producing analgesia is significant side effects, most notably dizziness, drowsiness, and cognitive impairment primarily from activation of the CB1 receptors in the CNS. These tend to occur with higher doses given acutely and can be avoided with dose adjustments. Nonetheless patients with psychiatric conditions such as schizophrenia should likely not be given these compounds [11]. It is these side effects in combination with the modest analgesic benefits that have so far limited use of the cannabinoids for the treatment of pain. It is therefore seems a reasonable approach to target instead the CB2 receptors, which are either outside the CNS or are expressed on microglia in the CNS under pathological conditions such as neuroinflammation and injury [22, 23].

Studies of selective CB2 agonists in rodent models of inflammatory or neuropathic pain show a marked reduction in hyperalgesia, although reduction in acute pain is not consistent among compounds [12]. However, as with all animal studies, translation to clinical practice is not always consistent; while an orally administered CB2 agonist AZD1940 showed antinociceptive properties in acute and neuropathic pain in rat models, it was ineffective for acute pain models in man [24–26]. Nonetheless there is still much effort aimed at developing selective CB2 agonists (of which there are many undergoing preclinical testing) that have little activity at the CB1 receptor. However, none of the many such agonists are completely selective for CB2, so at higher doses CB1 receptors may still be activated. Hence, analgesia is desired at doses below those which activate CB1 receptors [22].

TRPA1 Antagonists

Another area of pursuit in novel approaches toward pain pharmacology is in the identification and development of TRPA1 antagonists. The transient receptor potential (TRP) channels in mammals are a superfamily consistent of 28 members within 7 families: V (vanilloid), M (melastatin), P (polycystin), C (canonical), ML (mucolipin), non-mechanoreceptor C (not found in mammals), and A (ankyrin) [27, 28]. The one receptor currently targeted in approved pain treatments, the TRPV1 (transient receptor potential vanilloid 1, aka the capsaicin receptor), was proven to be the receptor for capsaicin in 1990 and was cloned 7 years later [29]. Taking advantage of both its role in nociception and its ability to be desensitized by agonism, the TRPV1 receptor is the target of several treatments, including capsaicin containing creams such as Zostrix and patches (Qutenza). Unfortunately, these treatments have compliance issues due to the burning pain they initially induce, so on the surface it would appear that a TRPV1 antagonist would be a better option. It has proven difficult, though, to identify compounds with sufficient specificity to this cation channel exclusively, and those compounds that have been identified have demonstrated issues such as induced hyperthermia or excessively elevated thresholds to heat stimuli (raising concerns about self-injury through burns) [29]. Hence, there are continued efforts to identify further compounds that antagonize TRPV1 but also that antagonize the other TRP receptor channels that mediate nociception.

The TRPA (transient receptor potential ankyrin) family is notable in that in mammals, it has only one member: TRPA1 (which is not the case in invertebrates) [30, 31]. This receptor is highly expressed in nociceptors and subsets of the small-diameter fibers in the dorsal root and trigeminal ganglia among other sites [27]. The role of this receptor in normal physiology is unclear but may be a nonspecific "irritancy receptor" given all the data that shows TRPA1 agonists when injected produce all the signs of inflammation (with pain) [27, 32]. It has also been shown to be involved in airway inflammation (in mice) [33]. Numerous chemicals are capable of activating TRPA1 ranging from formaldehyde to endogenous substances like prostaglandins and nitric oxide, and even calcium can activate currents through the receptor [27]. The discovery of a link between a mutation in the TRPA1 channel and the condition of familial episodic pain syndrome further adds to the interest in targeting this receptor for analgesic compounds [34]. However, adding to some confusion on the receptor's role, anesthetics like etomidate, propofol, and isoflurane can all activate TRPA1 as well, although possibly by their chemical irritant rather than anesthetic effects [35]. Animal and human data regarding the role of TRPA1 in neuropathic pain (e.g., diabetic neuropathic pain) is even less consistent, depending on the model or condition being assessed [28]. Adding to the confusion/understanding of TRPA1, while focus has been on its peripheral sites and activities, these channels have been found to be expressed on central terminals of primary afferents in the CNS, raising questions on the best route of administration to target them [36]. Again, many of these data come from animal models that may or may not apply to human TRPA1 receptors, furthering the risk of investing in the development of an antagonist compound.

Challenges in targeting this receptor for analgesic compounds include the reporting by some groups that various pain models increase its expression, while others report either no change or a decrease in expression [27, 28]. Still, there is an active pursuit by many companies, and as a result, selective inhibitors of TRPA1 have been produced. A significant problem is that although TRPA has only one member (TRPA1), there is a notable divergence in its sequence between species. This species variability results in compounds that antagonize human TRPA1 but are inactive (or agonists) in the animal models critically needed to conduct preclinical studies [27]. In addition, TRPA1 has been found in other locations, such as the cochlea, raising concerns of side effects that may be borne out in clinical trials, although knockout animals showed no hearing impairment [37].

At least two compounds are being actively pursued as TRPA1 antagonists. Glenmark Pharmaceuticals of Mumbai, India, was noted to be developing an oral

TRPA1 antagonist, GRC-17536. Indications targeted for this compound include neuropathic pain and respiratory disorders [28]. As of December 2012, it has been registered for a phase II proof-of-concept trial in patients with painful diabetic neuropathy [38]. In addition, in January 2012 Cubist Pharmaceuticals and Hydra Biosciences (Lexington, MA) filed to initiate human studies with their TRPA1 antagonist CB189,625 (also seen as CB-625) [28]. Initial studies of oral dosing of CB-625 in healthy volunteers did not show loss of temperature sensation, and the company has stated that early trials will be to assess efficacy in acute postsurgical pain [9, 39]. Other companies continue to identify TRPA1 antagonist compounds, and only time will reveal which, if any, offer a reasonably safe and effective option for acute, chronic, neuropathic, or inflammatory pain states [40, 41].

Spicamycin Derivative

As an example of inadvertent drug discovery, a spicamycin derivative produced by *Streptomyces alanosinicus* was discovered during the identification of antineoplastic compounds. KRN5500 (DARA Biosciences, Inc) did not show efficacy as an antineoplastic agent during phase I trials, but a patient treated in the protocols experienced remission of a 20-year history of neuropathic pain secondary to IgA monoclonal gammopathy and Raynaud's disease after a single treatment. While relief of this pain was long standing, his upper quadrant pain from liver metastases did not improve, suggesting KRN5500 may be effective for neuropathic but not nociceptive pain [42]. In subsequent rodent studies, single-dose KRN5500 reversed hyperalgesia within hours and lasted up to 6 weeks. Again, there was no effect in inflammatory models or normal rats, suggesting activity only in neuropathic pain [43–45].

The mechanism of action for producing pain relief is unclear for KRN5500. It lacks activity at 87 studied G protein-coupled receptors, ion channels, and enzymes. It does inhibit acetylcholinesterase and fatty acid amide hydrolase enzymes, both of which can affect neuropathic pain, but the duration of relief far outlasts the half-life of the substance (0.6–1.5 h). This suggests a more disease-modifying mechanism [46].

In a phase IIa multicenter double-blind, placebo-controlled dose escalation study, 19 patients with advanced cancer suffering from refractory neuropathic pain were given KRN5500 IV in up to eight doses over 10 weeks. While nausea and vomiting were noted side effects, there was also a significant (24 %) decrease in baseline pain as measured 1 week after dosing [46]. Although showing promise, the small size, the lack of power for efficacy (it was primarily to test safety and tolerability), the higher initial pain scores in the KRN5500 group, and the continued use of (and lack of control over) prior analgesics render this very preliminary data. In a press release to Reuter's, it was noted that KRN5500 had been submitted to the FDA under orphan drug status to treat chemotherapy-induced peripheral neuropathy, following it's designation in 2011 as an FDA "Fast Track" medication [47].

Anti-nerve Growth Factor Antibodies

Although development of this new class of medication for pain control was slowed in 2010 by an FDA research hold, studies resumed following modifications to the protocols after FDA review in March of 2012 [48]. The delay in development related to concerns about this class of drug potentially contributing to osteonecrosis and with the resumption of studies that had stricter patient selection and greater monitoring for bone changes, some drugs that were in both phase I and II of development were apparently dropped [48]. This again demonstrates the enormous risk organizations take in pursuing new therapeutic targets in pain treatment. The drug furthest along in development appears to be tanezumab (Pfizer, formerly RN624), although other drugs have been or are undergoing development, including fulranumab (Johnson & Johnson, formerly JNJ-42160443/AMG-403). It is not clear whether other drugs will continue to be developed, however, e.g., REGN475/SAR164877 (Regeneron and Sanofi-Aventis) and medi578 (AstraZeneca) [49]. The impression by many after the FDA review was that this class of medication, while worth pursuing given the unmet needs in pain management, would not be in widespread use for either back pain or osteoarthritis as originally intended [48]. It may well be, however, that some of the adverse effects are more individual drug related rather than class related.

Nerve growth factor (NGF) is a neurotrophin released from target tissues that binds to receptors on the distal ends of axons innervating those tissues [50]. The receptor complex NGF binds to consist of two receptors: the tyrosine kinase-A (TrkA) and the p75 neurotrophin (p75^{NTR}) receptors. In early animal development, NGF plays a role in the development of peripheral small fibers involved in pain transmission as well as autonomic fibers. Mutations in the TrkA gene seem to contribute to the condition of congenital insensitivity to pain with anhydrosis (CIPA), which in addition to producing an inability to feel pain is associated with renal failure and mental retardation [49]. However, the rarer condition of congenital insensitivity to pain without anhydrosis has only a loss of deep pain perception with other sensory modalities left intact and is the result of a NGF abnormality that prevents its normal binding to the p75^{NTR} receptor while the TrkA binding is unaffected [51]. Since pain treatment cannot be targeted during human development, the role of NGF in the adult becomes more relevant.

Postnatal NGF seems to change its primary activity from neural development to one of being a critical component in neural sensitization. Intramuscular injections in man of NGF produce mechanical allodynia and hyperalgesia that seem resistant even to local anesthetic blockade of the muscle, with such hyperalgesia persisting for at least 7 days [52, 53]. Similar sensitization occurs quickly in local skin injections [54]. NGF has been found to be elevated in numerous conditions of chronic pain, including degenerative disc disease, endometriosis, prostatitis, cancer pain, interstitial cystitis, and others [49]. The mechanism of NGF neural sensitization seems to be via its TrkA receptor when it co-localizes with TRPV1 receptors (a cation channel which responds to thermomechanical and chemical stimuli) on nociceptive neurons. When the NGF binds the TrkA receptor, not only does it cause the TRPV1 receptor to lower its threshold to opening, it also increases the expression of the TRPV1 receptor. In addition to enhancing nociceptive neuron firing, NGF has also been found to upregulate genes in nociceptive neurons that can further facilitate CNS second-order nociceptive neurons [49].

Given NGF's role in developing hyperalgesic states, antagonism of it would seem a reasonable way to produce pain control in compatible conditions. Anti-NGF antibodies work by sequestering NGF thus preventing binding to its receptors, and they have demonstrated effective analgesia in several human and animal models of pains ranging from pancreatic pain to osteoarthritic pain [55, 56]. Tanezumab has been studied since 2004 and has proven more effective than placebo or naprosyn in studies of knee osteoarthritis, low back pain, and interstitial cystitis. These studies involved an intravenous infusion once or once every 8 weeks for multiple does, with duration of relief lasting for the entire period between infusions [49]. The optimal dosing, frequency, and duration of treatment are yet to be determined. Side effects were deemed to be minimal and did not result in significant patient dropout from the studies. These effects included arthralgias, headaches, myalgias, paresthesias, hypesthesias, and hyperesthesias [49]. Preliminary clinical studies with fulranumab suggest possible efficacy in painful diabetic neuropathy as well, but development is less advanced than tanezumab at this time [57].

However, in 2010 the FDA stopped development on the anti-NGF antibody class due to findings of significant progression of knee and hip osteoarthritis with evidence of bone necrosis following a phase III trial of tanezumab. This is not entirely unexpected given that patients with congenital insensitivity to pain without anhydrosis present frequently with fractures, bone necrosis, and neuropathic joint destruction due to the inability to feel deep pain [58]. It was unclear whether this could be a class effect or the effect of a single-drug entity or whether the effect was related to treatment at all (vs. progression of underlying disease or joint overuse due to effective analgesia). After the review of all anti-NGF data, it was recommended to the FDA by an independent panel that research and development of the anti-NGF agents continue, but that subject should be monitored for bone health, that target patients be those in whom no other analgesic options exist, and that NSAIDs should not be coadministered with the anti-NGF agents [59]. Given the challenges so far with these agents, even though tanezumab is in phase III development, it is difficult to predict when any of these drugs may be filed for approval [60].

Other Approaches

Given the business of drug development, not all information on novel molecules under investigation may be included in this chapter simply because it may not be publicly known. Further, given how quickly compound development can be discontinued depending on a single-study result or perceived risk/benefit/profit, many drugs mentioned here may never see phase III studies, let alone a filing for full approval by the FDA. The list of other approaches is not meant to be comprehensive but rather to be an insight into what efforts are being made in the area of novel analgesic drug development. Most of what follows are in phase I or early phase II at the time of this writing. One note should be made from this review: not a single one of these compounds is an opioid replacement. We are still primarily dependent for the treatment of acute (and possibly chronic) pain on a class of drug with its origins in a natural plant that has been used for six millennia. This alone should provide the insight on how difficult it is to successfully understand and fully treat pain.

- AYX1 is an oligonucleotide being developed by Adynxx (San Francisco, USA) to target acute and persistent postsurgical pain. It is believed to affect spinal cord sensitization via inhibition of transcription factor EGR1, an early growth response protein. Single intrathecal dosing is currently being evaluated in phase II trials [61].
- Adenosine agonists continue to be investigated for neuropathic pain, although targeting the A1 and A2 receptors carries risks of cardiovascular side effects owing to their presence in cardiac and endothelial tissue. The A3 receptor, however, is potentially showing benefit in animal neuropathic pain models [62].
- Gene therapy for cancer pain is being pursued by Benitec Biopharma (Sydney, Australia). Preclinical studies of lentivirus gene therapy vectors designed to control spinal cord sensitization are being conducted in patients with terminal cancer [63].
- CR4056 is an imidazoline (I2) ligand being developed by Rottapharm/Madaus (Brussels, Belgium). So far, two phase I clinical studies of tolerability and kinetics have been completed in healthy volunteers with phase II trials planned for 2013 [64]. It was found as a result of purely empirical observations that the endogenous imidazole receptor agonist, agmatine, has notable antihyperalgesic properties in both inflammatory and neuropathic pain. CR4056, a selective I2 agonist, has shown in animal models to be effective for acute visceral, inflammatory, and neuropathic pain as well as being synergistic to opioid analgesia [12].
- Blockade of the NaV1.7 voltage-gated sodium channel is of interest given its key role in peripheral transmission of nociception [65]. While several organizations are pursuing blockers to this channel, most are still in early phase development. XEN402 (Teva Pharmaceutical Inc and Xenon Pharmaceuticals, British Columbia, Canada) is a topical NaV1.7 and NaV1.8 channel blocker that in a phase II trial showed efficacy in treating the pain of post-herpetic neuralgia [66]. It has also shown efficacy in the treatment of erythromelalgia, a rare inheritable condition characterized by intermittent burning pain and erythema in the extremities known to be a result of a mutation in the gene SCN9A which encodes subunits of the NaV1.7 channel [67]. As of April 2013, XEN402 was granted orphan drug status by the FDA specifically for the treatment of the pain associated with erythromelalgia [68].
- p38 mitogen-activated protein kinase (MAPK) inhibitors are being developed since this enzyme phosphorylates intracellular proteins involved in signal

transduction and transcription factors that affect biosynthesis of inflammatory cytokines. Since inhibitors of cytokine action, such as anti-TNF-alpha treatments, reduce pain and inflammation of rheumatoid arthritis and lumbosacral radiculopathy, MAPK also seems a reasonable target to inhibit to control pain [69–71]. Animal models of neuropathic pain show a reduction in pain with MAPK inhibitors, including sciatic constriction, diabetic neuropathy, and capsaicin injection models [72–74]. At least two such inhibitors are being developed with pain indications: dilmapimod (SB-681323, GlaxoSmithKline) and losmapimod (GW856553, GlaxoSmithKline). Many others are being developed with indications ranging from the treatment of inflammatory diseases to cancer treatments. Unfortunately an early study of losmapimod in the treatment of patients with neuropathic pain did not show improvement versus placebo, nor did it show improvement of pain in patients with lumbosacral radiculopathy [75, 76]. However, as with most early development molecules, it continues to be pursued even for other indications, such as the treatment of acute coronary syndromes [77]. Oral dilmapimod, however, has shown efficacy, although modestly so, in patients with a variety of neuropathic pain forms in one early phase trial [69]. Lastly, in a trial of another MAPK inhibitor, oral talmapimod (SCIO-469), after positive preclinical trials, it was demonstrated to reduce acute postsurgical dental pain in patients in a preliminary study [78].

- Angiotensin II type 2 receptor antagonists have been shown to relieve symptoms of neuropathic and inflammatory pain in animal models [79, 80]. In patients with hypertension, pain sensitivity is unchanged with the use of beta blockers or diuretics, but enalapril has been shown to modify pain perception [81]. It has been shown that antagonism of the angiotensin II type 1 receptor produced blood pressure reduction, but that antagonism of the type 2 receptor had more of a role in providing relief of pain at least in neuropathic models [79, 82]. EMA401, an angiotensin II type 2 receptor antagonist, is under development (Spinifex, Melbourne, Australia) for chronic pain including neuropathic pain, and so far has shown positive results in a post-herpetic neuralgia phase II study and is being pursued for chemotherapy-induced peripheral neuropathy as well [83].

Summary

We have discussed potential pharmacologic agents in the management of chronic pain. The most promising drugs target the cannabinoid receptor, TRPA1 (in addition to the TRPV1) receptor, spicamycin derivative, nerve growth factor, and angiotensin II type 2 receptor antagonists. Further development of these novel drugs entails tremendous risks on the part of drug companies in terms of unproven efficacy and unforeseen side effects. Hopefully, newer drugs will be introduced in the future that are effective and with acceptable side effects.

References

1. Melnikova I. Pain market. Nat Rev Drug Discov. 2010;9:589–90.
2. Dworkin R, Turk D, Katz N, Rowbotham M, Peirce-Sandner S, Cerny I, Clingman C, Eloff B, Farrar J, Kamp C, McDermott M, Rappaport B, Sanhai W. Evidence-based clinical trial design for chronic pain pharmacotherapy: a blueprint for ACTION. Pain. 2011;152:S107–15.
3. McQue K. Newron's ralfinamide fails for Katie McQue neuropathic pain. SCRIP World Pharmaceutical News. 7 May 2010. http://s3.amazonaws.com/cuttings/cuttingpdfs/9547/217f d9e47def65479dc4933329b5eb24.pdf.
4. Schmidt W. 6th annual pain therapeutics summit. Oct 2013. www.painresearchforum.org/ news/22419-filling-pain-drug-pipeline.
5. ClinicalTrials.gov Identifier: NCT01693692, Sponsor Theravance, first received Sept 20, 2012. http://www.clinicaltrials.gov/ct2/show/NCT01693692.
6. PRNewsire. KemPharm, Inc. Receives notice of allowance for novel pain drug candidate, KP201. 3 April 2013. http://www.prnewswire.com/news-releases-test/kempharm-inc-receives-notice-of-allowance-for-novel-pain-drug-candidate-kp201-201233571.html.
7. Campbell CM, Kipnes MS, Stouch BC, Brady KL, Kelly M, Schmidt WK, Petersen KL, Rowbotham MC, Campbell JN. Randomized control trial of topical clonidine for treatment of painful diabetic neuropathy. Pain. 2012;153(9):1815–23. doi:10.1016/j.pain.2012.04.014. Epub 2012 Jun 8.
8. Reichenbach S, Wandel S, Hildebrand P, Tschannen B, Villiger P, Egger M, Trelle S, Juni P. Cardiovascular safety of non-steroidal anti-inflammatory drugs: network meta-analysis. BMJ. 2011;342:c7086. doi:10.1136/bmj.c7086.
9. Talkington M. FDA advisory panel gives the green light to restart NGF antibody trials. Pain Research Forum. 13 March 2012. http://www.painresearchforum.org/news/14439-fda-gives-green-light-restart-ngf-antibody-trials.
10. Fowler PD. Aspirin, paracetamol and non-steroidal anti-inflammatory drugs. A comparative review of side effects. Med Toxicol Adverse Drug Exp. 1987;2:338–66.
11. Kraft B. Is there any clinically relevant cannabinoid-induced analgesia? Pharmacology. 2012;89:237–46.
12. Li JX, Zhang Y. Emerging drug targets for pain treatment. Eur J Pharmacol. 2012;681:1–5.
13. Lichtman AH, Martin BR. Spinal and supraspinal components of cannabinoid-induced antinociception. J Pharmacol Ther. 1991;258:517–23.
14. Richardson JD, Aanonsen L, Hargreaves KM. Antihyperalgesic effects of spinal cannabinoids. Eur J Pharmacol. 1998;345:145–53.
15. Liu C, Walker JM. Effects of a cannabinoid agonist on spinal nociceptive neurons in a rodent model of neuropathic pain. J Neurophysiol. 2006;96:2984–94.
16. Jaggar SI, Hasnie FS, Sellaturay S, Rice AS. The anti-hyperalgesic actions of the cannabinoid anandamide and the putative CB2 receptor agonist palmitoylethanolamide in visceral and somatic inflammatory pain. Pain. 1998;76:189–99.
17. Valenzano KJ, Tafesse L, Lee G, Harrison JE, Boulet JM, Gottshall SL, Mark L, Pearson MS, Miller W, Shan S, Rabadi L, Rotshteyn Y, Chaffer SM, Turchin PI, Elsemore DA, Toth M, Koetzner L, Whiteside GT. Pharmacological and pharmacokinetic characterization of the cannabinoid receptor 2 agonist, GW405833, utilizing rodent models of acute and chronic pain, anxiety, ataxia and catalepsy. Neuropharmacology. 2005;48:658–72.
18. Kraft B, Frickey NA, Kaufmann RM, Reif M, Frey R, Gustorff B, Kress HG. Lack of analgesia by oral standardized cannabis extract on acute inflammatory pain and hyperalgesia in volunteers. Anesthesiology. 2008;109:101–10.
19. Buggy DJ, Toogood L, Maric S, Sharpe P, Lambert DG, Rowbotham DJ. Lack of analgesic efficacy of oral delta-9-tetrahydrocannabinol in postoperative pain. Pain. 2003;106:169–72.
20. Holdcroft A, Maze M, Dore C, Tebbs S, Thompson S. A multicenter dose-escalation study of the analgesic and adverse effects of an oral cannabis extract (Cannador) for postoperative pain management. Anesthesiology. 2006;104:1040–6.

21. Borgelt L, Franson K, Nussbaum A, Wang G. The pharmacologic and clinical effects of medical cannabis. Pharmacotherapy. 2013;33:195–209.
22. Pertwee RG. Targeting the endocannabinoid system with cannabinoid receptor agonists: pharmacological strategies and therapeutic possibilities. Phil Trans R Soc B. 2012;367:3353–63.
23. Atwood BK, Mackie K. CB2: a cannabinoid receptor with an identity crisis. Br J Pharmacol. 2010;160:467–79.
24. Groblewski T, et al. Pre-clinical pharmacological properties of novel peripherally-acting CB1-CB2 agonists. In: 20th annual symposium on the cannabinoids. Research Triangle Park: Int. Cannabinoid Research Society; 2010, p. 37.
25. Kalliomäki J, Annas P, Huizar K, Clarke C, Zettergren A, Karlsten R, Segerdahl M. Evaluation of the analgesic efficacy and psychoactive effects of AZD1940, a novel peripherally acting cannabinoid agonist, in human capsaicin-induced pain and hyperalgesia. Clin Exp Pharmacol Physiol. 2013;40:212–8.
26. Kalliomaki J, Seqerdahl M, Webster L, Reimfelt A, Huizar K, Annas P, Karlsten R, Quiding H. Evaluation of the analgesic efficacy of AZD1940, a novel cannabinoid agonist, on postoperative pain after lower third molar surgical removal. Scan J Pain. 2013;4:17–22.
27. Fanger CM, del Camino D, Moran MM. TRPA1 as an analgesic target. Open Drug Discov J. 2010;2:64–70.
28. Radresa O, Dahllöf H, Nyman E, Nolting A, Alberta JS, Raboisson P. Roles of TRPA1 in pain pathophysiology and implications for the development of a new class of analgesic drugs. Open Pain J. 2013;6:S137–53.
29. Trevisani M, Gatti R. TRPV1 antagonists as analgesic agents. Open Pain J. 2013;6:S108–18.
30. Clapham DE. TRP channels as cellular sensors. Nature. 2003;426:517–24.
31. Montell C. Drosophila TRP channels. Pflugers Arch. 2005;451:19–28.
32. Lennertz RC, Kossyreva EA, Smith AK, Stucky CL. TRPA1 mediates mechanical sensitization in nociceptors during inflammation. PLoS One. 2012;7:e43597. doi:10.1371/journal.pone.0043597.
33. Nassini R, Pedretti P, Moretto N, Fusi C, Carnini C, et al. Transient receptor potential Ankyrin 1 channel localized to non-neuronal airway cells promotes non-neurogenic inflammation. PLoS One. 2012;7(8):e42454. doi:10.1371/journal.pone.0042454.
34. Kremeyer B, Lopera F, Cox JJ, Momin A, Rugiero F, Marsh S, Woods CG, Jones NG, Paterson KJ, Fricer FR, Villegas A, Acosta N, Pineda-Trujillo NG, Ramirez JD, Zea J, Burley MW, Bedoya G, Bennett DL, Wood JN, Ruiz-Linares A. A gain-of-function mutation in TRPA1 causes familial episodic pain syndrome. Neuron. 2010;66(5):671–80.
35. Matta JA, Cornett PM, Miyares RL, Abe K, Sahibzada N, Ahern GP. General anesthetics activate a nociceptive ion channel to enhance pain and inflammation. Proc Natl Acad Sci U S A. 2008;105(25):8784–9.
36. Kosugi M, Nakatsuka T, Fujita T, Kuroda Y, Kumamoto E. Activation of TRPA1 channel facilitates excitatory synaptic transmission in substantia gelatinosa neurons of the adult rat spinal cord. J Neurosci. 2007;27:4443–51.
37. Corey DP, Garcia-Anoveros J, Holt JR, Kwan KY, Lin SY, Vollrath MA, Amalfitano A, Cheung EL, Derfler BH, Duggan A, Geleoc GS, Gray PA, Hoffman MP, Rehm HL, Tamasauskas D, Zhang DS. TRPA1 is a candidate for the mechanosensitive transduction channel of vertebrate hair cells. Nature. 2004;432(7018):723–30.
38. A clinical trial to study the effects GRC 17536 in patients with painful diabetic peripheral neuropathy (painful extremities due to peripheral nerve damage in diabetic patients). Clinicaltrials.gov, identifier NCT01726413. Updated and verified as of December 2012 by Glenmark Pharmaceuticals Ltd, India. http://www.clinicaltrials.gov/ct2/show/NCT01726413?term=GRC-17536&rank=2.
39. Business Wire. Cubist reports fourth quarter and full year 2012 financial results. www.thestreet.com. 23 Jan 2013.
40. SBIR/STTR, Department of Health and Human Services. Analgesics targeting TRPA1 for treatment of chronic pain. Tracking number R43DA031516, solicitation year 2011. Principal investigator Herz, J of Algomedix, Inc. www.sbir.gov/sbirsearch/detail/368227.

41. Nyman E, Franzén B, Nolting A, Klement G, Liu G, Nilsson M, Rosén A, Björk C, Weigelt D, Wollberg P, Karila P, Raboisson P. In vitro pharmacological characterization of a novel TRPA1 antagonist and proof of mechanism in a human dental pulp model. J Pain Res. 2013;6:59–70.
42. Borsook D, Edward A. Antineuropathic effects of the antibiotic derivative Spicamycin, KRN5500. Pain Med. 2004;5:104–8.
43. Kobierski L, Abdi S, DiLorenzo L, Feroz N, Borsook D. A single intravenous injection of KRN5500 (antibiotic spicamycin) produces long term decreases in multiple sensory hypersensitivities in neuropathic pain. Anesth Analg. 2003;97:174–82.
44. DiLorenzo L, Kobierski L, Moore KA, Borsook D. A water soluble synthetic Spicamycin derivative (San-Gly) decreases mechanical allodynia in a rodent model of neuropathic pain. Neurosci Lett. 2002;330:37–40.
45. Abdi S, Vilassova N, Decosterd I, Feroz N, Borsook D. The effects of KRN5500, a spicamycin derivative, on neuropathic and nociceptive pain models in rats. Anesth Analg. 2000;91:955–99.
46. Weinstein S, Abernethy A, Spruill S, Pike I, Kelly AT, Jett LG. A Spicamycin derivative (KRN5500) provides neuropathic pain relief in patients with advanced cancer: a placebo-controlled, proof-of-concept trial. J Pain Symp Manag. 2012;43:679–91.
47. Reuters Press Release. DARA BioSciences announces submission of KRN5500 to FDA for orphan designation. 29 Nov 2012.
48. Dolgin E. Panel backs pain drug studies with new safety checks. Nat Med. 2012;18:472.
49. McKelvey L, Shorten G, O'Keeffe G. Nerve growth factor-mediated regulation of pain signaling and proposed new intervention strategies in clinical pain management. J Neurochem. 2013;124:276–89.
50. Davies AM. Regulation of neuronal survival and death by extracellular signals during development. Embo J. 2003;22:2537–45.
51. Covaceuszach S, Capsoni S, Marinelli S, Pavone F, Ceci M, Ugolini G, Vignone D, Amato G, Paoletti F, Lamba D, Cattaneo A. In vitro receptor binding properties of a "painless" NGF mutein, linked to hereditary sensory autonomic neuropathy type V. Biochem Biophys Res Commun. 2010;391:824–9.
52. Gerber RK, Nie H, Arendt-Nielsen L, Curatolo M, Graven-Nielsen T. Local pain and spreading hyperalgesia induced by intramuscular injection of nerve growth factor are not reduced by local anesthesia of the muscle. Clin J Pain. 2011;2011(27):240–7.
53. Svensson P, Castrillon E, Cairns BE. Nerve growth factor evoked masseter muscle sensitization and perturbation of jaw motor function in healthy women. J Orofac Pain. 2008;22:340–8.
54. Rukwied R, Mayer A, Kluschina O, Obreja O, Schley M, Schmelz M. NGF induces non-inflammatory localized and lasting mechanical and thermal hypersensitivity in human skin. Pain. 2010;148:407–13.
55. Zhu Y, Colak T, Shenoy M, Liu L, Pai R, Li C, Mehta, Pasricha PJ. Nerve growth factor modulates TRPV1 expression and function and mediates pain in chronic pancreatitis. Gastroenterology. 2011;141:370–7.
56. Shelton DL, Sutherland J, Gripp J, Camerato T, Armanini MP, Phillips HS, Carroll K, Spencer SD, Levinson AD. Human trks: molecular cloning, tissue distribution, and expression of extracellular domain immunoadhesins. J Neurosci. 1955;15:477–91.
57. Wang H, Romano G, Frustaci ME, Sanga P, Ness S, Russell L, Fedgchin M, Kelly K, Thipphawong J. Analgesic efficacy of fulranumab in patients with painful diabetic peripheral neuropathy in a randomized, placebo-controlled, double-blind study. Neurology. 2013;80 (meeting abstract):S58.002.
58. Minde J, Toolanen G, Andersson T, Nennesmo I, Remahl IN, Svensson O, Solders G. Familial insensitivity to pain (HSAN V) and a mutation in the NGFB gene. A neurophysiological and pathological study. Muscle Nerve. 2004;30:752–60.
59. Carey K. Anti-nerve growth factor drugs exonerated. Nat Biotechnol. 2012;30:298.
60. Loftus P. J&J delays plans for arthritis drug as FDA continues hold on testing. Wall Street J. 2013. http://online.wsj.com/article/BT-CO-20130207-714849.html.

61. Clinicaltrials.gov. Study to evaluate safety/efficacy of a single pre-op dose of AYX1 injection to treat pain after knee replacement surgery. Identifier NCT01731730, verified March 2013.

62. Chen Z, Janes K, Chen C, Doyle T, Bryant L, Tosh DK, Jacobson KA, Salvemini D. Controlling murine and rat chronic pain through A3 adenosine receptor activation. FASEB J. 2012;26:1855–65. doi:10.1096/fj.11-201541. Epub 2012 Feb 17.

63. Zou W, Song Z, Guo Q, Liu C, Zhang Z, Zhang Y. Intrathecal lentiviral-mediated RNA interference targeting PKCγ attenuates chronic constriction injury-induced neuropathic pain in rats. Hum Gene Ther. 2011;22:465–75. doi:10.1089/hum.2010.207. Epub 2011 Feb 26.

64. Rottapharm website. http://www.rotta.com/en/service/rd/areTerap/pain.html.

65. Ossipov M. The perception and endogenous modulation of pain. Scientifica. 2012:561761, 25 p, Hindawi Publishing Corp. http://dx.doi.org/10.6064/2012/561761.

66. GEN. Teva Enters Up-to-$376 M deal for xenon pain drug. 11 Dec 2012. http://www.genengnews.com/gen-news-highlights/teva-enters-up-to-376m-deal-for-xenon-pain-drug/81247756/.

67. Goldberg YP, Price N, Namdari R, Cohen CJ, Lamers MH, Winters C, Price J, Young CE, Verschoof H, Sherrington R, Pimstone SN, Hayden MR. Treatment of Na(v)1.7-mediated pain in inherited erythromelalgia using a novel sodium channel blocker. Pain. 2012;153:80–5. doi:10.1016/j.pain.2011.09.008. Epub 2011 Oct 28.

68. Wall Street Journal. Teva gets orphan drug designation for XEN402. 2013 April 23.

69. Anand P, Shenoy R, Palmer J, Baines AJ, Lai RK, Robertson J, Bird N, Ostenfeld T, Chizh BA. Clinical trial of the p38 MAP kinase inhibitor dilmapimod in neuropathic pain following nerve injury. Eur J Pain. 2011;15:1040–8.

70. Redlich K, Schett G, Steiner G, Hayer S, Wagner EF, Smolen JS. Rheumatoid arthritis therapy after tumor necrosis factor and interleukin-1 blockade. Arthritis Rheum. 2003;48:3308–19.

71. Cohen SP, Bogduk N, Dragovich A, Buckenmaier 3rd CC, Griffith S, Kurihara C, et al. Randomized, double-blind, placebo-controlled, dose-response, and preclinical safety study of transforaminal epidural etanercept for the treatment of sciatica. Anesthesiology. 2009;110: 1116–26.

72. Sweitzer SM, Medicherla S, Almirez R, Dugar S, Chakravarty S, Shumilla JA, et al. Antinociceptive action of a p38alpha MAPK inhibitor, SD-282, in a diabetic neuropathy model. Pain. 2004;109:409–19.

73. Ji RR, Gereau 4th RW, Malcangio M, Strichartz GR. MAP kinase and pain. Brain Res Rev. 2009;60:135–48.

74. Obata K, Yamanaka H, Kobayashi K, Dai Y, Mizushima T, Katsura H, Fukuoka T, Tokunaga A, Noguchi K. Role of mitogen-activated protein kinase activation in injured and intact primary afferent neurons for mechanical and heat hypersensitivity after spinal nerve ligation. J Neurosci. 2004;24:10211–22.

75. Ostenfeld T, Krishen A, Lai RY, Bullman J, Baines AJ, Green J, Anand P, Kelly M. Analgesic efficacy and safety of the novel p38 MAP kinase inhibitor, losmapimod, in patients with neuropathic pain following peripheral nerve injury: a double-blind, placebo-controlled study. Eur J Pain. 2013;17:844–57. doi:10.1002/j.1532-2149.2012.00256.x. Epub 2012 Dec 14.

76. GlaxoSmithKline study register, Study No: KIP113049, completed August 2010, http://download.gsk-clinicalstudyregister.com/files/42c7fc18-27c2-461e-9464-378441578185.

77. Melloni C, Sprecher DL, Sarov-Blat L, Patel MR, Heitner JF, Hamm CW, Aylward P, Tanguay JF, DeWinter RJ, Marber MS, Lerman A, Hasselblad V, Granger CB, Newby LK. The study of LoSmapimod treatment on inflammation and InfarCtSizE (SOLSTICE): design and rationale. Am Heart J. 2012;164:646–53.e3. doi:10.1016/j.ahj.2012.07.030. Epub 2012 Oct 16.

78. Tong SE, Daniels SE, Black P, Chang S, Protter A, Desjardins P. Novel p38α mitogen-activated protein kinase inhibitor shows analgesic efficacy in acute postsurgical dental pain. J Clin Pharmacol. 2012;52:717–28.

79. McCarthy T. EMA401 for treating neuropathic pain. Drug Discovery and Development. 2012 Dec 4. www.dddmag.com/articles/2012/12/ema401-treating-neuropathic-pain.

80. Chakrabarty A, Liao Z, Smith PG. Angiotensin II receptor type 2 activation is required for cutaneous sensory hyperinnervation and hypersensitivity in a rat hind paw model of inflammatory pain. J Pain. 2013;14:1053–65. doi:10.1016/j.jpain.2013.04.002. Epub 2013 May 30.

81. Guasti L, Gimoldi P, Diolisi A, Petrozzino MR, Gaudio G, Grandi AM, Rossi MG, Venco A. Treatment with enalapril modified the pain perception pattern in hypertensive patients. Hypertension. 1998;31:1146–50.
82. Wexler R, Greenlee W, Irvin J, Goldberg M, Prendergast K, Smith RD, Timmermans P. Nonpeptide angiotensin II receptor antagonists: the next generation in antihypertensive therapy. J Med Chem. 1996;39:625–56.
83. Press Release. PR Newswire, United Business Media. 27 Mar 2013. www.marketwatch.com/story/ spinifex-receives-15m-in-rd-tax-incentive-for-research-activities-related-to-the-discovery-of-treatments-for-pain-2013-03-27.

Index

A

AABB. *See* The American Association of
    Blood Banks (AABB)
Abnormal ventricular repolarization, 754
ABW. *See* Actual body weight (ABW)
Acetaminophen. *See also* Aspirin
    absorption, 436
    chemical structure, 160
    with codeine, 135
    and COX-2 inhibitors, 441
    description, 155
    distribution, 437
    dosing, 134, 156
    drug class and mechanisms, 155, 156
    effective pain reliever and antipyretic, 155
    elimination, 437
    fever reduction, 435
    gastrointestinal adverse effects, 435
    hepatotoxicity, 131
    hydrocodone, 125, 130, 132
    inhibition, 435
    IV form, adults and children, 155–156
    manufacturers, 131
    NSAIDs, 156
    opioids, 124, 131, 140
    osteoarthritis and prophylaxis, 156
    preterm neonates, 440
    rectal, 440
    side effects/black box warnings, 135, 157
Acetazolamide
    chemical structure, 254
    hyperglycemia, 336
    metabolic alkalosis patient, 240
    oral and parenteral forms, 244
    osteomalacia, 248

ACTH. *See* Adrenocorticotropic hormone
    (ACTH)
Activated clotting time (ACT), 401, 404, 611
Actual body weight (ABW), 666–667
Acute lung injury (ALI), 665
Acute pain management
    buprenorphine, 120
    butorphanol, 119
    fentanyl, 119
    hydromorphone, 119
    morphine, 119
    nalbuphine, 120
    opioid agonists/antagonists, 116–118
    pharmacokinetics and
        pharmacodynamics, 112
    therapy, 112
Acute respiratory distress syndrome (ARDS),
    276, 648, 665, 711
Adenosine agonists, 867
Adjuvants
    analgesic therapy, 92
    benzodiazepine, 106
    injectable non-insulin, 328
    pediatrics, 704
    pharmacologic agents, 422
Adrenocorticotropic hormone (ACTH), 318,
    320, 493–494
Adverse Event Reporting System (AERS), 806
Albuterol
    injectable insulin, 336
    QT prolongation, 757, 758
    short-acting beta-2 agonists, 224, 298,
        308, 647
    structure, 231
    sympathomimetics, 222

A.D. Kaye et al. (eds.), *Essentials of Pharmacology for Anesthesia,
Pain Medicine, and Critical Care*, DOI 10.1007/978-1-4614-8948-1,
© Springer Science+Business Media New York 2015